"Katherine Carson and Susan Polis Schutz have done a monumental service to the public with **Take Charge of Your Body.** At last — a book for women of all ages written by experts who are compassionate and dedicated to providing accurate information."

George M. Ryan, Jr., M.D. Past President, American College of Obstetricians and Gynecologists

---

"Socrates admonished us to 'know thyself.' Schutz and Carson are appropriately telling women to 'Take charge of your body.' Men, the church and legislative bodies have controlled women's feminity, sexuality and reproductivity long enough. It is time women assume these important responsibilities. This is a beautifully written and authoritative compendium that will allow women to understand the uniqueness of being a woman so that they can really take charge of their bodies."

Charles E. Flowers, M.D. Chairman of the Department of Obstetrics and Gynecology at the University of Alabama. Vice-President of the American College of Obstetricians and Gynecologists

---

"This book is an indispensable guide for all of us. Understanding how to 'Take charge of your body' will influence us in taking responsibility for our lives."

Donna deVarona Two-time Olympic Gold Medalist. Member of the President's Council on Physical Fitness and Sports. National Television Sports Commentator

---

"For years most women were afraid to articulate their own fears to their doctor. Thank heavens this curtain of ignorance has been lifted. Congratulations to Susan Polis Schutz and Dr. Katherine Carson. They tell it like it always should have been told."

Virginia Graham, Television Personality

Take Charge
of Your Body

Take Charge of Your Body

2,300 most asked questions from women
of all ages, answered by a woman doctor.
Includes ten important ways to improve
your health and happiness.

Susan Polis Schutz
Best-selling author

Katherine F. Carson, M.D.
Fellow of the American College
of Obstetricians and Gynecologists

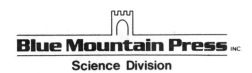

Blue Mountain Press INC.

Science Division

Library of Congress Number: 83-071746
ISBN: 0-88396-199-7

The following poems by Susan Polis Schutz have previously appeared in Blue Mountain Arts publications:

I want to wake him; Copyright © Continental Publications, 1974. *I had a discussion; Whenever anyone sees me now; A doctor to Avoid If You Are Busy; I am a prisoner; Will our baby; Cesarean Section; Cesarean Stigma; I can't believe it; Jared Polis Schutz; Oh My God; Today I woke up;* and *Postpartum Blues;* Copyright © Continental Publications, 1976. *If you make; It is marvelous; It is so important; If you know;* and *This life is yours;* Copyright © Continental Publications, 1978. *We had a beautiful little girl; Many women;* and *Today's woman;* Copyright © Stephen Schutz and Susan Polis Schutz, 1980. *What more beautiful sight; We cannot listen; My Son; You deserve the best;* and *Love is;* Copyright © Stephen Schutz and Susan Polis Schutz, 1982. *At thirty-nine I realized; To my daughter; I know that lately;* and *You are a woman;* Copyright © Stephen Schutz and Susan Polis Schutz, 1983. All rights reserved.

Manufactured in the United States of America

First Printing: October, 1983

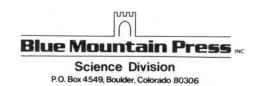

Blue Mountain Press INC.

Science Division

P.O. Box 4549, Boulder, Colorado 80306

DEDICATION

Dr. Katherine F. Carson dedicates this book to her daughters, Ruth, Helen and Sylvia.

Susan Polis Schutz dedicates this book to beautiful Jordanna Polis Schutz and all women who want to better themselves.

ACKNOWLEDGMENTS

Susan Polis Schutz and Dr. Katherine F. Carson wish to thank:

Stephen Schutz, Susan's husband, for his ideas, direction, help, and love.

George West, Katherine's husband, for listening to Katherine's typewriter in the wee hours.

Patricia Wayant, Blue Mountain Arts editor, for her enormous help in every aspect of the book including gathering and sorting questions, preparing the index, as well as editing and proofing the entire book.

Dr. Purvis Martin, Dr. Eugene Appel, Dr. Diana Barrows, Mark Solo (Director of Planned Parenthood of San Diego), and Kathy Sheehan for their review of various chapters of this book.

Susan's third baby, who observed it all in utero.

We wish to thank some of the many people that helped type and prepare the manuscript: Shirlee Goetz, Diane Gilmore, Nancy Brown, Evelyn Booth, Sylvia Kantor, Faith Hamilton, Doug Pagels, Gary Morris, Bob Gall, Patty Brown, Nancy Trachtenberg and Karen Ram.

You Deserve the Best

A woman will get only what she seeks
You must choose your goals carefully
Know what you like
and what you do not like
Be critical about what you can do well
and what you cannot do well
Choose a career or lifestyle that interests you
and work hard to make it a success
Enter a relationship that is worthy of
everything you are physically
         and mentally capable of
Be honest with people, help them if you can
but don't depend on anyone to make life easy
or happy for you
Only you can do that for yourself
Strive to achieve all that you like
Find happiness in everything you do
Love with your entire being
Make a triumph
of every aspect
of your life

— Susan Polis Schutz

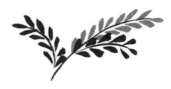

INTRODUCTION

Two hours before I gave birth to my first child, I found out that I needed to have a cesarean delivery. Since this was to be done immediately, I had no time to prepare myself, and what proceeded was something like a nightmare. I was put into a cold, little cement room, all alone. I was so scared that I asked my doctor to give me ether so that I wouldn't know what was going on. When I finally woke up, I was too groggy and weak to see my son. I had an intravenous needle in my arm for over twenty-four hours and could not eat solid foods. I felt miserable and thought that I was truly sick! Not once did it dawn on me that I had had a baby.

Five years later when I had my daughter, I had another cesarean delivery. This time I requested a spinal (an injection of anesthesia into the spine). I was numb from my chest to my feet; my mind was perfect. After the anesthesia was given, I was talking to my husband who was sitting right next to me. Within ten minutes I saw my beautiful baby girl being born. After another seventeen minutes I was moved to the recovery room, perfectly alert, sipping a glass of ginger ale. After one hour in the recovery room, I was back in my regular hospital room with my baby and family, but without any intravenous needle. We were all ecstatic.

Why was one birth experience so miserable and the other so beautiful? How could there be such a difference? The answer is that in the years between having my son and daughter, I learned how to take charge of my body. Also, many hospitals finally gave into some of the demands of obstetricians and their women patients.

As soon as I knew that I was pregnant for the second time, I interviewed five doctors until I found the one who I felt cared about me as a woman and agreed with my philosophy. One of the doctors that I interviewed said to me, "Will your career stop when you have your baby?" I said, "Of course not. As soon as I feel better I will return to work." He then said, "Then why are you bothering to have a baby at all?" I immediately crossed him off my list of doctors. I finally chose a doctor, Dr. Katherine Carson, with whom Stephen and I spoke for a long time. Everything that Dr. Carson does is for my convenience and happiness, not hers. Now I was given choices in every aspect of the childbirth, and it was up to me to learn enough to make the best choices. I couldn't believe how many tales I had heard from various friends and acquaintances about childbirth. I needed to learn enough to distinguish between fact and fiction. So I read everything about childbirth that I could. I then felt ready to speak with my doctor. We discussed the pros and cons of my choices and outlined a definite plan for the birth of my child. I even spoke with the anesthesiologist to help alleviate my fear of the pain that the large needle would cause. Fear often is the result of not understanding something, as was the case with me. The anesthesiologist explained that he would first numb the area, and he assured me that I would not feel the spinal injection, and I did not.

Childbirth is merely one example of why taking charge of your body is so important. There are hundreds of other situations where decisions have to be made by you about your body, such as birth control, illnesses, menstrual problems, menopausal problems, or perhaps simply how to keep your body healthy to function at its optimum. It is very easy to find someone who wants to control your body—your doctor, your family, your church, your friends, your boyfriend, and many others—but if you are to live a life that you control, you had better not let anyone control your body other than yourself. You must learn how it functions, what is normal, what is abnormal. You need to make intelligent choices concerning your body. Your choice of a doctor is very important. It is wise to choose a doctor when you are in good health before anything is wrong, because it will be much harder to do so if you are under pressure. But choosing the right doctor is not enough. In order to take charge of your body, you must have a background of knowledge so that you can make decisions and choices that are right for you. The purpose of this book is to give you this background of knowledge.

For *Take Charge Of Your Body,* we gave a thousand women a form that asked them to list questions about their bodies that they most wanted to know the answers to. We expected that each woman would ask several questions, but the response was phenomenal; most women needed additional paper to ask all their questions. They really wanted to know a lot of things about their bodies, but they did not want to bother their doctors all the time. I know how they felt because when I was pregnant, I remember calling Dr. Carson so many times. On one particular occasion I said, "I'm really sorry to disturb you, but my heart is beating loudly. Is this normal?" Her response always made me feel better, and I told her how I wished that there were one book where I could look these things up so I wouldn't have to call her so often. That was when we decided to create such a book.

What a need there is for this book and what a great person to coauthor the book with! Dr. Katherine Carson doesn't just treat problems, she treats the woman as a whole. In addition to having very high professional credentials and enormous experience, she has delivered over 6,000 babies and has counseled over 25,000 women. She understands things because she is a woman. She had three daughters after she was thirty-five years old. She has a very active career and understands the stress, strains, and pleasures that can occur in a woman's body. She lectures to thousands of women each year about breast cancer and how so many men withdraw sexually from their wives after finding out that they have this disease. Last year, Dr. Carson found out that she had breast cancer. She had a mastectomy and later had reconstructive surgery, while missing only three days of work for each surgery. She discusses in this book how she and her husband, George, were drawn even closer together after this experience. When Dr. Carson writes, counsels her patients, or lectures to groups, she includes her own personal experiences in addition to her medical expertise.

Take Charge of Your Body answers medical questions in a scientific, yet humanistic way. It is written for the woman who wants to control her own life and her own body. It is organized into chapters that discuss and answer questions in depth about certain subjects: everyday good health; menstruation; breasts, breast cancer, and other problems of the breast; birth control; sex; how to get pregnant; normal pregnancy and choices in childbirth; women's diseases and surgery; menopause; and body abuse. Each subject is broken down into smaller categories for quick reference. We have parenthetically defined all scientific terms. A great deal of time was spent preparing the index. We hope that if you have a specific question, you will find the answer quickly and easily by referring to it. Also, if you read the Foreword you will have a better idea of how to use this book, and will learn what we consider to be ten important ways to control your body and increase your health and happiness.

These questions were created by women like yourself and answered by a very caring woman doctor; they were edited and organized by me. My poems on various feelings that we all have are interspersed throughout the book to emphasize the totality of women. We hope that *Take Charge Of Your Body* will help you to take charge of your body.

Susan Polis Schutz

Ten Important Ways to Control
Your Body and Increase Your
Health and Happiness

Take Charge of Your Body will inform you of what goes on in your body and what you can do to control it. Read the sections that concern you, but keep the book handy, because you will be interested in other topics in the future. This book is not a substitute for your doctor. It will, however, give you the knowledge to make choices that are right for you.

Take Charge of Your Body is the source for hundreds of ways in which you can control your own body and increase your health and happiness. Below are ten particularly important facts that we have selected for you to learn about, which could have a major impact on your life. All of these topics are discussed in detail in this book.

1. Did you know that one out of every eleven women will get breast cancer, and that 90 percent of breast cancer is discovered by women themselves? Many of these women could have discovered their condition earlier, thereby greatly improving their chances for being cured. If you learn the simple self-examination technique described in this book (refer to Chapter 3, questions 528 through 533 and the illustration on pages 132 and 133) and spend merely one minute each month doing it, it will enable you to detect a cancerous lump early enough so that you will be able to help choose your method of treatment and possibly cure yourself and extend your life.

2. Did you know that by not having children you increase your chances of getting breast cancer, cancer of the uterus, cancer of the ovaries, endometriosis (small cysts), and fibroids? (Refer to Chapter 8, questions 1811, 1828, 1848, 1852, 1853, 1866, and 1872.)

3. Feelings of depression, lethargy, anxiety, cramps, headaches, indigestion, craving sweets, and sleeplessness before menstruating are felt by 40 percent of menstruating women who are not on birth control pills. You are normal, not "crazy," if you feel these things. Society is finally recognizing this as a genuine, uncomfortable syndrome called premenstrual syndrome. Now there is research being done to discover why premenstrual syndrome occurs and what type of medication can cure it. Did you know that the latest research shows that your diet may be paramount in preventing premenstrual syndrome? (Refer to Chapter 2, question 431.) Read the section on premenstrual syndrome (Chapter 2, questions 380 through 388 and 425 through 430) and learn to enjoy your female cycle.

4. You probably know that smoking increases your risk of lung cancer, but did you know that recent research has shown that smoking also contributes to heart attacks, bladder cancer, peptic ulcers, chronic bronchitis and, after menopause, the thinning of your bones (osteoporosis)? In order to take charge of your body you should not smoke. (Refer to Chapter 1, question 178 and Chapter 10, questions 2295 through 2299.)

5. Choose the age and time at which you want to have children. Some women want to have children right after high school. Many are now waiting until their mid-thirties, after they have established themselves in careers. You can control when you get pregnant. The pill is the most effective method of birth control, but you must decide whether you want to take it. You must learn about all the methods of birth control, how effective each one is, and what the risks are. Then you are controlling your body. (Refer to Chapter 4 on Birth Control.)

6. Did you know that 60,000 women die each year from broken bones due to the thinning of their bones (osteoporosis), which almost always occurs after menopause? In comparison, 36,000 women die each year from breast cancer. Recent breakthroughs in research have led to an effective medication to prevent this disease, yet few people know about this. Even your doctor may not tell you about it unless you ask. (Refer to Chapter 9, questions 2093 through 2096, 2145 and 2166.)

7. Thousands of women risk their lives because they want to deliver their babies at home. They want their relatives and friends there. But there is a safe way of doing it that is not widely talked about—delivery in a home-like atmosphere in an "Alternative Birth Center" in a hospital. Many hospitals have this, but you must ask about it. They do not advertise it. (Refer to Chapter 7, questions 1538 and 1659 through 1661.)

8. Did you know that about 10 percent of women never have an orgasm? Most of these women could learn to have one if they wanted to. (Refer to Chapter 5, questions 1227 through 1283.)

9. Did you know that as you get older your fertility rate goes down, so that it will take you longer to get pregnant? When you are twenty, it might take you about four months to get pregnant, but when you are thirty-five, you could expect it to take more than eight months to get pregnant. (Refer to Chapter 6, questions 1371 and 1464.)

10. Did you know that you may have had a sexually transmitted disease and received treatment from a doctor without even knowing that you had such a disease? This is because many doctors are afraid to offend their patients by telling them what they have and how they caught it. If you develop a pelvic or vaginal infection other than a yeast infection and your

doctor treats you and your sex partner, you should realize that you have one of the sexually transmitted diseases, such as gonorrhea or chlamydial infection. You must be persistent with your doctor so that you will get specific answers and understand exactly why and how you contracted the disease. (Refer to Chapter 8, questions 1892 through 1989.)

Susan Polis Schutz

TABLE OF CONTENTS

CHAPTER 4. BIRTH CONTROL

CHAPTER 7. NORMAL PREGNANCY AND CHOICES IN CHILDBIRTH

CHAPTER 9. MENOPAUSE

CHAPTER 10. BODY ABUSE

AUTHOR BIOGRAPHIES

INDEX

Chapter 1

Everyday Good Health

This life is yours
Take the power
to choose what you want to do
and do it well
Take the power
to love what you want in life
and love it honestly
Take the power
to walk in the forest
and be a part of nature
Take the power
to control your own life
No one else can do it for you
Take the power
to make your life happy

— Susan Polis Schutz

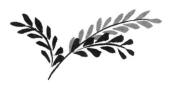

EVERYDAY GOOD HEALTH

Ten Commandments

1. Learn how to self-examine your breasts; you are the one in the best position to find breast cancer in time for a cure.

2. Take care of your body as well as you would your car: feed it, run it, solve its problems, learn how it works, and give it checkups. No one else's name is on the pink slip.

3. Take the mystery out of menstruation; control it if you wish. Learn how healthy and important it is to have your female cycle.

4. Decide whether and when you will have a baby, and choose the birth control method that works best for you.

5. Arrange for the method of delivery that is best for you, but combine it with first-class safety in the hospital. The hospitals can meet all your needs; make demands.

6. Take responsibility for your orgasms; learn to please yourself as well as others sexually.

7. Sexually transmitted diseases are not usually serious, but they may control and annoy you until you control them.

8. Make your own surgical decisions with the assistance of your doctor, and in accordance with **your** health goals, lifestyle, religion, ethics, comfort, and plans, not the doctor's.

9. Put as much effort and planning into your last twenty-five years as you did your first twenty-five, and enjoy them; don't just call them menopause. Lots of people helped care for you during your first twenty-five years, but after fifty you are on your own. Get all the help you need.

10. Nurture yourself at least half as well as you nurture your children, your husband, your parents, and everyone else. You would not let them be sexually abused, battered, hungry, overworked, or drugged. Love yourself as you do your neighbor, and let your neighbor help you when you need help.

EVERYDAY GOOD HEALTH: HOW TO TAKE CHARGE OF YOUR BODY

1. In medical matters, my doctor is in charge; in sex, my partner is usually in charge; at home, my parents or my husband take charge of what is good for me. How can I take charge of my own body?

You must learn to act as your body's owner. Surveys have shown that people have a different attitude toward men and women and treat the two sexes differently, but it doesn't have to be that way. Find out whether or not your doctor is making decisions about your body for your own good and no one else's. Make sure that the doctor's idea of your role in life is not affecting any of his decisions for you. To take responsibility for yourself, you must have knowledge, so acquire it. Do not consider it wrong for women to know something about sex. You are the world's expert on your own sexual functions. After you are eighteen, you are legally the only person who is competent to make decisions regarding your body.

2. I am under eighteen years old, what can I do to take charge of my body?

If you are under eighteen, find out about the laws in your state regarding contraception, abortion, treatment for sexually transmitted diseases, and qualifications for an emancipated minor (a minor who is self-supporting, married, or living away from home). Find out diplomatically how your parents really feel about important issues, instead of assuming that you already know how they feel because they must be like all other parents. You may be surprised. Regardless of your age, you are still your body's owner, so you must act as its owner.

3. Dr. Carson, what is your philosophy on a woman controlling her body, and how do you incorporate this into your practice?

Because of their reproductive capacity, women in the past have been enslaved by others in society who wanted to control childbearing for their own purposes, philosophies, and religions. In the last few years women have realized this, but they need help in their struggle to gain control over their own bodies, so that they can make their own decisions regarding the use of their bodies. To do this, women need knowledge, not only of their own bodily functions, but also of alternatives in medical treatments. If a woman says to me, "You're the doctor!" and then tries to tell me that I should make a decision for her regarding her body, I tell her that she is the patient, and I am only a consultant whom she has selected to help her carry out her wishes. I have a great deal of information and will even make recommendations and provide reasons for the different alternatives, but you always know more about yourself, your life style, goals, and attitudes than anyone else can ever learn. Therefore, you must make any final decision. You even have the legal right to refuse all medical care for yourself if you so desire. I always talk to

EVERYDAY GOOD HEALTH: HOW TO TAKE CHARGE OF YOUR BODY (Continued)

my patients before any examination, including follow-up visits and annual checkups. I give them choices in contraception, styles of delivery, and diagnostic tests. I provide them with reasons for diagnoses, treatments, and their alternatives, and I offer reprints of articles and booklets on subjects that affect them.

EVERYDAY GOOD HEALTH: MAINTAINING A HEALTHY BODY

4. What part does a healthy mind play in maintaining a healthy body?

Perhaps the most important function of a healthy mind is to take action to solve a problem concerning the body; an unhealthy mind may deny or ignore the problem. The mind is the part of the body that acts as the control computer that organizes the action of the whole. If it breaks down, so will something else it controls. We are just beginning to understand how much influence the mind—and our emotions as well—can have on the immune system. Some researchers claim that all problems start with stress and that the role of the mind is being understated. A healthy mind can control our lifestyles and environment, and that can certainly affect our health. Smoking, drinking, drug abuse, poor nutrition, imbalance between rest and exercise, tensions (sexual and otherwise), and reproductive control or chaos are all situations that develop out of our lifestyles and environment.

5. What can I do to keep my body free of disease?

Value and nurture your mental health and happiness. Include exercise and good food in your daily routine, and stay within five or ten pounds of the normal weight for your height (according to insurance tables, not those given in diet programs). Avoid abuse of your body by cigarettes, alcohol, drugs, too little sleep, too much work, or sex with too many partners. Get regular medical examinations, but also seek medical help for any problem you can't solve. Prevent infections by avoiding intimacy with people who may be ill.

6. Is a good, healthy diet a preventative for disease?

Yes, a healthy diet can be a preventative for disease. That explains why a high standard of living with a good food supply is associated with a reduction in diseases, especially infectious diseases. Starving people can die of minor infections, like measles, while healthy people usually will not. If the food supply is too good, however, and there is too much fat and too many calories, other problems arise, such as coronary heart disease. Of course, a really "healthy" diet will not overdo fat and calories.

7. Are some people more prone to disease than others? Are some more immune?

Yes. Some people carry genes that make certain diseases almost in-

EVERYDAY GOOD HEALTH: MAINTAINING A HEALTHY BODY
(Continued)

evitable. Others simply have a very poor immune system, which does not protect them from disease. Children born this way do not live long without intensive treatment. Some adults who suddenly develop a poor immune system are diagnosed to have AIDS (acquired immune deficiency syndrome), which is frequently fatal. Perhaps when immunity is studied more, knowledge will be gained about how to avoid more diseases.

**EVERYDAY GOOD HEALTH: FORMS OF HEALTH CARE—
HOLISTIC AND PREVENTATIVE**

8. What is "holistic health care"?

With holistic health care, the person is treated as a whole, instead of considering only the diseases, disorders, and symptoms that may be present. It is wellness-oriented and balances mind, body, and spirit. Environment, lifestyle, and relationships are considered in the treatment. It provides information for patients that enables them to take responsibility for decisions to optimize their health. Holistic health care is democratic and tolerant, not authoritarian. It provides "tender loving care." It is what every physician has been taught, but sometimes forgets or neglects to do.

9. What is preventative medicine?

Preventative medicine is health care designed to prevent problems rather than treat them, or else to find them early enough so that they can be treated more successfully. Pap smears, breast examinations, physical checkups, blood tests, mammograms, EKGs (elektrokardiogramm), exercise programs, weight control, vaccines, and all health education come under the category of preventative medicine. Medical insurance, however, will not pay for this kind of medical care.

**EVERYDAY GOOD HEALTH: HOW TO SELECT AND
INTERVIEW A DOCTOR**

10. How can I find a doctor who is right for me?

If you only have one doctor in your town, then you haven't much choice, unless you are willing to travel. If you belong to a health care group that restricts your selection to a panel of doctors or does not allow you a choice at all, you may need to learn how to adjust to your doctor in order to obtain the best care. But if your financial status, location, or medical insurance allows you to choose from a wide variety of physicians, then there are several methods for selecting the right doctor. Talking with your friends

EVERYDAY GOOD HEALTH: HOW TO SELECT AND INTERVIEW A DOCTOR (Continued)

will give you an impression of the personality of their doctors, but you must remember that most patients like their doctors. Asking for a referral from the staff at a local hospital you admire is a good beginning, because hospital staffs are constantly reviewed for quality. Asking your medical society for referrals helps eliminate some doctors who have been ousted for serious problems, but it also eliminates good doctors who do not want to pay dues to the medical society. If you have time and money, you can interview all the doctors on your referral lists and choose the one you like best. If you have lots of time, you can use your annual checkup for this purpose. If you need a doctor for a special purpose, you can get referrals from special groups interested in that particular field. An example of one such group is the Planned Parenthood clinics who select doctors who will do abortions in the manner that you want, in either the office or the hospital. Childbirth Education Associations can tell you which doctors like natural childbirth methods, fathers in the delivery room, Leboyer method, Alternative Birth Center rooms, siblings present during the birth, or fathers in the cesarean section room. Mental Health Associations can refer you to psychiatrists who deal with problems, such as drug abuse, incest, or sex therapy. A family practitioner who understands your lifestyle can be the best source of general care and can also refer you to specialists when you need them, matching them with your needs and personality.

11. How do I find a doctor if I have no money or insurance?

If you are truly in need and apply through your local welfare office, most states can provide a form of federally sponsored Medicaid in which state and national funds help pay for your medical care. States that do not participate in Medicaid may also have some minimal welfare care available. If you are in a true life and death emergency, no hospital or emergency room will turn you down. If your income places you in the category between welfare and private care, then you may select a community clinic, often called a "free" clinic, although fees may be requested of some patients. The caretakers there may not always be doctors, but may be nurse practitioners or other licensed health workers who are practicing according to the procedure designed by the physician who is in charge of the clinic. Feminist health clinics, which cater to women, often do not have full-time doctors. However, they may do well in helping you to know your body and to learn to care for it. These community clinics still provide better care than depending on a friend's diagnosis and advice for treatment.

12. How should I interview a doctor in order to select one?

Interviewing doctors may be expensive. Some pediatricians or young

**EVERYDAY GOOD HEALTH: HOW TO SELECT AND
INTERVIEW A DOCTOR** (Continued)

doctors who are new in practice are willing to give free time for interviews in order to build their practice. However, in most cases you are going to pay for a first office visit to find out what the doctor is like. To actually go through a history and physical examination, as well as to talk about your desires for health care, is a better basis for selection than just asking the doctor a few questions. Paying for your visit also puts you on a better footing, especially with a busy physician. Make a list (but not too long) of the most crucial questions that you need answered to decide if this is the doctor for you. Attitudes toward childbirth styles, working mothers, premarital sex, abortion, contraception, sterilization, and discussion of sexual difficulties can be crucial to your future care, yet can be distorted by the doctor's religious or moral convictions. You should find out how the doctor feels on those issues that are important to you. I once suggested that each woman ask her doctor's opinion of the Equal Rights Amendment. If you both are for it or both against it, then your decisions affecting sexual freedom, job disability, and even hysterectomy may be more aligned. Some doctors are so worldly and tolerant that they can adjust to a woman of any cultural or religious background, but some are not. Languages spoken may be crucial, too. In a crisis, many people revert to their native tongue. Another very important thing is to find out how much experience the doctor has had with your particular problem. The more experience, the better.

13. What is the best way to find a doctor in an emergency?

In urban areas, the hospital emergency room is best in emergency situations, since a doctor is already there on duty to start your care. A list of physicians and specialists willing to take a new case for further care and follow-up later is also available there. However, when using an emergency room, you should have a real medical emergency, not just an old problem that you can't stand any longer. In rural areas or small towns, the County Medical Society is a good referral agency in an emergency. The local hospital can also refer you, even if it does not have an emergency room. After hours and as a last resort, there is the yellow page section of the telephone book, where physicians are listed according to their specialty.

14. When is a "second opinion" advisable?

When your doctor's plan of treatment is exactly what you want to do, you do not need a second opinion. But when the doctor's plan involves something you would like to avoid, usually some form of surgery, then you will probably want a second opinion. If it turns out to be the same as the first, you may feel better adjusted to the course of action. You will be more confused if the second opinion is different from the first, but then at least

EVERYDAY GOOD HEALTH: HOW TO SELECT AND INTERVIEW A DOCTOR (Continued)

you will realize that you have a choice of action. If your doctor refuses to do or prescribe something you definitely want, then you also have the option of trying elsewhere. However, if there is an acute emergency, it is usually not wise to try to seek a second opinion.

EVERYDAY GOOD HEALTH: CHECKUPS

15. How often should I have a complete checkup?

The American Cancer Society and the American Medical Association both recommend that you have a complete checkup, including a Pap smear, every three years if you are an adult between the ages of eighteen and fifty, are in good health with no problems found on previous checkups, and have had at least two consecutively normal Pap smears if you are sexually active. If you have engaged in sex since your early teens, have multiple partners, or have had herpes, venereal warts, or a teenage pregnancy, then you are in a high-risk group for cervical cancer, and it is very important that you have a Pap smear at least once every three years. The American College of Obstetricians and Gynecologists advises women to have annual checkups and Pap smears. Due to developmental changes, babies and children under sixteen years of age need checkups varying from monthly to annually. After fifty years of age, all organizations recommend annual checkups, including an X-ray of the breasts (mammogram). If any problem or disease is encountered, your physician may also recommend more frequent visits. You should seek medical care for any problems that warrant it, and women should examine their breasts every month for lumps or other abnormalities. Men should examine their testicles monthly. If you are on any prescription medication, by most state laws, an annual checkup must be done in order to renew the medication.

16. If I have a physical examination each year, can I be reasonably sure that my doctor will spot any disease that might be forming?

"Reasonably sure" is difficult to define. Your doctor will have a better chance of spotting a disease in progress if you are accurate and detailed in describing any changes in how you feel or symptoms that are unexplained. Elaborate laboratory tests and X-rays, electrocardiograms, stress tests, sonograms, and neurological tests are too expensive to do on everyone each year, nor could anyone tolerate all the tests needed to check for all diseases at one time. However, some of these may be indicated by the symptoms you tell your doctor. If you are silent during your examination, the doctor can only identify problems that can be seen, tumors that can be felt, or abnormal cells by way of the Pap smear. Your breast check must be done by you every

EVERYDAY GOOD HEALTH: CHECKUPS (Continued)

month, because in three months a lump can form and grow beyond a surgical cure. You must also see the doctor sooner than your scheduled checkup if you have significant new symptoms. If present, high blood pressure, diabetes that is out of control, cancer of the cervix, breast cancer, large tumors, and enlarged livers will probably be found during your annual examination. This makes a checkup worthwhile, but certainly not all diseases will be found.

EVERYDAY GOOD HEALTH: SELECTING A GYNECOLOGIST

17. How do I go about finding a good gynecologist?

Asking your friends for recommendations is not a bad idea, because by listening to them you may be able to decide whether you would or would not like their doctors. You can also call your local medical society for a referral, and they will give you names of three doctors of whom they approve in your area. An even better way to find a gynecologist is to call the hospital that you think is the best one in your town and ask for a referral. Hospitals keep an even closer eye on doctors than the medical society. If you already have a family physician, ask him or her for a recommendation. At that time, you can also describe what kind of gynecologist you would like to have. The phone book is probably a referral list of last resort, since anyone with a license can be listed there.

18. How can I find a gynecologist who will listen to me?

Talk to your friends about their experiences, because word-of-mouth is still probably the best recommendation. Then you can check on the doctor's qualifications through your local major hospital or medical society. Prepare yourself with knowledge, and review the purpose of your medical visit, so that you know what you want to accomplish. Taking your partner or husband with you to the visit does not always work, because the doctor may talk to him instead of you, but your partner could ask your questions for you if you are too shy. Through your questions show the doctor that you are really interested in your body, in your problems, and certainly in any diagnoses or treatments. Show that you are willing to assume responsibility for yourself and for the outcome of your choices. This actually lifts a burden from the doctor's shoulders. Insist on talking to the doctor before you are examined. Doctors are trained to interact with patients and to respond to their expressed needs. If you are not satisfied during the interview, leave before the examination. You will usually not get a bill. However, if you request free

EVERYDAY GOOD HEALTH: SELECTING A GYNECOLOGIST
(Continued)

time for an interview to select a physician, you may be refused by a qualified, sensitive, responsive physician who is very busy.

EVERYDAY GOOD HEALTH: VISITS TO THE GYNECOLOGIST, CHOICES IN GYNECOLOGY

19. When should I go to a gynecologist?

You should see a gynecologist if your general or family practitioner refers you to one because of a special problem that he or she cannot solve. This referral might come from an internist or from any other doctor you might see. If you feel that you have a problem with heavy bleeding, menstrual pain, contraception, childbearing, sexual dysfunction, vaginal discharge, or a breast lump that your present doctor is not solving, then you should also see a gynecologist. If you have no other physician, you might choose to have a gynecologist as your sole physician. A gynecologist can give you your regular checkups and also refer you to other specialists when you have a problem, such as heart disease or bone fractures, which he or she cannot handle.

20. Do I have a choice in what will happen during a gynecological exam?

You can ask to have a discussion before you are examined. You can request a breast examination if it is omitted. If you have a problem with your breasts or you are over fifty years old, ask for a mammogram (breast X-ray), just as you have learned to ask for a Pap smear. Bring a mirror and ask to see your cervix during the pelvic exam. Bring up contraception for discussion and action, or for referral if religion interferes. Ask to discuss sterilization, if you are interested in this. Discuss any sexual problems that you are having, or ask for a referral to a sex therapist. Ask why you need a checkup more often than the recommended three years needed for the Pap smear. If a hysterectomy is planned, discuss the removal or retention of ovaries and the appendix, too. Ask for alternatives to any treatment that is recommended, medicines as well as surgery, and possible complications and side effects. If you have an unwanted pregnancy and want an abortion, ask for one or for a referral for one. If none is forthcoming, go to a Planned Parenthood clinic for a referral. If your doctor says that it is too late for an abortion, get a second appraisal, as this may just be a matter of opinion. If you are having a baby, ask about preparation classes; if significant other persons are allowed at delivery, even if a cesarean section is done; about rooming in with the baby, even for twenty-four hours a day; about early discharge after delivery; the availability of alternative birth rooms; different methods of childbirth, such as Lamaze, Leboyer, and Bradley; and anything else that you are in-

EVERYDAY GOOD HEALTH: VISITS TO THE GYNECOLOGIST, CHOICES IN GYNECOLOGY (Continued)

terested in including in your birth experience, especially choices of anesthesia. Most doctors will be pleased that you are interested in your examination and treatment. You should care more about your body and give it more thought and consideration than anyone else in the world. He or she may be the doctor, but **you** are the patient.

21. How can I stay in the best of health between visits to my gynecologist?

Your gynecologist will give you instructions to follow between visits. Get regular exercise, maintain a good diet, and make some provisions for happiness. Be observant of your body, and call for help or special examinations between visits if something unusual occurs that you cannot easily explain. Avoid infections. The idea of avoiding infections used to receive a lot more consideration than it does today, probably because everyone trusts antibiotics to cure every infection. The publicity about genital herpes has brought attention to the fact that antibiotics do not always work.

EVERYDAY GOOD HEALTH: PELVIC EXAMINATION AND PAP SMEAR

22. What should a doctor check me for during a pelvic exam?

During a pelvic examination, your doctor will check the lips (labia) around your vagina and the clitoris for abnormalities or difficulties, such as skin changes, infections, or tumors. In addition, you will be checked for: vaginal wall changes; the condition of your cervix; position, size, shape, and any tumors of your uterus; condition of your tubes; size, shape, and the occurrence of any cysts or tumors on your ovaries; abnormal tenderness or pain; and discharge. The opening of your vagina will be checked for tightness or looseness. You will be given a Pap smear, and laboratory cultures will be taken for any suspected infections. The size of your pelvis is important for childbearing plans, and the condition of your hymen is important if you are planning intercourse, so both of these will be checked. Your anus and rectum should also be examined for small ulcers (fissures), hemorrhoids, or rectal problems.

23. What is a Pap smear?

A Pap smear is a sample of cells scraped from the cervix. These are put on a slide and sent to a pathologist where they are stained and examined for cancer cells or abnormal cells that may become cancerous. Dr. George Papanicolaou, for whom the Pap smear is named, discovered that in this way cancer of the cervix can be found while it is in a curable stage. Today the smear also picks up infections of the cervix so that they can be treated. It

EVERYDAY GOOD HEALTH: PELVIC EXAMINATION AND
PAP SMEAR (Continued)

reveals abnormal changes in the cervix that can be studied by biopsy and treated in the office long before they become cancer. In this way, cancer of the cervix can actually be prevented.

24. Why should I get a Pap smear?

The purpose of getting a Pap smear is to find and treat cancer of the cervix while it is in an early stage, long before you have symptoms of bleeding or pain. It also indicates conditions of the cervix that might develop into cancer of the cervix. In this way, cancer of the cervix is totally prevented by minor office treatments or a partial excision (conization) of the cervix in the hospital, and hysterectomies are avoided. The number of women with cancer of the cervix in the United States has actually been reduced in recent years. Thanks to Pap smears, cancer of the cervix is a preventable disease.

25. At what age should girls start having a regular Pap smear and pelvic examination?

A Pap smear is necessary shortly after a girl has had her first intercourse. If she delays intercourse to a later age, then she can delay the Pap smear. However, if her mother had taken DES (diethylstilbestrol) during pregnancy, she not only needs a Pap smear, but she also needs a special examination shortly after she begins menstruation (see "Women's Diseases and Surgery"). If a girl has problems with menstruation, such as not starting menstruation by the age of fourteen, bleeding too much or too often, or if she can't insert a tampon, then she needs a pelvic examination as well. She also needs one before marriage or before starting sexual activity, so that contraception can be discussed and planned. Any problems about childbearing can also be assessed at this time. If there are no problems or she has no sexual activity, then she can delay having a pelvic exam until she is eighteen, when she will not need parental consent.

26. Is there anything that I should or shouldn't do before having a Pap smear or a pelvic examination?

The most important thing that you should **not** do is douche for a day or two prior to an examination. Most gynecologists don't think you should douche at all, but even those who do recommend it will tell you not to do it before an examination. It washes out the cells needed on the Pap smear and also the discharge that is needed to diagnose a problem. It would be best to avoid examinations during menstruation because that prevents study of the discharge, and sometimes it results in a poor Pap smear. Intercourse the night before presents the doctor with sperm and semen in the discharge.

EVERYDAY GOOD HEALTH: PELVIC EXAMINATION AND
PAP SMEAR (Continued)

27. What can women, especially young women, do to calm their fears during a pelvic examination?

Many young women are scared of being hurt during a pelvic examination, particularly if it is their first such exam. One way to avoid this fear would be to place your own finger in your vagina, in order to prove to yourself that it does not need to be painful. If you can insert a tampon without pain, then the small speculum used for a first pelvic examination, which is the same size as a tampon, need not be painful. If you can learn to bear down when inserting a finger, tampon, or even a penis into your vagina, then you can learn to bear down during a pelvic examination. In this way, you can avoid the pain that occurs if you tighten up.

28. What can a gynecologist do to make my examination easier?

Doctors can try to keep on schedule with their appointments. They can have a relaxing waiting room to ease apprehension, and they should always talk to their patients before touching them. Examining rooms should be kept at the best temperature for being nude. Speculums can be warmed prior to use, and coverings can be kept over the metal stirrups so that bare feet won't get cold. Gynecologists should use a small speculum for virgins or women with a small vaginal opening who are relatively inexperienced in sexual intercourse, and they can ask the woman to bear down as the speculum is inserted, so the muscles around the vagina will open instead of close. They can show the woman as much as possible about herself, using mirrors if needed, and also explain things as the examination proceeds. They can take time.

29. How often should I have a Pap smear and pelvic exam?

The American College of Obstetricians and Gynecologists advises you to have a Pap smear and pelvic exam annually. The American Cancer Society advises this every three years, after you have had two consecutively normal Pap smears, until age sixty-five. The Consensus Conference, convened to answer this question by the National Institutes of Health, could not decide on exactly how often Pap smears should be done. They advised one every one to three years. Women who are virgins do not need a Pap smear, but a pelvic examination is still necessary to determine the existence of tumors and cysts. Very sexually active women with multiple partners have a higher risk of cancer of the cervix, so Pap smears for these women are more important. They certainly should not be delayed more than three years.

EVERYDAY GOOD HEALTH: SELF-EXAMINATION OF THE PELVIC AREA

30. How do I give myself a pelvic self-examination?

Lying on your back, you can insert a speculum into your vagina and adjust it so that it will stay open. Then you can hold a mirror in front of it with a good light at one side. In this way, you can see your vagina and cervix. You can insert one or two fingers and touch the cervix, which feels like the end of your nose. With your other hand you can feel your lower abdomen, but it is difficult to feel your uterus or ovaries in this way.

EVERYDAY GOOD HEALTH: GROWTH AND DEVELOPMENT— THE EARLY YEARS

31. At what stage does the fetus take on its sex?

At fifteen weeks from conception, the fetus develops ovaries and female genitalia, or testicles and male genitalia. Before that time, you cannot tell one sex from another just by looking at the fetus. You would have to grow the cells and identify the chromosomes to determine the sex; if they are XX, it is a girl, and XY is a boy. This is one thing that amniocentesis, a prenatal test, can accomplish.

32. What causes "growth spurts," and when do they occur?

Growth is fairly steady until puberty. In girls, puberty occurs the year prior to menstruation, and in boys, it occurs the first year of testosterone production or beard growth. The hormones that first produce puberty stimulate the growth of the long bones, adding four or five inches to height in one year. This is what is often called a "growth spurt." Then the same hormones close the growth centers of the long bones, and no more growth in height occurs.

33. What causes muscle aches and pains, sometimes called "growing pains"?

There is no such thing as a natural growing pain. Rheumatic fever is the actual diagnosis for what people used to call growing pains. It was an arthritis caused by a reaction to a streptococcal infection in children and young adults, and it had serious effects on the heart. Other specific problems around the knees and even injuries or unusual activity can cause pain, too.

34. Are diet and exercise more important when I'm young and my body is still developing?

Yes. If nutrition and activity are missing at the crucial times of the growth spurt or spinal column development, the effects can be lifelong. No amount of nutrition or exercise can make up for it later. Children need good

EVERYDAY GOOD HEALTH: GROWTH AND DEVELOPMENT—
THE EARLY YEARS (Continued)

food and time for play and exercise as much as they need a good education.

35. Do certain parts of the body develop faster than others?

Sometimes one breast develops faster than the other one in girls. Sometimes bones grow long, but the muscles do not develop until years later. Height generally comes before the hips broaden in girls.

36. Is it true that girls develop and mature faster than boys? If so, why?

Yes, this is true, because the sex hormones are produced several years earlier in girls than they are in boys. That explains how it happens, but why? Perhaps it happens this way in order to make females fertile as quickly as possible so that they can reproduce sooner in order to continue the species. Many fertile females are required for reproduction, but not as many males are needed, partly because men are fertile for many more years than women.

37. At what age does most growth occur?

In women, the greatest growth in height occurs in the year prior to the onset of menses, at approximately the ages of eleven or twelve.

38. At what age does growth stop?

Two years after the onset of menses in girls, at approximately the age of fourteen, nearly all growth in height stops. In boys, this occurs later, at sixteen to eighteen years of age.

39. At what age is the body fully developed?

At age twenty-five, the body is fully developed: the bones, muscles, and hormonal status are completely mature, all growth centers are closed, and calcification is complete. That is why weight charts are given for age twenty-five.

40. What sorts of things that would indicate "abnormal" growth or development should I look for in my children?

There are about a dozen books written by Arnold Gesell about infants' and children's development that are good guidelines for this information.

41. Do young broken bones mend faster and better than bones that are broken later in life?

Actually, bones in children are sometimes so soft that they bend, rather than break. This is called a greenstick fracture, and it does heal rather rapidly. However, real breaks in children heal at about the same rate as they do in older people.

You Deserve the Best

A woman will get only what she seeks
You must choose your goals carefully
Know what you like
and what you do not like
Be critical about what you can do well
and what you cannot do well
Choose a career or lifestyle that interests you
and work hard to make it a success
Enter a relationship that is worthy of
everything you are physically
         and mentally capable of
Be honest with people, help them if you can
but don't depend on anyone to make life easy
or happy for you
Only you can do that for yourself
Strive to achieve all that you like
Find happiness in everything you do
Love with your entire being
Make a triumph
of every aspect
of your life

— Susan Polis Schutz

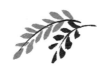

EVERYDAY GOOD HEALTH: GROWTH AND DEVELOPMENT— THE LATER YEARS

42. At what age is a woman considered to be in her best physical condition?

Between the ages of twenty-five and thirty-five, a woman is probably in her best physical condition, especially from a medical viewpoint. For a ballet dancer, this age is much younger, and for a physician it is older, from a professional viewpoint. Socially and intellectually, it can be much older.

43. What changes are likely to occur in the body, particularly the reproductive system, as a woman ages?

Aging of the reproductive organs starts when the ovaries begin to fail. First, they fail to release an egg, and then they fail to produce any estrogen at all. When this happens, the ovaries become smaller, menses stop, and the uterus begins to shrink, along with any fibrous tumors it may have in it. The vagina becomes thinner, drier, more tender, and also shrinks, especially if you are not having regular intercourse. The lips (labia) around the vagina become shorter and thinner, and the tissues that support the vaginal walls become weaker. The breasts become more dense and smaller, and there is less supporting tissue. Hot flushes occur with most people to some extent, but these may disappear after a while.

44. What are some of the other physical changes likely to occur as a woman ages?

As a woman ages, her skin becomes drier and, of course, wrinkles appear. Brown spots develop on her hands, arms, and other areas that are exposed to the sun. Hair becomes thinner and turns grey. The cornea of the eye becomes flatter; therefore, it becomes harder to read at a close distance. Most people lose about one inch in height, due to the flattening of the discs in their spines, and some develop a curved back because of collapsed vertebrae. This happens especially in menopausal and postmenopausal women who do not take certain hormones and it is usually worse in thin, fair-skinned, blue-eyed people. The skin turgor also lessens, so that you can pick up the skin on the back of your hand, and it will stay for awhile in a peak formation.

45. What happens to my bones as I get older?

As estrogen decreases, and especially if the amount of calcium and vitamin D in your diet decreases or exercise lessens, bones lose their density, and the actual substance that forms the center of the bone (the matrix) begins to disappear. A small strain can then cause a fracture, especially to the wrist and hip. Twenty-five percent of women have such a fracture by the age of eighty.

46. Will my bones become more brittle as I get older?

Bones fracture more easily with age because they lose their substance

EVERYDAY GOOD HEALTH: GROWTH AND DEVELOPMENT— THE LATER YEARS (Continued)

and density, especially calcium. With men, this does not usually begin to happen until they are eighty or older, but with women it can occur within five years after menstruation stops. The loss usually occurs at a rate of 1½ percent per year, so that in ten years, 15 percent of the bone is lost, and they look almost transparent on X-rays. As a result, 600,000 women per year in the United States break their hips following even a minor fall or accident.

47. Will vitamins or minerals help to reduce bone loss?

Yes. Vitamin D and calcium are essential in preventing bone loss, although they will not prevent it completely unless estrogen is taken as well. Bone loss is more rapid in fair, blue-eyed, slender women, and much less severe in dark, brown-eyed, overweight women. It is less likely with exercise, and occurs more often in people who are sedentary. Weight bearing exercise, such as running, walking, and tennis, will also help, but an activity like swimming will not.

48. Will hormones help lessen the pains of aching bones?

Yes. Hormone replacement therapy that includes estrogen and progestin, and sometimes testosterone (male hormone), too, seems to arrest the bone loss and reduce the pain associated with arthritis as well. However, it does not actually change the course of arthritis. You may also need to take progesterone to make the estrogen safe if you still have your uterus.

49. Do people really begin to shrink in size as they age?

Yes, even men generally lose at least an inch as they age. This is mostly due to the settling and flattening of the discs, the cushions between the vertebrae, in the spine. If thinning of the bones occurs, the vertebrae collapse even more. This produces a humpback curve.

50. I've never really felt my age. I'm fifty years old right now and quite active. Will my body let me know when it's time to slow down?

If you really listen to your body, you will not ignore chest pain, shortness of breath, unexplained fatigue, or unusual feelings that should remind you that a physical examination and consultation with your physician are needed. You may eventually need to slow down your fast pace, but not the good, outdoor, physical exercise. Most aging people slow down too much when it comes to regular, beneficial, physical activity. If you were inactive, sudden unaccustomed exercise might be hazardous without a checkup first.

51. Why do women outlive men?

According to cardiologists, testosterone causes a change in the blood fats that makes men subject to coronary heart disease, so they tend to die at an earlier age. Estrogen seems to protect women from that. After women lose

EVERYDAY GOOD HEALTH: GROWTH AND DEVELOPMENT— THE LATER YEARS (Continued)

estrogen at menopause, they have more androgens (male-type hormones), but never as much as men have all their lives. A complete answer to this question is not known, and it is probably worth a lot more research.

EVERYDAY GOOD HEALTH: HEREDITY

52. How can members of the same family look so different, especially in size and shape?

The thousands of genes and combinations that are selected when the sperm and egg unite create a unique individual every time fertilization takes place. In this country, there is such a varied genetic background that even siblings can look entirely different. In countries where less mixing occurs, people look more alike. Most people in the United States have at least four nationalities, if not several races, in their backgrounds.

53. Are body size and shape hereditary?

Yes, body size and shape are primarily hereditary. However, well-fed children grow taller and bigger than starving ones, and exercise builds the muscles that contribute to shape.

54. What aspects of the body, such as breast size or susceptibility to disease, are inherited?

The answer to that question is not known. More and more evidence is being found that indicates diseases are hereditary; even the location of the disease on the chromosome is being found. For example, the C6 chromosome carries the diabetes disorder and the hyperthyroid disease. Certainly the smallest details of the body, even facial expressions, are obviously hereditary. Twin studies, where each twin has been raised in a separate environment, are used to point out hereditary aspects of development, especially diseases that affect both twins. Someday, screening for diseases, especially cancer, may be limited to just those persons who have the right heredity for them.

55. What kinds of diseases are hereditary?

As more and more is learned about genetics, it is disturbing to find that genes for certain diseases are actually located on certain chromosomes. Juvenile diabetes is located on the C6 chromosome. Diseases that involve severe degeneration, such as sickle cell diseases, muscular dystrophies, Tay-Sachs, and Huntington's chorea, are inherited and so severe that many people would use abortion to avoid them if they were prenatally detectable. Even hormonal patterns, fibroids, and endometriosis (small cysts) have a family tendency. Changing the hormones by taking birth control pills could

EVERYDAY GOOD HEALTH: HEREDITY (Continued)

make a difference. Breast cancer, ovarian cancer, uterine cancer, colon cancer, and heart attacks have hereditary tendencies, but they have not yet been located on the chromosomes, and the list gets longer every day with new research. Perhaps in the future genetic engineering will help to change the course of some of these diseases, but this is not true of the present.

56. Are most diseases hereditary?

No, most diseases are still infectious. However, some fatal diseases, such as cardiovascular disease and cancer, may be more hereditary than environmentalists would like to think. Since we cannot change the heredity of those already born (at least not yet), we must work on the environmental factors of diet, smoking, and exercise to modify the risk of hereditary diseases.

57. If a certain disease, such as cancer or heart disease, is common in my family, what can I do to lessen my chances of developing the same disease?

Since heart attacks (cardiovascular disease that includes strokes) are the most common cause of death in the United States and cancer the second most common, your family history is bound to include one or the other. If you will learn whatever you can about factors that increase and decrease your risk of familial diseases, then you can change as many of these factors as possible without sacrificing all that you value in your lifestyle. For example, sunscreens can protect your skin if you know skin cancer occurs in your family. If heart attacks abound in your relatives, it is more dangerous for you to smoke. Mammograms can find your breast cancer at an earlier stage than your mother could. You can also ask for more frequent tests and examinations so you can catch and treat the disease early.

EVERYDAY GOOD HEALTH: ANATOMY AND BODY SHAPE

58. Please describe, illustrate, and explain the reproductive system and all of the other parts of both the male and female bodies.

There are many well-illustrated books that do this in great detail. *Gray's Anatomy* is an excellent source to answer your question.

59. Why are there so many different sizes and shapes of women?

Every person has forty-six chromosomes and thousands of genes. When the sperm and egg unite, these combine in a multitude of variations to produce a unique individual. With the availability of worldwide travel, all races of people from different countries have intermingled. Nowhere has there been more intermingling than in the United States, also known as the melting pot of the world. How dull it would be if we were all alike.

60. How is a woman's anatomy specially suited for reproduction?

The most basic requirement for survival of a species is that the male and

EVERYDAY GOOD HEALTH: ANATOMY AND BODY SHAPE
(Continued)

female be attracted to each other so that sexual activity will ensue. Our nervous system accomplishes that. Our clitoris and labia, the lips around the vagina, are equipped with genital bodies that give us sensual pleasure. Our vagina is constructed to accommodate the male penis. The cervix allows the sperm to swim up the uterine cavity into the tubes, where they wait for a fertile egg. Ovaries are cycled to produce an egg each month, and the open end of the fallopian tube is attracted toward that part of the ovary where the egg comes out. It then catches the egg, and as the egg is swept down the tube by millions of tiny cilia toward the cavity of the uterus, the sperm penetrates it. A few days later, when it has divided many times, it implants itself in the wall of the uterus, which is prepared by estrogen and progesterone to let it dig in. The muscle of the uterine wall stretches and grows to accommodate the enlarging fetus. When it is mature and large enough, labor usually starts by some complex mechanism that is, as yet, unknown. The cervix of the uterus dilates to the size of the baby's head. Responding to sensations of pressure in the pelvis, the mother pushes the baby's head out of her vagina and pelvis and into the world. The bones of the pelvis are shaped differently in women than in men, providing a wider opening for the baby's head to come through. Hormones secreted in pregnancy, such as relaxin, make it even larger by loosening the joints of the pelvis. After birth, the mother holds her baby in her arms, and the baby suckles her nipple, where, in a couple of days, milk will be produced. Another generation survives.

61. How does the shape of my pelvic area affect my ability to have children?
You can have children no matter what the shape of your pelvis, but they may have to be born by cesarean section. The male pelvis is shaped like a valentine, with the backbone jutting forward so that there would be little room for a baby's head. The female pelvis is more oval and deep, with plenty of room between the backbone and front pubic bone for a baby's head to pass.

62. Will my anatomy change after childbirth?
Yes. During pregnancy the bones of your pelvis spread, and they do not ever really return to their prepregnancy size. If you have a vaginal delivery, the opening to your vagina is either stretched or stitches are taken in a cut (episiotomy) so that it is not as small as it was before you had a baby. The opening to the cervix is also wider after a vaginal delivery than before you had a child. Some other changes that may or may not occur after childbirth include varicose veins, stretch marks (striae) on your abdomen, separated rectus muscles in the abdominal wall, and a change in the contour of your breasts and color of your nipples.

EVERYDAY GOOD HEALTH: ANATOMY AND BODY SHAPE
(Continued)

63. Is it healthy for a woman to have a little fat on her body?

A little fat is necessary for women to menstruate and be fertile. Therefore, if you consider fertility to be healthy, then it is healthy for a woman to have a little fat on her body. If you have no need for reproduction, menstruation, or ovulation, then a little fat is not required. Ballet dancers have no fat and they are quite healthy, but they might also be infertile. If you are underweight and want to have babies, then you may have to gain some fat.

64. What percentage of a woman's body should be fat?

For fertility, you must have 12-15 percent body fat. During pregnancy, the percentage of fat must rise if you are to have a healthy baby and then breast-feed. To be an athlete, you may have to have less body fat and, therefore, give up your fertility.

65. Are certain areas of a woman's body more prone to fat deposits than others?

Yes, and that is what makes them look like women. In both men and women, fat is first deposited on their abdominal walls, as this is apparently the easiest place for it to go. In women, the next areas in which fat is deposited are their hips and thighs, and then their breasts. Only when fat is extreme does it go to the arms and back. If a man is given female hormones, his fat will also deposit on his hips and thighs, and he begins to look like he has breasts, too. If you give a woman testosterone (male hormones), her weight gain will be more muscular, especially in her back and shoulders.

66. Why are women so heavily built in the hips and thighs?

It is easier for a woman to carry her fat on her legs and buttocks, which are constructed for greater strength than are her arms and back. On the hips and thighs, the fat is also not in her way as much when she is active. Fat that accumulates in her breasts tends to get in her way and also inhibits her ability to run and jump. Men have no similar need for fat and are, therefore, more lean. Muscles make a man's shoulders large, not fat.

67. What has been and is currently considered a perfect figure for women and men?

The "perfect figure" varies from decade to decade. The flapper of the twenties was flat chested, while the "pin-up girl" of the forties was supposed to have very long legs for her body. During the fifties, a woman with a large bosom was popular. Today, it is popular to be slim. Unfortunately, people look down on "female fat." Fat is, indeed, a feminist issue. The "perfect man" does not seem to change as much. He remains broad shouldered, lean hipped, and not too muscular.

EVERYDAY GOOD HEALTH: ANATOMY AND BODY SHAPE
(Continued)

68. What percentage of people have perfect bodies or figures?

Judging from television, movies, and chorus lines, you would think that almost 100 percent of people have perfect bodies. But if you watch people on the street, you see that this is not the case. Of course, the answer to this question depends upon your opinion of ideal body measurements and contours, and also the age at which you judge this.

EVERYDAY GOOD HEALTH: COMPARISON OF THE MALE AND FEMALE ANATOMIES

69. What are the fundamental differences between the male and female anatomies?

A testicle is what makes a male. Only if a testicle is present in the embryo fetus will the anatomy begin to look like a male: developing a penis and scrotum, instead of a clitoris, vulva, vagina, and uterus. If an ovary is present, then the embryo fetus is a female, whether it develops all the other anatomy or not. So, the fundamental difference between the male and female anatomies is that men have testicles and women have ovaries. All other things can be defective, absent, or unusually small.

70. What are the fundamental similarities between the male and female anatomies?

Even though size, shape, and hairiness are different, all of the structures of the two sexes, excepting the reproductive organs, are exactly the same. The bones, muscles, nerves, blood vessels, digestive organs, liver, spleen, and brain are the same in both the male and female anatomies.

71. Are there any differences between the male and female anatomies that would cause differences in emotional responses?

The differences in emotional responses between men and women are usually attributed to the sex hormones coming from the ovary and the testicle. All other hormones are the same between the sexes, as is the brain. But if you give estrogen to the male and testosterone to the female, you don't change their emotional responses, perhaps because previous experiences have already established the pattern. Research has shown that the speed of the transmission of nerve impulses across the gap between nerve endings (the synapse) in the female brain is faster than in the male.

72. Can women handle hard labor jobs, such as factory work, without injuring their bodies?

Some of the hardest labor jobs that women handle are housework,

EVERYDAY GOOD HEALTH: COMPARISON OF THE MALE AND FEMALE ANATOMIES (Continued)

cleaning, moving furniture, chasing and lifting children, grocery shopping (lifting bags and water softener is hard work), and gardening. Yet this is all considered women's work. Many "hard labor" jobs would not be any worse for a woman's body than doing all of these jobs at home. At least when you have a paid job, you think more carefully about how you will lift and accomplish the work, and you strengthen your body so that you can do the job. At home, you think it just comes naturally, but really you should train yourself for home work, too. The worst prejudice is to assume that all men are capable of hard labor, and all women are not. That is not true. Some men can't handle hard labor jobs, and many women can. Conditioning the body for physical activity is the primary solution for women who want a hard labor job. The good pay that many of these jobs offer gives the motivation to women to condition their bodies so that they will succeed. They must also learn to do the work correctly. Still, many men can't do heavy lifting because they have back problems, and many women can't because they have pelvic relaxation problems from having large babies. It is an individual problem and decision, and has nothing to do with a person's sex.

73. Should women avoid lifting heavy objects?

Women who have had children vaginally should avoid lifting heavy objects. This is especially true of women who had their vaginas stretched by large babies, particularly if they did not have the advantage of an episiotomy. The reason for this is that no matter how correctly a woman lifts to protect her back, the pressure on the vaginal opening makes the bladder and rectum protrude, and the uterus comes down and sometimes out of the vagina. This is more true as you get older, particularly after menopause when hormones no longer keep the tissues strong. However, since not all women have had babies, it is not right to make laws that restrict women from lifting because all women do not have this problem. Each woman must determine for herself whether her body will be damaged by heavy lifting. Most of the lifting around the home is done by women regardless of this problem, especially lifting children. In fact, some of the worst damage in older women occurs when they care for and lift their invalid husbands who are bedridden. Perineal muscles can be exercised to strengthen the flow of blood to the pelvis so this will not happen so much. These are called Kegel, or squeeze, exercises. This is very important after delivery, but can be done all your life, especially at the moment of lifting.

74. Are there any differences between male and female anatomies that would cause a difference in physical responses?

Women are more limited than men due to their smaller stature, more

EVERYDAY GOOD HEALTH: COMPARISON OF THE MALE AND FEMALE ANATOMIES (Continued)

delicate bone structure, and smaller muscle mass. The carrying angle of their arms is more pronounced, affecting how they throw a ball. Usually their legs are relatively stronger than their arms, compared to men. When they lift objects it produces great abdominal pressure, and their vaginas tend to bulge, especially if they have had children to stretch the supports around the vagina. Last of all, the presence of tender breasts can limit the amount of pounding a woman's chest walls can stand.

75. Is it true that women have a greater endurance than men?

It is certainly true that women live longer than men. The main difference between the two sexes may simply be the greater incidence of coronary artery disease in men and, therefore, more heart attacks. Men are capable of greater bursts of strength and speed, but, perhaps because of their lower energy output, women can last longer in some tasks. With athletic training, the differences tend to become smaller.

76. Is there any difference between the male and female brains?

The difference between the male and female brain is still under intense study. Some reports have indicated that there is a greater speed of transmission at the gap between the nerve endings (the synapse) in the brain of the female. Some researchers have interpreted this to mean that women are therefore more flighty or intuitive, rather than fast thinking. In babies of the same birth weight, girls generally have higher intelligence test scores at ages five, seven, and nine, according to a British study.

77. How does the center of balance vary between men and women?

The weight distribution is usually heaviest in the chest, shoulders, and arms of the male, but in the hips, thighs, and pelvis of the female. Of course, this is not always true.

78. Do men and women have the same basic bone structure?

Yes, the number, function, and placement of the bones in men and women are the same. However, the pelvis is usually shaped differently and the total height is usually, but not always, greater in men.

79. Are women's vital organs in the same place as men's?

Of course they are. Size, shape, and weight of the organs vary, but the locations are the same.

EVERYDAY GOOD HEALTH: "ABNORMAL" ANATOMY

80. What would be considered "abnormal" anatomy?

There are many variations in anatomy; however, a variation is con-

EVERYDAY GOOD HEALTH: "ABNORMAL" ANATOMY
(Continued)

sidered abnormal only if it interferes with body function. For example: most people are brunette, yet it is normal to have blonde or red hair, too. It is abnormal to be albino (white hair, pale skin, and pink eyes) because it interferes with body function, since these people cannot withstand sunlight. Most people have a second toe that is longer than their great toe, yet approximately 11 percent have a great toe that is longer than their second toe. This is not considered abnormal, because people with both types of toes walk equally well. A club foot is abnormal because it interferes with walking.

81. What kinds of abnormalities in women's anatomy might cause future problems, such as with childbirth or menstruation?

There are many different kinds of abnormalities that might interfere with childbirth and menstruation. A pelvis that is too flat from front to back or too small overall will make childbirth by a cesarean section necessary. A double vagina and/or a double uterus can interfere with intercourse. It can also limit the growth of the fetus to one portion of the double uterus so that a very premature delivery occurs. A blind uterus, which has no opening, can menstruate anyway and cramp with pain. A transverse septum that divides the vagina into two cavities can prevent menstruation and pregnancy, as will a hymen that has no opening (an imperforate hymen). A uterus that is absent from birth will do the same, but there will be no discomfort. An absent vagina can be surgically produced before intercourse occurs, but a uterus cannot be produced or transplanted. Absent ovaries interfere profoundly with development. The clitoris is never absent, and a retroverted uterus does not interfere with functions at all.

EVERYDAY GOOD HEALTH: COPING WITH A BODY THAT YOU DISLIKE

82. How do I cope with a body that I dislike?

Whether or not you like your body is not a matter of taste or beauty, it depends upon how you feel about yourself. If you love yourself, then you are fond of even the obvious faults, because they are yours. If you don't love yourself, then you find fault with your body, even if the world finds it beautiful. Many people dislike their own name! If you don't like your body, then you must work on your self-esteem.

83. Is it common for a person to be ashamed of his/her body?

Yes, this is a common problem, but the reason for it is not because there is something wrong with the person's body. It depends upon whether they

EVERYDAY GOOD HEALTH: COPING WITH A BODY THAT YOU DISLIKE (Continued)

grew up surrounded with love, so that it is natural for them to love themselves. Surveys show that more women are ashamed of their bodies than men, and more women have a poor self-esteem. More men are proud of being men, than women are proud of being women.

84. If I am ashamed of my body, what can I do to feel more comfortable with myself?

You can give your body some assistance. Accomplish skills with your body that will make you proud of the way your body functions. These can be dancing, running, skiing, or even weight lifting. These activities can improve the appearance of your body as well. Dressing with care and consulting a hair dresser or make-up specialist can really help, too. Do not be afraid to spend money on yourself! A healthy diet can help if you are over- or underweight and can also help solve complexion problems. Dermatologists (skin doctors) can be helpful. Plastic surgery is not beyond the realm of possibility if you have a correctable flaw and if you can afford it. Being comfortable with yourself is very important.

85. How would you assure women who are concerned about their figures that "the world needs every size and shape"?

Women today really do not depend upon their size and shape for survival, fulfillment, advancement, or success, although not all of them know that yet. It is far more important that you be able to give and receive love, and that you are able to use all of your talents and powers. Advertising, television, and movies have not yet caught up with what is really happening, and young women sometimes still have the attitude that their looks are all important. With exercise and diet, you can have a good body that functions well for you, and if your face expresses your emotions, then it is functioning, too. A pretty face and a shapely body won't even get you a place in a Broadway musical without the ability to sing or dance. Men have always been valued for their abilities. Now women are starting to be valued for what they can do.

EVERYDAY GOOD HEALTH: VAGINA

86. What is the function of my vagina?

The function of the vagina is for intercourse and the delivery of babies.

87. Where is it located?

It is located between the bladder and the rectum.

88. Does the size and shape of the vagina vary from woman to woman?

Yes, it does. For this reason, diaphragms have to be fitted for each

EVERYDAY GOOD HEALTH: VAGINA (Continued)

woman individually. The size and shape of the vagina also changes with childbearing, but even before that they are different.

89. Is it normal to have extra skin around the vagina?

Yes. The skin around the vagina is folded up into lips. The small lips (labia minora) are closest to the vagina. These elongate at puberty and even more with pregnancy, and turn dark at the edges. Sometimes the minor lip is missing or is a very short fold on one side. The large lips (labia majora) are just outside the minor lips, and these have a pubic-type of hair growing on them. Right at the opening of the vagina is the hymen. After first intercourse, the hymen still exists, but it is broken into little pieces that feel like bumps around the opening, or it is stretched out.

90. Is it normal to have occasional itching and swelling around my vagina? If yes, why?

Yes. It is a normal reaction of skin to swell when it is rubbed a lot and to itch, especially if it is moist. Therefore, wearing tight pants can produce this reaction. Even sexual intercourse (coitus), especially if it is prolonged or if you are not very lubricated, can cause itching and swelling without any infection being present at all.

91. It hurts whenever my husband and I have intercourse. Is it possible that his penis is too large for my vagina?

No. If the pain you are experiencing is at the opening of your vagina, it is the opening that is small, not the vagina. The vagina is more than adequate in size for any penis, provided you have developed as far as puberty; the vagina of a child would be too small. The problem occurs at the entrance to the vagina, at first in the form of a hymen, which may be dilated or torn, and then in the form of a muscle-tightening reaction around the opening, called vaginismus. By squeezing the muscles tightly closed, the opening is then too small for the penis. This is a natural and unconscious reaction to something that was painful in the last sexual experience, and it becomes a vicious cycle. You can learn to overcome this reflex by bearing down to release the perineal muscles. You can also consult your doctor or sex therapist for help with this problem.

92. Is this a common problem?

Yes, it is. Women sometimes allow painful intercourse to occur, and then the next time they try it the muscles tighten without their intending to do so. Most sex therapists find this to be one of the most common reasons they are consulted. If it is not a long-standing problem, it can be reversed in a fairly short time with proper instruction.

EVERYDAY GOOD HEALTH: VAGINA (Continued)

93. Is there a physical reason why some women are unable to use tampons?

Yes. The vagina in some women has been so enlarged by childbirth that it cannot hold in a tampon. Virgins can have such a small opening in their hymen or a band across the middle of their hymen that it will not admit even a small tampon without first being stretched.

94. Is it possible to have my vagina enlarged?

Yes, it is possible, but not advisable. Since it is only the entrance to the vagina that can be too small due to muscle action, you would have to cut the muscles themselves, and then control would be lost. Cutting other tissues to enlarge will not help because the muscles can still close tightly. Instruction on how to gradually admit larger and larger dilators is far more effective and much less expensive.

EVERYDAY GOOD HEALTH: VAGINAL DISCHARGE

95. Is it normal to have a discharge between periods?

Yes, it is normal. The lining of the vagina constantly sheds and combines with mucus from the glands to form a discharge. Usually bacteria grow in the vagina and are also present in the discharge.

96. Why do I have mucus discharges between menstrual periods?

The vaginal discharge changes throughout the menstrual cycle in response to hormone production. It has a very delicate and specific function. There is very little discharge after the menstrual flow, but at mid-cycle, when ovulation is about to occur, the discharge becomes very clear and stringy, especially right in the opening of the cervix. This kind of discharge allows sperm to penetrate more easily by helping them to enter the uterus at the right time for getting pregnant. After ovulation, the discharge becomes thick and pasty. This type of discharge is hostile to sperm and does not permit entry any more.

97. What causes mucus discharge between periods?

The most mucus is produced by glands that are located around the cervix at the time of ovulation. Some mucus is produced all the time by glands located around the cervix and around the opening of the vagina as well.

98. What are these discharges made of?

The vaginal discharge consists of: cells shed by the vaginal wall, the cervix, and endocervix (the opening of the cervix); mucus from the glands around the cervix and the Bartholin's glands; as well as mucus and fluid that are secreted by the vaginal walls when you are sexually aroused. It normally

EVERYDAY GOOD HEALTH: VAGINAL DISCHARGE (Continued)

contains a mixture of bacteria, especially Doderlein's bacillus, lactobacillus, and others.

99. What color and consistency should a normal discharge be?

Normally this varies throughout the cycle. The discharge is scant in the first half, then thin and watery mucus during mid-cycle when ovulation occurs. After ovulation, it becomes thicker and creamy white in color, like paste or whipped cream. Grey, yellow, and green are abnormal colors that would suggest infections.

100. Should I worry if my discharges are quite heavy?

No, because the normal quantity varies a lot. If you are under tension or are sexually aroused, there will be a greater quantity of discharge. If you have an infection, there will be itching, burning, discomfort, or a foul odor. Then you should worry enough to seek a medical examination.

EVERYDAY GOOD HEALTH: DOUCHING

101. Is douching harmful?

Eighty percent of gynecologists consider douching to be harmful, because it introduces substances and bacteria into the vagina that do not belong there. It also changes the bacterial flora and may encourage yeast infections, since it can remove the normal bacteria that resist yeast. It can be drying and irritating to the mucosa lining, depending upon which douche powder or solution you use, and it is generally unnecessary for cleanliness.

EVERYDAY GOOD HEALTH: HYMEN

102. What is the purpose of the hymen?

Perhaps the hymen serves to keep sand and other foreign objects out of the vagina of a little girl as she sits on the beach, for example. The adult vagina cleans itself by the production and passage of discharge, but the little girl has no such defense. Of course, some people would say that the hymen serves to tell who is a virgin and who is not, but it is not very accurate for that purpose.

103. What physical changes occur in a young girl the first time that she has sexual intercourse?

Whether the girl is young or old, first intercourse will either tear or stretch her hymen to the size of the penis that enters it, unless it has been previously dilated by some other method. No other physical changes really take place.

EVERYDAY GOOD HEALTH: CLITORIS

104. Where is the clitoris?

The clitoris is located where the labia minora, the small lips of the vagina without hair, come together above the vagina and above the urethra. It is a small tubular structure above the pubic bone, whose end is covered by a fold of tissue or a hood, which can be pulled back in order to see the end of the clitoris.

105. How big is the average clitoris?

The average clitoris measures one inch long and one-quarter inch in diameter.

106. How can I see it?

Take a mirror and hold it up in front of your vaginal area. Spread the lips of your vagina open, and you will see the little end of your clitoris peeking out of the hood. If you can bend over far enough, you can also see it directly without using a mirror.

107. What is the function of the clitoris?

The sole function of the clitoris is for sex. It is richly endowed with nerve endings, and transmits the stimulation that leads to orgasm. Although it is usually too sensitive to touch directly, nearby touch is effective. During coitus, the labia minora wrap around the penis and with each thrust pull the hood back and forth over the clitoris, giving it stimulation that leads to orgasm. Of course, mere mechanical action is not effective, and must be combined with all of the other methods of sexual arousal.

EVERYDAY GOOD HEALTH: UTERUS

108. What is my uterus?

It is your womb, inside of which a fertilized egg can attach and develop into a baby.

109. Where is my uterus?

Most women have an anteflexed uterus; that is, one that tilts forward at a right angle to their vaginas. It usually rests against the back wall of the bladder.

110. What is a prolapsed or dropped uterus?

After childbirth, especially with a large baby or in certain families where the tissues are inherently loose, the ligaments that hold the uterus in place remain stretched. The uterus drops farther into the vagina than before, sometimes dropping so far that it appears at the opening of the vagina where you can see it. In severe cases, it comes completely out of the opening of the vagina and hangs out several inches, especially when there is straining, walk-

EVERYDAY GOOD HEALTH: UTERUS (Continued)

ing, or lifting taking place. When the woman lies down, it goes back in. Heavy lifting contributes to the uterus dropping out, but it is not the whole cause.

111. I've been told by my doctor that I have a retroverted or tipped uterus. What does that mean?

In most women, the top (fundus) of the uterus leans forward toward the bladder, but in about one-third of women it leans back toward the rectum. This is what your doctor means by a retroverted or tipped uterus. Sometimes it leans only partially back, and this is called mid-position.

112. If I have a retroverted or tipped uterus, will I have any trouble becoming pregnant?

No, this will not interfere with your getting pregnant. The vagina is closed, and the walls touch each other when nothing is in it. This brings the sperm up against the cervix, no matter what position the uterus is in. In the South Sea Islands, the midwives noticed that the women who had children more often had a uterus that was tipped back, so they associated it with fertility and manipulated the uterus of women who couldn't get pregnant until it was in the retroverted position. They thought it would make the women fertile. They were just as wrong as the tale told here that the tipped uterus is less fertile. The only problem it can produce is that it can hurt during intercourse if it is tender, since it is in the direct line of the thrust.

EVERYDAY GOOD HEALTH: HORMONES

113. What are hormones?

Hormones are substances that are produced by glands in one part of the body, but have their action and effect in another part of the body. Some hormones are testosterone, estrogen, progesterone, cortisone, insulin, oxytocin (Pitocin), epinephrine (Adrenalin), growth hormone, prolactin, and many others with more complicated names. The list continues to grow as new ones are identifed.

114. Do men and women have the same hormones?

Most of the hormones, such as thyroid, growth hormone, and cortisone, are the same, while the sex hormones are mainly different in quantity. Men have some estrogen in small amounts, and women have some testosterone in small amounts. In some diseased states, if a woman produces a lot of testosterone, she can become defeminized or masculinized. If a man has a disorder that produces a lot of estrogen, he develops breasts, fat over his hips and thighs, if he has fat at all, and suppression of testosterone production. Since men do not release eggs, they cannot form a corpus luteum (a small

EVERYDAY GOOD HEALTH: HORMONES (Continued)

yellow body that forms after ovulation) that makes progesterone, so progesterone is unique to women, but women only have it when they ovulate.

115. Why do women need hormones?

All plants and animals require hormones to survive. Each hormone has its own function; some are essential to life and others are just beneficial. Women need the benefits of estrogen and progesterone, the female hormones produced by the ovaries, to develop the secondary sex characteristics of breasts, body contours, and feminine appearance, as well as the uterus to maintain a pregnancy. Women can survive without estrogen and progesterone, but not as well. They particularly need these hormones to maintain calcium in their bones, normal skin, a moist and nontender vagina, and normal bladder function.

116. How do hormones affect my growth and development?

Growth and development are almost entirely controlled by hormones, and the pituitary gland is the leader. Thyroid and growth hormone maintain the growth of the body. Gonadotropins from the pituitary cause the ovaries (or testicles) to develop and produce the hormones that create the adult female (or male) appearance; they also help to stop growth. Insulin and the adrenal hormones are necessary for the maintenance of life. Their action and interaction are really quite complicated, making a fascinating study.

117. Does the amount of hormones in my body vary from day to day, or is it always the same?

It varies. Thyroid is one of the more stable ones, while cortisone varies with the time of day. It is different during the day than it is at night. Many of the pituitary hormones that control the sex hormone production change every hour and a half, and of course, the estrogen and progesterone vary according to the menstrual cycle. Epinephrine (Adrenalin) can even change depending upon the state of stress and excitement.

118. How does my hormone level change during the menstrual cycle?

During menstrual flow, production of estrogen and progesterone falls to a low level and almost ceases. Following menses, estrogen is produced by the ovaries, with a sudden spurt in production at the time of ovulation. This is followed by the addition of progesterone production from the ovaries, as well as increased estrogen production. Fourteen to sixteen days after ovulation occurs, this hormone production from the ovaries stops, and menses follow.

119. Will the amount of hormones in my body change as I grow older?

Yes, indeed. The very definition of menopause is the reduction of female hormones, so that menstruation no longer occurs. Growth hormone is produced primarily in children and young people until they reach their full

EVERYDAY GOOD HEALTH: HORMONES (Continued)

growth. If a pituitary tumor produces it in later life, this is a serious disorder, called acromegaly. If estrogens occur in a very young girl, this is usually called precocious puberty, although it may also be caused by a serious ovarian tumor.

120. How do hormones affect my mood?

It is not an accepted medical fact that hormones affect your mood. The biochemistry of moods involves far more than just hormones. Because premenstrual syndrome (PMS) occurs at the time of their cycle when women have the highest hormone production, it has been attributed to the excess hormones. It has also been attributed to a deficiency of hormones by some people, but this is denied by others. Likewise, birth control pills are associated with mood changes in some women, but not most others.

121. Do hormones directly influence the growth of fatty tissue?

The thyroid hormone controls the rate of metabolism, which is the burning of energy-containing tissues. Adult onset of hypothyroidism is associated with fat that is very hard to lose without taking thyroid. Unfortunately, most overweight people have normal thyroid action, but they should have a test to be sure of that. Estrogen and testosterone control the distribution of fat in women and men, but do not control the quantity. Women get fat on their hips; men get fat on their bellies. When the fat is extreme, men and women begin to look alike.

122. Are hormone pills safe?

Hormone pills are relatively safe, but nothing is absolutely safe. Whether hormones are safe depends upon which hormone you are asking about and the state of your health. Doctors try to weigh the risks and benefits with you every time they prescribe a medication. They should discuss the use of hormones with you, relative to your particular situation. What is safe for one person may be quite risky for another. You have to consider the dangers to your health involved in not taking the hormones, too.

123. Are the hormones in my body the same as those sometimes prescribed by the doctor?

Prescription hormones are not identical to those produced in your body, but they function in a similar way. Sometimes the way in which they function is not similar enough; sometimes it is better. The natural extractions of hormones used are not pure; the synthetic ones may only function similarly in one way and not in another. The body converts prescription hormones into other compounds, which are sometimes more similar to the hormones produced in the body. There is hope in the future that a synthetic hormone can be produced that is exactly what the body should have. An example of a synthetically produced hormone that works very well in the body

EVERYDAY GOOD HEALTH: HORMONES (Continued)

is human insulin. It is now produced by a bacteria whose genetics have been changed by genetic engineering, and it works better for the patient than any insulin extracted or produced before.

EVERYDAY GOOD HEALTH: GLANDS

124. What is the function of glands?

All of the functions of the body are influenced or controlled by glands. There are many different kinds of glands, but what they all have in common is that they secrete something. Endocrine glands secrete a hormone that works somewhere else in the body, while other glands secrete something that works nearby. The entire breast is a modified sweat gland that secretes milk. Salivary glands make saliva in the mouth to start digesting food. The pancreas secretes pancreatic juices that digest food and also insulin which works all over the body to metabolize carbohydrates.

125. What are the names of the glands that influence sexual development?

The hypothalamus is not a gland, but it is the base of the brain that causes the pituitary gland that is located just below it to secrete (or not secrete) gonadotropins that cause the ovaries to produce estrogen. Estrogen then produces its effect on the breasts, uterus, vagina, labia, and in fact the entire body to make it look feminine. Further secretions by the pituitary cause ovulation, and then the ovaries can produce progesterone, too. The adrenal gland produces androgens (male-type hormones) that cause the growth of pubic, underarm, and body hair.

126. Where are the glands located which influence sexual development?

The pituitary gland is located at the base of the brain, in the middle of the head, almost between the eyes but a little lower. The ovaries are on each side of your pelvis, attached both to the uterus and to the side wall of the pelvis by ligaments, but movable in position. They lie alongside the fallopian tubes, so their eggs can go into the tubes. They are usually just above your groin on each side, but sometimes lie in the middle of the pelvis behind the uterus. When you are pregnant, they rise out of the pelvis along with the growing uterus to which they are attached. The testicles, of course, are in the scrotum of the male, the sac just below the penis. If they are not there, then they may be "undescended," which means they lie along the groin or back inside the abdomen like the ovaries do. They do not work well here, and often become cancerous.

127. Can glands which do not function properly be a cause of obesity?

If the thyroid gland is underfunctioning, it can cause obesity, and so can injuries to the hypothalamus. Stein-Leventhal syndrome, or polycystic

EVERYDAY GOOD HEALTH: GLANDS (Continued)

ovaries, is also often associated with obesity. However, most obesity is caused by overeating and underexercising.

128. Could problems with my glands be a cause of breast cysts?

Yes, glandular problems can be a cause of breast cysts. If your ovaries do not ovulate, resulting in constant estrogen stimulation without progesterone, there is a greater incidence of fibrocystic breasts. If thyroid function is altered so that it prevents ovulation or prolactin produced from the pituitary prevents ovulation, then indirectly, they are also the cause of breast cysts.

129. Are thyroid problems common in women?

Thyroid problems are more common in women than in men. They also seem to recur in families.

130. What is hypothyroidism?

Hypothyroidism is a condition in which your thyroid gland produces too little thyroid for the body to function properly. Your metabolism is too slow, your heart beats slowly, and sometimes the heart function is not at all efficient, so that heart failure can occur. Sleepiness prevails, your eyes become sunken in appearance because the lids are partly closed, reflexes are slowed, constipation increases, you are constantly too cold, weight gain occurs even with less eating, and sometimes the face swells with a thick fluid.

131. What is hyperthyroidism?

Hyperthyroidism is a condition in which your thyroid gland produces too much thyroid for your body to handle. Your metabolism is too fast, your heart beats too quickly and becomes exhausted, insomnia prevails, your eyes stare, tremors develop, bowel movements occur too often, perspiration occurs because you are constantly too warm, weight loss occurs even with increased appetite and eating, and in severe cases death can result from heart failure.

132. Are thyroid nodules (or enlarged thyroid glands) common in women?

Thyroid nodules are certainly not normal and must be investigated every time they occur. They may be due to inflammation (thyroiditis), overactivity (hyperthyroidism), underactivity (hypothryoidism), or even cancer of the thyroid, which actually is more common in women than men. There are many tests and treatments for all of these conditions.

133. What are lymph nodes?

Lymph nodes are glands that produce lymphocytes, which are part of the white cells in our blood that fight disease. There are many lymph nodes located throughout the body. They are part of the lymph circulation system, which returns extra-cellular fluids to the blood stream. You can feel them

EVERYDAY GOOD HEALTH: GLANDS (Continued)

swell and become tender in your neck when you have a sore throat, or even in your elbows when you have mononucleosis. They also trap cancer cells that drain along lymph channels, and can become large and nontender.

134. Where are the lymph nodes located?

Common places that you can feel lymph nodes when they are enlarged are in the groin, draining infection from your feet, and in the neck, draining infection from your teeth and throat. These cannot be felt when they are not enlarged. Lymph nodes also exist along the intestinal tract, lungs, pelvis, arms, legs, scalp, chest well, and in fact, throughout the body.

135. Why do lymph nodes sometimes become enlarged?

Most of the time it is because they are draining infected areas. Lymph nodes trap and fight infection in the node, producing an increased amount of lymphocytes to do so. Less often it is because cancer cells have found their way from the original cancer to the lymph node and have taken up residence there and are growing.

136. What are the signs that my lymph nodes are not functioning properly?

When lymph nodes are enlarged and tender, they are involved with fighting infection from their territory, but that is indeed their proper function. They may even remain large, but less tender, for two or three weeks after such an infection occurs. If they are in your neck, look for infection in your teeth, throat, or even ears. If they are at the nape of your neck and you have a red rash, you might have rubella (German measles). If they are in your groin, look for an infection from cutting your toenails, going barefoot, or even an infection on your labia, the lips around your vagina. If they are on your elbows or elsewhere, you can have a blood test to check for mononucleosis. If your nodes are large and nontender, there is more likely to be something seriously wrong, so let your doctor check for the cause. One particularly important node is the one in your neck just above your collar bone, because it drains infections from the abdomen. Sometimes a biopsy has to be done to find out why the lymph node is large.

EVERYDAY GOOD HEALTH: APPENDIX

137. What does my appendix do?

Your appendix has no known beneficial function in man. It can get infected and fill with pus, causing appendicitis, or an infected appendix can rupture causing peritonitis (infection) all over the abdomen. You should have it removed (an appendectomy) before it has gone this far.

138. Where is the appendix located?

The appendix is located on the right side of the abdomen, low in the

EVERYDAY GOOD HEALTH: APPENDIX (Continued)

pelvis, almost to the groin, which is the crease where the thigh is attached. It is found at the beginning of the large colon, where the small bowel enters.

EVERYDAY GOOD HEALTH: HAIR

139. What causes dry hair? Oily hair?

Thyroid function may have more to do with the texture of hair than anything else. When it is low, the hair is dry and fine. The type of skin you have also affects your hair. If you have oily skin (seborrhea) and a lot of acne, you will have scalp trouble and oily hair, too.

140. What will make my hair look better?

Good nutrition helps to make good hair. Sun and wind dry out the hair and scalp. Permanents and bleaching tend to weaken the hair, but new hair will grow back normally. Keeping your hair clean will make it look better.

141. How and why does the texture of my hair change when I am pregnant?

Sometimes your hair becomes better and stronger because you take care of yourself better and eat better when you are pregnant. In other cases, it becomes dry and fine because your thyroid is relatively low, or you do not eat enough for both you and your baby. There is no consistent change in hair texture for women in pregnancy.

142. What causes hair loss?

As children develop, their hair becomes thicker until maturity, about the age of twenty-five. After that, the hair usually becomes gradually thinner, becoming markedly thin after the age of seventy-five. This varies with heredity and severe illnesses. Patchy baldness, where the hair leaves one spot and not another, is called alopecia areata, and is attributed to nervous causes. It is usually temporary. Permanent baldness on the crown is hereditary in males. If a woman becomes bald in this way, she should be tested for testosterone production. If she has the heredity for this type of baldness and takes testosterone, she can become bald. Some chemotherapy for cancer produces temporary baldness, and radiation can produce permanent baldness.

143. Is it normal to lose a little hair each time I brush or shampoo?

Yes, this is normal. In some seasons you will lose more hair than in others, due to periodic shedding.

144. Is there any way to permanently remove unwanted facial hair?

Yes. Electrolysis is performed by licensed technicians, and permanently removes the hair it treats. There is no guarantee that you will never grow new hair again, but if you do, a subsequent treatment can remove that, too. It is available in private offices and beauty parlors, as listed in your telephone

EVERYDAY GOOD HEALTH: HAIR (Continued)

book. Shaving, bleaching, and plucking to remove hair consume a lot of time and are only temporary.

145. Why do some women develop more hair on their legs and pubic area than others?

In some women, it is completely hereditary that they have a lot of hair, even though they have very few male hormones (androgens) in their bodies. Other women actually produce more male hormones (androgens) from their ovary and adrenal glands. Sometimes birth control pills are used to suppress the ovary, or cortisone is used to suppress the adrenal gland. When excess body hair (hirsutism) is extreme, there may be a tumor of the ovary or adrenal gland producing these hormones. If so, the clitoris will enlarge too. This requires medical examinations, tests, and perhaps surgical removal of the tumor. Fortunately, these conditions are very rare.

146. When I get older and my hair turns gray, will my pubic hair also change color?

Yes, eventually this will happen, but probably not at the same time. The gray hair on your head will come first. Pubic hair is not the same kind of hair as that on the head, nor is it under the same controls.

EVERYDAY GOOD HEALTH: SKIN

147. Why does my skin dry out as I get older?

People are born with beautifully moist skin. The main drying agent is the sun, and next is the wind. The portions of skin that are kept shielded from these agents do not dry out as much as the exposed areas. However, as we get older, there is also some drying caused from a lack of estrogen, which keeps some water content just beneath the skin when we are younger. Poor nutrition also contributes to dry skin, especially if there is a deficiency of vitamins A and D. The best agent to prevent drying is a sunscreen. You can either use the liquid kind that you apply to your skin or a mechanical one, like a good hat. You could also simply stay out of the sun.

148. What can I do about the scars on my face that are the result of acne when I was younger?

You can consult with a dermatologist or plastic surgeon regarding your problem. They are specialists who can do skin abrasions or planing to diminish your scars. Often the results are very good.

149. I've heard that putting vitamin E on blemishes will help them heal and prevent scarring. Is this true?

Even some plastic surgeons report that this is true, but scientific in-

EVERYDAY GOOD HEALTH: SKIN (Continued)

vestigation does not seem to bear them out. The enthusiasm for vitamin E is widespread, but that does not mean it is deserved.

150. What can I do about the rash that I sometimes develop as a result of shaving my pubic area bikini style?

You can apply a topical hydrocortisone, now sold over the counter, to the skin after shaving, which will reduce the redness. Washing with medicated soap, such as Phisohex, to keep the bacteria count down also helps. Even applying an antibiotic cream, like bacitracin, to the skin reduces the little infections that occur in the hair follicles that have been cut. You could also shave less closely.

151. What causes age spots, also called liver spots?

These are caused by the sun. In some people, although certainly not in all, the action of the sun on the skin produces spots of brown pigmentation on the hands, arms, and other exposed areas, including the face and neck. The condition becomes worse with age. With continued usage and application, some creams can fade these spots. Some of these are available by prescription, and others are sold over the counter. It takes months of application, however, and if you still expose your skin to the sun, there may be no improvement.

152. Is it true that wearing nylon undergarments prevents the skin from breathing and are therefore unhealthy?

Unlike some reptiles, humans have very little respiration through their skin; they breathe with their lungs. However, they do have perspiration. Since nylon does not absorb moisture well or allow much air circulation to evaporate the sweat if the nylon clothing is tight, it may cause more problems in cooling the body. If the clothing is loose, air circulates anyway and does its job. In temperate climates this is not really a problem, but in the tropics, cotton becomes important.

EVERYDAY GOOD HEALTH: THE IMPORTANCE OF GOOD POSTURE

153. How important is good posture?

Good posture is essential for avoiding backaches and other muscle and bone aches and pains. You do not even breathe well when you have poor posture. Good posture also makes other people think you feel well, even if you don't. Being happy, proud, and having a good self-image are probably the best ways to promote good posture. Exercises that train your body for good posture habits will also work well.

EVERYDAY GOOD HEALTH: THE IMPORTANCE OF SLEEP

154. How much sleep do I need to stay healthy?

Recent studies have determined that eight hours is the average amount of sleep you need to stay healthy, but this is not a general requirement. There is a great deal of variation. If you do not feel well when you get less than eight hours of sleep, then you should try to get eight hours and see if this makes you feel better.

155. What is the best position for sleeping?

The best position for sleeping is on your side. The small of the back is too curved, or swayback, when you sleep on your back or on your stomach. In pregnancy, it is crucial that you sleep on your side after the seventh month, not only for your back, but also to allow circulation to your uterus and your baby. It is also essential that you turn over and move about in your sleep, to avoid prolonged pressure on one spot.

156. Is broken sleep as restful to the body as continous sleep?

If the dream cycles are interrupted, the sleep is not as restful. Most sleep varies from deep to light, with dream sleep occuring at least every ninety minutes. This is called REM sleep, in which there is rapid eye movement with the eyes closed. Without REM sleep, you are not as rested, regardless of how long you sleep. Many sleeping pills eliminate REM sleep, so there is a feeling of fatigue the next day. Sleep that is interrupted at some time other than during the dream cycle, is as restful as it would have been without the interruption.

157. Why does sex before sleeping lead to a very deep, sound sleep?

If the sex involves orgasm, this relaxes the body and discharges the whole nervous system so that sleep is promoted. If no orgasm occurs with sex, sleep may be hard to induce. Adults sometimes forget that orgasm promotes sleep and try sleeping pills instead.

158. Is the night sleep cycle our natural cycle?

In general, the daylight environment is more stimulating to wakefulness and the dark night more conducive to sleep, but this can be changed, so it is not inevitable. When you travel to another time zone, it takes a long time to convert your sleep cycle to the new hours of darkness. It takes time to convert the metabolic and hormonal systems of the body, especially cortisone, when there is jet lag. However, night workers, for instance, can learn to sleep in the daytime if they try long enough.

EVERYDAY GOOD HEALTH: THE IMPORTANCE OF A DAILY BOWEL MOVEMENT

159. How important is a daily bowel movement?

The Egyptians thought it was very important to have a daily bowel movement, but modern medicine deems it to be unnecessary. Regular elimination is essential, but regular can mean every other day, or every day. It should be at consistent intervals. Many healthy people have a bowel movement once a week, and some once a month. The problem to avoid is hard stools that are painful and difficult to pass. Bran or other roughage included daily in your diet can prevent this from happening. Chronic constipation (hard stools) can lead to hemorrhoids or even bowel cancer. Bran and roughage can prevent the bowel cancer that is so common to Americans who have relatively soft diets. Laxatives should rarely be used, except in unusual situations, because chronic, harsh laxatives can lead to diverticulosis. This is a common disorder after the age of fifty, in which swelling occurs on the colon, like blisters on a tire, that can become infected and rupture.

EVERYDAY GOOD HEALTH: EXERCISE

160. How important is exercise to having a healthy body?

Our muscles absolutely require use to keep fit. Our heart is a muscle that needs to be worked vigorously in order to keep the blood vessels that serve it, the coronaries, in proper condition. Our nervous system is also better toned if we occasionally do something besides sit and worry. Even our digestive system has less constipation if we provide for daily exercise. Our lungs expand and clear out inactive areas that remain unexpanded when we do not exercise. Our skin improves with the circulation that accompanies exercise, provided we do not get too much sunburn with the exercise. Bones retain their calcium only if we exercise; calcium leaves bones when we just lie in bed. Of course, if our daily work involves exercise, then we do not have to make a special effort to obtain it.

161. What kinds of physical activites are not good for a woman's body?

Lifting is probably more damaging to a woman's body than to a man's. Lifting puts pressure on the support structures of the vagina, and if a woman has had a vaginal delivery, these may be already stretched. Heavy lifting can produce bulging of the bladder and rectal walls through the vagina or lowering of the uterus, called prolapse. Both sexes develop back difficulties from lifting, but women are at a greater disadvantage because their sacroiliac joints are loose and more liable to strain than the rather solid joints of men. Women who have had babies have even looser sacroiliac joints.

EVERYDAY GOOD HEALTH: EXERCISE (Continued)

162. Have women athletes been known to suffer any physical problems which relate directly to their being women?

Many women athletes stop menstruating while they are active, but this is hardly suffering.

163. What impact does strenuous exercise have on the female body?

Research in this area has just begun. Frequent strenuous exercise can lead to the loss of menstruation altogether as a result of the loss of body fat, and perhaps through the loss of other body mechanisms. Exercise in pregnancy has always been recommended in a light way but is now being studied in detail. Early results show that moderate exercise during pregnancy is not harmful. It may be some time before strenuous exercise is studied in pregnancy; however, most doctors do not recommend it.

164. How much can exercise determine a woman's build?

A woman's bone structure does not change once she is mature, but her posture changes with exercise. Muscles to support good posture need help. Distribution and reduction of fat with an increase in muscle give a different appearance to the body but do not change the build.

165. Is it possible to build up my bust size through exercise?

Exercise will improve your posture so that your breasts look larger when you stand with your chest held up and out, instead of slumped, but they are not actually larger. The pectoral muscles of the chest can become larger and, therefore, lift the breasts up, but the breasts themselves are not larger. You can notice this in male athletes or body builders, who have large chest muscles.

166. Why are women's muscles shaped differently than men's?

The muscles throughout a woman's body are exactly the same as those in a man's body. They are just smaller in size to fit a woman's smaller body, and they may be less developed according to her lifestyle. The distribution of fat in the body along with the shape of the pelvic bones and the angles of the joints, especially the hips and elbows, make a woman's shape look different from a man's.

167. Are women's muscles capable of achieving the same strength as a man's?

Probably not. Some women can build their muscles so that they have even greater strength than some men, but if you compare the strongest men with the strongest women, the strength of the women will be less. Some women have taken testosterone, the male hormone, to build their muscles, and it really does increase muscle size and strength. In the United States, using hormones in this way is considered cheating in athletic competitions. The bone structure of women is smaller and cannot support the muscles that

EVERYDAY GOOD HEALTH: EXERCISE (Continued)

larger-built men can support, although most women can improve the strength of their muscles more than they imagine. Working out with weights has become popular for women today.

168. What kinds of exercise are good for women who need to lose weight in problem areas, such as the thighs, waist, and stomach?

For the thighs: running, bicycle riding, dancing, and floor workouts in which the leg is raised from the floor while you are on your side are all good exercises. For the waist, you can go swimming and do floor exercises in which twisting the waist is emphasized, such as side bends. For the stomach, try swimming, sit-ups, and floor exercises where you lie flat and then raise your legs.

169. Is aerobics a good method of exercise for women?

Yes, because women like it. You will do something you enjoy much longer and more often than something that is boring. Aerobics conditions your heart and your entire cardiovascular system, as well as your muscles and posture.

170. Is there any danger in getting my heart rate going very fast, as with aerobics?

Yes. With a very rapid heart rate, the efficiency can be so poor that the blood does not circulate to the brain, causing you to faint. Also, if the coronaries do not have time to fill and nourish the heart muscle, a heart attack can occur. A treadmill test is a test of exercise to see what the heart does at a high rate. If you are in doubt or have heart problems, ask your doctor to do a treadmill test before beginning your exercise program. Most young women who are not obese, diabetic, hypertensive, or do not smoke have few heart troubles. However, after the age of fifty, more care is needed because the incidence of coronary artery disease increases.

171. Is lifting weights a good conditioning program for the female anatomy?

In men and women, lifting builds muscles, particularly of the upper torso, but it does not condition the heart. Running, jogging, or cycling do that much better.

172. Is jogging a good exercise program for women?

Jogging is good for conditioning the heart and for keeping weight down, but when done often enough, it can lead to cessation of menses. This is not really harmful unless you are trying to get pregnant. Jogging can be harmful to old knee injuries or back problems. Women who have had vaginal support stretching from having large babies may also find that they lose their urinary control while running, but then any exercise activity can cause that. When you are swimming, you just may not notice it as much.

EVERYDAY GOOD HEALTH: EXERCISE (Continued)

173. Can jogging cause problems in women?

Too much jogging seems to stop ovulation and menstrual periods in women. If this is so severe that estrogen completely disappears, it can become a problem. However, jogging does not stress the pelvic floor, as lifting does.

EVERYDAY GOOD HEALTH: DIET AND NUTRITION

174. What is a proper diet?

A proper diet contains enough calories for your energy needs, without producing weight loss or gain, if you don't need to change. For nonpregnant and nonlactating young, adult women who are active, this usually consists of about 2100 calories a day. It should contain fifty grams of protein, enough roughage to control elimination, all the daily minimum requirements for vitamins and minerals, and it should be attractive and palatable. Teenagers need more calories, and older women need much fewer.

175. Do I need to change my diet during menstruation?

Many doctors have recommended that women change their diet to six small, protein meals per day during the week before menstruation to help cope with premenstrual syndrome. Since these problems usually disappear with menses, a change in diet is not really necessary then.

176. Can vitamins make up for a poor diet?

Vitamins are only one part of your dietary requirements and can only make up for vitamin deficiencies. A poor diet may also require more protein, calories, iron, roughage, or even fats.

177. Does a vegetarian diet fulfill a woman's special needs?

A well-balanced vegetarian diet can fulfill a woman's needs until she becomes pregnant. Then she must have some vitamin B12 if she wants to have a healthy baby. If she is an ovolacto vegetarian, and includes eggs and milk in her diet, there will be no problem. A strict vegetarian, however, needs a B12 supplement during pregnancy.

178. Are vegetarians less likely to develop serious diseases, such as cancer, due to the absence of meat in their diets?

The National Academy of Sciences issued a report on "Diet, Nutrition, and Cancer" that showed a strong correlation between diet in affluent societies, like the United States, and cancer of the breast, uterus, and colon. The Academy found that people changed their patterns of cancer when they migrated to new countries. They also found that exposure to pollutants in industrialized societies is not a significant cause of cancer, although the long-term effects may not yet be clear. According to the report, one-third of all cancers could be eliminated by a proper diet, and another third if everyone

EVERYDAY GOOD HEALTH: DIET AND NUTRITION
(Continued)

stopped smoking. The strongest relationship with diet was between cancer of the colon, rectum, and breast and consumption of a high, total-fat diet, that includes meat and animal protein. The Academy specifically condemned alcohol and foods that are smoked, salt-pickled, or salt-cured. They found the best foods to be fruits, vegetables, and whole-grain cereals.[1] So, if they are right, vegetarians would be better off. However, this theory has not been entirely accepted.

179. What is a low-cholesterol diet?
It is a diet which has a low content of cholesterol, a blood fat that is sometimes correlated with hardening of the arteries (arteriosclerosis) and coronary heart disease. Eggs, dairy products, meats, and animal fats are high in cholesterol.

180. When is a low-cholesterol diet recommended?
If you have a blood test that shows a high cholesterol level and your doctor finds that it could be influenced by dietary control, then a low-cholesterol diet is recommended. This can be particularly important if your doctor finds that you need to control your cholesterol due to advancing arteriosclerosis or an actual heart attack. It is not recommended that all people, especially women, avoid all cholesterol because most people are not coronary risks. This is a much greater problem in men than women. However, it is recommended that people reduce the total animal fat in their diet and that they not be overweight. Sometimes being overweight affects the blood cholesterol more than diet.

EVERYDAY GOOD HEALTH: VITAMINS AND MINERALS

181. Is it possible to take too many vitamins?
Vitamins A and D are not easily passed through the body. Too much of them can cause bone and skin disorders or even death, especially in children. The B and C vitamins are water soluble, and extensive intake is simply cast off into the urine so no harm is done.

182. Are there any particular vitamins and minerals which women are likely to be deficient in?
Because they menstruate and lose iron in the blood loss, women are more likely to be deficient in iron. Primitive women menstruated very little, spending most of their time breast-feeding with no menses. Pregnancy is a drain on iron stores, too. Red meats and green vegetables contain iron, but if

[1] Gloria Hochman, "The Diet That May Have Licked Cancer," *San Diego Union,* 19 April 1983, p. Dl.

EVERYDAY GOOD HEALTH: VITAMINS AND MINERALS
(Continued)

you can't eat these, iron tablets can be purchased over the counter and taken. During pregnancy, women also have a noticeably increased need for folic acid. It is often added to prenatal vitamins; after delivery, this need disappears.

EVERYDAY GOOD HEALTH: WEIGHT LOSS AND GAIN

183. How do I determine the normal weight I should be?

Most women decide if they are overweight by the tightness of their clothes or how they feel. However, the latest insurance company tables are an excellent reference for this, too. Another way to determine your ideal weight is to calculate 112 pounds for a height of five feet, and then add or subtract 4 pounds for each inch you are over or under that, by the age of twenty-five. Subtract 1 pound for each year under twenty-five you are, but subtract nothing for being older. Large frames can add 5 pounds, and small frames subtract 5 pounds. When using weight tables, be sure that you do not read your weight from one which allows two inches for heels. If you do use such a table, then add two inches to your real height. Do not use charts from diet books or salons. They are in the business of weight control.

184. Why do some people gain weight easily, yet others can eat and never gain an ounce?

The energy output of people is much different than it appears when you watch them for a short time. Tensions burn energy. Frequency of eating may be impressive, but if the calories are low, people won't gain weight. Your weight gain or loss depends on the calories taken in and the calories burned off. Both are hard to observe without actually counting calories. There is some variation in metabolic rates, especially with young people who burn calories more rapidly than old people, but within the same age group, the rate is usually similar, unless thyroid disease is present.

185. Are weight problems inherited?

Yes, to some extent weight problems are controlled by metabolic processes and hormonal patterns, which may be inherited. Eating habits are also learned at the family table.

186. How are weight gain and loss related to changes in my body's metabolism?

Most people's metabolism does not change very much. It gradually slows down from the day you are born, when it is at its highest point. However, sometimes abnormal function of the thyroid gland can make the weight go either up or down. If the thyroid is hyperactive, weight will go down because you burn energy faster; if it is hypoactive, weight will ac-

EVERYDAY GOOD HEALTH: WEIGHT LOSS AND GAIN
(Continued)

cumulate because you burn it so slowly. Replacement thyroid can correct thyroid deficiency, but treatment for overactive thyroid is more complicated.

187. Why are more women overweight than men?

This is probably because most women are in charge of food preparation. Men's overweight problems are usually the result of consuming too much beer and other high-calorie drinks, which are normally more available to them than to women. Women are more condemned for being fat in our society, while overweight men are more tolerated. The fat woman draws more attention than the fat man. Men are usually not judged on their bodies. Some fat is beneficial to women, making them fertile and, after menopause, producing estrogen to alleviate hot flushes and thinning bones. Men have no similar need for fat.

188. What is the safest way to lose weight?

Gradually. If you eat fewer calories than you burn up, you will lose weight. The problem is that when you eat less, you do less; when you do more, you eat more, so your weight may not go down. Two main facts about dieting are: protein tends to curb your appetite for a long time, at least four hours, and several meals a day are less likely to make you gain weight than the same number of calories eaten in one meal per day. So several small protein meals is the best way to lose weight. Protein with a little fat will sustain life, although you may still need vitamins, especially vitamin C.

189. Is counting calories the best way to diet?

Calories must always be restricted to lose weight, unless you change your energy output or exercise enormously. Counting them, however, may not be the best way to reduce them. Certainly, limiting calories to a certain number does not necessarily mean that you have taken in adequate protein, minerals, vitamins, or roughage. One method of determining the calorie intake that will allow you to lose weight is to count the calories you are eating while you are overweight. Then you know that you have to reduce your intake below that level, without decreasing your activity level, in order to lose weight.

190. What are starch blockers? How do they work?

Starch blockers are an extract of a bean that interferes with the digestion of starch in the digestive tract. Some people experienced discomfort and gas when using them. They were withdrawn from the market, because they had not been properly tested for safety and effectiveness.

191. Could I harm my body by dieting?

Yes, indeed. Nutritionally insufficient diets for rapid weight loss can

EVERYDAY GOOD HEALTH: WEIGHT LOSS AND GAIN
(Continued)

tear down muscle and sometimes produce weakness due to a low potassium level that brings on irregularities in heart rate. Dieting can be carried to extremes, like anorexia nervosa, and lead to death. Being chronically very underweight can interfere with most of your body's functions. Dieting when you are overweight is less harmful than dieting when you are underweight, but many women diet who are already underweight. Dieting while you are pregnant can be very harmful to the fetus. Dieting can also interfere with your mental functions and produce an irritability that interferes with your social functions.

192. How much weight can I safely lose in one week?
You can safely lose 2½ pounds per week, or 10 pounds a month, without tearing down muscle in the process. If you lose weight slowly like this, you are more likely to keep it off, because you are learning a new eating pattern that you can continue for a long time.

193. What are the hazards of extreme weight gain or loss?
The answer to this question would fill a volume. Both extremes can stop menstruation and fertility. Weight gain can increase your chances of high blood pressure, heart attack, and diabetes. Morbid obesity (one hundred pounds overweight for five years) can strain your heart and your lungs, as well as your back. Extreme weight loss can reduce your resistance to all infections, deteriorate your muscles, interfere with your mental functioning, produce heart irregularities, slow down all body systems, and produce death from starvation.

194. Why do I always lose weight in my breasts first whenever I go on a diet?
Perhaps this is because your breasts are the only places where you have fat to lose. More than likely, it is because you do not want to lose weight there, so you notice it far sooner than you would if it were on your hips, where you want to lose fat. Women value fat in their breasts more than on their hips. Actually the first place that fat is found or removed is on the abdominal wall.

195. Why did I start gaining weight after I reached the age of thirty?
Your metabolic rate lowers gradually and does not suddenly change at the age of thirty. There must have been some difference in your lifestyle and dieting pattern at that age to account for your weight gain.

196. Why is it harder to lose weight the older I get?
As you age, your metabolic rate decreases, so that you burn fewer calories per day. Therefore, you should take in fewer calories per day. This is

EVERYDAY GOOD HEALTH: WEIGHT LOSS AND GAIN
(Continued)

true even if your activity level is the same. However, the biggest problem is that as you get older you allow yourself to do less and you have less physical activity, without reducing your food intake.

197. How does being overweight affect sexual enjoyment?

Some of the best long-term sexual relationships I have known about have been between men and women weighing over two hundred pounds each. Perhaps this is because they do not lie back and look beautiful, but actually put some effort and activity into their sexual relationship. On the other hand, when couples are undergoing sex therapy and are asked to lie together nude in a warm private room as part of the sensate focus exercises, they often report afterward that they discovered they were too fat. These are people who have hidden and ignored their bodies for some time and are just beginning to discover them again. If you are ashamed of your body, it is difficult to permit someone else to love it. Many people with perfectly good bodies are quite ashamed of them, so it does not correlate with being overweight. If your partner puts you down for being overweight, then you will suffer. If you dislike his being overweight, then your sexuality will also suffer.

198. Does a thin person experience more enjoyment during sex than an overweight person?

In general, no. A thin person may be more attractive to the other partner, and this pleases the partner, but it does not mean this person will enjoy sex. Sometimes, people who are thin and weak do not have the energy to participate in sex. The public prejudice shown toward people who are overweight is one that should not be allowed; yet, many people feel free to express such prejudice without condemnation from anyone. There is a general obsession with fatness and thinness in our society.

199. Is it possible to lose weight during sex? If so, how many calories will I burn up?

Any activity will help you lose weight if it burns calories. If you are active in sex, the energy expended is similar to that expended in walking up a flight of stairs. This comparison has been used to determine whether heart patients can participate in sex. If they can climb stairs, they can have sex. The calories expended during sex depend, of course, upon how you participate and whether it lasts very long. An estimate would be that about three hundred calories are burned up for fifteen minutes of sex.

200. What is cellulite?

A writer invented the term "cellulite" for the small folds that cover the

EVERYDAY GOOD HEALTH: WEIGHT LOSS AND GAIN
(Continued)

female body, especially on the thighs and buttocks. These are formed by water and fat just under the skin.

201. How can I get rid of cellulite?

The only way to get rid of cellulite would be for you to turn into a man. Female hormones retain fat and water under the skin. This is what makes a woman soft to touch, and not hard like a man's surface. If you starve yourself enough, you will quit making female hormones and the cellulite will disappear, but so will you eventually. You should hail cellulite as a badge of femininity, something men don't have.

EVERYDAY GOOD HEALTH: ANOREXIA NERVOSA, BULIMIA
(Anorexia Nervosa and Bulimia also are discussed in Chapter 10,
Body Abuse)

202. What is anorexia nervosa?

Anorexia nervosa is a disorder that usually occurs in young girls when they start dieting to lose weight. They carry this dieting so far that they almost do not eat at all, losing weight down to severe levels that may cause death. They stop menstruating when nutrition is bad enough, and their thyroid and other hormone functions slow down in an effort to try to conserve energy. Usually deep psychotherapy and hospitalization is required to save the girls' lives and reverse the process. The original dieting can start from someone's chance remark that the girl is getting too fat. The deep-seated causes are, of course, more than that.

203. What causes anorexia nervosa?

Different causes have been proposed for anorexia nervosa, and these are probably slightly different for each case. Since it occurs almost exclusively in women, usually young, it must involve a female-related problem. This culture builds a disgust for fat into its values, and sometimes a disgust for being female. Thinness in women is idealized in movies and on television, and clothes seem to be designed only for those who are thin. Many actresses who are bulimics or anorectics may die of their disorder in the midst of stardom. Some people have suggested that the fragile, tuberculous heroine of the nineteenth century has been carried over into the Twiggy of today.

204. What is bulimia?

The original meaning of bulimia was overeating in vast amounts. Today it means binge overeating, followed by self-induced vomiting to keep from becoming fat. The numbers of women with this eating disorder are ris-

EVERYDAY GOOD HEALTH: ANOREXIA NERVOSA, BULIMIA
(Continued)

ing, especially on college campuses and among performers. Many groups are being formed for psychotherapy to help these women who are usually intelligent, attractive, and successful females. Part of the problem is our culture and its emphasis on being thin. The overeating is a rebellion against the requirement to diet, which is compensated for by vomiting. One theory is that it is caused by a conflict between wanting to be a male (thin) and a female (fat). A properly functioning, fertile female will have water retention and at least 12 percent body fat. The rejection of all fat is a rejection of femaleness. Women with bulimia do not often face death as do the women with anorexia nervosa, since they usually keep their weight at about normal and seldom deprive their body completely of nutrition. Their problems are centered around how they feel about the overeating and vomiting, paying for the overeating, and also some heartburn caused by the vomiting itself. Some women with this disorder reduce the vomiting and use exercise, such as running, to keep their weight down. Others resort to laxatives. Our whole culture should review the importance of being thin, and perhaps reevaluate its ideals.

EVERYDAY GOOD HEALTH: BACKACHE

205. What is the most common cause of backache?

Poor posture and poor body mechanics in activities or work, such as leaning over to make beds or to lift children, are the most common causes of backaches. High heels can contribute to poor posture by promoting swayback in standing and walking. Swayback is an increased forward curve in the lower back. Poor back position during sleep also contributes to backache, especially if the lower back is curved, as it is when you sleep on your stomach.

206. Are back problems common in women?

Yes, they are. There are several factors that contribute to a woman's backaches. One is that her sacroiliac joints remain loose and unfused throughout her life, and are therefore easy to strain. In men, these become solid joints. Women also have loose ligaments around their knees, and they tend to stand with them locked in a hyperextended position curving backward. This makes them swayback in the lower back to compensate, which strains their back. Pregnancy makes the joints even looser and more unstable. It also weakens the abdominal muscles. Women, in general, do not athletically develop their abdominal muscles, and therefore do not have the strength in them to stand up and work efficiently. You need good abdominal muscles to protect your back from strain. Perhaps the biggest factor con-

EVERYDAY GOOD HEALTH: BACKACHE (Continued)

tributing to women's backaches is that they never learn how to lift heavy objects, or even light ones. Women tend to lean over to lift groceries, babies, children, and furniture, and that is the wrong way. They should learn to lift things by bending their knees and holding their backs straight.

207. Why does my back hurt when I menstruate?

Uterine contractions in menstruation or in labor are often felt as pain in the back, even though there is nothing wrong with the back. It is caused by a radiation of the uterine pain. If you have a real back defect, it usually hurts worse during menses, probably due to the prostaglandin released with menstruation. Aspirin is a fairly good antiprostaglandin that can relieve both menstrual cramps and backache. Heat on the affected area helps, too, as well as rest.

208. I have a small frame and large breasts. Could this be contributing to my backache?

Yes, especially if you have a high backache between your shoulders. The pressure caused by heavy breasts and supporting bras makes a groove in the shoulders. This makes a curve in the back at the level of the shoulders and the neck. Reduction breast surgery can be done to correct the problem and will even be covered by federally funded programs, if five pounds or more is removed from each breast.

209. Does continuous backache pain usually indicate a more severe problem?

It is not the duration or severity of pain which indicates a more severe problem, but the development of nerve symptoms, such as numbness or weakness in the leg. Pain which can be felt down the leg may just be severe radiating pain, but numbness and weakness of the muscles can indicate pressure on a nerve root in the back. This could lead to possible destruction and paralysis. Medical therapy may include muscle relaxants, traction, surgery, or more recently papain injections, which are all substitutes for surgery.

210. How can I relieve backache pain?

You can stop aggravating the pain by maintaining good posture with a flat back and buttocks tucked in. Pretend that you are holding a penny between the cheeks of your buttocks as you stand and walk and that you will drop the penny when you stop pinching the cheeks. Do not lean over from the waist to do anything, but rather bend your knees and squat to lift or even pick up a paper from the floor. Lie down on a hard surface on your back, bend your knees, and put your feet flat on the surface. Flatten your lower back and lift your tailbone slightly, over and over. This is a pelvic-tilt exercise

EVERYDAY GOOD HEALTH: BACKACHE (Continued)

that relieves low backaches at the lumbosacral area. It also relieves sacroiliac strain. Sleep on your side with your hips bent, so your back will be straight. Use heat (hot shower, hot water bottle, heating pad) to relax the muscle spasm. Get plenty of rest. Aspirin is excellent for pain relief, but if it bothers your stomach, use an antacid with it or get a coated aspirin. If all this doesn't work, see your doctor for help. You may have more than strain. Back pain that is caused by kidney infections occurs above the waist, and is usually accompanied by fever.

211. Should I see a chiropractor about my backache?

Doctors of Medicine (M.D.s) who diagnose and treat backaches are usually better qualified than chiropractors. If you have a severe disc problem, you can be injured by a chiropractic manipulation. If there is numbness or weakness, such manipulation is more dangerous. Orthopedists, neurologists, and neurosurgeons are specialists who have spent years training in the treatment of backaches. You may not be a aware of them because they do not advertise as chiropractors do. Some states do not even license chiropractors.

EVERYDAY GOOD HEALTH: ANEMIA

212. What does it mean to be anemic?

If you are anemic, this means that you do not have enough red blood cells in your body to carry the oxygen you need to function. Hemoglobin is the substance in the red blood cells that carries oxygen from the lungs to the tissues where it is used. The ideal measurement of hemoglobin in the blood is usually 14.5 grams. You are anemic if it is 10 grams or less.

213. What causes anemia?

Most anemia in women is caused by losing too much blood during menstruation and not eating enough iron in your diet to replace the blood that is lost. If your menstrual flow is normal or light, but you do not eat enough iron and protein to manufacture the red blood cells, you may still be anemic. If you have inherited a certain kind of anemia, such as sickle-cell anemia, then taking iron will not help. Sometimes anemia comes from being very ill with an infection that suppresses the bone marrow. Sometimes it comes from having leukemia.

214. Is anemia common during childbearing years?

Yes. Anemia becomes common in girls at the onset of menstruation, and it continues to be common until they reach menopause, whether they have children or not. If you are on birth control pills, there is a remarkable reduction in anemia, because of the reduced blood loss at time of menses.

EVERYDAY GOOD HEALTH: ANEMIA (Continued)

215. Does anemia result from multiple pregnancies?

Yes, it can. The drain of iron from the body during the nine months of pregnancy is greater than it would be with menstruation, so you need more iron during pregnancy. You may also lose perhaps a pint of blood with your delivery, and will have to make up for that, too. If you have one baby right after the other, then you must have an excellent diet and probably an iron supplement as well, in order to not be anemic after you have had three or four children.

216. Is anemia more common in women than men?

Yes. If men are anemic, the cause must be hereditary, or else it comes from some abnormal bleeding, such as a bleeding ulcer. Since these things are uncommon, few men are anemic. Women have about four hundred menstrual periods in their lives, and they lose a lot of blood as a result. Also, all over the world women do not eat quite as well as men. Some women give the best piece of meat to their husband and the rest to their children, leaving only small pieces for themselves. Another reason for women being more anemic is because of their constant dieting to be slender.

217. How do I know if I am anemic?

A blood test is the only way you can tell you if you are anemic. However, you might suspect that you are anemic if you are pale, tired, bleeding heavily, dieting, and getting every infection that comes along. But until you take a blood test to measure your hemoglobin and count the red blood cells or measure the hematocrit, this is only a suspicion.

218. How does anemia affect my body and vital organs?

Anemia makes you feel tired; that is why it is called "tired blood." When you are anemic, your heart has to work extra hard to circulate enough oxygen around the body because the blood is thin. The heart has to pump more blood faster. All the tissues suffer, even the brain, so you may have trouble with your memory and learning. It is harder to recover from surgery or an injury when you are anemic, and much harder to fight infections. Your appearance may or may not be pale, but your skin will not seem ruddy and robust.

219. Why are teenage girls so often anemic?

Teenage girls do not ovulate regularly, and when they do not ovulate, their menstrual cycle is quite heavy, with clots, and occasionally prolonged bleeding. Such bleeding can certainly make girls anemic. This used to be called "the green anemia" because the girls were often so pale that they looked green. Teenage girls are also notorious for not eating well, partly out of concern that they should be thin and not allow their bodies to develop.

EVERYDAY GOOD HEALTH: ANEMIA (Continued)

They do not eat enough red meat or green vegetables to replace the iron they lose with menstruation. They also do not eat enough protein to make a good ovulatory hormone cycle with a lesser menstrual flow.

220. What sort of foods should I eat if I am anemic?

For an iron deficiency anemia, which most women have, you should eat foods that are rich in iron and protein, the building blocks of red blood. Red meats contain a lot of iron, and pale meats, like fish, contain less iron. Green vegetables contain iron, and the greener they are, the more iron they contain. Some other foods are also rich in iron. However, if your anemia is not due to bleeding or poor diet, a diet rich in iron will not help. Hereditary anemias will not improve with an iron-rich diet.

221. What is the best treatment for anemia?

The most common anemia, iron deficiency anemia, is produced by too much bleeding or too little iron in the diet. It is best treated by taking iron orally. Iron is obtainable over the counter and does not require a prescription. You can use plain ferrous sulfate, if it does not give you too much constipation or diarrhea. If it does, try another form of iron. If your anemia is not due to an iron deficiency, you will have to follow the advice of your doctor about the particular kind of anemia you have. Of course, another approach to treating anemia is to stop the blood loss that is causing it. Birth control pills reduce the blood loss with menstruation, so most women taking birth control pills are not anemic. Recent surveys show that this is one of the benefits of taking the pill.

EVERYDAY GOOD HEALTH: WATER RETENTION

222. What causes water retention?

Female hormones cause water retention. It is heavier just before menses, when hormones are high, and certainly during pregnancy. Water retention is worse when the body is always held in a vertical position, whether sitting with the feet up or standing, because the kidneys actually work harder to rid the body of water when they are in a horizontal position. If you stand or sit all of the time, the kidneys retain water to keep circulation going in your head. Many women lie down very little so their feet tend to swell. Running seems to be better for this than sitting or standing. If men have water retention, something is really wrong with their heart or kidneys. With women, it is normal.

EVERYDAY GOOD HEALTH: HEADACHE

223. What causes headaches? Are they ever a symptom of disease?

The most common cause of headaches is tension. However, the

EVERYDAY GOOD HEALTH: HEADACHE (Continued)

number of other causes is very great, including such things as dental problems, jaw problems, problems of the bones in the back of the neck, injuries that produce bleeding in the brain, or even brain tumors. Diseases which cause headaches range from the common cold, sinus problems, and any illness accompanied by fever to serious problems, such as high blood pressure, toxemia of pregnancy, and expanding aneurysms of blood vessels in the brain. Not every headache, of course, needs to be studied by a neurologist, but if it is unexplained and persistent for a long time and a general checkup does not find the cause, you should be referred to a neurologist. A brain tumor can occur at any age, even in children. Migraine headaches, which have a special pattern that starts with visual changes, are inherited and are often cyclic just before menses.

224. How are headaches affected by cyclic hormonal changes?

Tension headaches that occur in the week before menses are common. They are aggravated by the premenstrual syndrome, as well as by water retention. Sometimes, water retention also aggravates migraine headaches. Headaches during menstruation may be a reaction to painful cramps. During the rest of the cycle, headaches are probably unrelated to hormones at all.

225. What is the best remedy for a headache?

Since most headaches are caused by tension, relaxation is probably the best remedy. Learning to relax, even for a few minutes, is an art that you can use to relieve headaches. If there is not an opportunity to do this, aspirin may provide the relief you need until you can find the time and place to relax. Of course, if your headaches are due to sinus problems, sinus medication may be much more effective. If headaches are the result of an allergy, such as those caused by chocolate, antihistamines may help, too. The best remedy depends upon the cause of the headache.

226. What is a migraine headache? How does it differ from an ordinary headache?

A migraine headache is a vascular headache in which blood vessels in the brain constrict, and then dilate and throb. Usually there is an aura (a sensation) that precedes the headache. Characteristically it takes the form of a visual change, like seeing odd lights or parts of things, for a few minutes before the headache actually starts. Nausea may accompany the headache, and vomiting may actually relieve it. Many people think that any severe headache is a migraine, but other types of headaches can be much more severe and long lasting than a migraine. Migraines seem to be inherited. They are especially aggravated by hormonal changes and often appear with pu-

EVERYDAY GOOD HEALTH: HEADACHE (Continued)

berty and disappear with menopause. They are frequently one-sided. Migraines are more likely to be aggravated by birth control pills than any other type of headache.

227. What is the best remedy for a migraine headache?

Ergot preparations, available by prescription from a doctor, can relieve or even prevent migraine headaches, if they are taken early enough, especially during the visual changes that precede the headache. Migraines may also be prevented by taking some other drugs, such as propranolol (Inderal). Otherwise, medications used for any headache can be used for pain relief; strong ones that are prescribed by a doctor are usually recommended.

EVERYDAY GOOD HEALTH: STRESS

228. Is there a way to get more in touch with my stress, in order to stop tension headaches, for example?

Learning to relax can stop your stress reaction. Laughter can be a good medicine, too. Biofeedback is another way; it uses a machine to show you that you can learn to relax.

229. What is the best way to deal with stress?

The ideal way to deal with stress is to solve the problem that brings on the stress. But since that is not always possible, as it may require major changes in your life, the next best method is to modify your reactions to stress. Conscious relaxation works better than rigid self-control. Avoidance of minor aggravations, such as a vaginal itch, can leave you enough power to cope with major aggravations, so at least solve minor problems. You can observe your stress reactions and learn just what brings them on. If the source cannot be changed or avoided, rapid relaxation can avoid the stress effects on the body. You need to feel that you have the right to seek an activity that relaxes you and relieves stress. All work and no play makes Jill very tense.

230. Can the way I walk, sit, or hold my body be a cause of tension?

It is more likely to be a result of tension, not a cause. However, tight shoes, high heels, tight clothes, a tight head band or hair pins, or even a complicated hairdo can produce tension by prolonged discomfort. When there is a choice, you should choose comfort over style and beauty to reduce your stress.

231. How does stress affect a woman's body?

Stress reaction is primarily muscle tension, usually found in the back and neck, but sometimes found all over the body. It can also involve increased activity of the intestines and stomach, producing colitis and ulcers. It

EVERYDAY GOOD HEALTH: STRESS (Continued)

can tighten the bronchi of the lungs, producing the wheezing of asthma, or it can constrict all of the blood vessels causing high blood pressure. Neck and scalp tension can convert into a headache. Hives and swelling can appear, without an allergic reaction even being present. Sweating, a racing heart, or even shaking may result. Dizziness, hyperventilation (overbreathing), mental confusion, or loss of consciousness, as with fainting, can be methods of coping with stress. Some people develop little jerking motions or "tics." A twitching eyelid is an example.

EVERYDAY GOOD HEALTH: DEPRESSION

232. What causes depression? Is it entirely a mental state?

Depression is not just caused by being sad, especially after an event that should sadden you; that is a normal reaction. It is not just a mental state either. It is a condition in which your activity level becomes very low, and you feel you can't do anything anymore, not even get out of bed. You avoid social contacts and can't go to work. You lose your appetite and can't sleep, waking in the middle of the night to worry. Depression certainly involves a mental state, but it is also an organic state, with many changes occurring in the chemical state of the body. The effective treatments for depression in the past have been both chemical and physical, in the form of antidepressant medications and electroshock treatments. Of course, psychotherapy is needed for anyone who has such a problem, but it is not enough. The cause of depression is found within the body chemistry. It is probably inherited and only possibly triggered by events. The real cause of depression is not known.

233. When does depression become a serious problem?

When suicide is contemplated, threatened, or attempted, depression is a very serious problem. When it ruins your work or your relationships with others, it is also serious.

234. When should a person who is overly depressed seek professional help?

When a depressive state is so severe that it interferes with school, work, or child care, or it is threatening marital and family relations, help should be sought. Psychiatrists are specialists in treating depression. They are familiar with all the antidepressants that are used to treat depression, and the psychotherapy needed as well. With professional help you need not lose a year at college, your job, or your husband. It is very expensive **not** to treat depression. Mental health clinics that are state supported are available in urban centers with referrals for those patients who cannot afford private psychiatric care or whose insurance does not cover it. Call your Mental Health Association or any hotline for help.

EVERYDAY GOOD HEALTH: DEPRESSION (Continued)

235. What can I do to overcome my depression?

Throughout your life, you must learn techniques to relieve your mild depressions. This can be remembering activities that release energy for you, perhaps camping outdoors or playing the piano. These are different for everyone, and it is your job to notice what activities work for you. It is part of self-preservation to do things that make you feel good. Do not expect anyone else to cure your depression, except perhaps professional help. Husbands and family would like to help, but they can only follow your directions as to what you need. If your depression worsens no matter what you do, seek professional help. It is much better than ruining or taking your own life.

236. Does my hormonal level affect depression or my many moods?

It is difficult to separate whether your moods change your hormones, or your hormones change your moods. There are definite hormonal and other chemical changes that occur in a very depressed person. The menstrual cycle involves mood swings which are pronounced in some women, especially if the women are already in a general depression. But general depression is not due to the menstrual cycle or even being female. Men get depressed, too. Part of women's problems is that they spend a lot of time solving their families' problems, but don't feel they have the right to take action to solve their own problems. If women felt more responsible for their moods, they would do things to improve and control them. Women should not helplessly ride the roller coaster of mood swings. They must find and use techniques that reduce their lows and even diminish their highs, if they get too high.

EVERYDAY GOOD HEALTH: VARICOSE VEINS

237. What causes varicose veins, and why do women have them more than men?

Varicose veins are dilated veins, in which the valves are no longer capable of holding the blood and pushing it back to the heart. They usually occur in the legs and are often worse on the left side. The tendency for varicose veins is inherited. It is brought out by excessive standing and sitting, and by pregnancy. Women acquire varicose veins most while they are pregnant. Sometimes varicose veins improve after delivery, but they seldom disappear.

238. Is there any way to prevent varicose veins?

Walking and running, instead of standing and sitting, helps to prevent varicose veins. But the best way would be to choose your parents, so you won't inherit them. Support hose and elastic stockings bring relief from

EVERYDAY GOOD HEALTH: VARICOSE VEINS (Continued)

discomfort, but do not prevent the veins from getting worse. Avoiding pregnancy is effective in preventing them, too.

239. How are varicose veins surgically removed?

While the patient is under anesthesia, small incisions are made in the leg where the veins branch. Then a loop is passed down the vein, stripping it free to the next branch, and removing it in sections. The scars of these incisions may not look better than the varicose veins, but they feel much better. You should have surgery when your veins are very uncomfortable, not because you don't like the way they look.

EVERYDAY GOOD HEALTH: HEMORRHOIDS

240. What are hemorrhoids, and why do women have them more often than men?

Hemorrhoids are dilated veins around the anus, sometimes bulging outside and sometimes hidden inside. They can hurt, itch, or bleed. Women develop them as a result of pregnancy and delivery, which explains why they are more frequent in women. Of course, men and women with no children may also develop hemorrhoids from heavy lifting or straining with a bowel movement, especially with constipation.

241. What is the best treatment for hemorrhoids?

Avoiding constipation or diarrhea helps to avoid the aggravation or even formation of hemorrhoids. Tub baths decrease the itching and irritation. Many over-the-counter creams and suppositories will also relieve itching, pain, and bleeding. If you cannot get relief, then seek medical help or even surgery from a special doctor who treats hemorrhoids (a proctologist), a general surgeon, or your family doctor.

242. Do hemorrhoids ever go away?

They may seem to go away, but really don't. Six weeks after delivery, the hemorrhoids that were so bad during pregnancy do not bother the mother at all, but when examined, they are still there. They are collapsed and shrunken, and even lie inside the rectum instead of bulging out the anus. They may no longer be a bother, but they still exist.

243. When would hemorrhoids need to be surgically removed?

If your hemorrhoids have not subsided within a few months after having a baby, you may need surgery. If they develop without pregnancy and continue to produce itching, pain, and bleeding, despite normal stools and local treatment for a few weeks, you may also need to have them removed (a hemorrhoidectomy). If they do not bother you at all, then you do not need surgery, no matter how large or ugly they are.

EVERYDAY GOOD HEALTH: HEMORRHOIDS (Continued)

244. Does anal sex cause hemorrhoids?

Anal sex may not be the cause of hemorrhoids, but it certainly aggravates and irritates them.

EVERYDAY GOOD HEALTH: ARTHRITIS

245. What is arthritis?

Arthritis is pain in a joint, no matter what the cause.

246. What causes arthritis?

Gouty arthritis is caused by too much uric acid, so crystals are actually deposited in the joint. Rheumatoid arthritis is an inflammation of the joint which causes redness and swelling, and later deformities. Osteogenic arthritis forms extra bony nodules. An example of osteogenic arthritis is the nodes that may develop on the last joint on the fingers, called Heberden's nodes. These are often seen in older people. It can also cause extra calcifications in the joint which can be seen in an X-ray. Infections by bacteria in the joints can also cause an arthritis.

247. Is there a cure for arthritis?

Antibiotics can cure infectious arthritis, but a damaged joint is still left. Gout can be controlled by diet and by medication, which lowers the uric acid in the blood stream. Aspirin and other antiprostaglandins, as well as cortisone and other anti-inflammatory agents can bring relief and change the course of rheumatoid arthritis. Similar results can be obtained for the relief of pain in osteogenic arthritis, while exercise, heat, and physical therapy can help to prevent or delay some deformities. Surgery can help some joints to function better. Joints, especially the hip, can also be replaced, with metal joints.

EVERYDAY GOOD HEALTH: HEART ATTACKS

248. How can I take care of my heart in order to reduce my chances of a heart attack?

Exercise that speeds up your heart rate, like running, jogging, swimming, or tennis is the best method. Keeping your weight within ten pounds of normal is also helpful. Following a diet that is not very high in fats is important. Treating any high blood pressure before it strains the heart is a good idea. Having a heart checkup and following the medical advice you receive regarding your heart becomes more important as you get older. Avoiding smoking is extremely important if you want to take care of your heart.

249. Do hormones protect a woman from heart attacks?

Yes, and that explains why women have fewer heart attacks than men.

EVERYDAY GOOD HEALTH: HEART ATTACKS (Continued)

Estrogen tends to increase the high-density lipoproteins that protect women from heart attacks, but progesterone tends to push it the other way. Fortunately, the estrogen is present more of the time and usually supersedes the progesterone effect. Testosterone lowers the high-density lipoproteins, which must explain why men have more heart attacks. This is a good reason for women to not take testosterone. They would lose their advantage.

250. Are heart attacks common among women?

In premenopausal women, heart attacks are almost rare, while at that same age in men, they are becoming a major problem. Only after menopause do women become more subject to heart attacks, but they never catch up to the frequency with which this occurs in men.

251. Are heart attacks more likely at a certain age?

Heart attacks in women become more likely after menopause. However, in women who smoke, have diabetes, high blood pressure, or who are overweight, they become more likely after the age of thirty-five. If these women also take birth control pills, this aggravates their chances of a heart attack a little more, so such women are usually refused contraceptive pills after the age of thirty-five. A blood test, called a coronary risk profile, can be taken to determine the risk of heart attack. It measures the types and levels of fats in your blood, cholesterol, and high- and low-density lipoproteins. If the lipoproteins are in a good ratio between high and low density and your cholesterol is not too high, your risk of heart attacks is less, even if you are overweight and over thirty-five.

252. Are my chances of having a heart attack greater if there is a history of heart attacks in my family?

As a woman, if the heart attacks in your family were in men, then you will not be at a higher risk. If the relatives with heart attacks were women, especially if they were associated with high blood pressure and diabetes, your risk becomes higher.

253. What causes a heart attack?

A heart attack occurs when the arteries that supply the heart narrow. A clot of blood forms in the narrow opening that is left, so that the blood vessel can no longer supply the heart muscle with blood. Without blood, the heart cannot function properly, and pain usually occurs.

254. Are there any warning signs that a heart attack is about to happen?

Chest pain and pressure under the breastbone, located in the middle of the front of the chest, is called angina. It often occurs during exercise. When this begins to happen frequently with less and less exertion, a heart attack may be imminent. Sometimes there is no warning at all. Chest pain, with

EVERYDAY GOOD HEALTH: HEART ATTACKS (Continued)

pain going into the left shoulder and arm, is also a significant sign of coronary blockage, which may lead to heart attack. Sometimes people think they have bursitis in their left shoulder or a simple stomachache, but if these symptoms are aggravated by exercise, they should be checked.

EVERYDAY GOOD HEALTH: EFFECTS OF AGING

255. Is there any way to delay the aging process?

Mankind has been looking for a way to do this for centuries. Female hormones, estrogen and progesterones, can delay the special aging problems that occur with menopause. Sunscreens and other protection from the sun and wind can delay the aging of skin. Exercise, good nutrition, happiness, and avoiding disease can do their part in keeping us young. But the real hope is that we can find something to prevent the special aging of the brain, called senility. Research goes on, but results are not yet forthcoming.

Chapter 2

Menstruation

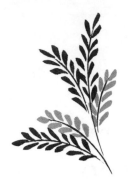

It is so important
to choose your own
lifestyle
and not let others
choose it for you

— Susan Polis Schutz

If you know
who you are and
what you want and
why you want it
and if you have
confidence in yourself and
a strong will to obtain your desires and
a very positive attitude
you can make
your life
yours
if you ask

— Susan Polis Schutz

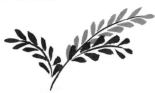

MENSTRUATION

How can you be in charge of your body if you are "cursed" with bleeding and cramping at unpredictable intervals throughout your life? Menstruation has been called a "woman's sickness," the "monthly period" (even when it was not even remotely monthly), a "woman's time," or just "menses." All over the world, the onset of this cyclic bleeding has been the sign of a girl's entrance into womanhood. Instead of being celebrated, however, it is hidden, denied, even shunned by others, male and female. In Africa, menstruating women are kept apart from others in a special hut while they bleed. In America, girls sometimes stay home from school for fear their heavy bleeding might show through their clothing or because they can find no relief from the cramps that disable them. Are we better off? We can be if we take action.

To conquer menstruation, you must first learn all about it and understand it, thus dispelling all fears. Then you can decide to let it occur naturally, while enjoying and observing all its unpredictable qualities. Or you can assume hormonal control, such as with the birth control pill, and have it come only when you want it, or perhaps not at all. For the first time in the history of womankind, you can be in charge of the process of menstruation.

What is the process of menstruation? In simple terms, during a few days every month, blood and the mucus lining of the womb, or uterus, are passed out of the vagina and onto a tampon or pad. After a few days, menstruation stops and a new lining begins to grow in the uterus, making a fresh place for a possible pregnancy to grow. If pregnancy does not occur, this lining, too, is cast away and a new one started next month. This process occurs only in human beings, macaque monkeys, and a few other primates. Other mammals have a cycle without bleeding at all or only with ovulation, as in dogs.

What brings all this about? At puberty, around age twelve, our pituitary gland, which is found at the base of our brain, begins to secrete hormones that stimulate our ovaries to produce estrogen, then release a developed egg, and finally secrete progesterone, another female hormone. These hormones cause the lining of the uterus to grow thick and luxuriant, so that a fertilized egg can implant there. When the ovaries have produced a sufficient amount of hormones, a feedback mechanism in the pituitary gland turns off the stimulating hormones and the ovaries temporarily stop producing. Without a pregnancy, the thick lining then shrinks down to being very thin and part of it sheds along with blood from the open blood vessels found in the uterus. This is the fluid that is expelled during menstruation. After a few days of this, the pituitary gland again begins to work, because the hor-

MENSTRUATION (Continued)

mones are now gone. The ovaries again secrete their hormones, a new lining grows over all the raw areas, and bleeding stops.

The pituitary gland, in turn, is controlled by secretions from the hypothalamus, a portion of the brain found just above the pituitary gland. Yet, more recent research suggests that, after all is said and done, the ovary is the one that controls the whole cycle! Wrong. You can control it all, if you decide to take the action necessary to do so.

MENSTRUATION: WHAT IS IT? WHAT IS IT NOT?

256. What takes place in other areas of my body during menstruation?

The hormone levels of estrogen and progesterone drop rapidly. The fluid retention that the hormones caused in your body leaves the tissues, so that swelling (edema) of the premenstrual phase disappears. The prostaglandins (substances locally produced in the tissues that can cause cramps) released in your uterus cause your intestine to cramp and even produce diarrhea or vomiting. Your breasts become less tender because of the reduction in stimulating hormones.

257. What were some of the "old wives' tales" about menstruation?

The ancient Jews thought that intercourse with a menstruating woman was a mortal sin. Strict orthodox Jews today still follow this rule. The blood of the flow was supposed to have great powers, causing evil of all kinds to befall those associated with a menstruating woman. The women in this condition were hidden or kept apart. More recently it has been said that a bath or swimming, while menstruating, will stop the flow and cause great pain, that a permanent wave given at this time will not take, that exercise is harmful, or that the milk from the breast of a menstruating woman will upset the child who drinks it. Of course, none of these things are true. Although it is not the most fertile time of your cycle, it is also not true that you are safe from getting pregnant by intercourse during menses.

258. What is the origin of the word "menstruation"?

It comes from the Latin word menstruus, meaning monthly.

259. Why is menses often called the "monthly sickness"?

The primary reason is that it occurs monthly, and the secondary reason is that the bleeding and pain which occurs are often mistakenly associated with sickness.

MENSTRUATION: BLOOD—WHERE DOES IT COME FROM? HOW IS IT REPLACED?

260. Where does the blood that is expelled during menstruation come from?

It comes from your general blood circulation. It leaks out through the holes in the blood vessels of the lining of your uterus left when the lining sheds off. The blood on your pad may have been in your brain a few minutes before.

261. Is the blood that comes out during menstruation the same as the blood that flows through our bodies?

Yes, it starts out exactly the same, because it comes out of the blood vessels in your uterus. It looks different by the time you see it, because it has

MENSTRUATION: BLOOD—WHERE DOES IT COME FROM? HOW IS IT REPLACED? (Continued)

been partly dissolved by enzymes in the uterus and has been combined with shreds of endometrial (inner surface of the uterus) lining cells, as well as secretions, such as prostaglandins from the uterus, and other secretions and cells from the cervix and vagina.

262. Where does all the blood go, if it does not come out?

There is no accumulation of blood that is later discarded with menses. Your blood circulates constantly, and it only leaks out with menses because there are holes in the blood vessels in the uterus. If the lining is thin and the holes are small, then little blood leaks out. Instead, it stays in your body where it circulates and keeps you from becoming anemic. Women who are taking birth control pills are seldom anemic, because they lose little blood with menses. Women who bleed heavily cannot seem to eat enough red meat and vegetables in order to get enough iron to keep up their blood supply. These women should probably also take iron orally.

263. How does the body replace the blood that is lost during menstruation?

Iron, protein, and various vitamins necessary to build blood cells are absorbed from your intestinal tract (if you eat enough). They are used in the marrow of your bones to form new blood. This takes several weeks, so you are usually forming blood all the time in your bones.

264. Are toxins released during menstruation?

No. A toxin is some kind of poison, but there is no poison in menstruation. An excess of prostaglandins may seem like it must be a toxin, since it produces cramps, nausea and vomiting, but it is not really harmful. The toxin in "toxic shock syndrome" comes from the Staphylococcus aureus bacteria (a bacteria that grows in grapelike clumps, commonly found on the skin), not from menstruation.

MENSTRUATION: BLOOD COLOR AND MAKE-UP

265. What does the blood released during menstruation contain?

First of all, it contains pure blood, just like you would see if you stuck your finger with a pin. Then it contains blood breakdown products, because the substance that prevents clots in your menstrual flow is dissolving the blood. In addition, it contains bits and pieces of the endometrium, the lining of the uterus. It also contains secretions, such as prostaglandins (substances locally produced in the tissues that can cause cramps) and their breakdown products. It is not pure enough blood to use for a blood count or for a transfusion. It is not very fresh.

MENSTRUATION: BLOOD COLOR AND MAKE-UP (Continued)

266. What color should the blood be?

There is great variation between women and sometimes between cycles. The best menstruation is actually the least flow, so the best color would be a dark wine color or almost black, indicating a very slow flow and, therefore, little blood loss. Bright red blood means a very rapid flow and, therefore, a lot of blood loss, and it is not as healthy for you. You are more likely to become anemic with a bright red flow than with a dark red or almost black flow.

267. What does it mean if my blood with menses is really dark, almost black?

It means the blood is flowing very slowly and, therefore, not very much blood loss. This is a good sign, not a bad one. Normal acid in the vagina turns the blood dark when it seeps instead of rushes through. It also means that you probably have a lot of progesterone that makes the blood loss less, either because you ovulated well or because you took birth control pills that contain a lot of progesterone.

MENSTRUATION: AGE OF ONSET

268. What is the most common age to start menstruating?

The average age for the first menses for girls in the United States is twelve years old. The youngest is nine and the latest age is about eighteen. Fifty years ago, the average age was fourteen. In developing countries, girls often do not start menses until they are sixteen.

269. How important is it to begin menstruating before the age of fifteen?

It is only important in that if it does not occur, it is time to let a doctor study the situation and find out why it has not occurred, in case something needs to be treated or corrected. If there is nothing wrong and menstruation can be expected later, nothing need be done.

270. Is there a correlation between breast development and the onset of menstruation?

Yes, breast development begins about two years before menstruation. Breast development is stimulated by the same hormones that eventually bring about menses.

MENSTRUATION: SYMPTOMS OF FIRST MENSTRUATION

271. What are the warning signs that a young girl is about to begin her period?

Breast development for at least two years and attaining the weight of

MENSTRUATION: SYMPTOMS OF FIRST MENSTRUATION
(Continued)

about one hundred pounds should warn a mother that her daughter is about to begin menstruating. This usually occurs at the age of twelve, but if she is large, it will be earlier and if she is very petite, it will be later.

272. Is abdominal pain in young girls a sign that menstruation is about to begin?

No, abdominal pain is not a sign of the onset of menses. If a young girl has a stomachache before she menstruates for the first time, she is probably ill.

MENSTRUATION: FACTORS INFLUENCING AGE OF ONSET OF MENSTRUATION

273. Why do some girls start to menstruate when they are nine years old and some when they are sixteen years old?

Recent research has shown that this is because the hormones that produce menstruation do not appear until a girl reaches a total weight of a little over one hundred pounds. Girls in underdeveloped countries who are undernourished may not start menses until they reach sixteen years old, because it is not until then that they weigh over one hundred pounds.

274. What effect does race, climate, and genetics have on menstruation?

It previously was thought that race, climate, and genetics controlled menstruation, but now it is known that it is the influence that these have on growth and nutrition that affects menstruation.

275. Why do girls in the United States start menstruating at an earlier age than they did fifty years ago?

Girls in the United States today are bigger and healthier than they were fifty years ago. They have fewer childhood diseases to interfere with their growth and development, and there is no shortage of food for them to eat, so they reach a weight of over one hundred pounds at an earlier age. Fifty years ago, girls were smaller due to the ravages of childhood diseases, which are now widely prevented through the use of immunizations and antibiotics.

276. Why does the start of menstruation depend on weight?

Apparently, there must be at least 12-20 percent body fat before enough estrogen is supplied to work with the ovarian hormones to produce menstruation. Fat produces estrogen by converting certain adrenal hormones into estrogen. It is partly for this reason that girls who weigh over one hundred pounds, but exercise so much that they have almost no fat, will still not menstruate. Ballet dancers, gymnasts, and even runners are good examples.

MENSTRUATION: FACTORS INFLUENCING AGE OF ONSET OF MENSTRUATION (Continued)

277. Is it true that active women begin menstruating early?

No. Menstruation onset has been correlated with size, weight, and especially with percentage of body fat, and activity would tend to reduce body fat. The genetics of your family are also involved.

278. What part does heredity play in menstruation? Am I likely to start my period at the same time that my mother did?

Yes, but heredity affects menstruation in indirect ways. You inherit your type of body and its growth pattern, but you learn nutrition and eating habits from the family you live with. Onset of menses is controlled more by nutrition, body weight, sports, running, and body fat than it is by heredity. Immigrants from countries where menses start late find their daughters starting menses earlier in America where they are well fed and grow to one hundred pounds at an earlier age than their cousins in the old country. The age at menopause seems to correlate even more closely with heredity, perhaps because the mechanism that controls how fast the eggs are destroyed is inherited. But since good health and nutrition also tend to prolong the menstrual life, women usually menstruate a year or two longer than their mothers did.

MENSTRUATION: FLOW AND AGE

279. Will my menstrual flow increase or decrease with age?

This depends on the level of progesterone that your ovaries are producing. Ovaries are capable of producing a lot of estrogen without releasing an egg or progesterone, and it is progesterone that reduces the menstrual flow, because it makes the lining of the uterus less thick. As teenagers, women often have a very heavy flow and even pass clots. This is because they are not yet releasing eggs, ovulating, or producing progesterone. The same thing also happens to women who are in their forties and find themselves bleeding as heavily and sporadically as their teenage daughters. The natural time for the lightest flow is from ages twenty-five to thirty-five, which is the time that women are most fertile and are producing the highest levels of progesterone. This light flow often frightens women into thinking that they are running out of hormones and becoming menopausal, when actually it shows that they are quite healthy and fertile.

280. If menstruation begins at an early age, does that also mean that menopause will begin earlier?

No, it does not. Some years ago it was a medical myth that if you started menstruation early, you menstruated longer (very unjust!). But, according to computer studies, that is not true.

MENSTRUATION: FLOW AND AGE (Continued)

281. Why do some women menstruate until they are in their fifties and some women until their forties?

How long you menstruate depends upon how healthy you are and the other mechanisms in your body that control how fast the eggs are destroyed in your ovaries. Not all your eggs are released at ovulation time, they are mostly destroyed without ovulating at all. Medical science has not yet determined just what controls this rate. With some women, it is so fast they run out of eggs at the age of thirty-five; with others, they still have some at sixty. (See Chapter IX, "Menopause," for further discussion.)

MENSTRUATION: TYPES OF PROTECTION

282. What type of protection absorbs the blood the best?

For heavy menstrual flow, pads are best because they hold the blood better than tampons. Tampons may allow blood to flow by them if you are flowing fast. Larger, more absorbent tampons help some women since the wider tampons allow less blood to pass by them, but with clots and heavy flow, a back-up pad may be needed as a safety measure. When flow is light, tampons work well and allow greater sports activity.

283. What is the best protection to use at night to eliminate leakage?

A double pad should hold the flow, so you can sleep a long time. If you have more flow than that, you really have a problem that may need attention.

284. Is it safe to wear a tampon at night?

If you want to minimize any risk from toxic shock syndrome*, you are advised to wear a pad rather than a tampon at night. However, since toxic shock syndrome is rare, you could do what is most comfortable and take your chances. (*Toxic shock syndrome is covered in more detail in Chapter VIII, "Women's Diseases and Surgery.")

285. My vagina seems to itch every time I menstruate. Could I be allergic to sanitary napkins?

You don't have to be allergic to be irritated by sanitary napkins. The surfaces can be irritating, and if they are perfumed, the irritation may be even worse. Changing the pads often or putting a tissue next to your skin can help. The itching also could be due to a yeast infection.

286. Besides pads and tampons, what other methods of protection are available?

Long ago women really wore cloth napkins, which is why they are called sanitary napkins today. Some women still wear a folded cloth. There

MENSTRUATION: TYPES OF PROTECTION (Continued)

was a type of cervical cap (trade name Tussaway) that women put in place for a long period of time because it would hold a lot of flow. It is not on the market now and probably will not come back for fear that anything left in the vagina for a long time can cause toxic shock syndrome. Women also use the diaphragm to avoid as much blood as they can, in order to have intercourse during menstruation. Sponges made to be worn in the vagina are sold in some places for absorption of blood.

287. How can I prevent the worst horror of all horrors - leaking menstrual blood through my clothes?

There probably is not a woman alive who has not had this happen at some time in her life. Some women live in such terror of this possible event that they wear a tampon at all times. Some girls will not go to school because they flow heavily and are not allowed to leave class to change pads. They are afraid of just such a "horror." Some women stay home for the first two or three days of menstruation because they are afraid of such a leak, not because they are in any discomfort. Such fear interferes with our education, our work, and our social lives. Why are we so horrified? It is a normal function. Is it because we think it is like losing control of urine or feces? But we have no control over menstrual flow. Until we change our reaction, the best prevention is frequently changed double protection (or a red dress!).

288. Is there any truth to the myth that if you use a tampon you are no longer a virgin?

No. The normal opening in the hymen is big enough to insert a finger or a tampon without stretching or tearing it, and a virgin is someone who has not had her hymen stretched or torn large enough to be able to insert a penis. The hymen can be stretched or torn, but it takes something larger than a finger or a tampon to do this. Since a penis is much larger in diameter than a finger or a tampon, insertion of a penis will require stretching or tearing of the hymen in order to make the opening large enough.

289. Is it okay to use tampons the first time I menstruate?

Yes, but you should definitely practice inserting one before the big day.

290. How do I know what size tampon to use?

The size you need depends upon how heavy your flow is and how often you are willing to change tampons. Super is for heavy flow, junior for light flow. It does not depend on whether you are a virgin. The opening in the hymen is naturally large enough for super, as well as junior tampons. Of course, the smaller size is easier to insert, but you will have to do it more often because it will absorb less blood.

MENSTRUATION: TYPES OF PROTECTION (Continued)

291. How do I insert a tampon?

For the first time, lie down on your back with your knees up and your feet flat on the bed. Spread your vulva apart with your left hand and find the opening of your vagina with the index finger of your right hand. Insert this finger as far as you can to convince yourself there is room for a tampon. Then prepare the tampon for insertion (unwrap it and be sure the string is in the proper place). While straining down (to open the vagina), insert the tampon just like you did your finger. Get it in all the way, so that you can't touch any part of it except the string. You can do this with an applicator or with just your fingers holding the tampon, depending on which kind you bought.

292. Is it easier to insert a tampon with your fingers or with an applicator?

Different people have different reactions. If you have a psychological problem with touching yourself, you will be better off with the applicator.

293. Is it easier for a woman who is not a virgin to insert a tampon than a woman who is a virgin?

Certainly. After the hymen is stretched or torn large enough to make room for a penis, it will also be easier to put in a tampon.

294. Why can't I seem to get a tampon into my vagina?

Sometimes women are afraid to put enough pressure in the right place to insert a tampon. Try to put your finger in first so you know where the tampon is supposed to go. If you can't even get your finger in, you may have been born with a small abnormality, such as a hymenal band (a small pink band of tissue going across the middle of the opening), a cribriform hymen (a covering with only pinholes in it, instead of a finger-size opening), or just a very small opening. To wear tampons in this case, you may have to have help from your doctor to make your hymen opening as large as normal.

295. Are tampons for everyone?

Of course not. Some women flow too heavily to be able to use them. Some have an abnormal hymen and can't insert them. But most women are more comfortable using them than they are with external pads. They are an absolute necessity if you want to participate in most sports, especially water sports. But be sure to change your tampons frequently.

296. I'm worried about toxic shock syndrome*. How often should I change tampons?

After 1976, coincidentally with the change in tampons from cotton to synthetic material, the first case of toxic shock syndrome was reported. Changing your tampon several times a day and wearing a pad at night (since

MENSTRUATION: TYPES OF PROTECTION (Continued)

you don't want to wake up at night to change) is the general advice from the Center for Disease Control on this subject. Also, if you must wear a tampon, use the regular kind that needs to be changed more often rather than the super absorbent kind, which you would keep in your body for more hours. (*Toxic shock syndrome is covered in more detail in Chapter VIII, "Women's Diseases and Surgery.")

297. Does a tampon cause blockage if I am clotting?

No, unfortunately, they usually do not even block the vagina enough to keep the clot from coming out on its own. They certainly do not block the uterus. Some tampons, such as the OB brand, are shaped in a way that makes a clot less likely to fall out. Rely brand tampons also were excellent in this respect, but they were taken off the market. Perhaps because they did too good a job in keeping everything in the vagina, they became associated with toxic shock syndrome.

298. Are deodorant tampons safe?

Yes, but some people are sensitive and allergic to many chemicals and may be irritated by deodorant tampons.

299. Are some women allergic to the deodorants used in some tampons and pads?

Some women experience irritation even if it is not a true allergy. Most of the time, however, their vaginal itching is really caused by a yeast infection, rather than reaction to a deodorant. If the skin under your arm gets along fine with a deodorant, the skin around your vulva should, too.

300. Are certain types of tampons more likely to cause cramps than others?

Tampons do not cause cramps. If the tampon is only halfway into the vagina, it will cause discomfort at the opening, but not uterine cramps. It is not in the uterus and does not block the flow from the uterus. Therefore, it cannot cause cramps.

301. Is using the wrong size tampon a potential danger?

No, but it is annoying to have blood flow past a tampon that is too small and get on your clothing. It also may be more difficult to insert the larger tampons.

302. Is it possible for a tampon to slip into the uterus?

No, the opening into the uterus, the cervix, is too small to admit a tampon, except for a few days immediately after you have had a baby.

303. If I wear a tampon when I go swimming, why doesn't it absorb water from the pool?

When you swim in a pool without a tampon, the pool water cannot cir-

MENSTRUATION: TYPES OF PROTECTION (Continued)

culate into your vagina, unless your opening is very loose from bearing children. Normally, the walls of the vagina are closed, especially at the entrance. When the tampon is properly placed high in the vagina, only the string extends out through the opening and certainly some water will be absorbed on the string, but not much in the vagina. It is a closed place, except when you open it.

304. Are natural sponges, which are sold in health food stores for menstrual protection, safe to use?

None of the natural sponges have been certified by the Food and Drug Administration (FDA) for this use, although a synthetic sponge recently was approved for menstrual protection. Another type of synthetic sponge also was approved for contraceptive use.

MENSTRUATION: MENSTRUAL CYCLE—WHAT IS NORMAL AND HOW TO CHART IT

305. What percentage of women have a "normal" twenty-eight-day cycle? Should I be worried if my cycle is not regularly twenty-eight days?

Thirteen percent of adult women have twenty-eight-day cycles most of the time. Another 12 percent of adult women have twenty-nine-day cycles and another 11 percent have twenty-seven-day cycles. So 36 percent of adult women have a cycle close to twenty-eight days. Of course, if you vary a week or so shorter or longer you are still normal, but you cannot make a calendar by your cycle. If your menses are coming as often as every two weeks or you skip more than three months, you probably should look into the problem to see why.

306. How can I chart (predict) my cycle?

Keep a record on your calendar of the first day of each menses. If these are always twenty-eight days apart, then you can predict a menstrual period on the twenty-eighth day after the last one started. You will not always be right. If your length of cycle is never the same, sometimes twenty-one days and sometimes thirty-five, then there is no way to predict a period accurately. You can keep a temperature chart to determine ovulation, and predict menstrual flow fourteen days after the rise in temperature that showed ovulation. If you do not ovulate, there is no way to predict your menstrual flow.

307. Is it true that women who live in the same household or who are very close friends will have the same menstrual cycle and will menstruate at the same time?

No, studies do not really show this to be true. By chance, at least one-

MENSTRUATION: MENSTRUAL CYCLE—WHAT IS NORMAL AND HOW TO CHART IT (Continued)

sixth of women will be menstruating more or less in the same five days out of thirty. Close friends and families could react to some traumatic situation by stopping or delaying ovulation and after that recover and cycle at the same time. But surveys do not show this to be generally true.

MENSTRUATION: MENSTRUAL CYCLE—WHEN DOES OVULATION OCCUR

308. On what day in my cycle do I ovulate?

It is not easy to tell exactly when you ovulate. In general, you ovulate fourteen days before you begin to menstruate, so if your menses are very regular (twenty-eight to thirty days apart), it is likely that you are ovulating on the fourteenth to sixteenth day. If you menstruate every thirty-five days, then it is likely on the twenty-first day.

MENSTRUATION: MENSTRUAL CYCLE—HOW TO DETERMINE WHEN OVULATION OCCURS

309. Is there a test that can determine the specific day that I ovulate?

The only absolute way to be sure of the exact day is to actually see the egg come out of its follicle on the ovary, see the follicle collapse, and then see it form a corpus luteum. The corpus luteum is a small, yellow body that forms on your ovary in the spot where the egg was released. In learning to make test-tube babies, this is what scientists did, first by operating with a device called a laparoscope that allowed them to see inside the abdomen, and then by looking at the shadow of the ovary on a sonogram with an ultra-sound machine. They could see the follicle grow to 24 mm in diameter and then collapse immediately after ovulation. But these procedures are expensive. A basal temperature chart is the only inexpensive, practical way to find out, but it is only approximate. Test tape can also be applied to the cervix daily. When it turns blue, you have ovulated.

310. What is the best way to determine exactly when ovulation occurs? How do I do it?

One of the more reliable ways to determine whether you are ovulating is to keep a basal temperature chart. For this you need a special basal temperature thermometer, which is very sensitive and only has a range of 97-100 degrees. (A fever thermometer will not work, because it is not sensitive enough.) You put it in your mouth every morning when you wake up, before you get out of bed. Then after three minutes, record your temperature on a chart. Do this from the beginning of one menstrual period

MENSTRUATION: MENSTRUAL CYCLE—HOW TO DETERMINE WHEN OVULATION OCCURS (Continued)

to the beginning of the next one. If the first few days show a low temperature, like 97 degrees, then it rises above 98 degrees for two weeks, you have ovulated at that point where it changed and rose. If there is no pattern and it just goes up and down, then you probably did not ovulate. Detailed instructions come with the thermometer. If you are using test tape, applied daily to your cervix, it will turn blue when you ovulate. You can then expect menses fourteen days after this happens.

311. What kind of medical tests are there to see if I am ovulating?

A blood test to measure progesterone in your blood after the time you should have ovulated is one test. An endometrial biopsy, a sample of tissue taken from the lining of your uterus, can show the effects of progesterone, if you have produced it after ovulation. This is an office procedure that is sometimes painful and requires local anesthesia, usually a block. A fern test is done by taking mucus from your cervix and letting it dry on a slide. If you have not ovulated yet, it will dry with a fern formation, but if you have ovulated and progesterone is present, its consistency is changed, and when it dries there will be no fern formation. Infections, however, also can prevent the ferning, so the test is not perfectly reliable.

312. I have a heavy discharge around the time I ovulate. Is this normal?

Yes. One way to detect the time of ovulation is to study the type of discharge you have. It should be clear and stringy when you ovulate.

313. What type of discharge means that I am ovulating?

Your cervical mucus (discharge) is clear and scant the first half of your cycle. The day before ovulation, it becomes jelly-like and very stringy. You can string it out for inches, just like sugar syrup. After ovulation, it thickens and will not string at all, but becomes heavier. If you watch this closely, you will become very familiar with your own changes in cervical mucus. Of course, if you have a vaginal infection, you will have a yellow discharge all of the time, so you won't be able to recognize the clear ovulation mucus.

314. Is there a more scientific way I can study my own discharge to prove when I am ovulating?

Yes. You will need to look at your cervical mucus (discharge) with a microscrope under low power. You can study how it dries on a slide. To do this, touch your cervix with your finger and spread the mucus on a slide. If you are in the first half of your cycle when only estrogen is produced, the mucus will form a fern-like pattern as it dries. When you produce progesterone, in the second half of your cycle or after you ovulate, the pro-

MENSTRUATION: MENSTRUAL CYCLE—HOW TO DETERMINE WHEN OVULATION OCCURS (Continued)

gesterone prevents the fern formation and the mucus just dries in globs. If you watch this closely, you will become very familiar with your own changes in your cervical mucus. But if you have a vaginal infection, this mucus test won't work well.

315. I can tell the exact day I ovulate, because I have a very heightened sexual urge. Why is this?

Recent research shows that there is a sudden rise in testosterone and other androgens (male-type sex hormones) produced by the ovaries when ovulation occurs. Some women are very sensitive to these androgens and show an increase in sex drive (libido) at this time. Like other mammals, this genetically derived urge also tends to increase reproduction to preserve the species.

316. Do most women feel a sexual urge when they ovulate?

No, most women do not report an urge for sex with ovulation. Even though a rise in testosterone and other androgens could account for such an urge, sexual urges in most women are complicated by sexually arousing situations, culture, relationships, and tensions, so they do not notice the hormone rise.

MENSTRUATION: MENSTRUAL CYCLE—CRAMPS AT OVULATION TIME

317. What are "mittelschmerz" pains?

Mittelschmerz is German for pain in the middle; in this case, the middle of your menstrual cycle. The pain occurs when you ovulate, when the egg bursts out of the follicle cyst it was in and leaks out a little blood that irritates your pelvis, causing pain. When the blood absorbs, the pain is gone. Most people do not feel this at all, some women feel it every month, and others only on rare occasions. It can last a few minutes to several days. This is one of the pains that birth control pills prevent, because they prevent ovulation.

318. Why do I sometimes get cramps or feel pain as early as two weeks before I begin menstruating?

This is a sign of ovulation. When the egg bursts out of its follicle or cyst, a little blood leaks out of the ovary. When this has been observed through a laparoscope (a device which allows doctors to see inside your abdomen), a little blood is always seen and sometimes there is more than just a little. The more blood that is released into the abdomen, the more it hurts.

MENSTRUATION: MENSTRUAL CYCLE—MENSTRUATION WITH NO OVULATION

319. Can I menstruate, but not ovulate?
Certainly. We all do, once in a while.

MENSTRUATION: MENSTRUAL CYCLE—NO OVULATION

320. Why don't I ovulate?
Ninety-five percent of the time, it is because of poor nutrition or being underweight or overweight. If you are very fat, the fat produces so much estrogen that it prevents ovulation, just like taking hormones can. If you are thin and have only 5 percent instead of 12 percent body fat, you don't produce enough estrogen in your fat to make the ovulation cycle work. If you run, especially if you run a lot, the beta-endorphins (opiates or pain relievers) produced in your brain that give you a "high" from running also act to stop the mechanism of ovulation. It is also possible that you have a pituitary tumor, adrenal tumor, or even an ovarian tumor that is interfering with ovulation. Though this chance is small, it is worth checking out.

MENSTRUATION: MENSTRUAL CYCLE—OVULATION WITH NO MENSTRUATION

321. Can I ovulate without menstruating?
Yes, but only if you get pregnant from that ovulation. When you ovulate, you either menstruate two weeks later or you are pregnant.

MENSTRUATION: MENSTRUAL CYCLE—OVULATION AND PREGNANCY

322. Is ovulation the time that I am most likely to become pregnant?
Ovulation is the only time that you can become pregnant, as it is the only time that the egg leaves the ovary and enters the tube where it can be fertilized by the sperm waiting there.

323. Is the day I ovulate the only time I can get pregnant?
Technically yes, but practically speaking, no. Intercourse can place sperm in the vagina six days before ovulation, and the sperm can be still in the tube, lively as ever, just waiting to penetrate the egg when ovulation occurs. So intercourse in the week before you ovulate can cause pregnancy on the day you ovulate. Of course, intercourse in the twenty-four hours just prior to ovulation makes your chances of getting pregnant even better. After you ovulate it is too late, because the egg will not last long enough for the sperm to reach it by sex later that day.

MENSTRUATION: MENSTRUAL CYCLE—OVULATION AND PREGNANCY (Continued)

324. Can I get pregnant if I am not ovulating?

No, not that cycle, but you might ovulate the next cycle.

325. Are there any special circumstances, over which a woman would have no control, that would cause her to not ovulate and therefore not be able to get pregnant?

Because some problems do affect ovulation, a woman is less likely to become pregnant if she is starving, very overweight, emotionally upset, or acutely ill. It is a rather protective mechanism. Who needs a baby with those troubles?

MENSTRUATION: PREGNANCY AND BIRTH CONTROL

326. Is it possible to get pregnant during menstruation?

Yes. The sperm can enter the tubes and stay there for as long as six days. In the event of an early ovulation, the sperm could still connect with an egg and produce a fertilized egg. Thus, even though the most fertile time for a woman is really the week after menses, late in menses can be, too, so contraception should be used at all times. You also may have ovulation bleeding, which is difficult to distinguish from menstruation. This often fools women who are using the rhythm method of contraception.

327. I don't take birth control pills while I'm menstruating. If I want to have intercourse at this time, will I have to use another form of birth control?

No. Since ovulation is stopped when you start taking the pills, pregnancy will not occur from sex during menses, even though you are not actually taking the pills during the week of menses. However, if you do not start taking the pills after menses has stopped, then pregnancy could occur. The "menses" you have while you are taking the pill are really withdrawal bleeding from the pill, not true menses.

328. Does the fact that I've always had regular periods necessarily mean that I'm fertile?

No, but it is certainly more likely to indicate fertility than irregular periods. To be fertile, you also must have a normal cervix, vagina, uterus, and fallopian tubes that are open and functioning well. Unless you were born with an abnormality or had some infection or surgery to damage them, you are probably fertile. Regular periods suggest that you ovulate, but if you want to be sure that you are fertile, then you must prove this by a temperature chart, study of the cervical mucus, tests of your tubes, an endometrial biopsy, or by getting pregnant.

MENSTRUATION: PREGNANCY AND BIRTH CONTROL
(Continued)

329. Are there differences in fertility between women who have heavy periods and those with very light periods?

No, the heaviness of your period is not a reliable factor in predicting fertility. A very heavy period can occur when there is only estrogen production with no ovulation at all. A very light period can occur when there is not much estrogen production and no ovulation at all. But also, a woman with a very heavy period may be very fertile, as might a woman with a very light period. There is more correlation between having cramps and being fertile than with the flow. Menstrual cramps indicate that you ovulated two weeks before menses began.

330. If my period is late, how long should I wait before having a pregnancy test?

To use the home pregnancy test on urine or the urine test in a doctor's office, clinic, or laboratory, your menstrual period should be at least one week overdue in order to obtain about 95 percent accuracy with the test. You can get a blood test that indicates pregnancy as early as the week before you even miss your period. These are more expensive and are usually reserved for special problems.

331. When does menstruation return after pregnancy?

Half of the women who do not breast-feed will have a menstrual period by six weeks after delivery, and the other half will trail out until nearly all have menstruated within three months. If you breast-feed, the delay in return of menses is usually at least three or four months. If you are a slender girl with a low calorie intake, menses may not return until after you stop breast-feeding entirely.

MENSTRUATION: HEALTH AND HYGIENE

332. What are some of the general rules governing health, comfort, and hygiene during menstruation?

If your flow is not heavy and you do not have severe cramps, then the only rule is that in our civilization you are expected to wear some kind of pad or tampon to absorb the flow. You may be as physically active as you feel like being, bathe, eat as you like, and even be sexually active, if you desire. If you do not feel well, you should be allowed to avoid uncomfortable activities, use pain medication as needed, and curl up in bed with a hot water bottle, if that is the only way you find peace. Our culture doesn't really allow this; school, jobs, families, and husbands are far too demanding. So it might be better for you to use medication to feel as well as you can.

MENSTRUATION: PSYCHOLOGICAL FACTORS THAT AFFECT IT

333. Do any psychological or anatomical changes occur at the onset of menstruation?

This varies with the individual. Many women notice no psychological changes while others, who suffer pain with menses, might become apprehensive and depressed. Recent research suggests a drop in your endorphin level (morphine that occurs naturally in your body) with the onset of menses. This leaves you irritable and changes your bowel action from constipation to diarrhea. Anatomically, you may lose as much as five pounds of water weight, and your clothes may fit more loosely, because the gas in your bowel passes with the diarrhea. The lining leaves your uterus with the blood, and the corpus luteum on the ovary regresses and becomes small. The corpus luteum is a small yellow body on your ovary that formed in the spot where you ovulated and produced the large amounts of estrogen and progesterone for two weeks from ovulation to menstruation. Because the corpus luteum stops producing, the hormones stop and menstruation begins. When it stops, it shrinks in size. Breasts also may decrease in size and certainly in tenderness.

334. Can emotions interfere with my menstrual cycle?

Some menstrual irregularities can be attributed to emotions; however, if you have skipped a period, you should have a pregnancy test taken once or twice before you conclude that emotions are the reason for your irregularity. Emotions can interfere with all of the body's functions, so you should always try to be as emotionally well-balanced as you can be.

335. Why does tension cause my period to be late?

Tension can interfere with your hypothalamus (a portion of your brain) and its interaction with the pituitary in its production of hormones that cause the ovaries to ovulate. If it delays or prevents ovulation, your period can be late.

336. My period is very irregular, especially when I am worried about something. Could psychological problems cause me not to ovulate?

Yes, the reason you do not ovulate possibly could be psychological stress. The pituitary gland at the base of the brain is very much affected by this. Severe emotional tension, even if it is happy excitement, can interfere with the cycle. Travel often is the cause of an upset cycle. Most women who are subjected to extremely severe traumas will stop ovulating. Other traumas, such as marital stress, school exams, and family arguments, will stop some women from ovulating. Even a mild illness, like influenza, can interfere.

MENSTRUATION: EFFECTS OF DIET AND WEIGHT ON MENSTRUATION AND RATE OF FLOW

337. Does my body weight have any effect on how much or how long I bleed during my period?

How much you weigh and the percentage of your body weight that is fat are two very important factors involved in length and amount of flow. The fat promotes the production of estrogen, which increases the flow. If this is balanced with ovulation and a good production of progesterone, the flow will not be too long or too heavy.

338. I am overweight. Why do I seem to have my period all of the time?

Fat converts hormones from the adrenal gland into estrogen, and this estrogen makes a thick lining of the uterus, which can bleed for a long time. The best solution for you would be to normalize your weight, but this may take a long time, and you could bleed to death in the process. It would be better to get some temporary help with the control of flow until you lose the extra weight.

339. Could my diet cause me to stop menstruating totally?

Yes, extreme starvation causing malnutrition can cause you to stop ovulating and stop menstruating altogether, until your diet becomes sufficient to furnish what your endocrine system (glands) needs to get going again.

340. How can I help my body to ovulate, so that I will have a regular menstrual cycle?

Have a normal weight, have good nutrition, and allow some fat to accumulate on your body instead of exercising it all off. This will help regulate your menses. If you are within the first two years of menstruation, it is quite normal not to ovulate, at least not regularly. As you mature, it should become more regular and you should become more fertile.

MENSTRUATION: BLOOD LOSS—NORMAL AND HEMORRHAGING RATES OF FLOW

341. What determines the amount of blood I will lose during menses?

The blood loss is determined by the thickness of the endometrium (the lining of the uterus); whether it is secretory or not (secretory type only occurs after ovulation); the contour and shape of the internal wall of the uterus; whether or not it has been distorted by fibroids or other abnormalities; the presence of polyps; and the absence or presence of abnormal cell growth, such as cancer or precancerous changes. Estrogen makes the lining thick with a tendency to bleed heavily, but then progesterone makes it secretory with a tendency to bleed lightly.

MENSTRUATION: BLOOD LOSS—NORMAL AND HEMORRHAGING RATES OF FLOW (Continued)

342. Do changes in diet or exercise affect the amount of menstrual flow?

Yes. If your diet is so low that you are malnourished and you exercise so long and strenuously that you have no fat at all, you probably will have no menstrual flow. Some specialists have said that most menstrual problems would disappear if women had normal, nutritious diets and were normal weights. Diet and exercise certainly can do this for you, but you cannot do it just during the days you menstruate. It must be continued throughout the years that you menstruate.

343. What else contributes to how long and how much I flow during menstruation?

Ovulation is important. Another factor would be abnormalities of the uterus, such as fibroids, which can affect flow. Some things that do not affect flow are: bathing during menses, swimming in cold water, exercise, and sex.

344. How much blood loss is normal during menstruation?

The average menstrual flow for the entire period is 44 cc or about one-quarter cup. This can be translated into three to five pads (not completely soaked) or tampons each day for the first two days, then less for the next three days. On contraceptive pills, the average flow is half that much, measuring 22 cc. But, as in all biology, there is a great variation. Some women flow 400 cc (nearly a pint) each cycle, yet do not become anemic; others barely put a spot on a pad for a day or two, but they are normal and fertile.

345. When is bleeding from my vagina a hemorrhage?

Soaking six pads in an hour or passing clots larger than your fist several times an hour is an acute hemorrhage requiring immediate action. You should call a doctor or visit an emergency room. In either case, you will need to describe to your physician the extent of the hemorrhage, so you must count the number of pads that you soak. Clots don't soak into a pad, so they must be measured, in addition to the pads you have soaked. If the blood has gone onto the floor, you should be able to give the doctor an idea of the diameter of the puddle. Sitting on a toilet seat makes you bleed even more, just because that position holds everything open, so lie down with a pad or towel and stay near a phone. However, lying down masks the rate of bleeding. The vagina fills with blood, and then releases a pint of blood when you get up. So don't lie down too long.

346. How many days should my flow be heavy?

Most women normally have a heavy flow for only two or three days,

MENSTRUATION: BLOOD LOSS—NORMAL AND
HEMORRHAGING RATES OF FLOW (Continued)

and the heaviness of the flow is not more than five pads or tampons a day. If it is longer or heavier than that, you are more likely to become anemic. The rest of menstruation is a much lighter flow.

347. I know I'm not hemorrhaging, but my period is very heavy and it lasts a long time. What should I do?

Menses that soak ten pads a day and bleed ten days per cycle are too much to tolerate for many months. Even though this is not an emergency or a hemorrhage, some diagnostic tests and/or treatment procedure should be scheduled. Bleeding for more than two weeks at a time is another reason for a visit to the doctor, but it is not an emergency, unless you are bleeding so heavily that you think you may be hemorrhaging (please see previous question).

348. Is it normal to become weak in my legs when I lose a lot of blood?

Yes, it is normal with a real hemorrhage, but not with ordinary menstruation, because you do not lose a lot of blood. It is the prostaglandins (substances locally produced in the tissues) that cause nausea, diarrhea, weakness, and faintness along with the cramps. Faintness can be felt as a weakness in your legs.

349. Should I assume that I'm anemic just because I have a heavy menstrual flow?

No, but it would be wise for you to consult a physician and have your hemoglobin level checked for anemia. You can, at least, find out if you should be taking iron. Your doctor also may want to take additional measures to diagnose the cause of your heavy flow and treat it. If you find that you are not anemic (tired blood), you may wish to take further steps to curb the flow just because it is inconvenient, as well as abnormal.

350. Is there any way to reduce the length of flow, especially if it lasts ten days?

Yes, that is what gynecology is all about. First, do what you can to have a normal diet and weight. Then it would be best to find out why your period is lasting ten days, because that is exactly the length that most physicians consider too long. If they find that you are not ovulating and not producing any progesterone, you can either take progesterone (alone, or in a birth control pill) or do something to ovulate. If it is because you have a polyp, cancer, or a precancerous lining, a D & C (dilatation and curettage—a surgical procedure in which the uterine wall is scraped) will tell you about that. A pelvic examination may show you have fibroid tumors, and if they are bleeding this much you are going to have to deal with them. Perhaps you

MENSTRUATION: BLOOD LOSS—NORMAL AND HEMORRHAGING RATES OF FLOW (Continued)

are just spotting ten days from a cervicitis, a bleeding area on the cervix. Find out and take action. That is just too long to tolerate menstruation.

351. What is the normal rate of flow when a woman is on birth control pills?

A total blood loss of 22 cc is normal on the pill, compared to 44 cc off the pill. This amounts to one or two small tampons a day for one to three days. Sometimes the flow is only a little brown spotting for a day or two.

MENSTRUATION: IRREGULAR CYCLE

352. What would cause my periods to suddenly become irregular after being regular for a long time?

Irregularity is usually caused by a change in ovulation or stopping ovulation altogether. Approaching menopause can do that, but at younger ages it is more likely to be due to tension and emotional upsets. Weight loss and a change in the amount of exercise, especially running, also can change ovulation. Very frequent heavy periods can be due to growing fibroids or even to cancer of the uterus, and they must be investigated. Of course, you must always think of pregnancy when bleeding is irregular.

353. Why is my flow inconsistent, some months light and others heavy?

If you ovulate some months and not others, it will vary like that, and this is the most sensitive variable. However, every developing follicle is a little different from the previous one, and the hormones produced also can be different and will produce a different flow. Some women are sure that when they ovulate from one ovary it is different than when they ovulate from the other. Some specialists think we alternate ovaries every month, but most do not agree.

354. My periods are very irregular. What are some of the signs I could look for that would indicate my period is going to start?

Many women would like a reliable sign of approaching menses so that they could be prepared. Most women depend on tender, engorged breasts and a few pelvic cramps to tell them to wear a tampon or pad soon. Others have absolutely no sign of oncoming menses until they see blood, so they carry a tampon or pad in their purse for many days before they use it. If you are not ovulating, then there is even less chance of any warning signs.

355. Is it common for college women to have irregular menstrual cycles?

I've never seen a study comparing college women to others, but I think it might be true that they ovulate less often. Ovulation can be inhibited by such things as travel, change in living arrangements, tension (such as that which examinations produce), and malnutrition, which runs rampant when

MENSTRUATION: IRREGULAR CYCLE (Continued)

girls leave home and eat and diet as they like.

356. Instead of every month, I bleed every two weeks to every three months. Why are my menstrual periods so irregular?

The most common cause of such irregular bleeding is failure to release an egg (not ovulating). If you menstruate every twenty-eight days, or about once monthly, you are probably ovulating. If you are very irregular, you menstruate every two to three weeks or two to three months, you are probably not ovulating and not fertile—at least at that time. This is not reliable birth control, of course, because you might become fertile and ovulate the next month; so don't rely on irregular menstruation for contraception.

357. Do women with irregular cycles have trouble getting pregnant?

Yes. Difficulties with ovulation will make difficulties with getting pregnant, but any of the other causes of irregular bleeding also will interfere.

358. My period was very irregular at first. Then I started having sex, and it became more regular. Is there a connection?

No. Most girls start with irregular menses and then they become regular, even though they remain a virgin and sexually inactive. Time and maturity changed your menses, not sex.

359. How can I improve my heavy, painful, or irregular periods without going to a doctor or taking hormones?

Nutrition is under your control, and it can do a great deal to improve your menstrual life. If you flow heavily, eating foods that are rich in iron or taking over-the-counter iron tablets can keep you from being weak and anemic. A heavy flow also can occur as the result of not ovulating, and a high-protein diet can provide more of the materials needed to produce ovulation. Why not see a doctor to find out what is wrong? If you have cancer, fibroids, or an infection, you are delaying treatment.

360. How do birth control pills regulate menses?

They contain the hormone estrogen and a progestin that suppresses the pituitary from stimulating the ovaries into making any hormones or releasing any eggs. Therefore, the hormones present are mostly the hormones being taken by mouth. When you take the hormones, you don't bleed, and when you stop them, you bleed. You will be regular if you take them regularly. After you stop them altogether, you will go back to being your old irregular self. They only regulate you while you take them.

361. So many young girls are given birth control pills to regulate their period. What effect will this have on their fertility and growth in later life?

The most prominent endocrinologists (physicians who specialize in the

MENSTRUATION: IRREGULAR CYCLE (Continued)

glands, such as the pituitary) confirm that taking birth control pills to regulate menses will not hurt young girls' fertility or do anything to their growth pattern. Taking the pills simply controls their flow and does not interfere with their development. If they stop taking the pills, they may still have irregular menses. If their general health is good, weight normal, and nutrition good when they stop taking the pills, then they may have by that time matured to regular menses. Since there is no time limit on taking the pills, they still are able to use them later for contraception.

362. Can regulating my weight improve my irregular periods?

Most irregular heavy flowing could be improved by good nutrition and normal weight. Being overweight causes excessive estrogen to be produced in the fat, so by losing weight you could normalize menses. On the other hand, if you are underweight, you could eat more food and gain weight, and this perhaps could bring back menses that have disappeared.

MENSTRUATION: BLOOD CLOTTING

363. What causes clotting during menstruation?

Clotting during menstruation is caused when the bleeding is so fast that the mechanism that usually dissolves clots can't keep up with it. Blood from a cut on your finger clots very quickly, but menstrual blood is usually liquid. That's because there is an enzyme formed in the uterus that dissolves or digests clots into liquid blood, which is easier to pass through the cervix. It doesn't work fast enough for some heavy bleeding, which appears as clots.

364. Is some clotting normal during my period?

Most women do not have clots with their menses at all, because they bleed slowly. If you normally have clots, it is normal for you, because you bleed fast. It just indicates more blood loss.

365. Does the pill affect clotting in the menstrual flow?

Yes, if you are taking contraceptive pills, clotting may disappear because the flow is less. It also may disappear as you mature. It is an entirely different question as to whether the pill affects the clotting of the blood within blood vessels of the body, such as in the legs. Elaborate studies have shown some connection between the pill and phlebitis (inflammation of a vein) and thromboembolism (blockage in a blood vessel), which can be fatal, though they are rare (1 in 25,000). But this is an entirely different problem of clotting than clots passed with menstrual blood. Menstrual clots are not dangerous.

MENSTRUATION: EFFECTS OF BIRTH CONTROL METHODS USED DURING MENSTRUATION

366. What are the effects of the pill on menstruation?

In general, the combination-type contraceptive pills (those which contain both estrogen and progesterone) reduce your flow to half, make your period regular if the pills are taken regularly, and reduce the cramps that occur with menses. There also is a birth control pill containing only progesterone that does not regulate menses at all. It is taken constantly and often is associated with irregular menses and spotting.

367. Why do birth control pills make my flow lighter?

The newer birth control pills are high in progesterone and low in estrogen. Consequently, they produce a uterine lining that is quite thin, which reduces menstrual flow. For women taking these contraceptive pills, there is little bleeding at the end of their cycle, and occasionally it is non-existent.

368. After I stopped taking birth control pills, my period became heavy and long. Why?

When you started birth control pills, your period became short and light. The average amount of blood lost in menses on the pill is half that of normal menstruation, 22 cc instead of 44 cc (about one-eighth cup instead of one-fourth cup). Periods off the pill are expected to be heavier and longer than on the pill. If you have been on the pill for a long time, you may not even remember how your periods used to be. And, of course, they could have changed. Pill periods are lighter because they contain a lot of progestins compared to the amount of estrogen. If the pills had very little progestins and a lot of estrogen, your flow would be heavy.

369. Could the use of a copper IUD cause my periods to stop? Why?

This has been well studied, and there is nothing about a copper IUD that could stop your periods. It can make your periods longer and heavier, but not stop them.

370. What are the effects of the IUD on menstruation?

The IUD (intrauterine device) has a tendency to increase the flow and the length of menstruation. It also increases the cramps as well as spotting during your cycle.

371. Why does my period get heavier with an IUD?

The presence of the IUD produces a foreign-body reaction or inflammation in the lining of the uterus where it lies, and this inflammation makes more bleeding by causing the destruction of small blood vessels. It also acts as an irritant to the muscle and makes it contract more, producing more

MENSTRUATION: EFFECTS OF BIRTH CONTROL METHODS USED DURING MENSTRUATION (Continued)

cramps. You can imagine the mechanical rubbing of the IUD against the small blood vessels, preventing them from healing.

372. Do any other birth control methods affect menstruation?

The diaphragm, jellies, condoms, foams, suppositories, and rhythm or abstinence methods of birth control have no effect on menstruation.

MENSTRUATION: SEX DURING MENSTRUATION

373. Is it okay to have sex during menstruation?

Yes. There is no special harm to the male or female from coitus during menses. Coitus after a miscarriage or after having a baby can cause an infection of the uterus because of its condition then, but during menses this is not true. However, you are not safe from becoming pregnant if you have sex during menstruation.

374. Whenever I have sex regularly, my period is regular; however, when I go without sex for a while, my period becomes very irregular. Why?

It could be that when you go without sex you build up enough tension to interfere with or at least delay ovulation.

375. Can girls who have not begun menstruating be sexually stimulated?

Yes. Human beings, from the time of birth, can be sexually stimulated. Society and culture have more to do with sexual development than hormones and puberty.

MENSTRUATION: ATHLETES, EXERCISE, AND MENSTRUATION

376. Will heavy exercise during menstruation increase my menstrual flow?

No. Your uterine muscle does not respond to exercise by contracting less. The rate of flow depends more on the lining that has built up in the uterus all month. While women who are experiencing cramps usually do not feel like exercising, it is not harmful to do so at this time.

377. Why do women athletes tend to miss periods?

There are two explanations given. One is that they have less than the 12 percent of body fat required to produce enough estrogen to ovulate. The other is that running makes the body produce its own pain relievers, called endorphins, and these interfere with ovulation.

378. Will swimming or cold water stop my flow?

No. This has been a myth for many years. It is all right to go swimming during menses; however, unless you wear a tampon, your blood-soaked pad

MENSTRUATION: ATHLETES, EXERCISE, AND MENSTRUATION
(Continued)

will certainly contaminate the swimming pool. It is for such sports as this that girls eventually learn to use a tampon instead of a pad.

379. Would I be more susceptible to fainting after a sauna during menstruation?

Yes, the prostaglandins released during menstruation can make you much more liable to fainting (syncope) even without a sauna. If you have a tendency to faint with menses, the sauna certainly could increase this tendency, because it dilates your blood vessels and, thus, draws blood away from your brain. Obviously, you should avoid things that make you faint. If you have never fainted with menses, then a sauna is not likely to make you do so.

MENSTRUATION: PREMENSTRUAL SYNDROME—SYMPTOMS, CAUSES, INCIDENCE

380. Is it true that athletes have less premenstrual tension?

It is generally accepted that exercise reduces tension, but there is no known survey on premenstrual syndrome (PMS) in athletes.

381. How many women suffer from premenstrual syndrome?

It is estimated that 40-50 percent of women who are not on the birth control pill and who are menstruating have premenstrual syndrome to the point that it somewhat interferes with their lives. About 10 percent of these women are completely incapacitated for one or two days every month.

382. Sometimes I am moody and uncomfortable before menstruating. Is this common?

Premenstrual syndrome (PMS) is a problem experienced by some women that has not yet been completely solved by medical science. Besides being moody, women also complain of anxiety, irritability, lethargy, depression, sleep disorders, crying spells, and even hostility a few days prior to their menstrual flow. Other women have headaches, especially migraines, or even seizures. Additionally, breast tenderness and swelling, abdominal bloating, constipation, and acne also may be associated with the syndrome. A few women experience all of these symptoms; some women only experience them sometimes. According to one study, 40-50 percent of women not on the pill experience premenstrual syndrome.

383. What is the cause of premenstrual syndrome?

The cause of premenstrual syndrome has been attributed to the accumulation of the hormones estrogen and progesterone, even though the levels of hormones in women with the symptoms are essentially the same as those without. Newer research attributes the depression to endorphins,

MENSTRUATION: PREMENSTRUAL SYNDROME—SYMPTOMS, CAUSES, INCIDENCE (Continued)

opiate-like substances that are produced in the brain. It is believed that a decrease in the level of opiate endorphins just prior to menses is the cause of irritability, or PMS. A British researcher found that progesterone is inadequate in PMS, and treated it with natural progesterone suppositories. Low blood sugar (hypoglycemia) has been blamed, and frequent small meals that are high in protein and low in sugar are used to prevent this. Water retention also has been thought responsible, and is treated with diuretics.

384. Why does premenstrual syndrome seem to worsen with age?

It is true that PMS worsens with age, but the cause of PMS really is not completely known, so the increase cannot be explained. It may be due to hormonal changes with age (decreasing progesterone), and it may just be that after a few years women become very aware of how their bodies are reacting. Perhaps they were ignoring it before. Probably as women approach menopause, progesterone decreases and PMS increases.

385. Are migraine headaches a symptom of premenstrual syndrome?

In a sense, yes, because women who have migraines have more of them premenstrually. To have migraines, you first have to inherit the tendency. But many women only have their first migraine with their first menstruation, and the migraines usually recur during the week just prior to menses. The explanation for this is that the increased number of hormones present just before menses retain fluid and dilate the blood vessels, aggravating the blood vessel expansion of the migraine-throbbing headache. This is why high-dose birth control pills also can aggravate and increase the frequency of migraine headaches. After menopause, these types of headaches often disappear. They also disappear during breast-feeding but are worse during pregnancy when hormones are in great supply.

386. I always crave sweets, especially chocolate, before I get my period. Why?

This has been in the limelight of recent research on premenstrual syndrome (PMS). It is theorized that during menstruation the body produces endorphins that change you in many ways. One change that may occur is that you become hypoglycemic (a condition in which there is a deficiency of sugar in the blood), so you crave sugar. To combat this, you can eat small, protein meals frequently throughout the day, which can prevent the drop in blood sugar and perhaps the craving for sweets.

387. Do most women like to feel the changes that take place in their bodies during the menstrual cycle, or would most women prefer to not feel them?

This all depends on personal preference. It is interesting that some

MENSTRUATION: PREMENSTRUAL SYNDROME—SYMPTOMS, CAUSES, INCIDENCE (Continued)

women like to feel the changes in their bodies during the menstrual cycle, while others complain bitterly about them. Of the women who complain, many do not want to feel the changes in their own cycles because they suffer from premenstrual syndrome and ovulation pain.

MENSTRUATION: PREMENSTRUAL SYNDROME AND SOCIETY

388. Why does society seem to frown upon a woman showing premenstrual syndrome?

One reason for this is that men cannot understand women's cyclic irritability. Another is that women demand of themselves that they behave at all times in a sweet, understanding, and tolerant manner, especially to their children and their husbands, even though they do not always demand the same treatment in return. If their life styles depend upon their being active, productive, assertive, and demanding, then they do well even during their premenstrual days. But if they feel that they are supposed to be passive, sweet, kind, responsive, self-effacing and non-demanding, then they have many problems in their premenstrual time, but do well in their postmenstrual days. Unfortunately, the characteristics women show in the postmenstrual time are considered best for the "feminine role" by a lot of people.

MENSTRUATION: PREMENSTRUAL BREAST CYSTS

389. How do you explain the presence of small lumps or cysts in my breasts just prior to menstruation?

Estrogen stimulates the accumulation of fluid in your breasts, especially in cystic areas, and sometimes quite large, clear cysts are produced that will disappear with menses. It is acceptable to wait until after your menstrual period before having a surgeon examine such a large cyst, because it may disappear. If it still is present after menses, then it is worth an examination and treatment, probably removing the fluid from the cyst in the doctor's office. Some research suggests caffeine is associated with cystic breasts. You can avoid coffee, tea, and colas to see if this is true for you.

390. How common are breast cysts?

Fibrocystic breasts are estimated to be present in about one-third of young American women, and in about two-thirds of premenopausal women. Large cysts are less common.

MENSTRUATION: PREMENSTRUAL AND MENSTRUAL CRAMPS AND INDIGESTION

391. Why do I get cramps before my period begins?

Sometimes prostaglandins (substances locally produced in the tissues) are produced several days before the flow actually starts, at which time some cramping begins. This serves as a warning to many women to prepare for menstruation.

392. Is it normal to get cramps during menstruation?

Yes. Since all women do not experience cramps during menstruation, they used to be considered "all in a woman's head." In fact, women who have cramps are normal, both psychologically and physically. They simply produce more prostaglandins, unless they have other problems, such as endometriosis (see next question).

393. Why do I get cramps during menstruation?

Women who experience cramps usually are producing a high level of a substance called prostaglandins in their uterus, and this is the reason for their cramps. Prostaglandins got its name because it was first found in the prostate gland of the male. When it is injected into a woman, she will experience cramps, nausea, vomiting, and even diarrhea. Similarly, women who have cramps with menses also are likely to have nausea, vomiting, and diarrhea. But cramps also may be due to the presence of a tumor, polyps, or endometriosis, a condition in which tissue from the lining of the uterus is found growing in other parts of the pelvis. A pelvic checkup would reveal these problems.

394. How much pain and cramping is normal during menses?

Most women have enough feelings of heaviness and pelvic discomfort to realize that they are menstruating before they ever see blood. This serves as a warning device so they can start wearing protection when those feelings begin. Some women also have enough cramps to warrant taking two aspirin, which relieves the cramps. Only 30 percent have pain that cannot be relieved by aspirin, and most of them are teenagers.

395. Are severe cramps a sign that something is wrong?

If you have severe cramps every time you menstruate and not in between menstrual periods and you have had them since a couple of years after you started having menses, there is probably nothing wrong. If you usually do not have cramps and then begin to have severe cramps, you may be having a miscarriage, not realizing you are pregnant. If you have more severe cramps than usual and they begin to worsen even after the menstrual flow has subsided, you are likely to have an infection. If your cramps worsen year

MENSTRUATION: PREMENSTRUAL AND MENSTRUAL CRAMPS AND INDIGESTION (Continued)

after year with every menstrual period you probably have endometriosis, especially if you also have pain between periods. A pelvic checkup can find out which is the case for you.

396. Is there a natural way to relieve cramps?

Heating pads and hot water bottles help relieve pain and also help you to lie still and go to sleep and forget about it. Exercise and good nutrition help you to have a healthy body and as good a balance of hormones as your genetics will allow, but they will not always relieve menstrual cramps. Pregnancy is natural, and it relieves cramps because there are no menses for nine months. It also changes the uterus so that it does not have as many sensitive nerve endings after delivery. Alcohol also is natural, and does reduce uterine contractions even in labor, as well as during menstruation. However, if you drink enough to relieve the cramps, you will have drunk too much and will hardly function doing anything else. The people who need help with cramps most, teenagers, would be breaking the law by drinking alcohol.

397. I've heard that the best remedy for relieving cramps is to just relax, maybe even have an alcoholic drink. Is this true?

Curling up in bed around a hot water bottle and going to sleep is a very fine remedy, but it doesn't get you through a class at school or through a day on the job. Narcotics, especially codeine, also may relieve the pain somewhat, but they will leave you sedated and not as alert as you should be for your daily activities. Even alcohol, wine, beer, or brandy actually will relax uterine contractions and relieve the cramps, but you could get drunk, and this is certainly not acceptable. Aspirin or other over-the-counter medications help relieve cramps.

398. Why do my thighs and back hurt during menstruation?

The pain you are experiencing comes from the uterine muscle. When the pain is severe, it seems to radiate out in wide circles. Most women feel cramps low in their pelvis in the front, at the bottom of their abdomens, or on both sides just above where their legs insert. Others feel cramps in their lower backs and, in fact, say that they have a backache instead of cramps. A smaller group of women feel the ache in their upper thighs. In any case, there is nothing wrong with their thighs or backs. It just means that the severe pain spreads out. The same is true of labor during childbirth; it can be felt in the front, back, or thighs. This is called referred pain.

399. Why do I get backaches when I'm having my period?

Menstrual cramps, as well as labor pains, are felt by many women as pain in their backs, instead of or as well as pain in their fronts, low in the pelvis. This is called referred pain; that is, the pain actually originates in the

MENSTRUATION: PREMENSTRUAL AND MENSTRUAL CRAMPS AND INDIGESTION (Continued)

uterus but is felt by you as actually being in your back. There is probably nothing wrong with your back. If there is something wrong with your back, however, it will feel worse at this time, because all pain is aggravated during menses.

400. Are digestive problems common during menstruation?

With severe menstrual cramps (dysmenorrhea), there may be associated vomiting and diarrhea. These are all caused by prostaglandins, which some women produce in high quantity and others do not. If you are injected with prostaglandins you will vomit, have diarrhea, and have menstrual cramps. Perhaps 10 percent of women under twenty-five years of age at least have nausea, if not vomiting, during the first day of menstruation.

401. What can I do to relieve the discomforts of gas, cramps, and constipation associated with menstruation?

If you can't fasten your jeans, you can try taking an over-the-counter medication, like Mylicon, for gas. Three tablets a day should be enough to get the gas out. Models find that this is especially important for their jobs. Bran is a reliable and healthful laxative that also can help you. When your period starts, your bowels may become loose and may even approach diarrhea, which certainly will remove the gas and flatten the abdomen. Of course, constipation and gas are worse if there is a lot of emotional tension prior to menses.

402. Is it true that a decreased intake of salt before my period will help reduce the severity of cramps?

No. Decreased salt intake is intended to reduce water retention caused by hormones. This is related to premenstrual syndrome but not to menstrual cramps.

403. I've heard that my cramps will go away when I have a baby. Is this true?

It is not entirely true, although the cramps should be less. That tale got started because most women have had a baby by age twenty-five, and by age twenty-five, most women have stopped having severe cramps. Women who reach the age of twenty-five and have not had a baby also will find that they stop having cramps. The credit should not go to having a baby, but rather to just becoming mature. However, research has shown that the number of sensory endings in the uterus are destroyed during pregnancy, and not all of them are re-formed after the uterus returns to normal. So pain is reduced because there are fewer sensory endings in the uterus.

404. My cramps also are accompanied by a weak feeling. Does this have anything to do with a loss of calcium?

No. Without actually hemorrhaging, you do not bleed enough during

MENSTRUATION: PREMENSTRUAL AND MENSTRUAL CRAMPS AND INDIGESTION (Continued)

menstruation to lower your calcium level. If your calcium level were low, all of the muscles in your body would contract tightly, not just your uterus. This rare condition is called tetany.

405. Sometimes my flow stops during the middle of my period, yet I continue to have cramps, and later I bleed for a day or two more without cramps. Why?

The pattern of bleeding is quite variable among women. Many bleed a small amount for a day or so, then heavily for two days, then light again for one or two more days. The pattern you describe can occur when the prostaglandins produce such forceful cramps of the uterus that the flow stops entirely. Cramps are produced by a contraction in the uterus, which tends to shut off the blood vessels found in the uterine wall. Once the cramps or contractions subside a little, then a little more flow can occur. It also can occur when there is cervical stenosis, in which the cervix constricts or becomes narrow. In this case, the pressure of the flow has to build up to get through.

406. Does fertility have anything to do with cramps?

Yes. The production of prostaglandins is more likely to occur when a woman is fertile and has actually released an egg during her menstrual cycle. Since twelve-year olds produce estrogen but seldom produce an egg for the first two years, they usually do not have cramps. However, at the age of fourteen to sixteen, they do become fertile and ovulate; then the cramps begin, since they are more likely to be producing prostaglandins. Often teenage girls at this age think that there is something wrong with them when, in fact, they are more normal than before because now they are fertile. Unfortunately, the thought that the cramps mean that they are more fertile is not always comforting to learn at this time.

407. Will the severity of my menstrual cramps vary with age?

Yes. The most severe cramps usually occur during the teenage years and become less severe as you grow older, usually becoming mild by the age of twenty-five. Since cramps are attributed to the production of prostaglandins, as the amount of prostaglandins found in your flow decreases, then so does the severity of your cramps.

408. Is it okay to exercise if I am having cramps?

If you are having cramps that are not severe, and you are exercising in a physical activity that you enjoy and that takes your mind off the discomforts, then that is fine.

MENSTRUATION: PREMENSTRUAL AND MENSTRUAL CRAMPS AND INDIGESTION (Continued)

409. Are there any good exercises to combat the discomforts and cramps of menstruation?

Not specifically. Cramps do not come from a lack of exercise. Gymnastic teachers have taught stretching exercises for the pelvis for a long time, as if they could stretch the uterine muscle, but this is really impossible. Nowhere in medical science is there advice or a description of exercises for menstrual cramps and discomforts.

410. How long will my cramps, nausea, and diarrhea last during menstruation?

Usually these symptoms are worse on the first or second day of the menstrual flow, although they may continue for four or five days.

MENSTRUATION: MEDICATION FOR CRAMPS

411. What are all the new medications that claim to alleviate menstrual cramps?

In the last few years, several antiprostaglandins have been developed solely for the relief of menstrual cramps. These include Motrin, Anaprox, Naprosyn, and Ponstel, and they do not have the side effect of making you sleepy. Their only side effect is that they irritate your stomach, much like aspirin; however, this can be alleviated by taking them with food, such as milk. Since they are taken only one or two days each month, few people notice any other side effects and 70-80 percent find relief.

412. Do aspirin or over-the-counter drugs really help menstrual cramps?

If your cramps are mild, aspirin should help because it is a weak antiprostaglandin. Over-the-counter medications, such as Midol or Pamprin, also work for mild cramps, but 30 percent of women who experience severe cramping need a prescription medication.

413. Can taking calcium really help relieve cramps?

No. You already have a huge supply of calcium in your bones that your body can use at any time. People in the United States are well supplied with calcium since they drink milk and eat cheese. Taking calcium produces no change in menstrual cramps. Only pregnant women and women past menopause need to take calcium.

414. What is an antispasmodic? When is it used for menstrual cramps?

An antispasmodic is a muscle relaxant that will relieve spasms of the uterine muscle. The results of their use for menstrual cramps are not as good as anti-prostaglandins, but they have some merit. Vasodilan is a brand of antispasmodic that has been used to stop labor as well as to stop cramps by

MENSTRUATION: MEDICATION FOR CRAMPS (Continued)

stopping the contractions. Alcohol has been used as an antispasmodic the same way.

415. What do the new drugs that are being marketed for menstrual pain contain?

The new ones being developed all require a prescription, but they are effective in 70 percent of women. They contain antiprostaglandins, which reduce the prostaglandins in your uterus that give you the pain. Aspirin is an antiprostaglandin, but it is too weak to do enough for everyone. These other drugs previously have been used for arthritis, as has aspirin, so there is a lot of experience with their safety.

416. Are birth control pills effective in relieving cramps? If so, why?

Probably the most effective medication for relieving cramps is birth control pills. These work by reducing the uterine lining and the menstrual flow so much that there is very little prostaglandin production. Of course, it is a lot of trouble to take a pill every day for three weeks just to be comfortable for one day, but it can be effective. Taking birth control pills is a decision that you must make for yourself.

MENSTRUATION: TIREDNESS AND WEAKNESS

417. Why do I become extremely tired during menses?

Some women bleed so heavily during menses that they actually are weak from sudden blood loss. Others are tired from coping with the pain of menstrual cramps, or the vomiting and diarrhea that go with them. Just before menses, when the hormone level is high, many women have more energy, but this energy falls with menstruation. To some women, this drop in energy feels good, because they call the energy "premenstrual syndrome" when they are irritable. With menses, they become calm. Others call this being tired. There is a definite energy drop, no matter what you call it.

418. What can I do about the weak feeling that often accompanies menstruation?

If there is pain, nausea, or vomiting, you can take medication to relieve it, preferably antiprostaglandins type, such as aspirin or even prescription drugs, such as Motrin or Anaprox. If you are weak but there is no pain or excessive bleeding, you often can change your energy level by eating frequent, small meals, including protein and carbohydrates with each meal so you will have quickly available energy, as well as long-lasting energy. You also can think of things that you would like to do, and do them instead of the things you are supposed to do. It is surprising how much this will change your energy level.

MENSTRUATION: PREMENSTRUAL AND MENSTRUAL WEIGHT GAIN

419. Why do I gain weight before my period?

In the two weeks before your period, your ovaries produce a large amount of estrogen and progesterone, hormones whose nature it is to retain water in the body. The more you produce, the more water you retain, so that many women gain three to five pounds of water weight just prior to menses. After a day or two of menstrual flow, you lose this weight.

420. What can I do about water retention prior to my period?

For years, women have been advised to decrease the salt in their diets during the week before menses, and perhaps heavy salt eaters should do this, but it is a very difficult task and has very little chance of success. Diuretics (agents that increase urination) also have been used, although these usually just make you feel more washed out and weak, with increased leg cramps. A milder diuretic would be less harmful but less effective. Drinking water is a diuretic, but not very effective. The best advice is not to try to get rid of the water retention; it is a natural phenomenon and not harmful. It really is not the cause of discomfort before menses.

421. I feel very bloated before and even during menstruation. Is this because of water retention?

No. It is because of gas accumulation in your intestine, along with the constipation that usually occurs during the week before your flow begins. This bloating or constipation is attributed to the endorphins (opiates or pain relievers) that your brain produces before menses, which are constipating. Water retention is what weighs on the scale but is actually found in your hands, feet, and even your legs, but not in your abdomen.

MENSTRUATION: PREMENSTRUAL ACNE

422. Are pimples common before menses?

Yes, but especially with teenagers. Many women have acne that is unrelated to their cycle. However, even in girls who have clear skin, you may see a few signs of acne premenstrually.

423. What causes premenstrual acne?

Acne is related to androgens (male-type hormones) and progesterone. Androgens come from your adrenal gland as well as sometimes from your ovaries; progesterone comes from your ovaries after you ovulate and until you menstruate. Prior to menstruation, there is an increase in glandular activity and in oil production. If you already have oily skin, these conditions can lead to premenstrual pimples.

MENSTRUATION: PREMENSTRUAL ACNE (Continued)

424. Is there a cure for premenstrual acne?

Taking an estrogenic-type of birth control pill may help to clear acne for some women, but not for others. Dermatologists have many treatments for acne-type problems and also could tell you about any new treatments that are just being released. Most acne clears itself after the age of twenty-five, although this is not universal. But most teenagers cannot wait until they are twenty-five for their skin to clear up, and if they do they may have scars. Antibiotic solutions applied to the skin, or tetracycline taken orally, have helped many people. Cleanliness helps, and above all, try not to touch your face. Do not constantly use your fingers on your skin. You also should see a dermatologist before you get too many scars.

MENSTRUATION: PREMENSTRUAL SYNDROME—CURE, HELP, AND NEW TREATMENTS

425. Is there a cure for premenstrual syndrome?

Thus far, the most reliable treatment seems to be low-dose contraceptive pills. Some women who have used this treatment have improved greatly, although other women complain of feeling "premenstrual" all of the time when taking contraceptive pills. Vaginal progesterone suppositories are used in Great Britain and sometimes here. Frequent protein meals fight the hypoglycemia (deficiency of sugar in the blood) that often accompanies PMS. Diuretics reduce water retention. Antidepressants and tranquilizers have been found unsatisfactory in the treatment of premenstrual syndrome. Vitamin B6 has helped some women. Avoiding caffeine has helped many women overcome some of the PMS symptoms.

426. Is there anything I can do to make the changes that occur in my body during menses feel less intense?

You would probably feel much happier if you took birth control pills. On the pill cycle, you will have almost no premenstrual syndrome and certainly no ovulation pain.

427. Are there other medications that I could take, besides birth control pills, for treating premenstrual syndrome?

Diuretics have been used for this for a long time. Tranquilizers have been used for PMS, but there is valid criticism in giving so many tranquilizers to so many women. Prostaglandins have been considered a possible cause of PMS, but taking antiprostaglandins does not seem to alleviate the symptoms. Progesterone also has been used, even though women who experience the syndrome have not all been shown to be deficient. However, PMS is worse during premenopause when the progesterone level is declining.

MENSTRUATION: PREMENSTRUAL SYNDROME—CURE, HELP, AND NEW TREATMENTS (Continued)

Lithium, a potent antidepressant, has been prescribed by some psychiatrists, but this treatment seems to be too excessive for most women with the syndrome. Until the actual cause is found, women probably will remain in the dark as to the proper treatment. Adjusting your life to the cycle may be the best answer.

428. Where can I go for help for premenstrual syndrome?
    You can visit your physician, especially your gynecologist. You also can read about PMS in magazines, newspapers, and books. Psychologists are even organizing groups to cope with it. There is a National PMS Society, Box 11467, Durham, NC 27703, that you can join and receive new information from as it is obtained.

429. What are the newest treatments for premenstrual syndrome?
    The current, most frequent medical treatment is the use of natural progesterone suppositories, inserted into the vagina from the beginning of symptoms until it is time for menses. These are not manufactured for this purpose, and they must be made up by each individual pharmacist. This treatment was promoted by Dr. Katharina Dalton of England.

430. What research is currently being done on premenstrual syndrome?
    At this time, practically every medical school is doing research on premenstrual syndrome. To find out more, you could write to the Department of Health and Human Services, 5600 Ficher's Lane, Rockville, MD 20857; attention: H.F.D. 100. Perhaps your letter will even influence approving more research programs.

MENSTRUATION: DIET IN TREATING PREMENSTRUAL SYNDROME

431. Is diet important in treating premenstrual syndrome?
    Yes, it may be paramount. The symptoms of PMS are similar to hypoglycemia, a condition in which there is a deficiency of sugar in the blood. Blood sugar can be prevented from dropping by consuming six small protein meals a day, especially in the week or two before your menstrual period. Staying away from caffeine also helps some women.

MENSTRUATION: RIGHT AFTER MENSTRUATION

432. Once I'm over my menstrual period each month, I feel more at ease with myself. Is it normal to feel this way?
    Yes. Most women are calm, sweet, tolerant, and complain about

MENSTRUATION: RIGHT AFTER MENSTRUATION
(Continued)

nothing during the week after their menses. It is during this time that their nurturing of others is at its highest point. By contrast, men do not have such a tolerant period. Perhaps women disappoint their associates by not continuing this mood for the rest of the month. After ovulation, the high level of hormones changes the way they feel, making them less at ease.

MENSTRUATION: WHEN TO SEE A DOCTOR
DURING MENSTRUATION

433. When should I see a doctor regarding abnormal menstruation?
If you bleed almost every day of the month, even if it is light spotting, you should get help. If you bleed heavily, such as soaking ten pads a day, you should see a doctor to be sure you are not anemic from the blood loss. Irregular, very heavy flow also can indicate cancer of the uterus, especially if you are over forty, so tests must be done to be sure this is not the case.

434. At what age should a teenager seek medical help for regulating her period?
She should seek help whenever she considers that she has a problem. If the irregularity is there for more than two years after the onset of menses, she might consider that this is a problem. Menstruation really does not have to be regulated if there is no medical problem and if she is not trying to get pregnant. Heavy bleeding deserves attention, and lack of menses for six months after she had been regular for a while also needs an explanation. It is a good idea for any teenager to get a pelvic examination even if she has no problem, just to be sure everything is in order.

435. When does blood loss, such as spotting, become an emergency?
A healthy young woman is capable of giving a pint of blood at a blood bank with no harm to her health, so by the same count, she also can afford to bleed a pint without a real emergency. Spotting means a small amount of blood. Vaginal bleeding becomes an emergency when it is so fast that it drops your blood pressure, raises your pulse, and makes you feel faint. Soaking six pads in an hour or passing clots the size of your fist are examples of vaginal bleeding that are emergencies. Get help quickly; do not wait until the next day.

MENSTRUATION: BLEEDING BETWEEN PERIODS

436. What should I do if I am bleeding a little bit or spotting between menses?
Even though the blood loss is small and, therefore, is not a hazard to

MENSTRUATION: BLEEDING BETWEEN PERIODS (Continued)
your health, it is worth scheduling a checkup visit with your doctor. You should keep a record of the days you bleed, as the doctor will want to know this. Spotting frequently occurs when something is wrong with your cervix, such as an inflammation or a polyp.

437. Why do I spot about a week before my period, and then not actually start menstruating until a week later?

There could be many different explanations for this. One answer is that your uterine lining matures in one part ahead of the rest of it and, therefore, bleeds first. This is called irregular shedding. Another reason might be that you have a polyp (a small, usually benign growth) in your cervix that bleeds at a different time than menses. You also might have cervicitis (inflammation of your cervical glands) that bleeds easily, especially after intercourse. If it were two weeks before your period, it could be the blood escaping from the ovary at the time of ovulation, and going down the tube and out the vagina. Keep a record of the day you bleed. You should consult your doctor for your own special explanation.

MENSTRUATION: MISSING MENSTRUATION

438. What happens inside my body when I miss my period?

If you miss your period without becoming pregnant, your ovaries simply continue to develop follicles with eggs in them that are not released but that produce estrogen. The lining of the uterus continues to grow and become thicker. Your breasts may become more tender and swollen.

439. Is it dangerous to my reproductive system to skip a period?

Skipping up to six periods is not considered to be a sign of a dangerous problem. If you skip six periods (and are not pregnant), then you probably should seek medical advice and testing to be sure that you do not have a dangerous tumor. Such tumors eventually may cause headaches and reduce your range of vision, but it would be better to find them before that kind of damage occurs.

440. I haven't had my period for two years, yet my doctor says that I'm normal. Am I? Should I be worried?

You may be normal in every way except that you don't ovulate and, therefore, you are certainly not fertile during that time. If your doctor has run tests that prove ovulation is the only missing item, then you easily can become fertile by taking drugs that cause ovulation. So why worry? Well, sometimes those fertility pills cause twinning. If you don't mind twins, fine. If you don't want a baby now, you should perhaps take progestogens and have menses once in a while to prove that you can. You also should use con-

MENSTRUATION: MISSING MENSTRUATION (Continued)

traception, in case you suddenly start ovulating.

441. If I miss my period for a long time, does that mean that I am incapable of conceiving during that time?

Yes, provided that you are not already pregnant. You cannot conceive unless you ovulate, and if you ovulate, you will either have a menstrual period or be pregnant. This wisdom, however, applies to the past, but not to the future. You might ovulate tomorrow, even if you have not had menses for a year or two.

442. Why do some girls temporarily stop menstruating when they diet?

Nature has provided a shut-off mechanism, so that when there is inadequate food for a woman and, therefore, certainly inadequate food for her fetus, no pregnancy will occur. This happens quickly in some sensitive women, especially if they are not already fat. Twelve percent body fat is required for menstruation or fertility. You can see the survival value of this for women in times of famine; they would die long before the men if they had the drain of pregnancy, too.

443. Suppose I am a professional tennis player or I am planning my wedding and I really don't want my period to come on a certain date; is there something I can do to delay it?

The only way to succeed in delaying menses is to go on birth control pills after your previous menses and then take them longer than three weeks, maybe even five weeks, until you are past the certain date and don't mind having your period.

444. Should I take any precautions before I try to delay my period this way?

It would be wise to practice doing it several cycles before you need the delay. You also need to know how the hormones of the pill make you feel, because if they nauseate you, then that is worse than having your period.

445. I don't need to produce eggs or children anymore. Is there anything that can be done to completely stop menstruation, other than by surgery?

Yes, there is a progesterone known as Depo-Provera that can be injected at three- to six-month intervals that usually will stop menses in most women by the end of a year. This is appropriate if you are in your forties and are having trouble with bleeding, have no cancer, and never want any more children. Years ago, radiation treatments were used to stop aggravating menstruation in older women, usually in their forties, but the long-term result was to increase the incidence of cancer attributed to the radiation, so it is not done anymore. Younger women can take oral contraceptives continuously, and they will not menstruate.

MENSTRUATION: MISSING MENSTRUATION (Continued)

446. Are there any other methods I could try to delay menstruation temporarily?

Depo-Provera injections can delay menses for several months, but it is not recommended for this purpose.

447. Is Depo-Provera an approved method of contraception?

It has not been approved yet for contraception, because it is not easily reversible and can cause menses to disappear for years, even after you stop having the shots. Some Planned Parenthood groups use it exclusively for older women who want contraception and wish to avoid menses.

MENSTRUATION: BREAST-FEEDING

448. Why don't I menstruate when I am breast-feeding?

Some women do and others don't. Medical research has finally come up with an explanation for this. In all pregnant women, the pituitary gland secretes a hormone called prolactin, which makes the breasts produce milk and suppresses all estrogen from the ovaries. At delivery, women also lose weight suddenly. In women who are overweight and eat a lot of food while breast-feeding, menses will return in at least three or four months, when prolactin levels fall, because their body fat produces estrogen, and that sets the stage for ovulation. Underweight women who barely eat enough to produce the breast milk do not menstruate until sometime after they wean the baby. Therefore, in slender women, breast-feeding is relatively contraceptive, and in overweight women it is not contraceptive.

MENSTRUATION: EXPLAINING THE FACTS TO YOUR CHILDREN

449. How can I prepare my daughter for menstruation?

When you see her breasts develop and her weight reach one hundred pounds, it is time to discuss menstruation with her. She may be more interested in what pad to wear than the implications of menses for fertility and reproduction, but all aspects should be included. You might remember your own fears about menstruating, such as odor, being embarrassed about having your period, or about blood showing up on your clothes, among other things. A discussion of these topics and explaining to your daughter that all girls have these anxieties would help her better to adjust to her new body functions. There are many booklets printed for this purpose, but usually your own words and answering her questions are the best approach. If you have been educating your daughter since childhood about her body and all of its parts, this development will be no more difficult to explain than

MENSTRUATION: EXPLAINING THE FACTS TO
YOUR CHILDREN (Continued)

anything else. Most schools include a program at the sixth grade level, in time for the majority of girls who start menses at twelve.

450. What is a positive way to discuss menstruation with my daughter so that she won't be frightened?

Menstruation is really the badge of womanhood and can be celebrated as such. Surely all girls know at an early age that women have babies and men do not. Menstruation occurs as a preparation for the possibility of getting pregnant, and the ability of a girl to become pregnant should be honored as a stage in development, not a curse. There is no way to discuss menstruation without discussing pregnancy, although some schools do so.

451. How do you explain menstruation to a five-year old?

How you tell it depends on how much knowledge you already have given your child. You build on the vocabulary you know she has already. If she already knows about a uterus or womb, you explain that at puberty certain hormones make the womb ready for pregnancy each month. If pregnancy does not occur, the bed on which the tiny baby would lie to grow has to be remade and, in changing the coverings, blood is lost, which then comes out the vagina. A fresh bed is made every month.

Chapter 3

Breasts, Breast Cancer, and Other Problems of the Breasts

It is marvelous
being a woman
I love being a writer
I love being a mother
I love sharing my life with you
As a woman,
I can be happy
as long as I am able to
control my own mind, body and life
and choose my own role to follow
rather than having society
choose a role for me
I cannot ask for more
and would not settle for less

— Susan Polis Schutz

Today's woman —
strength
tenderness
self-knowledge
self-confidence
mental alertness
sensitivity
body awareness
physical boldness
softness
not afraid
to be
today's woman —
a person
in full control
of herself

— Susan Polis Schutz

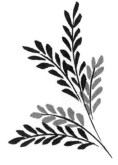

YOUR BREASTS

Your breasts belong to you. They are not the property of your husband or even your baby. You must take care of them and take charge of them.

Because you grew up as a girl without large breasts, at first they seemed a little strange, even embarrassing. The next embarrassment was that they were not the ideal shape that some male artist drew from his imagination. It was progress when the women's liberation movement burned the bra, because the bra tried to make everyone look alike and no one look natural. Women now feel free to wear nothing under their blouses and allow their real shapes to be detected. They also feel free to use an athletic, support-type brassiere when jogging or running because it gives them comfort, or they feel free to wear a bra all the time.

The main function of your breasts is breast-feeding. Babies still do best if started on their mothers' breast milk, so you can decide to breast-feed regardless of what other people say or think. Not only is it nutritious for babies, but they receive your antibodies that help them to fight infection. But if the process is miserable for you, you can decide that good nutrition can come in a bottle and stop breast-feeding. Breasts also are a source of sexual excitement. Many women are very concerned about the way their breasts look, though how they look doesn't affect the sexual arousal of their breasts, nor does it affect their breast-feeding capacities.

It is vitally important that you do your own monthly breast examination to check for cancer. Only you can find a lump in time to do something about it before it spreads. If you have any kind of problems with your breasts, or you are over fifty, demand a breast X-ray (a mammogram) annually, just as you learned to demand a Pap smear, to find cancer before it is a lump. If you have a family history of breast cancer, you must be extra careful to have frequent checkups and mammograms. When you or your doctor find a lump, do something about it, but select your consultants and surgeons with an eye to those who will cooperate with you in the decision as to what you do if you find it is cancer. The cure depends upon whether you remove the cancer before it has spread, not what type of surgery or radiation you use to do that. California has a law that requires surgeons to present alternatives in breast cancer treatment to their patients before any major treatment, although not before the biopsy. With a little assertiveness, you can get what you want anywhere. With almost 10 percent of women developing breast cancer, you could use all your influence to improve research in its prevention, detection, and treatment.

YOUR BREASTS (Continued)

After cancer treatment, use all your ingenuity and available assets to obtain the right prosthesis (artificial breast), clothes, or reconstructive surgery that you want. If sex difficulties seem to arise, get counseling for you and your partner to solve them before they become a habit. You are in charge.

BREASTS: GROWTH AND DEVELOPMENT

452. What is the average age at which a girl's breasts begin to develop?

The average age is ten years old, but this development just means the projection of the nipple. Occasionally this occurs as early as seven or eight, and as late as sixteen.

453. Is it common for a girl to be embarrassed when her breasts first develop?

Yes, of course. There are two reasons for the embarrassment. One is that breast development reminds the owner that she is a girl, and she must consider all aspects of her sexuality. The other is that with the sudden development of her breasts, she may feel that her breasts are defective, asymmetric, and inadequate, and she is not sure that her breasts will ever look right.

454. How do breasts develop?

The first stage in breast development is the projection of the nipples from the chest wall, but not the circular, colored areas (the areolae) around them. Next, small mounds form underneath, frequently feeling like a button on one or both sides, and the nipples and areolae darken. During the third stage, the breasts further enlarge, and the areolae remain smooth with the rest of the breasts. The fourth stage is the elevation of the areolae above the breasts, and lastly, the breasts become round or globular with erectile nipples, and small bumps (Montgomery's glands) appear around the areolae. By this time, the girl is usually menstruating. All the growth occurs in the ducts and not in the glands.

455. How much of my breasts is fatty tissue?

If you are not pregnant or breast-feeding, 90 percent of your breasts is fatty tissue.

456. For how long do the breasts continue to grow?

They usually grow for about two years before menstruation actually begins and continue to develop until you are about sixteen or eighteen years old. They then stay about the same size, except for weight gain and loss, until pregnancy occurs.

457. At what age are my breasts fully mature?

Most girls obtain the full mature stage of breast development by the age of sixteen, but that does not mean that your breasts will not increase in size after that. It means that the contour of your breasts is mature: the nipples are erect, the areolae are dark, and the shape is round, instead of a cone.

458. What does a mature breast look like?

A mature breast is round and smooth and has a dark, erectile nipple.

BREASTS: GROWTH AND DEVELOPMENT (Continued)

459. What are some of the changes that might occur in my breasts as I mature?

This all depends upon what happens in your life. Pregnancy makes the glandular portion of the breasts grow and enlarge. Breast-feeding makes the breasts produce milk in response to the suckling on the nipples, and this enlarges the breasts and the skin around them even further. When milk production (lactation) stops, the breasts may sag. Weight loss can make the breasts shrink, since breasts are mostly fat except during breast-feeding. Aging makes the tissue grow dense, and in some women the breasts shrink to almost flat again. In others, the breasts retain their shape, but become pendulous.

460. What can I do to keep my breasts firm and looking young?

Don't lose weight, but don't gain too much either. Don't get pregnant, and above all, don't breast-feed. Wearing a bra does not help at all. As you get older, you can take hormones.

BREASTS: FUNCTION

461. What is the true function of the breasts? Is it breast-feeding?

Any biologist would say that breast-feeding is the true function, because that is what makes us mammals, animals with glands that produce milk (mammary glands) to breast-feed our young. However, all other mammals have breasts that practically disappear, except for the nipples, when they are not actually breast-feeding. One main characteristic of human beings is that the women have large breasts beginning at puberty, not just with pregnancy. Therefore, perhaps another function of breasts is to serve as an identifying sex characteristic. In western civilized nations, less than half of the women who have children breast-feed, and then only for a short time.

462. Why are my breasts a source of sexual excitement?

There are little nerve endings called genital corpuscles in the skin of the labia (lips of the vagina) and in the nipples of the breasts. These have no other function except sexual excitement, so perhaps this is a function of the breasts.

BREASTS: SIZE AND SHAPE

463. What is the normal breast size?

If you measure your breasts with a tape measure over the nipples, going from top to bottom and then side to side, the average measurement is about

BREASTS: SIZE AND SHAPE (Continued)

25 cm by 20 cm, (10" by 8"). Manufacturers of bras say that a 34B is the most common size.

464. Are more women small chested or large chested?

Younger women are, in general, smaller chested and older women are larger chested. That is partly because younger women are more slender.

465. How will my breast size and shape vary with my age?

After you reach the age of sixteen to eighteen years, your breasts will stay about the same size, unless you experience weight gain or loss, or you become pregnant. With aging, the tissue becomes dense and withered, and sometimes fat accumulates there, which makes the breasts bigger. Depending upon this accumulation of fat, your breasts can become very flat or they can sag.

466. Besides an operation, what can I do to increase or decrease the size of my breasts?

A normal weight does not guarantee a normal breast size, but it is certainly worth the try. Some very slender girls have large breasts, but most do not. Some overweight girls have small breasts, but most do not. Proper posture and exercising the chest muscles that maintain good posture will make your breasts appear larger, because they will ride higher on your chest wall. Birth control pills sometimes enlarge breasts.

467. Is it normal to have one breast larger than the other?

Yes. In development one breast often gets ahead of the other, and many young girls think that their breasts are going to be very different, but when mature, they are almost equal. The right breast usually is larger than the left. The variation is one or two inches in diameter. Some women have virtually no breast at all on one side, but this is rare. Some women have breasts that are markedly different. Plastic surgery could help this.

468. Are women in other parts of the world as concerned with their breast size as women in the United States are?

It does not seem that women in other parts of the world are as concerned. Perhaps this is because breast-feeding is more common in other parts of the world. Italian women with large breasts do not seem particularly proud of them, and Orientals with their small, flat breasts seem unconcerned.

BREASTS: BRASSIERE

469. At what age should I begin wearing a bra?

There is a great deal of freedom to decide today if you want to wear a

BREASTS: BRASSIERE (Continued)

bra. Bras are not required for health reasons; nor does custom absolutely require them. Many young girls find them uncomfortable and refuse to wear them at all. Honesty and freedom are their passwords. Other young girls dislike the appearance of the breast bud when it first appears, and they wear a brassiere to cover it up. Girls with large breasts may find it more comfortable to wear a brassiere, especially when they are involved in active sports. They may like to wear a bra with some clothes and not with others. Girls with rather flat or undeveloped breasts often want to wear a brassiere to look fuller, either from the change in contour or because it is padded.

470. What effect does wearing a bra have on my breasts?

There is no proof that wearing a bra has any effect on your breasts, except while you are actually wearing it. Wearing a bra will prevent sagging while you wear it, but once you take it off, your breasts will still sag. If you are lactating and wish to stop the flow and leaking of milk, wearing an uplift bra will help reduce milk production.

471. What effect does not wearing a bra have on my breasts?

Not wearing a bra can make your breasts hurt more during running and other exercise, but there is no proof that wearing or not wearing a bra has any effect on your breasts.

472. Is it dangerous for large-breasted women to go without wearing a bra?

It is not dangerous, just uncomfortable.

BREASTS: EFFECTS OF PHYSICAL ACTIVITY

473. Is jogging harmful to my breasts?

No, there is no harm, although it may produce pain, especially with large breasts. An athletic brassiere may be necessary for comfort.

474. Can exercise of any kind be harmful to my breasts?

No. Exercise can improve your posture and help you to lose weight, both of which may help your breasts look better.

475. Are there any exercises I can do to increase my breast size? If so, what are they?

No. There is no exercise that will increase the actual size of your breasts, since there are no muscles in them. However, there are muscles under the breasts, and developing the chest muscles and good posture can make the breasts seem more prominent, even if they are the same size. A drooping, round-shouldered posture makes them look smaller. Some women stand this way to hide their large breasts; some are just so heavy chested that they can't help but stand this way.

BREASTS: CREAMS

476. Do creams that claim to develop the breasts really work?

Probably not. If a man used an estrogen cream, he might absorb enough to notice a change. Women already have so much estrogen that the amount in a cream would do nothing. Massage does nothing, either.

477. What do breast creams contain?

Most breast creams contain lanolin, which is intended to provide the oil the skin uses most to prevent dryness, flaking, and itching, especially during pregnancy. Creams are no longer allowed to contain estrogen without prescription.

BREASTS: OPERATIONS TO INCREASE/DECREASE BREAST SIZE

478. How dangerous are operations to increase or decrease breast size?

There is little danger that is life threatening, although bleeding and infection can follow, or an anesthetic accident is possible. The more frequent complication is just that the result can be less than what you expected, or the scars can be more prominent than anyone predicted.

479. Could operations to increase or decrease breast size cause or aggravate breast cancer?

No, and they also do not prevent it. It is not yet known if reducing the size of your breasts will reduce the risk of cancer.

480. What surgical procedures do doctors follow when increasing a woman's breast size?

Augmentation of the breast (making it larger) consists of an incision in the fold under the breast or around the nipple. This forms a pocket just over the chest muscle. A plastic bag of silicone is placed in the pocket and is sutured into place. The breast then lies on top of it.

481. Is silicone injected into the breasts harmful?

It is not directly harmful, but it can cause confusion. Ten percent of women develop breast cancer, and if there are hard lumps of silicone in their breasts, no physician can tell the lump from the breast cancer, so it may go untreated until it is too late. Silicone does not cause cancer; it hides it. It also can cause infections and skin problems later.

482. Are silicone injections still available to women in the United States?

No, they are not done in this country anymore, but because it is an inexpensive procedure, they are still done elsewhere. Many people consider silicone injections to be dangerous.

BREASTS: OPERATIONS TO INCREASE/DECREASE BREAST SIZE
(Continued)

483. What surgical procedures do doctors follow when reducing a woman's breast size?

To reduce the breasts, several incisions are required, which leave several lines of scars. The nipple is sometimes removed and placed higher on the chest wall, and a suitable portion of the actual breast tissue is removed.

484. Is breast-feeding still possible if I have my breasts reduced or increased in size?

Breast-feeding is quite possible if you have a placement of silicone in a plastic bag placed beneath your breasts to lift and enlarge them (augmentation). Each breast is still intact, but it is sitting on top of silicone. If you have a breast reduction, then breast-feeding usually cannot occur, because the ducts that carry the milk are cut when the nipple is transplanted to the center of the newly formed breast, and it no longer connects with the glands producing milk. Occasionally, breast reduction is done without moving the nipple, so breast-feeding can still occur.

BREASTS: SORENESS AND SWELLING

485. Why do my breasts hurt sometimes?

Many things are known to make breasts hurt. Changing estrogen levels during the menstrual cycle can produce tenderness. Birth control pills, especially those high in estrogen, can do this, although it is usually worse for the first two months after you begin taking them, and then less so. Exercise, especially without an athletic-type bra, can make the breasts hurt. Pregnancy can make them more tender, and so can breast-feeding. In addition, a condition known as fibrocystic breasts can cause tender cysts that will make breasts hurt more than normal. Rarely, an infection can make the breasts red, hot, and, tender, and you will have a fever, but this usually occurs only while breast-feeding. You should see your doctor if these symptoms occur. Sometimes there is no answer to this question.

486. What causes soreness and swelling of my nipples?

Estrogen is the main cause of soreness and swelling of your nipples. This first occurs at puberty when estrogen is first produced. It occurs at ovulation time when there is a surge of estrogen and again before menses for a week or so when estrogen production becomes high. Pregnancy makes estrogen production even higher, but with breast-feeding, the cause of soreness is not estrogen at all, since during this time it falls to low levels. The cause, then, is the suckling of the baby and the let-down reflex that happens when milk shoots into the nipple. Stimulation of your nipples in love-making

BREASTS: SORENESS AND SWELLING (Continued)

can get a similar reaction. High-dose estrogen birth control pills can cause this, too.

BREASTS: NIPPLES

487. Is it common to have hair around my nipples?

Yes, the average number of hairs around the areola, the dark circle around the projecting nipple, is about eighteen. Some women have none, and some have many more.

488. What is the proper color for the areola, the circular area around the nipple?

In the young girl, it is quite pink. With the increased hormones of maturity, it becomes darker, and with pregnancy it becomes quite dark. It may get lighter after delivery, but never quite as light as before pregnancy.

489. Why do some women have enlarged nipples?

There is as much variation in breasts and nipples as there is in body contours. However, pregnancy and breast-feeding tend to enlarge the nipples. Breast-feeding for several children makes even more of a change in the projection and size of the nipples.

490. Why does cold weather or touching my breasts cause my nipples to get hard?

Touching the breasts makes the nipples become hard and erect because this reflex assists the baby in suckling to obtain milk. Cold weather brings about the same reflex. It is the nipples that become hard, not the whole breast. This is the same muscle contraction that makes your hair stand up on your arm when you are cold.

BREASTS: INVERTED NIPPLES

491. What are inverted nipples?

They are nipples that turn in instead of out.

492. Are inverted nipples common? What kinds of problems do they cause?

Yes, they are common, and they often interfere with breast-feeding. The most common type can be pulled out with manipulation or the baby's suckling. Less common are inverted nipples that cannot be pulled out. Plastic surgery can correct inverted nipples.

493. Are inverted nipples a sign of disease?

If nipples have always been inverted, they are not a sign of disease. If they were normal and then became inverted, there could be a growing cancer pulling them in, and this should be investigated by a doctor. Inverted nipples cause problems with breast-feeding.

BREASTS: CHANGES DUE TO MENSTRUATION AND HORMONES

494. What changes occur in my breasts during menstruation?

Your breasts are the least stimulated for about a week after menstrual flow begins. This is why the best time for you to do your own breast self-examination is just at the end of menses. The tissue is then the least swollen or tender. As estrogen production begins and surges before ovulation, your breasts are stimulated to swell and become tender. From ovulation to menstruation they become increasingly swollen and tender, and then subside after menstruation begins.

495. How do birth control pills affect swelling in my breasts prior to menstruation?

If you are on birth control pills, the estrogen stimulation that occurs prior to menses is somewhat counteracted by the progesterone in the pills, and the total effect may be less stimulation to the breasts. For some women, the pills supply more hormones than they ever had before, and they have more swelling and enlargement, but less cystic formation. In general, there are fewer cysts and breast biopsies in women who are taking contraceptive pills.

496. Will breast pain and tenderness go away when I stop menstruating for good?

It is difficult to explain, but pain and tenderness do not go away as much as you would expect. The weight of the breasts can apparently still make them tender without hormones.

497. Does the amount of hormones a woman produces have anything to do with the size of her breasts?

Sometimes the amount of hormones you produce slightly affects your breast size, but there are other factors. Occasionally, girls take contraceptive pills and find that their breasts do enlarge, whereas other girls' breasts do not. During pregnancy, every woman's breasts enlarge, and hormones then are in enormous supply. Breast size also is correlated with fat and with heredity.

BREASTS: CHANGES DUE TO PREGNANCY AND LACTATION; AFTER PREGNANCY

498. What changes occur in my breasts during pregnancy and lactation?

Before pregnancy, the growth of your breasts is mostly in the ducts and fat. With pregnancy, it is in the glands. The milk-producing portion of your

BREASTS: CHANGES DUE TO PREGNANCY AND LACTATION; AFTER PREGNANCY (Continued)

breasts begins to grow, and with lactation, your glands actually produce milk, which again enlarges your breasts, changing hour by hour (feeding by feeding). The areolae become dark with pregnancy, lighten up a bit afterward, but are never again as light in color. Veins become prominent and blue, and often are mistaken for stretch marks (striae). These veins probably appeared at puberty, but they become red or purple in color during pregnancy, and then fade to white afterward.

499. Will breast-feeding cause my breasts to sag?

Yes. Any enlargement followed by a reduction in size stretches the skin and supporting ligaments, and they are not so elastic that they spring back, at least not completely. But this does not mean that anyone who breast-feeds will have breasts hanging down to her waist. By the fourth or sixth month, other food is added to the baby's diet, and this helps to prevent sagging because huge quantities of milk are no longer required. A good supporting brassiere will not prevent the sagging.

500. How does the size and shape of my breasts change during and after pregnancy?

During pregnancy, your breasts enlarge at least one cup and number size of a brassiere, mainly due to the growth of the milk-producing glands. Within forty-eight hours of delivery, milk is produced, and in 80 percent of women, it is released even if they do not let their babies suckle their nipples. When breast-feeding ceases, the breasts are reduced in size by the disappearance of the milk supply. After pregnancy, your breasts will sag, depending on how large they were stretched. They may be larger than before pregnancy as a result of simple growth that may have occurred, or they may be smaller because of sagging.

501. What changes occur in my breasts after pregnancy and breast-feeding?

Your breast size decreases by the amount of milk no longer produced, and a gradual reduction in your glandular tissue takes place. Since the skin cannot shrink, some sagging may occur. Your nipples lighten, but are darker than before. Stretch marks (striae) fade from purple or red to white and are less obvious, but they are still present.

502. Will my breasts be the same size after pregnancy as they were before?

Sometimes they are, but if you weigh more, they probably will be larger. If you weigh less, they probably will be smaller. They will likely change in shape, even if they are the same size.

BREASTS: CHANGES DUE TO MENOPAUSE

503. What changes occur in my breasts during menopause?

Menopause means the cessation of hormone stimulation, and so your breasts become less hormonally stimulated. They may reduce in size and turgor; the amount they decrease is controlled by hormone levels. The larger they were before menopause, the more they will sag. Some women, especially overweight women, produce a lot of estrone, an estrogen, in their fat, and their breasts change little. Other slender women have breasts that become very small and dense (atrophic). If a woman takes hormones for her menopause, she sees less change in her breasts than if she had not taken hormones. Some women notice a decrease as soon as they stop taking birth control pills.

BREASTS: SAGGING (PTOSIS)

504. What do sagging breasts look like?

The breasts are considered sagging (ptosis) if the nipples hang below the lower part of the contour of the breasts, the inframammary line.

505. What can be done to improve my sagging breasts?

Several things can help. Sagging shoulders and poor posture make sagging breasts worse. Even though there is no muscle in the breasts, exercise improves posture because it improves the base from which the breasts hang. Weight loss makes breasts sag, and weight gain can replace fat and make them look as though they sag less. There is surgery that plastic surgeons do to correct sagging (ptosis) of the breasts without using implants, and, of course, implants of silicone can raise the contour of the breasts as well as enlarge them.

506. Why do women in other countries, such as Africa, display such extremely sagging breasts? Is it due to breast-feeding?

In Africa, the baby is totally breast-fed, because no other proper food is available. As the quantity of milk becomes quite large, the breasts are enlarged so much that after pregnancy they can sag to the waist, especially after the tenth child. Pictures of such African women are sometimes misleadingly shown to advise women in more modern countries to wear a good supporting brassiere. The brassiere only helps to uplift breasts while it is worn.

BREASTS: STRETCH MARKS (STRIAE)

507. What can I do to prevent stretch marks on my breasts during pregnancy?

There is no known prevention. If you do not inherit them, you will not

BREASTS: STRETCH MARKS (STRIAE) (Continued)

get them. Stretch marks (striae) are an inherited defect in the elastic layer of the skin. In those women who have them, they indicate an inadequate elastic layer, so the skin breaks instead of stretching. Thus, they should be called break marks or nonstretch marks. If there is a lot of elastic tissue, the skin will stretch without breaking, and no mark appears. Many striae occur at puberty and just become more prominent with pregnancy, so avoiding pregnancy does not avoid them completely.

508. What can I do to get rid of stretch marks on my breasts?

Nothing, although plastic surgery on your breasts could be scheduled to remove as many stretch marks as possible. Whoever discovers how to prevent or cure stretch marks will make a fortune.

BREASTS: BREAST-FEEDING

509. Can a small-breasted woman successfully breast-feed?

Yes. If you think about it, you know that other mammals, such as dogs, cats, and even cows have no breasts, just nipples, until they deliver their babies. When suckled, the breasts form and get large with milk. Women are unusual in that they can have large breasts, even without breast-feeding. The same process works for all women, regardless of breast size. They go through pregnancy with some enlargement, and after delivery and suckling, the breasts enlarge more with milk. This can be so pleasing to the small-breasted woman that she breast-feeds for many months, because it is the first time she looks like other women in her clothes. It also may be the first time she hasn't worn a padded bra. In fact, there is more room for milk to expand the breast in the small-breasted woman than in the large one. The large breast may be so full of fat that there is hardly room for expansion with milk, and because the breasts are already large and heavy, the woman may resent the increased size with breast-feeding, along with the discomfort. Consequently, she may decide to stop breast-feeding very soon. However, the success of breast-feeding depends on how the baby suckles on your nipple and upon your response to that, not on the size of your breast.

BREASTS: HOW BREAST-FEEDING OCCURS

510. How do breasts produce milk?

During pregnancy, large quantities of estrogen and progesterone promote growth of the breasts, but they hold back the pituitary secretion of a hormone called prolactin, which stimulates milk secretion. At delivery, the hormone-producing placenta is removed, and the estrogen and progesterone levels fall. This frees the pituitary to produce prolactin, and in about forty-

BREASTS: HOW BREAST-FEEDING OCCURS
(Continued)

eight hours milk secretion starts in full force. Prolactin production also is aided by suckling, which stimulates production of the hormone oxytocin from the pituitary.

BREASTS: WHY AND HOW MILK PRODUCTION OCCURS

511. Are hormones related to milk secretion?

Yes. To secrete milk, the breast must first be prepared with estrogen and progesterone, and then stimulated with prolactin.

512. How does the pituitary gland produce milk?

The pituitary gland is responsible for producing the hormones called gonadotropins that tell the ovaries to produce estrogen and progesterone. These two hormones cause the breasts to develop and get ready for milk production. When estrogen and progesterone levels drop with delivery of the baby, the pituitary then produces prolactin, which stimulates the breasts to secrete milk. The pituitary gland also produces oxytocin, which causes the let-down reflex that shoots the milk into the nipples.

513. Will milk secrete from my breast after delivery even if I do not breast-feed?

Milk secretion will come automatically in most women. It occurs in 80 percent of women even if their babies never touch their breasts.

514. How is the milk carried from the glands to the nipple?

The glands at the end of the ducts (the acini) actually form the milk within the cell, and then a portion of the cell with the milk in it breaks off and goes down the ducts to the nipple. These are called apocrine glands. They don't just secrete, they break off, too.

515. How long after breast-feeding should milk remain in my breast?

Severe engorgement with milk lasts only about forty-eight hours after all breast-feeding is stopped, but the ability to squeeze the nipple and get a few drops of milk can last for a year or so. If the nipples continue to be stimulated, this will continue the secretion, so don't keep checking. Spontaneous leaking does not usually occur after six or eight weeks.

BREASTS: DISCHARGE AND ABNORMAL MILK SECRETION

516. Is discharge from my nipples normal if I am not pregnant?

Discharge is not really uncommon in the year or two after you have breast-fed a baby, and it can be continued by constant nipple stimulation in love-making, as can breast milk. However, if it occurs at other times, it needs

BREASTS: DISCHARGE AND ABNORMAL MILK SECRETION
(Continued)

to be investigated. It can result from chest trauma or chest surgery. If bloody, it can come from a little tumor in the ducts, called an intraductal papilloma.

517. What should I do if I have a discharge from my breasts?

You could have a Pap smear of the discharge done to see if the cells suggest a papilloma or even cancer. Papillomas can be removed from the nipple with a biopsy, which is minor surgery.

518. What does it mean if I have milk secretions from my breasts, and I am not pregnant?

Production of milk not connected with pregnancy (galactorrhea) can have many different causes. If the secretion is truly milk, that is, it really looks like milk even under a microscope, it can be caused from any nipple stimulation, especially sucking that sometimes is a part of love-making. Sometimes spontaneous milk secretion occurs if you take tranquilizers, especially one brand called Mellaril, because of their effect on the brain. A low thyroid function can cause the prolactin hormone to be high and result in milk secretion. When thyroid is given, the prolactin becomes normal, and the milk stops. Trauma or surgery on the chest wall is known to cause milk secretion. A brain tumor on the pituitary gland also can produce a large amount of prolactin, which causes lactation in the breast. Even when the tumor is so microscopically small that it really causes no other problem, it can still cause the breasts to leak milk. If it does this often enough, it also can interfere with menstruation and the ability to get pregnant. If the tumor grows large, it can press on other structures in the brain, especially the optic system, and interfere with vision, particularly the ability to see peripherally—to the side. Headaches also can occur.

519. How common is it to have milk secretions from my breasts when I am not pregnant?

Some milk secretions, without any interference in the pattern of menstruation, are quite common, since breast stimulation and use of tranquilizers also are common. An underactive thyroid (hypothyroidism) is not really unusual and can cause lactation, too. Brain tumors causing milk secretion and suppression of menstruation are quite rare. Very small pituitary tumors that cause some milk secretion are much more frequent, but they do not always require treatment unless they enlarge. It is wise to follow abnormal milk production with tests for many years.

520. What should I do if the milk secretion is very heavy?

You can take a blood test to see if you have an elevated level of the pro-

BREASTS: DISCHARGE AND ABNORMAL MILK SECRETION
(Continued)

lactin hormone. X-rays of the the bony seat of the pituitary gland at the base of the brain also may be done. If the milk production is heavy, then menses may be stopped altogether. This is called amenorrhea with galactorrhea (absence of menses with the production of milk, not connected with pregnancy). It should be investigated by your doctor.

BREASTS: PITUITARY TUMORS

521. How do I find out if I have a pituitary tumor?

If you have spontaneous leakage of milk and you are not pregnant or breast-feeding, you can have a simple blood test done to see if you have an elevated level of prolactin hormone. If it is normal or only slightly high, thyroid function can be checked by blood tests to see if that is the cause. Other causes also may be sought. If your prolactin level is fairly high or very high, X-rays of the skull or a CAT-scan of the brain (computerized axial tomography) can be done to locate the presence of a pituitary tumor. Eye tests can be performed to measure your ability to see well peripherally (in a wide field of vision). Consultations then occur with endocrinologists (physicians who specialize in glands, such as the pituitary) and neurosurgeons (brain surgeons) regarding whether treatment should be with a prescription drug called bromocriptine or with surgery.

522. Are pituitary tumors usually cancerous?

No, they are never cancerous and always benign. Pituitary tumors cause their harm by growing bigger and producing a hormone imbalance.

523. Do I need to have a large secretion of milk for a pituitary tumor to be present?

No, just a rather continuous secretion suggests the presence of such a tumor. More indicative of a larger tumor is the disappearance of menstruation, problems with vision, and headaches.

524. Should I stop taking birth control pills if I suspect that I have a pituitary tumor?

Yes, that way you can see if you still menstruate. If you are not menstruating, the possibility of a tumor is more serious.

525. Could I have a pituitary tumor if my level of prolactin is normal?

Yes, but it would be very rare. It would not be a prolactin tumor, but some other kind, that could still show on X-rays or a CAT-scan.

526. How do you treat a pituitary tumor medically?

If it is small, it may be controlled by a medicine, such as bromocriptine,

BREASTS: PITUITARY TUMORS (Continued)

or it may require no treatment at all, other than observation. If it is large, neurosurgeons can remove the tumor without destroying the entire pituitary gland. If radiation is used, the whole pituitary is destroyed.

527. What are the chances of survival with a pituitary tumor?

Chances are excellent if it is not too large to remove when it is first found. Even then, it sometimes can be reduced in size with medical therapy and then operated on. Fertility is restored if therapy is successful and menstruation returns.

BREASTS: SELF-EXAMINATION

528. How do I check myself for lumps?

Stand nude in front of a mirror. Look at your breasts for any dimpling, any place that seems to be pulled in. Notice whether the nipples point in the same direction that they always have and are not newly pulled in (inverted), instead of out. Look for any skin that resembles orange peel, or is flaking and scaling, especially on the nipples. Then lie down on your back, and put one arm over your head. With the other hand, holding it flat, feel the entire breast, going around it in a circle so you won't miss anything. Feel the nipple and the part of the breast that goes into your armpit. You can feel your ribs through your breast, so don't let them scare you. Remember how the tissue felt the last time you examined your breasts. You are looking for a lump that could be on the surface, or it could be on the inside. Then raise your other arm, and repeat on your other breast. Squeeze each nipple to check for discharge. If something worries you, check it out with your doctor. As an alternative, you can examine yourself in the shower with soap on your hands. This way, you are more conscious of the feeling of the tissue underneath and less conscious of the skin with the soap there. Checking yourself regularly is a good habit to develop.

529. How important is it for me to do my own breast examination monthly?

Breast self-examination once a month is still the best way to find breast cancer early enough so that it can be cured with minimal treatment. The cancer can advance too far between yearly doctor visits or mammograms, so it is essential that you perform your own exam monthly.

530. When is the best time to check my breasts for lumps?

The best time is just after menses when your breasts are less likely to have swelling, or just before you take your first pill if you are on hormone pills in a cyclic fashion, either for menopause or for contraception. If you have no menses and no hormone pills, just pick the same time every month. Then the breasts should feel about the same each time you examine them.

How to Examine Your Breasts
(This should be done once a month.)

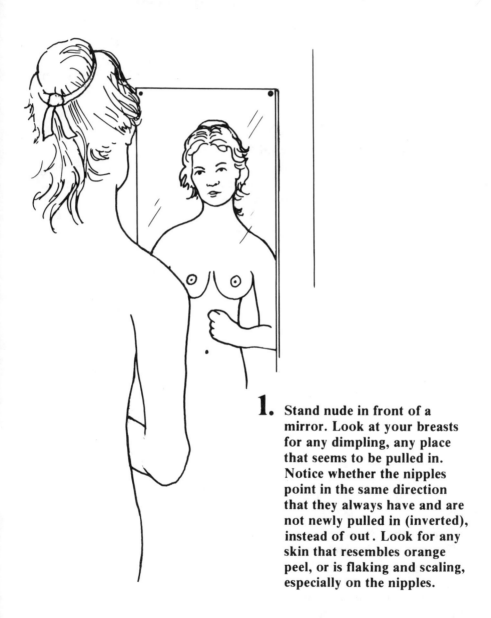

1. Stand nude in front of a mirror. Look at your breasts for any dimpling, any place that seems to be pulled in. Notice whether the nipples point in the same direction that they always have and are not newly pulled in (inverted), instead of out. Look for any skin that resembles orange peel, or is flaking and scaling, especially on the nipples.

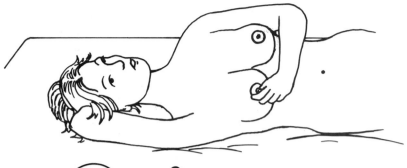

2. Then lie down on your back, and put one arm over your head. With the other hand, holding it flat, feel the entire breast, going around it in a circle so you won't miss anything. Feel the nipple and the part of the breast that goes into your armpit. You can feel your ribs through your breast, so don't let them scare you. Remember how the tissue felt the last time you examined your breasts. You are looking for a lump that could be on the surface, or It could be on the inside. Then raise your other arm, and repeat on your other breast. Squeeze each nipple to check for discharge. If something worries you, check It out with your doctor.

3. As an alternative, you can examine yourself in the shower with soap on your hands. This way, you are more conscious of the feeling of the tissue underneath and less conscious of the skin with the soap there. Checking yourself regularly is a good habit to develop.

BREASTS: SELF-EXAMINATION (Continued)

531. How often should I check myself for lumps?

Once a month is advised by the American Cancer Society. The habit can begin as soon as you have breasts and continue all through your life. You are never immune, but breast cancer is more frequent when you are in your fifties and sixties.

532. At what age should a girl start checking her breasts for lumps?

Probably as soon as she has breasts. To care for your body you should be familiar with all of it at all times. Children should be encouraged, instead of discouraged, to explore their bodies, including their breasts, as they form. There is no absolute age limit for breast cancer, but it is quite rare before the age of thirty. However, hard little oval masses (fibroadenomas) do occur in teenagers. They are usually removed, because you just can't be sure that they won't develop into cancer.

533. How often should I see my doctor for a breast examination?

If your breasts have always been normal with no problems, the American Cancer Society and the American Medical Association advise once every three years. The American College of Obstetricians and Gynecologists says every year. The primary advice is that you should do a self-examination every month. If you find a problem, take action to solve it by scheduling an examination by a physician. If you have fibrocystic breasts, a family history of breast cancer, or other problems, your physician will decide with you how often you need follow-up examinations or even tests for breast cancer, such as mammograms or thermograms.

BREASTS: LUMPS—CANCEROUS OR NORMAL?

534. When checking for lumps, how can I tell the difference between a potentially cancerous lump and the normal lumps found in my breasts?

The normal lumpiness is general throughout both breasts and does not have one dominant lump that is more pronounced than the rest. A potentially cancerous lump is not usually tender. It is hard, not very movable, does not have a clear cut edge, and may draw the skin in or pull the nipple to one side. However, if you have a lump, do not make your own decision based on these things. Even the best, most experienced surgeon needs a biopsy to know whether or not it is cancer.

535. My doctor says that it is normal for my breasts to feel lumpy. How will I know when I have a cancerous lump?

Breast tissue normally can feel granular, like it contains small cysts or lumps, but the cancerous lump is usually hard and nontender. If your doctor says your breasts are normal, examine them monthly, and get your fingers accustomed to how your breasts feel. Then if a change occurs, you will be

BREASTS: LUMPS—CANCEROUS OR NORMAL? (Continued)
more able to detect the change because your fingers will tell you so. A physician should check it for you, too.

536. Why do I have small lumps in my breasts prior to menstruation?

Most breasts swell and retain fluid within the breast tissue just prior to menses in response to estrogen stimulation, but some swell much more than others. This is certainly not the best time to examine them. The glandular portions of the breasts respond to hormones to prepare them for eventual breast-feeding in case of pregnancy. When menses occur instead of pregnancy, they regress for a while and wait for the next hormonal cycle to stimulate them.

537. If I discover a lump in my breast, what should I do?

You should call your doctor, or find one, and make an appointment for an examination. This is necessary just to calm your fear, if nothing else. If the lump disappears before the appointment, you can cancel. Some doctors make the appointment for just after menses because so many lumps disappear then, but if it is still present, the doctor will do something to diagnose it.

538. How does a doctor go about determining whether a lump is cancerous?

First, the doctor takes your history and your family history to determine if you are in a high-risk category. He or she examines your breasts, sometimes with a light (transillumination) to see if they are cystic. If the doctor thinks they are cystic, he or she may aspirate (drain) fluid from the cyst with a needle and syringe and send the fluid to the laboratory for a Pap smear to see if the cells are normal. If they are and the cyst does not recur, he or she may do nothing else. If it is solid, the doctor may do a breast X-ray (a mammogram). The doctor also will probably do an excisional biopsy under local or general anesthesia to see if it might be cancer.

539. Must all lumps in my breasts be removed, even if they are determined to be benign (not cancerous)?

It is difficult to determine absolutely that lumps are benign, unless they are removed and studied. Cysts are not always removed, but some of the fluid may be aspirated for study. It is a bad habit to leave solid lumps in, because then another doctor may have to prove that they are not cancer again. If biopsies and mammograms show nothing but fibrocystic areas, they will not be removed.

BREASTS: CYSTS

540. How can I tell the difference between a cyst and a lump?

That is not always easy. Even your surgeon may only be able to tell the

BREASTS: CYSTS (Continued)

difference by attempting to aspirate fluid from it. If fluid cannot be aspirated, it must be a solid lump. If it can be aspirated, it is a cyst. Shining a light through it can help to tell the difference, especially if it is large.

541. Should I see my doctor if I think I have a cyst?

Yes, a cyst can be a cancer, too, but it is less likely. You should see the doctor especially if the cyst remains after menstruation has passed.

542. Should cysts go away completely between periods, or should they just get smaller?

Some cysts disappear completely, but with fibrocystic breasts, they just get smaller. Some cysts are always present.

BREASTS: FIBROCYSTIC BREASTS

543. What is fibrocystic disease?

It is not really a "disease," but a condition that is present in almost 30 percent of American women at some time in their lives. It is a growth of cystic structures and dense fibrous supporting tissues that occasionally form rather large cysts, which are also painful. Since cancer also can occur in a cyst, they have to be investigated and at least aspirated (draining the cyst through a small hole) and the cells studied.

544. What is the cause of fibrocystic breasts?

There is no clear cause or cure. Caffeine may play a role. However, fibrocystic breasts are also thought to be a result of excessive estrogen compared to the amount of progestrone produced by women.

545. Are fibrocystic breasts painful and dangerous to my overall health?

They produce pain and worry and necessitate multiple aspirations and biopsies, but do not hurt your health in any other way, other than the fact that in certain cases involving large cysts, you may be more prone to breast cancer.

546. Why is caffeine thought to be a cause of fibrocystic breasts?

Recent studies seem to suggest, but do not prove, that women with fibrocystic breasts can improve their conditions if they eliminate caffeine, including coffee, tea, and soft drinks, from their diets. The percentage of women that improve is about 75 percent, so this does not apply to everyone. There also are people who have fibrocystic breasts who never touch caffeine, so it is not the sole cause.

547. Will cystic breasts eventually lead to cancer?

No, all cystic breasts do not lead to cancer. Fibrocystic breasts affect over 30 percent of all women in their reproductive years. Ten percent of all

BREASTS: FIBROCYSTIC BREASTS (Continued)

women get breast cancer, and according to many studies, the incidence of breast cancer is higher in women who have had fibrocystic breasts. Perhaps this association is just the same one that shows that women who have not had babies are more likely to get breast cancer. Women also are more likely to have fibrocystic breasts if they have not been on contraceptive pills for many years.

548. How does pregnancy affect fibrocystic breasts?

Pregnancies tend to make the condition better, and so does breast-feeding.

549. Do fibrocystic breasts tend to get better or worse after menopause?

They tend to improve after menopause, but not if estrogen, alone, is taken.

BREASTS: MOLES

550. Can small moles on my breasts be potentially cancerous?

All moles can be potentially cancerous, but they do not produce breast cancer. Moles on your breasts are no more likely to become cancer than moles anywhere else on your body, except on the palms and soles where they are more likely to become cancerous.

551. Should I have small moles on my breasts removed?

It is no more important than removing moles anywhere else. Any mole that becomes red, irritated, or seems to have small daughter moles growing around it is likely to be malignant and should be removed, but not just because it is on your breasts.

BREASTS: MASTITIS

552. What is mastitis?

This word is usually used to describe an infection of the breast caused by bacteria, in which an area of the breast becomes painful, red, and hard. The temperature rises very quickly to 103° or more and, if not treated, an abscess can form.

553. Is mastitis more likely to occur in women who are breast-feeding?

Yes, 95 percent of mastitis occurs in women who are breast-feeding. The bacteria that infects them comes from their babies' mouths. Occasionally a nonlactating breast also becomes infected after an injury or surgery, or from an infected hair follicle, pimples, or a boil on the skin that expands.

554. How do you treat mastitis?

You must take antibiotics, preferably the kind that will fight Strep-

BREASTS: MASTITIS (Continued)

tococcus or Staphylococcus bacteria, such as penicillin, as soon as possible as the main treatment. Heat in the form of hot packs or a shower helps carry the infection away. Pain pills might be needed as well for rest, because motion increases pain. Wearing a bra provides support and also reduces pain. Breast-feeding should continue, as it will not hurt the baby, and emptying the breasts is beneficial to the mother, helping to avoid abscess formation. An abscess occurs when the infection collects in a spot, comes to a head, forms a liquid center of pus, and must be drained by an incision into the abscess, which, of course, leaves a scar. Sometimes this cannot be avoided. It is best avoided by treating the infection quickly, before the abscess forms.

BREASTS: BREAST CANCER—AGE

555. Can breast cancer occur at any age?

Yes, but it is rare before the age of thirty.

556. At what age is breast cancer most prevalent?

The rate really increases after the age of forty and continues to increase through age seventy-five. The greatest numbers of breast cancers occur in women who are in their fifties and sixties, but that is because there are more women in this age group than there are in the seventies. Thus, the older you get, the more likely you are to develop breast cancer.

557. Dr. Carson, how old were you when you had cancer?

I was fifty-eight years old. This is almost the average age for breast cancer. I had had all my children after I was thirty-four. Babies after thirty-five don't protect you from breast cancer. Babies before thirty-five do. I was white, Caucasian, and living on the West Coast; this made me a higher risk than if I were Mexican, black, or living in the Midwest. I was overweight, and I usually ate the standard American diet. I was a low risk in that I had never had lumpy breasts, a breast biopsy, or fibrocystic breasts, and I had had a normal mammogram, although not recently enough.

BREASTS: BREAST CANCER—CAUSES

558. Are there any known causes of breast cancer?

Not really. The women exposed to the radiation of the atom bomb in Hiroshima had increased breast cancer, but this was enormous radiation. Women who had a lot of chest fluoroscopy X-rays for tuberculosis also had an increase in breast cancer. Women who have no children have more breast cancer than women who have many children. Countries with a low birth rate

BREASTS: BREAST CANCER—CAUSES (Continued)

have more breast cancer than countries with a high birth rate. Women with fibrocystic disease are more prone to breast cancer than women without. White women have more breast cancer than black women; East Coast women have more breast cancer than West Coast women. One of the highest rates is in Washington, D.C. No ones knows what all this means, and it does not give us a cause.

559. Is smoking a major cause of breast cancer?
No, smoking has not yet been linked to breast cancer.

BREASTS: BREAST CANCER—HEREDITY

560. Does a family history of cancer increase my chances of getting it?
Yes. If your mother, grandmother, sister, and aunt had breast cancer, and if it were on both sides of the family, then you have a high risk of getting breast cancer. If you just have a cousin with breast cancer in only one breast, the risk is less.

561. What are my chances of getting breast cancer if I don't have a family history of breast cancer?
In the United States in 1982, your chances of developing breast cancer were one in eleven.

562. Dr. Carson, did you have a family history of breast cancer?
Yes, three years before I had my mastectomy, my mother, who was eighty-three, had a mastectomy for breast cancer of a different type. I was taking care of her in my home at the time that I found my own cancer. When I told her I had a mastectomy, her reaction was, "That doesn't hurt very much."

BREASTS: BREAST CANCER—WARNINGS AND EARLY DETECTION

563. Are there any warning signs of breast cancer, besides finding a lump?
Skin changes, especially scaling on the nipple or dimpling like orange peel elsewhere; a retraction or pulling in, especially of the nipple; and a nipple discharge, especially if it is bloody, are warning signs of breast cancer. A bloody discharge from the nipple usually is a benign intraductal papilloma (a noncancerous lump), but it can signal a cancer.

564. Dr. Carson, how did you find out you had breast cancer?
Not in the usual way. I never had lumpy fibrocystic breasts, and my mammogram had been normal. Then one day, I had spontaneous bleeding from my nipple. All the patients I had ever had with a bleeding nipple had

BREASTS: BREAST CANCER—WARNINGS AND EARLY DETECTION (Continued)

had a benign intraductal papilloma when they had a biopsy, but they were younger women. My biopsy showed an intraductal carcinoma (a cancer) and a mammogram showed a positive lymph node under my arm, meaning the cancer in the nipple had spread to the node under my arm.

565. Can early detection of breast cancer really make a difference?

Yes. The difference is that survival is greater when cancer is found before it has invaded very far into the body (metastasized), that is, has travelled to another part of the body, such as to the lymph nodes or beyond. If the cancerous lump found is less than one-half inch in diameter, the survival rate is better than if it is an inch. If lymph nodes examined contain no breast cancer, survival is better. If only one lymph node has cancer in it, the chances or surviving are better than if four or five contain a spread of cancer. There is even a rare breast cancer called carcinoma in situ that is found only by accident when doing a biopsy for fibrocystic breasts or something else. It is really a cancer of the breast that has not even invaded yet. It can't be seen on mammograms, can't be felt, and can't even be seen by a surgeon, but the pathologist can see it under the microscope. With early detection of this kind of cancer, treatment can result in a 100 percent cure.

BREASTS: BREAST CANCER—WARNINGS AND EARLY DETECTION, THERMOGRAPHY

566. I have heard that there is a new way to detect breast cancer by taking the temperature of the breast. What is this all about?

Breast cancer is growing tissue that has a higher temperature than tissue that is not growing as rapidiy. There are many techniques that rely on this fact to detect portions of the breasts that are cancerous. Of course, infection and pregnancy also change the temperature of the breasts, but that is obvious. Thermography has been used for over twenty years to screen for breast cancer, but in comparison studies, thermography continues to miss breast cancers that mammograms find. Nevertheless, temperature-based studies continue to be used to follow up any abnormal disease states of the breasts and study them. Since there is no good solution to the problem of breast cancer, all scientific methods should continue to be tried. Any device that simply detects temperature changes has absolutely no harmful effects and can be used as often as you can afford it. Mammography is an X-ray and, therefore, involves radiation, although the new techniques of xerogradiography have far less radiation than the old mammograms. Mammograms are seldom done more than once a year, but if you could afford it, you could

BREASTS: BREAST CANCER—WARNINGS AND EARLY DETECTION, THERMOGRAPHY (Continued)

have your temperature checked daily. So far, thermography is not inexpensive, but perhaps future development will reduce the cost.

567. How successful is thermography in finding breast cancer?

It is not as successful as mammography, so the American Cancer Society and other medical organizations continue to recommend mammography as a screening tool for breast cancer. Reports do show that one-third of the women who have an abnormal thermography eventually develop breast cancer, but two-thirds do not. Just think how nervous that makes the other two-thirds who had an abnormal test, but did not develop breast cancer and possibly never will. Thermography misses breast cancer that mammography detects, and that makes it dangerous to have large numbers of women relying on thermography as their screening tool. Perhaps both tests should be used, if you can afford them, and abnormal thermograms could be a reason for you to have mammograms more often. The big advantage of thermography, of course, is that there is no radiation involved in the procedure; there is an effort to limit mammograms because of the radiation that is used.

568. Why is thermography important?

Thermography is a technique that has the possibility of being developed to detect breast cancer or follow any abnormal disease state of the breast, without radiating the breast. It is hoped that thermography will be perfected to the point that it is equal to or better than mammography, and then radiation could be avoided. But it definitely has not reached that point yet. Thermography can be recommended in addition to mammography, but it cannot yet find all the cancers that mammography can, so mammography cannot be eliminated.

BREASTS: BREAST CANCER—INCIDENCES OF BREAST CANCER

569. Is breast cancer likely to occur in women who have had children?

No, breast cancer is more likely to occur in women who have not had children. Statistics show that women with many children have less breast cancer, especially if they had their children before the age of thirty-five.

570. Is breast cancer more prevalent in larger-breasted women?

No one knows the answer to this for sure. Certainly breast cancer occurs in women with small breasts, but it seems reasonable to expect that more breast tissue would permit a greater chance of breast cancer. Men have very small breasts, and one in every one hundred breast cancers is in men. That would be about the right proportion, based on the amount of breast tissue in men as compared to women. Orientals have less breast tissue and a

BREASTS: BREAST CANCER—INCIDENCES OF BREAST CANCER
(Continued)

lower incidence of breast cancer, but, of course, there are other factors, too. Breast cancer increases in older women, and older women seem to have larger breasts.

571. Is the incidence of breast cancer among women in the United States increasing? If so, why?

Yes, the incidence of breast cancer has increased from one in twenty women to one in eleven women in the last twenty-five years. It is not exactly known why this has happened, but it could be because women have fewer children today than they did twenty-five years ago. It also could partly be because women are living longer and are not dying of other things.

BREASTS: BREAST CANCER AND BREAST-FEEDING

572. Do women who breast-feed their children have less of a chance of getting breast cancer?

In previous years the answer to this was yes, but now statistics show that what protects a woman from breast cancer is having children before the age of thirty-five, not particularly whether she breast-feeds them.

573. What should I do if I discover that I have breast cancer while I am still breast-feeding? What danger is there for my baby?

You will need to have a biopsy and surgical treatment, which will interfere with breast-feeding. Primarily, your baby is in danger of losing its mother. Of course, there is an increased risk of breast cancer in a woman if her mother had breast cancer, but not because she was breast-feeding at the time of the discovery. There are a few studies that suggest there is more likelihood of the daughter having breast cancer if she was breast-fed by the mother who later developed cancer, but these studies are not very convincing and should not be a reason to avoid breast-feeding. It might be a reason, however, for a woman who has had breast cancer not to breast-feed, although many of these women breast-feed anyway. It is not a settled question. In rats who breast-feed from a mother rat with breast cancer, there are more breast cancers. But we are not rats, and our breast cancers are quite different. If you were to discover breast cancer while you were pregnant, you could have surgery and still have a normal delivery and child.

BREASTS: BREAST CANCER—SPREADING

574. Can breast cancer spread to other parts of my body?

Yes, that is the problem. Even before you can find the lump, the grow-

BREASTS: BREAST CANCER—SPREADING (Continued)

ing cancer can spread to your lymph nodes, liver, bones, and lungs. Breast cancer spreads most often to your lymph nodes first, next to your bones, and then to your liver and lungs. Sometimes breast cancer is found by having a bone break, not because of a fall, but because the cancer that travelled from your breast to your bone and grew there caused it to break.

575. Is breast cancer painful?

Cancer in the breast does not produce pain, but cancer that spreads from the breast to a bone is quite painful.

576. If I have had one breast removed as the result of breast cancer, what are the chances of later getting cancer in my other breast?

Ten percent of women with cancer in one breast later get it in the other breast, according to some studies. The chances of this happening are so high that some women have the other breast removed to prevent the possibility and to facilitate reconstruction, which is then done on both sides.

577. What percentage of women who just had a cancerous lump removed later go back and have the entire breast removed?

Twenty to 25 percent later go back and have the entire breast removed, because the cancer has been found in another part of their breast.

BREASTS: BREAST CANCER IN MEN

578. Do men also get breast cancer?

Yes, but the relative incidence is that one in one hundred breast cancers is in men. This means that for every one thousand women, one man will develop breast cancer, but one hundred women will have it.

579. Is cancer in men easily cured?

Breast cancer in men is usually neglected and ignored for so long that it is not diagnosed early enough to have a good cure rate. Most of them are not cured.

BREASTS: BREAST CANCER TREATMENTS—MODIFIED RADICAL MASTECTOMY

580. What is the most common treatment for breast cancer?

The most common treatment in the United States today is a modified radical mastectomy.

581. What is a modified radical mastectomy?

A modified radical mastectomy means that the entire breast that contains the cancer is removed, as well as all the lymph nodes in the armpit

BREASTS: BREAST CANCER TREATMENTS—MODIFIED RADICAL MASTECTOMY (Continued)

(axilla) on that side. The muscle of the chest wall is not removed, as it was in previous years; therefore, the function of the arm is not so impaired.

582. Do most doctors recommend a modified radical mastectomy?

Yes. Today the most frequently recommended treatment for breast cancer is a modified radical mastectomy, as this is considered to have as good a cure rate as the former radical mastectomy, but it is less disfiguring.

583. How do other less extensive surgeries for breast cancer compare with the modified radical mastectomy?

Lesser surgery is not yet known to have as good a cure rate, but tests are being done on a national experimental basis to compare results in future years. A recommendation for less extensive surgery depends upon your cell type and the size of the cancer.

584. Is a modified radical mastectomy recommended most often for all breast cancers, or can other methods be just as effective?

Most doctors in the United States believe that a modified radical mastectomy is always necessary, because breast cancer starts in several places in the breast, not just in the one they find. The first place the cancer spreads to is the breast itself, so just removing the lump to the margin of the cancer that you can see doesn't mean it isn't somewhere else, even if an X-ray doesn't show it. Of those women who have just the lump removed (a lumpectomy), 20 to 25 percent come back within ten years and have the rest of the breast removed because of the recurrence in some other part of the breast. Of course, you can argue that therefore 75 percent did not have to have the rest of their breast removed, but in the 25 percent where it did recur, it could spread to the rest of the body and prevent their survival.

585. Dr. Carson, how long were you out of work after your modified radical cancer operation?

I cancelled three days out of my office schedule. My discovery occurred on a weekend, my biopsy was done on a lunch hour, and the mastectomy was scheduled for a midweek morning. I entered the hospital the previous night, a night I was supposed to meet as a member of the Executive Medical Board of the hospital. I put on the hospital gown and had all the tests. Then I got up, dressed, and went to the meeting. No one there knew. That is a good way to spend the evening before surgery. I had surgery on Wednesday and went home on Saturday. My surgeon was willing to treat my incision for me later in his office, which is located near mine, so I did not have to stay in the hospital for that. I went to work on Monday, as usual. Some other doctors

BREASTS: BREAST CANCER TREATMENTS—MODIFIED RADICAL MASTECTOMY (Continued)

were dismayed by my early return to work and called me the "iron lady," but it was very difficult to reschedule patients when my schedule was already full. My busy partner could not take over all of them. I felt happier returning to work, showing myself that this was not going to radically change my life. I continued to do surgery and deliver babies. All that is physically easier to do than housework anyway. People would ask, "How could you work after a mastectomy?" I replied, "I don't use my breasts very much in my work." I went back to using padded brassieres, at least on one side, as I had done in the past before I had children, and within a month I bought a really good, soft, plastic insert (a prosthesis).

586. Did the modified radical operation hurt? For how long?

No, not much. Of course, during the operation I was under general anesthesia. The main problems afterward were to stop vomiting, to learn to eat again, and to fight the nausea. The old radical mastectomy was really painful, because it removed muscles down to the bone and made it very difficult to move the arm with the few muscles that were left attached. There is really not much physical pain involved in a modified radical, because muscles are not removed. There is only a skin incision left and the edges of it are numb. Arm movement is not restricted, because all the muscles are there. I did not need pain pills after I got home three days later. The reconstruction, with the placement of the silicone under the chest muscle, was much more painful.

BREASTS: BREAST CANCER TREATMENTS—RADICAL MASTECTOMY

587. What is a radical mastectomy?

With a radical mastectomy, the entire breast that contains the cancer is removed, as well as the lymph nodes on that side of the armpit and the muscle of the chest wall, thus impairing the function of the arm.

BREASTS: BREAST CANCER—OTHER TREATMENTS

588. What other treatments, besides radical mastectomy and modified radical mastectomy, are available for breast cancer?

Lumpectomy, segmental resection, and radiation.

589. What are the newest treatments for breast cancer?

The lumpectomy is a relatively new treatment in the United States, even

BREASTS: BREAST CANCER—OTHER TREATMENTS
(Continued)

though it is an old treatment in Europe, especially Sweden. Lumpectomy is not yet proven to be as curative as the modified radical mastectomy, though studies on this are now being done. Another new approach is to do a mastectomy in such a way that reconstruction using silicone implants can be done later, even saving the nipple by transplanting it to the thigh and then back to the rebuilt breast. The advantage to this treatment is that it is less devastating to the psyche of the women and less disfiguring than the old radical mastectomy.

590. Dr. Carson, what treatment did you choose when you learned of your breast cancer?

I considered all the options, as I had always encouraged my patients to do. Many years before, I had been planning to go elsewhere for treatment if I ever had breast cancer, because no surgeon in my town would do anything but a radical mastectomy. I had been on television shows promoting modified radical mastectomy with a crosswise (transverse) incision and subsequent reconstruction of the breast. I also had fought surgeons until they agreed to do lumpectomies and radiation, if the patient so desired. Since my cancer was dead center in my nipple, a lumpectomy wouldn't have looked very good, and since I had one positive lymph node, the cancer had spread. I chose a modified radical mastectomy with a transverse incision, so I could later have reconstruction. Three months later I had the other breast removed, because it also had multiple polyps (papillomatosis) in the nipple and I had at least a 10 percent chance of developing another cancer. Also, it would at least have to have been reduced to match the reconstructed breast. Both, then, were reconstructed with silicone inserts. Later, I had excellent-looking nipples constructed using thigh skin.

591. Is there any other surgery or treatment that would be necessary after a mastectomy?

Though it has not been too common in recent years, reconstruction of the breasts and/or use of chemotherapy is happening more often every year.

BREASTS: BREAST CANCER TREATMENTS—LUMPECTOMY

592. What is a lumpectomy?

Removal of the lump with a clear margin around it is called a lumpectomy. It usually is combined with a lymph node dissection and radiation to prevent local recurrence.

BREASTS: BREAST CANCER TREATMENTS—SEGMENTAL RESECTION

593. What is a segmental resection?

Segmental resection removes a whole quadrant of the breast where the lump is located. The rest of the breast is then pulled over to fill the defect as much as possible.

594. How effective is segmental resection in curing breast cancer?

It is more effective than lumpectomy because it removes more tissue that could contain a recurrent cancer.

BREASTS: BREAST CANCER TREATMENTS—RADIATION

595. How often is radiation alone used in treating cancer?

Radiation alone has been carried out in less than 5 percent of patients with breast cancer. It has been used extensively in Sweden and Italy, but is rarely used in the United States, as it is thought that the cure rate is too low. Here it is done only in people who are too poor in health to withstand surgery, or who have such widespread cancer that a cure is hopeless, and it is just used to stop local growth.

596. What are the long-term effects of radiation?

There is concern that the radiation itself can cause some of the remaining breast tissue to become cancerous, since radiation is known to cause cancer. Sometimes cancer is found in the radiated breast later, and it is not clear if it is a recurrence or new cancer, perhaps caused by radiation. Possibly it is the latter since radiation to any part of the body in a large amount can cause leukemia to occur in later years. Skin changes, like a burn, also can be caused by radiation, but these are less likely to occur with modern radiation. Some cosmetic changes in the shape of the breast, such as the breast being smaller in size or positioned higher than the normal one, have been reported, although these changes are secondary to scarring.

597. How will my breast change in appearance after radiation?

If one breast itself is radiated, as in primary treatment or after a lumpectomy, it usually contracts and becomes smaller than the other breast.

BREASTS: BREAST CANCER TREATMENTS—CHEMOTHERAPY

598. When are other treatments followed by chemotherapy?

All treatments for cancer may be followed by chemotherapy if cancer is found in the lymph nodes or if the spread of cancer is detected.

599. What are the short-term effects of chemotherapy?

Short-term effects are nausea, vomiting, and loss of hair. There also can be a toxic effect on the nerves and the heart.

BREASTS: BREAST CANCER TREATMENTS—CHEMOTHERAPY
(Continued)

600. What are the long-term effects of chemotherapy?

Late effects of chemotherapy can include leukemia. There also is a reduction in the resistance to diseases.

BREASTS: BREAST CANCER—CURE RATE

601. What are my chances of dying from breast cancer?

Overall, if you have a biopsy that shows breast cancer of any level, your chance of surviving is about 50 percent; or, if one thousand women have any type of breast cancer, five hundred women will die. However, this greatly depends on how much cancer you have and what type of treatment you get. If you have a modified radical mastectomy and the lymph nodes have no cancer in them, and none is found elsewhere in your body, then your chances of survival are about 80 percent. If you have one to three nodes with cancer in them, your chances of living five years are 60 percent, and ten years, 40 percent. If you have more than three nodes with cancer, your chances of survival are less than that. If you add chemotherapy to your treatment, you improve your survival chances 10-15 percent. The survival record for lumpectomy and node dissection with radiation is not yet known in the United States, since it has not been done here very long.

602. How does the cure rate of the modified radical mastectomy compare with that of the radical mastectomy?

It has been shown that the cure rate with the less extensive, modified radical mastectomy is as good as it is with the disfiguring radical mastectomy.

603. Is there any treatment available today that is known to cure breast cancer completely?

The treatments for breast cancer are seldom called cures. Only the very early carcinoma in situ (a rare breast cancer) can be 100 percent cured by a simple mastectomy. All other breast cancers have cure rates.

604. What percentage of women who just have the cancerous lump removed (a lumpectomy), instead of a complete mastectomy, recover completely?

Whether you recover completely depends on whether the cancer had spread to the rest of your body before the lumpectomy was done. Your survival after lumpectomy, as compared to a modified radical mastectomy, is not yet known. It takes twenty years to find out, since women die of breast cancer as long as twenty years after they are treated. An experimental study on the treatment of breast cancer is now going on in the United States.

BREASTS: BREAST CANCER—CURE RATE (Continued)

605. How long after I have been treated for breast cancer must I wait before I can be reasonably sure that I have been successfully cured?

Ten years is the time usually given for a reasonable estimate of a cure, although five-year intervals are important, too. But breast cancer can be slow, and a woman can die as much as twenty years later from the same breast cancer.

606. How many new cases of breast cancer will be detected this year in American women?

The American Cancer Society estimates that 114,000 new cases of breast cancer will be diagnosed this year, and 37,000 victims will die.

BREASTS: BREAST CANCER—RECONSTRUCTIVE SURGERY

607. Is reconstructive surgery after a mastectomy advisable for everyone?

It is usually recommended for everyone who has had a mastectomy, but the variation is in when it is recommended, for immediately after surgery or later. Of course, it is not recommended if the woman's health is too poor for further surgery.

608. When is the best time to have reconstructive surgery done?

Some physicians advise women to wait a year, to be sure there are no local recurrences of cancer in the scar area before doing the reconstructive surgery. A few women have had the reconstruction done at the same time as their mastectomy, but many of these had to be removed because of the difficulty in healing. Reconstruction can still be performed even if the mastectomy was done many years ago with the wrong type of incision. Plastic surgery has been devised that uses flaps taken from the patient's back and plastic inserts to form a new breast. Sometimes a flap with fat from the tummy is used. Ideally, the plastic surgeon will be present or at least advise the surgeon who does the mastectomy about the proper incisions needed to make reconstruction possible later. Then when it is healed a few months later, the reconstruction can be done.

609. Dr. Carson, how much did your breast reconstruction cost?

I was covered by Blue Shield and went to doctors who accepted Blue Shield, so everything was paid for, except the added expense of a private room in the hospital for three days. The total cost varies from coast to coast and is probably less than you think.

610. How safe is reconstruction of the breast?

It is as safe as any surgery can be.

BREASTS: BREAST CANCER—RECONSTRUCTIVE SURGERY
(Continued)

611. What are some complications to be aware of with reconstructive surgery?

Sometimes it has complications, such as bleeding or poor healing, and has to be redone. Sometimes the result is less than ideal, becoming hard with fibrosis months afterwards, getting out of place, or being quite asymmetrical. It is hard to make one breast look like another one, so sometimes the other breast has to be reduced in size in order to match the reconstructed one.

612. How similar are reconstructed breasts to real breasts?

They are covered by skin, and if you heal well, the scars are minimal. You may have your own nipples transplanted, or you can have new ones constructed from skin of appropriate color. The silicone is placed under the chest muscles (pectoral muscles), so the surface is as soft and normal as are natural breasts. The contours can be like that of moderately small breasts, not large, pedulous ones. The nipples have little feeling in them. The breasts are perceived by women mostly as weight and bulk, and reconstructed breasts are perceived this way, too. You can go through a general physical, and the examiner may only think you had uplift breast surgery, not cancer surgery.

613. Does reconstructive surgery alleviate the emotional problems associated with mastectomy?

Yes, reconstruction can restore your body image to something more normal, so that you are not constantly reminded that you had cancer and were disfigured. You can dress without wearing an artificial breast (a prosthesis), and you can swim and do other sports without worrying about positioning the false breast. You can look as normal as someone who has had reduction breast surgery. You may feel much better than if you had a disfiguring lumpectomy followed by radiation, especially if the radiation were to cause other possible changes. Of course, you still know you had cancer, and reconstruction does nothing to increase your chances of survival. It just improves the quality of life.

BREASTS: BREAST CANCER TREATMENTS—ADJUSTMENT TO

614. How can I expect to feel if I am told that I have breast cancer?

According to an article entitled, "Mastectomy: Impact on Patients and Families," a patient's response to breast cancer is described in terms of stages. The first stage involves the woman's discovery of the symptoms which produces anxiety, denial, or avoidance. In the next stage, after cancer

BREASTS: BREAST CANCER TREATMENTS—ADJUSTMENT TO
(Continued)

has been diagnosed, the patient faces the prospect of surgery and is extremely afraid. After the operation, as the patient seems to get better, the patient goes through a stage of being angry, resentful, and depressed. She starts to think about facing other people, being deformed. As she figures out the meaning of her disability, she may move through a range of feelings from other-directed anger to self-blame. This really is a chronic disease, and the woman must, at this point, find a way to cope with it and get on with her life.[1]

615. How do most women feel after they have a mastectomy?

Physically there is not much pain at all, since there is simply a skin incision; no deep incisions are necessary when a radical mastectomy is not done. The surgery is not so major that a long recovery is required before most women can become physically active. Emotionally they are shocked to find that they can have something that can lead to their deaths, since they have always felt indestructible. After the minor physical discomforts and the major threat to their existence is considered, most women begin to wonder about their acceptance as female bodies by those with whom they are intimate—their husbands, their children, or in some cases their lovers or future lovers. Then they wonder about clothes, intimate apparel, swimsuits, nightgowns, and perhaps even reconstructive surgery for their breasts.

616. Do most women find it difficult to adjust to a mastectomy?

In general, the answer is yes. But the great difficulty in the past was in women who had a radical mastectomy, because the muscles to their arms were removed, and they could hardly raise their arms. They had to learn to move them using different muscles. With the modified radical mastectomy, the arm muscles are left in place, and the arm function is fine. The problem is no longer physical function, it is physical appearance, sexual functioning, and body image. A distorted body can be hard to live with. A prosthesis (artificial breast) makes the fully dressed woman look fine in public, but she is not always fully dressed during her life. Some women will not even look at themselves in the mirror after a breast is removed. Some will no longer let their husbands see them naked, and they avoid sexual exposure because they think they look so horrible. But the biggest problem they have to adjust to is the word **cancer.**

617. Do women get depressed to the point of suicide after a mastectomy?

Yes, they do. Several surveys show that 25 percent of women con-

[1] Elane M. Nuehring and William E. Barr, "Mastectomy: Impact on Patients and Families," *Health and Social Work,* 5 (1980), 51-8.

BREASTS: BREAST CANCER TREATMENTS—ADJUSTMENT TO
(Continued)

template suicide during the postoperative period. They are usually women with a high sexual interest and activity prior to surgery, who have more anxiety about sexual relationships while recovering. They also are the ones who are most interested in reconstructive surgery. Many women use more tranquilizers and alcohol after the mastectomy that they did before, even if they are not suicidal. One surgeon writes about how shattered he was when he lost three out of ten patients through suicide. He studied these cases and was told by the women's friends that their husbands had said they wouldn't go to bed with a "lopsided woman." One bought his wife an expensive car and got himself a girl friend. Another got a girl friend and was abusive and drank heavily. None of the couples were divorced. This surgeon feels all mastectomy patients go through a depression. He advises husbands to reassure their wives that they love them and that a change in body contour will not matter.

618. Dr. Carson, what was your reaction to knowing you had breast cancer?

My first reaction was one of fatalism. I thought, "So that is the way it's going to be." I had arranged that my biopsy would be done under local anesthesia on my lunch hour, so that I could return to work. While my surgeon was putting in the final sutures, he received the pathologist's report on the frozen specimen and told me the "bad news." I then thought that I would probably not live into old age as my mother did, and I was glad that my children were grown. I began to wonder how to tell my husband and how to arrange my next treatment. I did not cry. In the next hour, I returned to the maternity suite where I had two patients. I thought I would like to keep the problem a secret, so that it would not affect my practice. A woman colleague came up to the desk, not seeing me, and said, "I heard Dr. Carson had a breast biopsy today, but it's not on the schedule!" I looked up and said, startling her, "That's because it was supposed to be a secret!" I gave up on the secrecy.

619. Dr. Carson, how did you feel about losing your breast?

The appearance of my breast after the biopsy helped me to part with it with a minimum amount of grief. It was closed with temporary sutures, because surgery was already planned for the following week. It was black and blue, with small bloody areas (hemorrhages) under the skin from the surgery. I had really enjoyed having large, good-looking breasts, because I had had them for such a short time. I was flat-chested until I breast-fed a baby at thirty-six, and after that I looked normal. I enjoyed not wearing

BREASTS: BREAST CANCER TREATMENTS—ADJUSTMENT TO
(Continued)

padded brassieres for twenty years. But I looked at this marred breast as my enemy.

620. Dr. Carson, does not having breasts hinder your sex life?

Yes, it does. Although reconstructed breasts look pretty normal, the surgery does not restore the sensory feeling that used to be in the nipples. The feeling of weight and bulk, which is a great deal of the sensory perception of a breast, is there, but the surface nipple touch is gone. The nipples contain genital bodies, just like the vulva, and stimulation of them can bring about orgasm. Partner stimulation of breasts had become almost a ritual, satisfying to both of us, but now it is quite de-emphasized. Other activities are emphasized more, in compensation. Because I had seen so many problems of sexual difficulty after mastectomy and had even been involved in trying to get a research grant on this subject in the past, I was determined not to let that happen to me. By continuing activity at all levels of my life as soon as I was released from the hospital, I did not let a long period of sexual abstinence ensue. By being the aggressor, I allayed fears that I was not yet ready for sex. I had a good background for being able to have sex without much in the way of breasts when I was young and flat-chested.

621. What should I do to get back my self-esteem, after having one of my breasts removed?

Tell yourself how unnecessary a breast is. You didn't really use it for very much, and you probably have another one. You are far more important than a body part that was designed to feed a baby, although most people don't even use it for that anymore. If you really need good body contours to feel good, get them. Buy the most expensive prosthesis (artificial breast) and wear it. Find the undergarments you like best and adapt them to the prosthesis. Get beautiful nightgowns that make this possible. A special prosthesis that does not require a brassiere is made to wear with evening gowns. You are worth the expense of these items. In California and certain other states, insurance is required to pay for "mastectomy" items and clothes. If all this isn't enough, look into reconstruction of a new breast and nipple for yourself. If your other breast would be hard to match, reconstruct it, too. Many women have silicone inserts just to make their breasts look larger and more uplifted. You have a better reason to use silicone than they do. Insurance will pay for your reconstruction, too, at least in California. Do it for yourself, not for your husband or your lover. He will or should say he loves you without any plastic surgery. It will help you to face yourself, especially in the shower and in bed.

BREASTS: BREAST CANCER TREATMENTS—ADJUSTMENT TO
(Continued)

622. I am very depressed about my lack of breasts, even though the doctor told me my cure rate is excellent. What can I do?

First tell your doctor how you feel, and he or she may be able to arrange help for you. You can call the American Cancer Society, and someone from its "Reach to Recovery Program" can talk to you about your feelings. You can purchase a prosthesis and clothing that is appropriate. You can consider reconstructive breast surgery; just planning it with a plastic surgeon can give you hope about feeling better. It is always frightening to have the diagnosis of cancer, even if it is a small skin cancer, but as you become familiar with it, it becomes less frightening.

623. Dr. Carson, what did you learn from your breast cancer that you did not know before you had it when you were diagnosing other women's cancers? How was the adjustment different than you thought it would be?

I learned that it was much less painful than I had supposed it would be. I also learned that there is practically no disability resulting from the surgery. I had been involved in organizing the local chapter of the "Reach to Recovery Program" years ago, teaching mastectomy patients how to raise their arms again after the muscles were gone. That was really a problem. Now the main function of the program is to teach women how to dress with only one breast and how to keep their relationships, sexual and otherwise, functioning. I learned how to buy lingerie, bathing suits, and nightgowns that are adapted to a prosthesis and how to get insurance to pay for these mastectomy clothes. I also learned more about how to persuade women to go ahead with reconstructive surgery for their own self-image.

624. How many women who have a mastectomy have sexual problems afterward?

A United States study showed that 40 percent of the women had sexual problems in the early period following mastectomy and 33 percent of the women still had problems after one year. A 1980 British study showed that 50 percent of the mastectomy patients who were surveyed were found to have sexual problems, a figure that rose to 70 percent among those who had undergone both mastectomy and chemotherapy. A typical situation was described in *The New York Times* as "a woman, married for many years, who finds after her operation that her husband is remote and cold, unable to communicate his feelings or to comfort her. 'He hasn't touched me in two years,' she says bitterly."[2]

---

[2] Leslie Bennetts, "Breast Cancer and Sexuality," *The New York Times,* 1 March 1982, p. B6, col. 1. © by The New York Times Company. Reprinted by permission.

BREASTS: BREAST CANCER TREATMENTS—ADJUSTMENT TO
(Continued)

625. Do many women with mastectomies get divorced?

No, the actual divorce rate in the year following mastectomy is only about one out of twenty cases. What troubles most women is the fear of possible loss of affection and sexual responsiveness by the men in their lives. If men can accept the mastectomy, then women can, too.

626. Do single women fear mastectomy more than married women?

Their fears are different. They are afraid they will never find a partner because they feel unattractive to men.

627. How can I best recover psychologically after a mastectomy?

Some psychiatrists advise women to behave as though nothing unusual had occurred and to go on without any effort at adjustment. However, this can thwart communication of real feelings, leading to a breakup of the relationship or even the marriage. Counseling that includes the partner can facilitate recovery, especially sex counseling.

BREASTS: BREAST CANCER—MEN'S ADJUSTMENTS TO WOMEN'S MASTECTOMIES

628. Is there any place that I or my husband and I can go to help us adjust to my breast cancer and my lack of breasts?

The American Cancer Society sponsors a "Reach to Recovery Program" in every city. They will send someone to talk to you who has had cancer and has solved the many problems that cancer patients have. This program also includes counseling for you, your husband, and children to help them adjust to the problems. Call them for help. In some cities, there is a group called "Encore." "Encore" is a group of mastectomy patients who discuss the problems and solutions associated with mastectomy. Your hospital also may sponsor a group that helps fight the problems of cancer.

629. How do men respond to their partners' mastectomy?

The vast majority of men are supportive and worry about how they can help their partners, but some men become distressed, and the relationship suffers. Studies show that it is a bad sign if the man makes few visits to the woman in the hospital, if he avoids looking at the surgical scar, or if he delays resumption of sexual activity. Most men who react poorly to mastectomy also oppose reconstructive surgery because it means more suffering and hospitalization; they usually exaggerate the amount of pain. The men who do well in their adjustment to mastectomy think it is important to be involved in the decision-making process before the first surgery.

BREASTS: BREAST CANCER—MEN'S ADJUSTMENTS TO WOMEN'S MASTECTOMIES (Continued)

630. Dr. Carson, how did your husband react to your breast cancer?

Unfortunately, I didn't reach him first to tell him the results of my biopsy. He and my closest friends were sure my biopsy would be benign. He contacted my surgeon and demanded to know the results. When he heard, he cried, but not in front of me. He was concerned, more loving, and just showed the fear that he might lose something precious to him—me—not my breast. He went along with my desire to keep my practice going as if nothing had happened. A week after my surgery, we went to the beautiful Bonaventure Hotel in Los Angeles where I was scheduled for a medical meeting and he for a real estate meeting. We danced together at the banquet. I worried that my prosthesis was crooked, but he did not. We went to a football game the same weekend and I rooted with him for USC with my other arm. He was proud to tell people I had had the surgery the previous week and only took three days off from work. We have always had an energetic life together. We did not let it stop to grieve.

631. How do most men feel about a woman after she has undergone a mastectomy?

To some men, the sight and touch of a woman's breasts arouse them erotically. If the breasts are scarred, mutilated, or completely absent due to surgery, this type of man feels a tremendous loss and may, indeed, have to struggle with his sexual arousal in the absence of admiring and fondling the breasts. He may very much love his wife and want to stand by her, but can actually become impotent when viewing the loss. Adjustments can be made, sexual arousal can be modified, and he can overcome the problem. But it is a problem. Other men will stand by you and love you more than ever after a mastectomy.

632. How can I expect my husband to react after he sees me with no breasts?

His first reaction will be of concern when he sees a fresh surgical scar, which many people have a hard time looking at. Some women will not look at themselves in a mirror for a long time. Then he will show love for you, do things for you, and want to take care of you. The problems arise when, out of concern, he may avoid sexual advances for some time. When this is prolonged, he may have to admit that he's having a hard time with an erection. What happens after that may depend upon your response. You can withdraw or help.

633. What is a man's sexual reaction to a woman with a mastectomy?

According to an article in *The New York Times,* "Nobody knows how mastectomy affects a man in terms of sexual desire. It's a confrontation with

BREASTS: BREAST CANCER—MEN'S ADJUSTMENTS TO WOMEN'S MASTECTOMIES (Continued)

death, with illness and aging. It inhibits sexual drive. Men won't admit how affected they are. They feel terrible about it and they are saddened by it, but they may be physically turned off by it.''[3] The male may indeed develop sexual dysfunction because of his anxiety, his fear of hurting someone who is already hurt, and his actual shock on viewing the scar or the flat chest. He needs to be able to adapt to a new situation, even a new coital position, depending upon the woman's physical needs. If he already has problems, they become worse.

BREASTS: BREAST CANCER—CHILDREN AND FAMILIES

634. How do families of breast cancer patients adjust?

Some family members may experience guilt and despair. They may be afraid that the woman will die. The family will have enormous stress, in the same way that they would if the patient had any major debilitating disease.

BREASTS: BREAST CANCER—PREVENTIVE MASTECTOMY

635. My mother and sister had breast cancer, so I am a high risk. What could I do to prevent it?

Some plastic surgeons will remove the entire breast tissue, except for the nipple, and will insert silicone. This is done in cases where the woman has precancerous breast tissue, such as a severe fibrocystic condition called dysplasia (abnormal thickening), or papillomatosis (many small tumors in the ducts) is present. They could also do this for women, such as yourself, who are high risks because of family history. There is still some risk of cancer in the nipple, but most breast cancer would be prevented. This operation is called subcutaneous mastectomy. It is seldom recommended by a doctor, unless you demand that something be done.

[3] Ibid.

Chapter 4

Birth Control

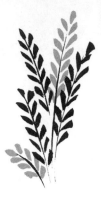

We cannot
listen to what
others want us to do
We must listen
to ourselves
Society
family
friends
do not know what
we must do
Only we know
and only we
can do what is
right for us
So start right now
You will need to
work very hard
You will need to
overcome many obstacles
You will need to go
against the better
judgment of many people
and you will need to
bypass their prejudices
But you can have
whatever you want
if you
try hard enough
So start right now and
you will live
a life designed
by you and
for you
and you will
love
your
life

— Susan Polis Schutz

BIRTH CONTROL

If you are not in charge of your reproductive organs, you have no control over your life. Without some effort at contraception, most women would have twenty or thirty babies in a normal lifetime. Margaret Sanger and others fought hard and endured imprisonment to set you free to control your own body through contraception.

The first control exerted by women, of course, was refusal of intercourse— abstinence. In medieval times, the prospect of having a lot of babies made the idea of joining a nunnery enticing. Abstinence, or at least periodic abstinence, is still the only method that is approved by several religions. But a lot of women today view sexual satisfaction as one of their rights, and this right includes the ability to have sex without pregnancy. Men have always had sexual freedom, curtailed only by their ethics or religion.

Women will only have complete sexual freedom when they have complete control over their ability to become pregnant. The perfect contraceptive has not yet been invented, but those available today are beyond the wildest dreams of women of a hundred years ago. You should learn about the forms of contraception. What you use, or whether you use anything, is your decision and yours alone.

BIRTH CONTROL: VARIOUS METHODS USED TODAY

636. What are the various methods of birth control available today?

The following birth control methods are currently available:

Combination birth control pills—contain both estrogen and progesterone, in high or low doses.

Minipill—contains only progesterone.

Intrauterine devices (IUDs), such as pure plastic devices or those with added copper or added progesterone.

Barrier methods, such as diaphragms, condoms, foams, jellies, creams, suppositories, and sponges.

Withdrawal, which is removing the penis before ejaculation.

Rhythm, calendar or symptothermal method, which is abstention from sex during the most fertile time of the cycle.

Abstinence, which is abstention from sex at all times.

Abortion, which is termination of any pregnancy that occurs.

Sterilization, which is tubal ligation or hysterectomy for the female, or vasectomy for the male. This is permanent.

Combination of two or more of the above methods, such as condom for the male and contraceptive foam for the female.

637. Which methods of birth control are considered to be preventive?

Barrier methods, such as the diaphragm or condom, and most types of birth control pills are considered to be preventive forms of contraception. The barrier methods prevent sperm from reaching the egg, while combination birth control pills prevent ovulation altogether. The minipill prevents sperm from entering the cervix and also prevents implantation.

638. Which birth control methods are considered to be abortive?

Only the IUD is considered to be abortive, although it really prevents implantation of the fertilized egg. The modern definition of abortion is the removal of an implanted embryo, so under that definition, the IUD is not abortive either. The new French pill (not available in the United States) is considered abortive, since it will dislodge an implanted embryo.

639. Which methods of birth control are used by most women today?

The methods of birth control used by most women worldwide are withdrawal and the rhythm method followed by breast-feeding. In the United States the most-used method is still the birth control pill.

BIRTH CONTROL: VARIOUS METHODS USED TODAY
(Continued)

640. How many people use each of the different birth control methods?

According to a 1978 family-planning clinic survey, the different methods of contraception used were as follows:

Pills	66%
IUDs	11%
Diaphragm	7%
Foams, Suppositories	5%
Condoms	3%
Sterilization	1%

But those are just the habits of people in a clinic. The World Health Organization estimated the 1978 worldwide use of contraception as follows:

Coitus Interruptus (withdrawal)	High, but unknown
Rhythm	Next highest, unknown
Prolonged lactation (breast-feeding more than six months)	50-100 million
Oral Contraceptives	50-80 million
Abortion	30-55 million
Sterilization	15-30 million
Condoms	15-20 million
IUDs	15 million
Diaphragms	2-3 million

641. What birth control methods are used by women in other countries?

All of the methods that we have here in the United States are also available in most other countries. The sponge and the cervical cap have been used in Europe for many years. Some herbs are used in China and vaginal salt is used in India, but these methods are considered to be mostly folklore by American physicians.

BIRTH CONTROL: ANCIENT METHODS, FIRST EFFECTIVE METHOD

642. What methods of birth control were used in ancient times?

Abortion and even infanticide preceded birth control, or the prevention of pregnancy, as a means of controlling the number of children who were born. A sea sponge was also inserted into the vagina, perhaps with salt, to prevent pregnancy.

643. What was the first effective method of birth control?

In the nineteenth century, the practice of withdrawal became widespread in France and then in Europe. This was the first method of birth control that really made a difference in the birth rate.

BIRTH CONTROL: WHAT TYPE OF CONTRACEPTION REQUIRES SEEING A DOCTOR?

644. What kind of a doctor do I see about birth control?

Your personal physician is probably your best source. If he or she is Catholic, and you prefer a birth control method other than the rhythm method, then you may seek an alternate physician. A gynecologist is specially trained in the treatment of women, especially in contraception, but general practitioners and family physicians are all excellent in this field. If your doctor will not discuss or provide contraception, inquire about his or her religion. Sixty percent of all Catholics use contraception, and many Catholic doctors will provide it. You may also go to a family-planning clinic or a Planned Parenthood clinic where you might see a nurse practitioner who is specially trained in the various birth control methods.

645. How important is it to have a physical examination and medical advice before deciding upon a particular method of birth control?

Medical examinations are not always necessary, although they may be important for girls who need to know that they are normal. They also provide a good opportunity for girls to bring up any problems about sexual activity that may be bothering them. If you cannot get a medical examination first, it is still best to use birth control devices, such as those available over the counter at a drug store.

646. Which forms of birth control require a medical examination and which do not?

Vaginal foams, suppositories, sponges, and jellies do not require a medical examination. Pills, diaphragms, and IUDs require medical examination and selection. They may also require fitting and insertion, depending upon which method is chosen.

647. Which birth control methods require a doctor's prescription?

All forms of birth control pills, diaphragms, IUDs (which must be inserted by a doctor or nurse practitioner), and Depo Provera shots (which are not readily available) require a doctor's prescription.

BIRTH CONTROL: CHANCES OF BECOMING PREGNANT; EFFECTIVENESS OF VARIOUS METHODS OF CONTRACEPTION

648. Which is the most effective method of birth control?

The combination birth control pill is the most effective method of birth control.

649. After the pill, which is the next most effective method of birth control?

After the pill, the IUD (intrauterine device) is the next most effective

BIRTH CONTROL: CHANCES OF BECOMING PREGNANT; EFFECTIVENESS OF VARIOUS METHODS OF CONTRACEPTION
(Continued)

method of birth control in actual use. Other methods, like the diaphragm, sponge, or condom and foam, may be theoretically very effective, but in actual use do not rate as effective, probably because they are occasionally omitted.

650. What is the effectiveness of the minipill?
The minipill is 97 percent effective.

651. What is the effectiveness of the high- and low-dose combination birth control pills?
Both are 99.9 percent effective if taken correctly. If you forget to take five pills, the effectiveness drops to 99 percent.

652. What is the effectiveness of the IUD?
It is 97 percent effective.

653. How effective is douching to prevent pregnancy?
It has been estimated that if you get up and quickly douche after coitus, this will be about 10 percent effective in preventing pregnancy. This percentage of effectiveness makes it hardly worth the effort.

654. What does 97 percent effective mean?
It means three pregnancies will occur in every one hundred women per year; 99.9 percent effective means one pregnancy will occur in one thousand women in one year. Ninety-five percent effective means five pregnancies will occur per one hundred women in a year, or fifty pregnancies per thousand women in a year.

655. What is the effectiveness of the diaphragm?
The diaphragm is 95 percent effective when it is used. Leaving it out once may permit pregnancy.

656. What is the effectiveness of spermicidal jellies, creams, and suppositories?
These are 80 percent effective if used. Failure to use them once may permit pregnancy.

657. What is the effectiveness of the rhythm method?
The rhythm method is 40-60 percent effective if your menses are fairly regular. It is less effective if your menses are irregular.

658. What is the effectiveness of the condom as birth control?
If it is used before any coitus, it is 80 percent effective. If it is only used before ejaculation, it is 50 percent effective.

BIRTH CONTROL: CHANCES OF BECOMING PREGNANT; EFFECTIVENESS OF VARIOUS METHODS OF CONTRACEPTION
(Continued)

659. What is the effectiveness of withdrawal as a birth control method?

Withdrawal is only 50 percent effective.

660. What is the effectiveness of using the sponge as a birth control method?

The sponge is 85-90 percent effective when it is used.

661. What are the chances of becoming pregnant if I don't use any birth control at all?

The chances of becoming pregnant in any one menstrual cycle are considered to be about 20 percent if you are normally fertile. The chances of becoming pregnant from any one episode of coitus depends upon when it occurs in your cycle. The chances of becoming pregnant in one year are about 85 percent.

BIRTH CONTROL: COSTS OF VARIOUS METHODS OF CONTRACEPTION

662. What is the cost of birth control pills?

Birth control pills cost around $8.00 to $10.00 or more per month, plus the cost of an annual medical examination.

663. What is the cost of an IUD?

An IUD costs $35.00 to $50.00 including insertion, plus a medical fee every one to three years, depending upon how long it lasts. The Progestasert is designed to last one year, while copper-filled IUDs, like the Cu-7 or Cu-T, last three years. Plastic ones, like the Lippe's Loop or Saf-T-Coil, have no time limit.

664. What is the cost of a diaphragm?

The diaphragm costs $15.00 to $25.00, plus a medical fee for fitting. If you have a baby, you will need to be refitted.

665. What is the cost of foam, spermicidal jellies and creams, and suppositories?

Foams cost approximately $7.00 per container. Jellies and creams cost about $6.00 per container. All three hold twelve to fifteen applications. Twenty vaginal suppositories cost about $8.00.

666. What is the cost of condoms?

Each condom costs between $.40 and $1.50 and can only be used once.

667. What is the cost of Depo-Provera shots?

They cost $10.00 to $15.00 each, plus a medical fee at three- to six-month intervals.

BIRTH CONTROL: COSTS OF VARIOUS METHODS OF CONTRACEPTION (Continued)

668. What is the cost of a sponge?

"Today" brand sponges cost $1.00 each and can be used for twenty-four hours.

BIRTH CONTROL: TEENAGERS

669. Which would be the most acceptable and easiest contraceptive for a teenage girl to use?

Usually, the low-dose combination contraceptive pill is the most acceptable. It is the easiest to use and the most effective. This is primarily because it prevents pregnancy so well. In addition, it regulates the irregular menses that are so characteristic of teenage girls, reduces their cramps and heavy flow, controls acne, and even helps to prevent VD, such as gonorrhea or chlamydial infection, from infecting and damaging their tubes.

670. I am a teenager. Which is the best birth control method for me?

There is no one method of birth control that is best for teenage girls. You should find the methods that you are most motivated to use, and then choose the most effective one. Some parents, on the other hand, feel that the best method is complete abstinence, since they do not even approve of marriage, much less sex, for their teenage daughters. By their standards, they are correct; however, they must consider that they live in a different world than their daughters.

671. When should I start using birth control?

When you start to have sex. It is best for you to decide which form of contraceptive you will use before you decide to have sexual intercourse or even engage in "heavy petting," which could go astray.

672. Which methods of contraception require parental approval?

Laws requiring parental approval of medical care for minors vary in their interpretation from state to state, and sometimes from doctor to doctor. However, all states permit the purchase of contraceptive foams, creams, jellies, suppositories, sponges, and condoms, if you are tall enough to "look over the counter." California has a special law that permits contraception in all forms, except sterilization, to be given to sexually active minors without parental notification or consent. Federal law encourages, but does not yet require, the family-planning clinics that it funds to involve a teenager's family in contraceptive planning. As of this writing, the regulation requiring parental notification if a girl is given a prescription for a contraceptive (pills, IUD,

BIRTH CONTROL: TEENAGERS (Continued)

or diaphragm) is being disputed in the courts. Telephone the clinic or the doctor's office and ask before you go.

673. I am a teenager, without very much money. Where can I go if I don't want anyone to know that I am seeking birth control?

If you do not want anyone to know that you are seeking birth control, you can ask your physician to keep it in confidence. If you are afraid of exposure or lack funds for a private physician, an alternative would be to contact a family-planning clinic, such as Planned Parenthood. If the clinic is federally funded, a recent federal regulation requires them to notify your parents. This regulation is now stopped in the courts in a battle, but you should make sure the clinic is not required to notify your parents. Anyone can go the drugstore and buy condoms for the male and contraceptive foam for the female, which is 95 percent effective if both are used in combination. They also help prevent venereal disease.

674. What about the side effects associated with the pill; aren't they dangerous to a teenager's health?

Teenagers are usually so healthy that the dangers associated with contraceptive pills are rarely incurred. The low-dose pills have few side effects, yet they are just as effective as the old high-dose pills. Some girls stop taking birth control pills because they gain weight, but the low-dose pills don't really cause that much weight gain. During the teenage years, you should and do gain weight regardless of whether or not you take the pill. Nausea is a side effect occurring in a few teenagers that is not dangerous, but can be avoided by taking the pill at bedtime or changing to a lower dose. Dark spots on the face (chloasma) can be cleared by a fade cream if they occur, and they can be prevented by using a sunscreen, preferably one in your make-up. Using a sunscreen also will help to prevent wrinkles. The benefits of using the pill generally outweigh the other side effects.

675. With all of the birth control clinics and information available today, why are there still so many teenage pregnancies?

That question is constantly being studied, and various answers appear. One explanation is that we give teenagers double messages: 1) "Be sexy, but don't have babies"; 2) "Effective forms of contraception are dangerous, and safe ones don't work." Another answer is that their sexual frequency is so low, approximately seven times per year, that they will not make a constant effort at birth control, such as taking the pills all of the time, and they often underestimate their fertility. Also, many adults think that by frightening teenagers away from contraception, they will frighten them away from sex. Obviously, this does not work. Many people who work in the family-planning clinics feel that if the girls could accept themselves as sexual people,

BIRTH CONTROL: TEENAGERS (Continued)

then they could take charge of their fertility and control it. Many still feel that they should not appear to be prepared for sex and that it should be an overpowering experience that sweeps them away.

676. Is the use of withdrawal among teenagers a major reason for so many teenage pregnancies?

No, the major reason is the use of no contraceptive technique at all. Teenagers often have premature ejaculations and a difficult time with withdrawal. It is mostly adult men who think withdrawal is a good technique; little do they realize that sperm in concentrated drops leak out long before ejaculation.

BIRTH CONTROL: WHICH IS SAFEST AND BEST FOR ME?

677. How should I decide which type of birth control is best for me?

This depends upon how much you do not want to get pregnant and which type of contraception you will use regularly. If you find yourself failing to use a method, especially a barrier method (such as a diaphragm), you should consider changing to one that does not require thought at the time of sexual activity, such as the pill or IUD. If you forget the pill more than five days per month, you should probably use something else. Acquiring the art of using a method is not very easy; it is really rather difficult. You can understand why the masses of the world use no contraception whatsoever. No one really likes contraception. They just like it better than pregnancy or no sex at all. It is also easy to understand why the IUD has been a popular method with the masses in South America. They just put it in and leave it there. The complications are no worse than their frequent pregnancies without it. It requires no action on anyone's part after it is in.

678. Is birth control safe for everyone?

This sounds like a simple question, but actually it has several different meanings. "Safe" can refer to the amount of danger to a patient's health, or it can mean the degree of effectiveness. The problem in answering this question is that in many cases, the method of birth control that is the safest for your health may also be the most dangerous as far as effectiveness. If pregnancy is a danger to your health, then the problem is compounded, because the safest birth control becomes unsafe in the overall sense of the word. Other factors relating to this question include: how easy the method is to use, and how easy it is to forget.

679. Are there any methods of birth control that would be considered safe for everyone?

The condom is one form of birth control that is relatively safe for

BIRTH CONTROL: WHICH IS SAFEST AND BEST FOR ME?
(Continued)

everyone, but it is also relatively ineffective. It certainly is safe for the health of the woman, perhaps even the safest form of birth control, since it also tends to prevent the spread of venereal disease. However, it does not prevent pregnancy as well as some of the other methods of contraception.

680. I have high blood pressure. Which method of birth control would be the safest for me?

High blood pressure makes pregnancy dangerous, so you need a method of birth control that is highly effective and that will not aggravate your blood pressure. Birth control pills aggravate blood pressure in about 5 percent of women. This is a complicated problem, and requires more information than just knowing your blood pressure is high. Consult your doctor, but make your own decision.

681. Can a doctor tell me which method of birth control is best for my body?

No. Your doctor does not know your total life pattern or motivation, even after a one-hour interview. You are in charge of your body, and you should use your doctor as a consultant to give you information, pros and cons, on various methods and why they would be a problem or well suited for you. Then you choose.

682. Are different methods of birth control better for me at different times in my life?

Yes, this is certainly true. The pill seems most adapted to young women with their intense fertility, lack of medical problems, and great exposure to venereal disease. Women who have had children and are monogamous are suited for the IUD but may continue the pill if they are healthy. Sterilization is certainly reserved for when you want no more children. The diaphragm is a reliable method for when you have a predictable sex pattern, and you are motivated enough to use it. Other barrier contraceptives, such as foams and suppositories, are good temporary measures at various times and places. These are available worldwide, over the counter, and would be good to use when you stop taking the pill for a month before you want to get pregnant. Abstinence can fill a spot in your life, too, especially when you are seriously ill.

683. Is it best to stick with one birth control method or to experiment with several?

You may need to try several methods before you find one that suits your life-style, likes, and needs, and which you are able to stick with. Changing methods often is not harmful unless you fail to use a method properly.

684. What is the best age for a woman to take the pill?

The best time for a woman to take contraceptive pills is between the

If you make your own goals
If you adhere to your own values
If you choose your own kind of fun
You are living a life made by you
If other people are telling you what to do
or if you are copying other people's ways
or if you are acting out a certain lifestyle
    to impress people
You are living for other people
    rather than yourself

People should not control you
You must control your own life

— Susan Polis Schutz

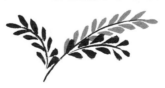

BIRTH CONTROL: WHICH IS SAFEST AND BEST FOR ME?
(Continued)

ages of fifteen and thirty-five. After thirty-five, you should take them only if you are a non-smoker and are in good general health.

685. Which is the best form of birth control for me to use after intercourse, if I didn't use anything before?

A very good protection, which is now being used, is to insert an IUD within seventy-two hours after intercourse, before the fertilized egg has a chance to implant. Another method, which some doctors suggest, is to use a high-dose birth control pill from the day after exposure until it is time for menses, with the hope that it will change the uterine lining so that the egg cannot implant. The "morning after pill" came into use many years ago and is about 98 percent effective. After an unprotected exposure to pregnancy, women are given 25 mg of diethylstilbestrol (DES) each day for five days, so it is really the "five morning after pills." However, it was discovered that taking DES in pregnancy causes vaginal cancer in the unborn child after she becomes a teenager, so the use of DES has stopped almost entirely. If it is taken and fails, an abortion should probably be performed.

BIRTH CONTROL: THE PILL

686. When and where was the pill first introduced?

The first large clinical trials, conducted on large numbers of women before the pill was on the market, were in Puerto Rico and Los Angeles in 1957. It was then released for general use by prescription in the United States in 1960.

687. Who invented the birth control pill?

Russell F. Marker, a chemist, discovered how to make large quantities of a progesterone from yams in Mexico. His process was not patented, and he eventually fell into oblivion, but his discovery is the basis for the ingredients of the pill. In 1950, the first chemical, norethindrone, was synthesized at the Syntex laboratories in Mexico. Gregory Pincus, long-time scientific consultant to G. D. Searle and Company in Chicago, was involved in the development that led to the marketing of the first pill, Enovid. The laboratories of Syntex actually developed the steroid hormones that were used and supplied other pharmaceutical companies throughout the world, who packaged them in their own formulas. Mr. Pincus and Dr. John Rock developed the clinical trials of the pill.

688. What are the ideal health conditions for being able to take the pill safely?

The ideal conditions are: that you are under age thirty-five, a non-

BIRTH CONTROL: THE PILL (Continued)

smoker, of normal weight, not sun sensitive, not easily nauseated, not diabetic, not hypertensive, never have headaches, and menstruate normally. These conditions are usually met by most women under thirty-five.

689. Is the pill more dangerous for women over forty years old?

Yes. It is more dangerous for women over the age of forty to take the pill, especially if they already have medical problems, such as high blood pressure, diabetes, obesity, smoking, and other conditions. The threat of clots (thromboembolism) and coronaries also increases with age and is somewhat more frequent in women who are using the pill. Pregnancy, however, is also dangerous to the health of these women.

690. Are there any advantages to women over forty years old in taking the pill?

Yes, there are advantages to women over forty taking a low-dose pill. Their menses are regulated, and they avoid the hemorrhages that often require a D & C (dilatation and curettage) during these years. Being on the pill for eight or ten years reduces the incidence of endometrial cancer of the uterus and ovarian cancer, both of which are problems in women over forty. Many women are adamant about their decision not to get pregnant at this age because of the risk to their health and possible abnormalities in the baby, so they enjoy the high protection of the pill. They often feel better on pills than they do on their own irregular cycles of hormone production. So, if you are over forty, do not smoke, are not hypertensive, diabetic, or obese, then although the risk of a coronary is still increased by the pill, it may be worth the risk if you do not have an extensive family history of coronaries. It would be well advised to have your blood levels of lipoproteins (blood fats) checked by a blood test. It can be your informed decision to take the pill.

691. When must I start taking birth control pills?

Birth control pills must be started after a normal menstrual period, after the delivery of a baby, after a miscarriage or abortion, or, if you are not having menses, after your doctor has assured you that you are not pregnant. The most important consideration before you start taking the pill is that you are not pregnant at the time at which you begin. If you want to be sure of not getting pregnant, you should also start them prior to having intercourse.

692. How long should I be taking the pill prior to sexual intercourse in order to be sure of not getting pregnant?

You are 97 percent safe from pregnancy the day after you first start taking the combination pill, provided you start right after a menstrual period. The following month, your safety from pregnancy increases to 99.9 percent. The minipill is 97 percent effective at all times.

BIRTH CONTROL: THE PILL (Continued)

693. When can I start taking birth control pills?

You can safely start within five to eight days of the beginning of a menstrual period. This means you can start on the fifth day of your menstrual flow (the old way) or on the Sunday following the beginning of your menstrual flow (the new way). If you start to menstruate on Sunday, you begin the pill on the following Sunday. If you start to menstruate on any other day, Monday through Saturday, you still start the pill the following Sunday, even if it is the next day. This way your flow will be mid-week, and you will always start a new box of pills on Sunday. It is easy to remember.

694. What should I do if I discover that I've forgotten to take one or more of my pills?

If you take two pills each day until you catch up to where you should be, then this should reduce the chances of pregnancy. If you stop the pills and wait for a menstrual period before restarting, you are likely to become pregnant from the sperm received before you stopped the pills.

695. What happens to my body when I forget to take my birth control pills?

At first, the hormone level in your body begins to drop, because you stopped taking the hormone, and this usually results in the loss of the lining of the uterus in the form of spotting or bleeding. Then the ovary recovers from its suppression and begins to form a follicle for an egg to ovulate, which takes one or two weeks, depending upon how far the follicle got before you stopped the pill. After it ovulates, you either become pregnant or have a menstrual flow two weeks later.

696. Are all of the different brands and types of birth control pills the same, or is one better to use than others?

No, not all brands of birth control pills are the same. Deciding which one is better depends upon which one suits you the best. There are three types of birth control pills: the high-dose combination, the low-dose combination, and the minipill. The high-dose pills have different amounts of progestin (progesterone) and estrogen than do the low-dose birth control pills. The minipill has only progestin (progesterone).

697. What does the high-dose combination contraceptive pill contain?

It contains 80 to 100 mg of estrogen and 1 to 2½ mg of progestin. Twenty or twenty-one days of pills are taken during your cycle.

698. What is the low-dose combination contraceptive pill made of?

It is made of 30 to 50 mg of estrogen and 1 mg or less of progestin. Twenty or twenty-one days of pills are taken during your cycle.

BIRTH CONTROL: THE PILL (Continued)

699. What is the minipill made of?

The minipill is made of only progestin. One pill is taken every day throughout your cycle.

700. How do birth control pills alter my body's chemistry?

Chemistry is a rather broad term. Birth control pills do not alter all of the chemistry and biochemistry of your body. They alter the steroid hormone levels of estrogen and progestins and they suppress the ovarian function. Some of these changes are far reaching—sometimes the effects are beneficial; sometimes they are not.

701. Do any chemical changes occur in my blood when I take the pill?

Yes, chemical changes in your blood can occur as a result of taking birth control pills. Some of the elements in the blood that are subject to chemical changes include: glucose, cholesterol, lipids, circulating thyroid, and many others. You would not be aware of these changes unless you happened to have a blood test, so it is important to inform your doctor that you are taking the pill, especially if you are having a blood test, as this information is necessary for correct interpretation of the test.

702. Are the hormones found in birth control pills the same as those that are sometimes prescribed during menopause?

The hormones prescribed for menopause are estrogens and progestins. These hormones are also found in birth control pills, but they are not the same. In general, the menopause hormones are much lower in dosage, and the progestin is much weaker.

703. Could birth control pills be taken during menopause to control the problems and symptoms?

Birth control pills will control the symptoms and problems of menopause, but most physicians feel that they contain hormones that are too high in dosage. In older women, this would increase the chances of a heart attack. In young women whose ovaries have been removed, birth control pills would be fine to control the symptoms of menopause.

704. How does the pill hormone cycle differ from my own natural cycle?

Estrogen is only produced during the first half of your own cycle; on the pill, both estrogen and progesterone are present during the entire cycle. In your own cycle, there is an estrogen and a luteinizing hormone (LH) surge mid-cycle, but this is absent during the second half of your own cycle. On the pill, you just gradually accumulate more estrogen and progesterone throughout the three weeks you are taking the pills, and there is no mid-cycle surge.

BIRTH CONTROL: THE PILL (Continued)

705. How does the pill prevent ovulation?

It supplies the estrogen and progestin to the blood stream that goes to the pituitary gland and, by a feedback mechanism, convinces the pituitary gland that there are enough hormones, so it stops signaling the ovaries to produce hormones. The ovaries stop producing hormones by stopping the development of the little cyst or follicle that contains the egg, so that it is never released. Instead, it just wastes away or forms a little white scar.

706. Are birth control pills safe for women who have breast cysts?

Yes. They are also beneficial, because they tend to reduce fibrocystic breasts, and by reducing the cysts, they help to avoid the biopsies that are sometimes necessary. Pills prevent other benign lesions of the breast as well.

707. How will I know if the pill I am using is the right one for me?

If you feel no different after you take them than you did before and you can detect no change, the pill you are using is the right one for you because it matches your own hormonal pattern. However, you often want to accomplish other things than just contraception: you may want to reduce acne, increase breast size, reduce menstrual flow, regulate the timing of the flow, and reduce mentrual cramps. To accomplish these, you may have to try several different types of birth control pills. You should report to your doctor or clinic any changes that occur and change the pill according to their directions until you have obtained the best possible result. All forms of the pill keep you from becoming pregnant. Of course, you should also change pills when noxious side effects, such as nausea or vomiting, occur.

708. Have the newer forms of the pill succeeded in eliminating water retention?

Lower doses have reduced, but will never absolutely eliminate, water retention. All female hormones make women retain water, whether you take them artifically or produce them on your own. Only if all of your female hormones are removed, as by surgical removal of the ovaries or by menopause, will water retention go away. Water retention is a harmless, feminine trait; don't try to get rid of it.

709. Does going off the pill make a woman extra fertile?

Not really. Most women do not realize how fertile they really are, and it is common for them to underestimate their chances of becoming pregnant. That is why women take so many chances with getting pregnant, and have to have a million abortions per year. Women should consider themselves extremely fertile until proven otherwise. The first month in which you stop using any contraceptive, you will have a 20-25 percent chance of getting pregnant.

BIRTH CONTROL: THE PILL (Continued)

710. Is it absolutely necessary for a woman to have a medical examination before being given birth control pills?

Of course, the pill will certainly work without the medical examination. Throughout the world, in overpopulated countries, it is given without any medical examination or supervision. There it is felt that the few dangers of the pill are far outweighed by the elimination of many pregnancies and the serious dangers of pregnancy. In the United States, a prescription is given only after a medical examination by a physician, because it is felt that it is far safer to administer it that way, and people can afford to do so. In Hong Kong, cards containing a month's supply of birth control pills are sold over the counter. The cards include instructions printed in six different languages and cost only one dollar.

711. Besides reducing the incidence of ovarian and uterine cancer, does the pill help to combat any other diseases, such as arthritis or colon cancer?

It does not help to combat colon cancer; only eating bran daily can do that. Those who have been on the pill for ten years do exhibit a decreased incidence of rheumatoid arthritis. Endometriosis (small cysts) is reduced or even prevented by the pill. Ovulation cysts, which have caused so much surgery for women, are completely prevented. Anemia is prevented, because there is so little blood loss. There is a reduction of benign tumors of the breasts, usually fibrocystic, in women on the pill, so there are far fewer biopsies of the breasts. It also prevents venereal disease, such as gonorrhea and chlamydial infection, from going up into the tubes and ovaries and forming abscesses (pelvic inflammatory disease). You may still get the venereal disease, but it is not so bad or so damaging to your female organs. The fact that taking the pill for at least eight to ten years reduces the incidence of ovarian and endometrial (uterine) cancer by half is indeed good news. Previously, the only way to prevent these two forms of cancer was to have a lot of babies.

712. Can I safely go back on the pill after I've discontinued using it for a while, perhaps one year?

Yes. There is no danger in starting and stopping pills, except for the danger of getting pregnant while you are off the pill. Many servicemen's wives and fishermen's wives go off and on the pill several times during the year when their husbands are away for several months. Some may even go off for years at a time. However, if your husband is only gone a few weeks, it isn't worth the trouble of stopping and hoping a menstrual period will occur just at the right time, so the pill can be started again before your husband returns.

BIRTH CONTROL: THE PILL AND ITS SIDE EFFECTS

713. What physical complications accompany the pill?

If you are healthy, usually no complications accompany the pill. The pill has been studied extensively for twenty-five years, and therefore a great deal is known about it. If you listed the complications associated with aspirin, it also would be frightening. The most common occurrences with the pill are a reduction in menstrual flow and cramps. The most common objectionable symptom is nausea. This is very infrequent on the low-dose pills but still possible, especially on the first cycle. Breast tenderness and enlargement, especially in young girls, is sometimes aggravating. Dark spotting on the face when in the sun, called chloasma, occurs in about 5 percent of women, who are sun sensitive. Perhaps one woman in ten thousand has an actual clotting problem, usually in the legs, that can result in a clot traveling to her lungs (embolism), which can be serious.

714. What percentage of women experience side effects from the pill?

There is a different percentage of women for each side effect. The majority of women experience no side effects, except for the reduction in menstrual flow.

715. How long can I take the pill before my chances of incurring harmful side effects increase?

Most of the side effects occur in the first month you take them. Clots and embolisms are as likely the first month as they are the twentieth year. The only rare side effect that seems to occur after years of use is the benign tumor of the liver (hepatoma). Increase in coronary heart attacks is more frequent as you become older, especially after you reach thirty-five, and if you begin to smoke heavily, become diabetic, hypertensive, or very overweight. If you have these problems, it doesn't matter how long you have been on the pill as much as it does how old you are.

716. What are the consequences of taking the pill for over eight to ten years?

There are good and bad consequences. Some of the best consequences are a reduction in the risk of cancer of the uterus (endometrium) and cancer of the ovary. These are significant. However, there are also bad consequences. The possibility of the occurrence of a benign tumor of the liver (hepatoma) is increased when you take the pill for a longer period of time and perhaps by taking higher doses of estrogen as well. This hepatoma will reverse itself when the pill is stopped, but if it is not discovered and you do not stop the pill, the tumor can rupture or hemorrhage and result in death. This condition is very rare, with perhaps a total of two hundred cases reported in the United States. If you do not take the pill at all, this tumor is extremely rare. This is one of the reasons for you to have an annual physical examination if you are on the pill.

BIRTH CONTROL: THE PILL AND ITS SIDE EFFECTS
(Continued)

717. When I'm on the pill, my breasts are very tender, I feel bloated, and I'm irritable. Why?

You are sensitive to the estrogen in the pill. Estrogen makes your breasts tender, and slight nausea produces gas in your bowel, or bloating. The irritability is harder to account for, unless it comes from the slight nausea or breast pain. Irritability during premenstrual tension also is hard to explain and may be due to the same reasons. Perhaps your pill has too high a dosage of estrogen for you. You could try a lower-dose estrogen pill, or the minipill, which contains no estrogen at all.

718. Why do I gain weight when I'm taking birth control pills?

If the steroid hormones in the pill are greater in quantity than those that you usually produce, you will retain more water than usual, and this accounts for the extra weight you see on the scale. If the pill nauseates you slightly, and you discover that eating frequently makes the nausea go away, then you will eat frequently and gain weight. Taking estrogen and progesterone tends to make women gain weight slightly, but not more than five pounds. If the pill contains a greater quantity of these hormones than you normally produce, you will have an even greater tendency to gain weight. Contraception is often started at the same time as a change in life style and a change in eating style, which may produce a weight gain.

719. What percentage of women gain weight when they take the pill?

Actual studies show that one-fourth of the women who take birth control pills lose weight, another one-fourth gain weight, and the rest stay about the same. This is especially true of the new low-dose pills.

720. I understand that there is a newer version of the pill that is safer. Is this true?

It is probable that all of the low-dose pills that contain 35 mg of estrogen are safer than the older pills that contained 50, 80, or 100 mg of estrogen. However, you may be referring to the minipill, which has no estrogen at all. Because it contains no estrogen, it may be safer to your health and have fewer side effects, but it is not as effective in preventing pregnancy. However, it is a good choice for women who cannot tolerate estrogen.

721. Have any long-term problems arisen in women who took the early high-dosage birth control pills?

If these women developed gallstones while they were on the high-dose pills, then they will still have an increased tendency to have gallstones. Some studies also indicate that an increased tendency for coronaries is present for many years afterward, but these are very small in number.

BIRTH CONTROL: THE PILL AND ITS SIDE EFFECTS
(Continued)

722. Have any problems arisen among the children of women who took the early high-dosage birth control pills?

No. Problems have not occurred in children of women who took the early high-dosage pills. Limb defects were reported in six male children of women who took the pill **while** they were pregnant, but these had been attributed to the progesterone in the pill; newer studies deny that there is any connection at all.

723. Is it a must to go off the pill periodically in order to let my body "rest" from the effect of the pill?

No. There is no reason to do this. If you do, you run a great danger of becoming pregnant, because you probably are not skilled at using other contraceptives. If you have developed some medical problem, it may be advisable to go off the pills to see if the problem is affected, but only if your doctor thinks it may be related. And then, if it is not related, you should go right back on. Your body does not "rest" when you go off the pills; it "rests" while you are on them. When you go off, it goes back to work producing the hormones you have been supplying for the body. Another reason given for going off the pills is to see if your body still works—if you still ovulate and menstruate. If you consider yourself to be in menopause, this is one way to find out.

724. Will my period come right back after I stop taking the pill?

Yes, most women will have a period within six weeks. A delay in resuming menses after stopping the pills (post-pill amenorrhea), occurs mostly in women who had irregular menses before they took the pill. However, menses will return sooner or later by themselves. If you are in a hurry, they can be brought back sooner by fertility pills.

725. Can the pill cause future problems in childbearing, such as physical or emotional problems with the baby or problems in pregnancy?

No. The pill has no effect on pregnancy or the child if the mother stops taking it prior to getting pregnant. Studies indicate that fertility, childbearing results, and malformations are not influenced, decreased or increased, by the pill.

726. Does the birth control pill make it harder or easier to reach orgasm?

No survey has ever really been done on the effect birth control pills have on orgasm. Most sex therapists have found that patients who do not want a baby have a better sexual response and reach orgasm more easily when they are confident that they will not become pregnant and are,

BIRTH CONTROL: THE PILL AND ITS SIDE EFFECTS
(Continued)

therefore, more relaxed about their bodily function. Thus, a woman's sexual responsiveness depends upon how she feels about getting pregnant and not what method of contraception she is using. Women who would really like to have a baby, but are forced by their partner or by economic circumstances to take the pill, are often less sexually responsive. These women also are less responsive when they use an IUD or any other reliable method of contraception. Women who are taking the pill because they do not want to get pregnant, which is why the majority of women take them, probably are more sexually responsive.

727. Does the pill affect other parts of my body? For instance, I was told that hormonal changes caused by the pill can change the shape of my eyes, thereby making it difficult to wear contact lenses. Could this be true?

The estrogen and progestin hormones affect all parts of the body, and therefore the pill can, too. The shape of your eyes is not actually changed, but the secretions and tearing of your eyes may be slightly different. This has been blamed for the difficulties among contact lens wearers. However, many people who are not on the pill also have problems tolerating contact lenses, and many people on the pill wear contact lenses with no problems at all. You might want to make sure that your lenses fit properly.

728. Will birth control pills prevent VD?

No, birth control pills do not prevent VD, but they do tend to keep the infection in the vagina and out of the tubes, thus preventing a complication of VD, called pelvic inflammatory disease.

729. Can the pill cause an abnormal Pap smear?

No, abnormal Pap smears are not caused by the pill. Pap smears show changes in the nucleus of the cell. Infections cause this, not birth control pills. It also can come from having sex. This is why women who do not have sex do not ever need a Pap smear.

730. Are birth control pills more dangerous for smokers?

Yes, but the real danger is smoking. Women who smoke greatly increase their chances of having a coronary more than women who just take the pill. But taking the pill and smoking, too, is more dangerous than just smoking.

731. Is it all right to take birth control pills if I have a thyroid problem?

Yes. There is no thyroid problem that is affected by taking birth control pills. Some of the thyroid tests are affected by being on the pills, and your doctor may want you to stop taking them just while you are being tested, but not necessarily while you are being treated.

BIRTH CONTROL: THE PILL AND ITS SIDE EFFECTS
(Continued)

732. If there is a history of cancer in my family, should I take birth control pills?

If there is a history of ovarian cancer or uterine (endometrial) cancer, then you should take birth control pills for at least eight to ten years just to protect yourself from having these kinds of cancer that do tend to be hereditary. There is no cancer that would make it necessary for you to avoid using the pill. Breast cancer is common—one out of ten women develop it—but it is not a reason to avoid birth control pills. There is no increase in breast cancer among women who are taking the pill.

733. Have there been any proven links between use of the pill and cancer?

No, there has been no documented evidence linking any form of cancer to the use of birth control pills. However, there may be some indirect explanations for this link. Cancer of the cervix occurs only in sexually active women, and since few people use contraception without having sex, this form of cancer is more common among women who use contraception than it is among Catholic nuns, for instance. Active young women tend to be out in the sun a lot and are most likely to take the pill. Such women also seem to have a few more skin cancers (melanomas) than indoor sedentary people. There is no evidence of an increase in breast cancer among users of the pill. There is a documented reduction in the incidence of ovarian cancer and uterine (endometrial) cancer among women who have used the pill for at least eight to ten years during their lives. This good news has only been publicized in the last two years.

734. Does the pill cause strokes in women?

There is no longer found to be an increase in strokes, hemorrhages, or brain clots in women who are on the pill. Earlier surveys suggested this was true, but later, larger studies, such as the Kaiser Study, did not show an increase. Perhaps this is because now the pill is no longer given to women who are likely to have strokes, such as women with severe hypertension or diabetes. The doses are also smaller now.

735. Does the pill cause depression in some women?

Yes. It also relieves premenstrual syndrome depression in some women by changing to a steady hormone supply, instead of a sudden surge at the end of their cycles. Depression on the pill has been studied and is sometimes related to frustration associated with the desire for children; when this is true, even the IUD causes depression. But some depression seems to be related to the progesterone that is present all month long in women who are taking the pill, in higher quantities than the women themselves produce. Sometimes the woman was depressed anyway, but now talks about it, because she can point to the pill as a casual factor.

BIRTH CONTROL: THE PILL AND ITS SIDE EFFECTS
(Continued)

Even yeast infections can be transmitted from a partner, according to some doctors.

740. Are headaches still a common side effect of the pill?

Yes, but less than they used to be with the high-dose pills. Headaches are common, and certainly can occur without being a side effect of the pill. Only if headaches occur in the week just prior to your period, when the hormones are high, do they relate to the pill, especially if they are migraine in type. People who have this side effect can change to the minipill, which is a small dose of progestin taken every day, not in a cycle. It is 97 percent instead of 99.9 percent effective, but that is better than any other birth control method.

741. Why does the pill make me dizzy?

If the pill makes you nauseous and tired and especially if these symptoms cause you to not eat, then you can become dizzy because of hypoglycemia (low blood sugar). Eating frequently can overcome this, but it can also possibly make you fat. If you eat small portions of high-protein meals, you can solve both problems.

742. Have there been any long-term studies on the pill that prove that it is a safe form of birth control?

The original studies and trials that began in 1957 are still continuing, so they have now been underway for twenty-seven years. So far the studies show pills to be safe. In fact, the current medical literature concludes that the beneficial results far exceed the infrequent bad results for most women. Some women have a higher risk for these bad results and are excluded from taking the pill. This is the main benefit of having a medical examination before taking the pill.

743. Why does the pill make my breasts bigger?

If it makes your breasts bigger (and it certainly doesn't always do that), it means that the hormones in the pill are in greater supply than the hormones you usually produce; therefore, they stimulate the growth of the ducts and other tissues, as well as fat deposition. If you gain weight on the pill, this is even more likely.

744. Do birth control pills cause varicose veins?

No, they do not cause varicose veins, and they do not make them worse. But people who have varicose veins are more likely to develop clots and embolisms (clots traveling to their lungs) than people who don't, and pills slightly elevate your chances of this. The elevation is so small that if you are not over thirty-five and overweight it is usually ignored.

BIRTH CONTROL: THE PILL AND ITS SIDE EFFECTS
(Continued)

736. Isn't it dangerous to tamper with hormone levels, as the pill does?

To assume this attitude is to say that mankind should never practice medicine or do anything to control their bodies. There is danger in everything you do. It might be dangerous not to have babies all the time, because not having babies may lead to endometriosis, fibroids, ovarian cancer, uterine cancer, breast cancer, and anemia. But having babies all the time is leading the world, as well as individual lives, to disaster.

737. What would happen if I took too high a dose of hormones?

The first symptom would probably be nausea and vomiting, although high doses are sometimes well tolerated. High dosages of hormones are considered to increase certain bad side effects of the pill, mainly increased clotting with embolism, increased coronary artery disease, increased facial spotting (chloasma), and increased water retention and its symptoms.

738. Does taking birth control pills stimulate hair growth, particularly on the face, arms, and legs?

No. The result is just the opposite. All birth control pills tend to suppress ovarian production of testosterone and testosterone-like compounds (male hormones) that increase hair growth on the legs, arms, and face. Some do a better job than others, because they contain more estrogen or the progestin that they contain is more effective in this way. There is one pill available in Europe, but not yet in the United States, marketed as "Diane," that will almost completely eliminate excess hair on the face, chest, and arms, as well as get rid of severe acne. Hopefully, this pill will soon be available in the United States for women who suffer embarrassment from excessive body hair.

739. Does the pill create more mucus in the vagina and therefore make it easier to get a vaginal infection?

There has been much discussion of this, but the idea that the pill causes vaginal infections is probably dying out. It certainly can change the consistency of the vaginal discharge, and for this reason it was blamed primarily for an increase in yeast infections (fungus, Monilia or Candida albicans). But little girls with no hormones at all have terrible yeast infections, as do postmenopausal women, and women who stop taking the pill do not have fewer infections. It is drastic to treat a yeast infection by discontinuing a very good contraceptive. It is better to treat the yeast infection directly and prevent it by taking vaginal medication than it is to stop the pill. The pill is associated with intercourse, and intercourse makes a yeast infection feel terrible. All other vaginal infections are completely unrelated to the pill, but very much related to infection during intercourse from an infected partner.

BIRTH CONTROL: THE PILL AND ITS SIDE EFFECTS
(Continued)

Even yeast infections can be transmitted from a partner, according to some doctors.

740. Are headaches still a common side effect of the pill?

Yes, but less than they used to be with the high-dose pills. Headaches are common, and certainly can occur without being a side effect of the pill. Only if headaches occur in the week just prior to your period, when the hormones are high, do they relate to the pill, especially if they are migraine in type. People who have this side effect can change to the minipill, which is a small dose of progestin taken every day, not in a cycle. It is 97 percent instead of 99.9 percent effective, but that is better than any other birth control method.

741. Why does the pill make me dizzy?

If the pill makes you nauseous and tired and especially if these symptoms cause you to not eat, then you can become dizzy because of hypoglycemia (low blood sugar). Eating frequently can overcome this, but it can also possibly make you fat. If you eat small portions of high-protein meals, you can solve both problems.

742. Have there been any long-term studies on the pill that prove that it is a safe form of birth control?

The original studies and trials that began in 1957 are still continuing, so they have now been underway for twenty-seven years. So far the studies show pills to be safe. In fact, the current medical literature concludes that the beneficial results far exceed the infrequent bad results for most women. Some women have a higher risk for these bad results and are excluded from taking the pill. This is the main benefit of having a medical examination before taking the pill.

743. Why does the pill make my breasts bigger?

If it makes your breasts bigger (and it certainly doesn't always do that), it means that the hormones in the pill are in greater supply than the hormones you usually produce; therefore, they stimulate the growth of the ducts and other tissues, as well as fat deposition. If you gain weight on the pill, this is even more likely.

744. Do birth control pills cause varicose veins?

No, they do not cause varicose veins, and they do not make them worse. But people who have varicose veins are more likely to develop clots and embolisms (clots traveling to their lungs) than people who don't, and pills slightly elevate your chances of this. The elevation is so small that if you are not over thirty-five and overweight it is usually ignored.

BIRTH CONTROL: THE PILL AND ITS SIDE EFFECTS
(Continued)

736. Isn't it dangerous to tamper with hormone levels, as the pill does?

To assume this attitude is to say that mankind should never practi medicine or do anything to control their bodies. There is danger everything you do. It might be dangerous not to have babies all the tim because not having babies may lead to endometriosis, fibroids, ovari cancer, uterine cancer, breast cancer, and anemia. But having babies all t time is leading the world, as well as individual lives, to disaster.

737. What would happen if I took too high a dose of hormones?

The first symptom would probably be nausea and vomiting, althou high doses are sometimes well tolerated. High dosages of hormones are co sidered to increase certain bad side effects of the pill, mainly increas clotting with embolism, increased coronary artery disease, increased fac spotting (chloasma), and increased water retention and its symptoms.

738. Does taking birth control pills stimulate hair growth, particularly on t face, arms, and legs?

No. The result is just the opposite. All birth control pills tend to su press ovarian production of testosterone and testosterone-like compoun (male hormones) that increase hair growth on the legs, arms, and face. Son do a better job than others, because they contain more estrogen or the pr gestin that they contain is more effective in this way. There is one available in Europe, but not yet in the United States, marketed as "Diane that will almost completely eliminate excess hair on the face, chest, a arms, as well as get rid of severe acne. Hopefully, this pill will soon available in the United States for women who suffer embarrassment fr excessive body hair.

739. Does the pill create more mucus in the vagina and therefore mak easier to get a vaginal infection?

There has been much discussion of this, but the idea that the pill ca vaginal infections is probably dying out. It certainly can change the sistency of the vaginal discharge, and for this reason it was blamed prim: for an increase in yeast infections (fungus, Monilia or Candida albicans). little girls with no hormones at all have terrible yeast infections, a postmenopausal women, and women who stop taking the pill do not fewer infections. It is drastic to treat a yeast infection by discontinuing a good contraceptive. It is better to treat the yeast infection directly and vent it by taking vaginal medication than it is to stop the pill. The associated with intercourse, and intercourse makes a yeast infection fee rible. All other vaginal infections are completely unrelated to the pill very much related to infection during intercourse from an infected pa

BIRTH CONTROL: THE PILL AND ITS SIDE EFFECTS
(Continued)

745. Could taking birth control pills cause high blood pressure?

In about 5 percent of the women who go on birth control pills, their blood pressure rises; when they go off, it comes down again. It is not a permanent change, but it is dangerous enough to warrant using another method of birth control.

746. Why does the pill cause blood clots in some women?

The pill changes the clotting mechanism in the blood just slightly, but enough to make a serious difference in about 1 in 25,000 women on the pill. Some studies do not show an increase in clots traveling to the lungs (thromboembolism) in thousands using the pill, and others do. It is not a settled question.

BIRTH CONTROL: THE PILL, MENSTRUATION, AND SPOTTING

747. Is it common to occasionally miss a period when taking birth control pills?

Yes. On the old high-dose pills, it was estimated that one in two hundred women would miss a period each month. With the low-dose pills, which are available now, it seems to be more frequent. There is no harm to the health in missing a period, but it makes women wonder if they are pregnant. In designing pills, many researchers thought it would be good to eliminate periods partially or altogether, but they realized women would have to have a lot more pregnancy tests if they did.

748. Why do I spot if I'm a few hours late taking my pill?

You may be on such a low-dose pill, that missing a boost of hormones by only a few hours lets the lining of the uterus start to shed. You also may have a raw place on your cervix that bleeds more easily than the rest when the hormone level drops. It is not dangerous to spot, just messy. You can have your cervix checked, change the pill, or even have a D & C (dilatation and curettage) to find out if you have a polyp inside your uterus, which bleeds easily when your hormone level drops.

749. What is breakthrough bleeding with the pill?

It is a small loss of blood (spotting) during the twenty-one days when you are taking the pill, even though the pill is designed so that you will not bleed at all. It can be due to some problem in your cervix or uterus that is unrelated to the pill, or it can be because the dosage of the pill is so low that your hormone level drops a little, especially at mid-cycle when you take the tenth pill.

BIRTH CONTROL: THE PILL, MENSTRUATION, AND SPOTTING
(Continued)

750. How will taking birth control pills change my menstrual cycle?

If you have a light flow for three days every twenty-eight days, your cycle will not really change. If you have any other pattern of flow, it will usually change to a light flow for three days every twenty-eight days, if you take the pills correctly. If you have severe cramps, they will be reduced. If you have absolutely no feeling with menstruation, you may for the first time feel some mild cramping with the pill periods.

751. When I am on the birth control pill, I can't tell where my body is in my menstrual cycle. For instance, I used to always know when I ovulated; however, when I am on the birth control pill, I can't tell. Why?

The reason that you can't tell where you are in your menstrual cycle when you are on the pill is because you no longer have your own menstrual cycle. You do not feel ovulation because the pill suppresses ovulation, nor do you feel the surges in hormones that you used to have. Instead, you just feel a steady increase in hormones from taking the same pill every day.

BIRTH CONTROL: THE PILL AND PREGNANCY

752. Why do some women have a difficult time getting pregnant after using birth control pills for a considerable length of time?

Women who have been on birth control pills do not have a harder time becoming pregnant than women who have been on any other form of contraception for a considerable length of time. Time makes women older, and women older than thirty-five have a decreased fertility, regardless of what contraceptive they used. If they also have acquired infections that harm the reproductive organs, these must be overcome before they can get pregnant. Women who have been on any good contraceptive may not realize they are not very fertile, because they have never tried to become pregnant before. Many times it is the male partner's problem that makes it hard for the woman to become pregnant. Infections and other problems that have gone uncorrected can reduce his fertility and sperm count. If you have not used a contraceptive for four months and are not pregnant, you should speak to your doctor about this.

753. If I've been taking birth control pills for a while, how long will I have to be off of them in order to get pregnant?

Four months off the pill, with adequate sexual activity, will get 80 percent of women pregnant. It is suggested that you have at least one menstrual period on your own without the pills before you try to get pregnant. This is because you will have a more accurate due date based on your own menstrual period, rather than one based on a pill withdrawal period. It is not

BIRTH CONTROL: THE PILL AND PREGNANCY (Continued)

because getting pregnant this soon would be harmful to the baby. There is no increase in miscarriages or malformations even if you get pregnant right after stopping the pill.

754. How long after I stop taking birth control pills should I wait before getting pregnant in order to assure no birth defects in my unborn child?

Birth control pills do not cause birth defects in a baby, so there is no amount of time required for this. There also is no way to assure there will be no birth defects in your child. However, it helps if you have no birth defects in your family history or in the father's family. Also, while trying to become pregnant and while you are pregnant, you can avoid taking medication, alcohol, caffeine, and cigarettes, and you can eat well, take plenty of B vitamins, and undergo no anesthesia or X-rays.

755. What danger would there be if I started taking birth control pills and later discovered that I was actually pregnant at the time? Could birth control pills cause birth defects in my baby?

There is really not much danger at all. The progesterone in the pill was previously given to prevent miscarriage, and the estrogen was given to stop bleeding in early pregnancy. Actually neither one worked very well, but no great harm occurred, as long as the estrogen was not DES (the "morning after pill"). There was one study of six boys with limb defects whose mothers had had some progesterone during early pregnancy, and for a while it was blamed as the cause, but subsequent large studies of progesterone and even estrogen given in early pregnancy (other than DES) show that there is no increase in abnormalities of the baby. There have been pregnancies in which women have taken the pill for as long as seven months of their pregnancies, and the baby has been just fine. It is certainly a waste of money to buy pills to prevent pregnancy when you are already pregnant. Therefore, you should start birth control pills when you are sure that you are not pregnant, such as right after a menstrual period, or right after delivering a baby, or a miscarriage, or an abortion. It is also recommended that women not take birth control pills or any other medication while pregnant unless approved by their physician.

756. Does the pill cause multiple births?

No, age causes this. The older you are, the more likely you are to have multiple births. If you use the pill as you get older and before you have children, there will be an increase in multiple births due to age, but not due to the type of contraception.

757. What are the chances of never being able to have children as the result of taking birth control pills?

Never being able to have children does not occur as a direct result of

BIRTH CONTROL: THE PILL AND PREGNANCY (Continued)

taking birth control pills. However, the danger that something will happen to make you irreversibly infertile increases the longer you live. It also increases if you have sexual intercourse with many different partners, making you likely to get venereal disease, especially pelvic inflammatory disease (PID).

758. Have there been any reported problems among the children of women who took birth control pills right up to the time of becoming pregnant?

No. At first there were studies that suggested an increase in twinning and an increase in miscarriages among women who took birth control pills right up to the time of becoming pregnant. However, subsequent studies indicate a perfectly normal incidence of both twins and miscarriages.

BIRTH CONTROL: THE DIAPHRAGM

759. How does the diaphragm work?

The diaphragm works by covering the cervix and the whole top of the vagina with a round plastic sheet that has a tight rim, is covered with spermicidal cream, and fits against the vaginal walls. It prevents sperm from reaching and entering the cervix before entering the tubes and fertilizing the egg. You should leave it in place for eight hours after intercourse, since sperm die in the vagina in six hours, especially with the spermicidal jelly there.

760. How can I maximize the effectiveness of my diaphragm?

Follow these directions:
1. Have it well fitted, and refitted if you gain or lose weight or get pregnant.
2. Use it every time!
3. Insert it less than one hour before coitus.
4. Use a good cream or jelly around the rim and in the center.
5. Check for proper placement.
6. If you have coitus a second time, check the placement and add more cream or jelly.
7. Leave it in for at least eight hours after the last coitus.
8. **Do not** douche. Douching forces sperm up into the uterus on a jet stream, even if they were too weak to swim there alone.
9. Use a condom, practice withdrawal, or even abstain from intercourse during your fertile time.

761. Can the diaphragm be as effective as the pill if used conscientiously?

No. Nothing is as effective as the conscientious use of the combination contraceptive pill, which has only 0.1 percent failure rate. That is why it has brought about a sexual revolution. Other contraceptives always have al-

BIRTH CONTROL: THE DIAPHRAGM (Continued)

lowed pregnancies, and when abortion was illegal this really changed the pattern of women's lives. A conscientious diaphragm user will still have to face a 5 percent chance of pregnancy each year (five out of one hundred women per year will get pregnant). An unwanted pregnancy now can be terminated by a legal abortion, but you must add to the cost of the diaphragm the cost of a possible abortion. If you do not want an abortion and do not want a child under any circumstances, you will have a problem with using the diaphragm for contraception due to its 5 percent failure rate.

762. How can I be fitted for a diaphragm?

You will need to have a pelvic examination performed by a physician or specially trained nurse practitioner. They will place fitting diaphragms or rings into your vagina until they find one that fits properly, so that it will work and be comfortable. You should then learn to insert and remove it, and you should be checked to be sure that you are doing it right. This can be done in a private physician's office or in a contraceptive clinic.

763. What sizes do diaphragms come in?

The size is measured by the diameter of the ring, ranging from 60 mm to 95 mm. (25 mm is equivalent to about one inch.)

764. What is the average, or most common, diaphragm size?

The average diaphragm size is 75 mm.

765. Will the size of my diaphragm ever change?

If you gain or lose twenty-five pounds or have a baby, your diaphragm should be refitted, regardless of how long you have had it. If you were fitted as a virgin, it should be refitted in a few months after you begin sexual activity, because your vagina may have enlarged. Of course, if it has failed, it should also be refitted.

766. How often must I be fitted for a diaphragm?

There is no regular interval for a diaphragm fitting. If you were fitted after you were sexually active and your diaphragm has never failed, and if you have not had a baby since you were fitted, or gained or lost twenty-five pounds, you probably still wear the same size.

767. How much does a diaphragm cost? How many should I have?

The cost depends on where you go to get it. It may be free in a subsidized contraceptive clinic. The cost of a diaphragm in a drug store ranges from $10.00 to $15.00. You might want one spare in case your other one tears, especially while you are traveling.

768. How can I check to see if my diaphragm is okay?

Look for tears near the rim, and fill it with water to see if it leaks. Tears

BIRTH CONTROL: THE DIAPHRAGM (Continued)

usually occur because your fingernail catches the diaphragm near the rim when you remove it from your vagina. If this happens, be sure to get a new diaphragm before the next coitus.

769. How long does a diaphragm last?

With proper care, a diaphragm should last at least two years. Of course, if you seldom use it, it will last much longer.

770. What is the difference between the various kinds of diaphragms available today?

Some are flat when folded. These are best inserted with a plastic holder to be sure they go behind the cervix, especially if the rim is soft. Some have a spring in the outer ring to hold the shape firmly; others arc or bow when folded so they will go behind the cervix with ease. Some diaphragms fold in any direction, others fold only in one direction, which makes them hard to remove if they turn around inside the vagina.

771. Are there any disposable diaphragms on the market today?

No. With features such as a spring in the rim, they probably are too well made to be produced cheaply enough to be disposable.

772. How do I put in a diaphragm using the hand method?

Most women are taught the hand method of insertion for the arcing type of diaphragm. When folded, these form an arc or bow, instead of folding flat. First you cover the inside, outside, and rim of the diaphragm with spermicidal jelly or cream. Then fold the diaphragm, point it downward into the vagina, just as you do a tampon, and push it all the way in, tucking the rim up behind the pubic bone. Feel the cervix with your longest finger, and see that it has rubber over it. If not, remove the diaphragm and try again. If it hurts, you should also remove it and try again.

773. What kinds of diaphragms are best inserted with a plastic inserter?

Diaphragms that are flat when they are folded can best be inserted with a plastic inserter. The inserter fits into the diaphragm and keeps it extended so that you can be sure of placing it behind the cervix.

774. How do you apply the cream or jelly with the diaphragm?

Squeeze out about an inch of spermicidal jelly or cream, and spread it with your fingers all over the top, bottom, and rim of the diaphragm. You do not need to completely fill the cup with jelly or cream, but just be sure that there is plenty there.

775. What does the jelly or cream do?

It kills sperm that escape past the diaphragm rim before they reach the cervix. It also lubricates the vagina for coitus.

BIRTH CONTROL: THE DIAPHRAGM (Continued)

776. How long must I keep the diaphragm in after intercourse?

Your diaphragm should be kept in for eight hours after intercourse. Most sperm live six hours in the vagina, but some may live longer. If you remove the diaphragm right away, live sperm will still be able to enter your cervix, and you can get pregnant. Perhaps that is another reason diaphragms fail: long-lived sperm!

777. If I have intercourse a second time, should I insert more cream vaginally?

Yes, but only after checking to see that the rim of the diaphragm is behind your pubic bone and the rubber covers the cervix. Then leave it in another eight hours after the second coitus.

778. What is the proper care of the diaphragm?

The diaphragm should be washed with soap and water after each removal, and stored in its case. Do not use powder, lanolin, or cold cream soaps, such as Dove, on it. Do not worry if blood leaves stains on the material.

779. Does the size of a diaphragm increase after I have a baby?

Yes, your vagina is usually enlarged by the passage of the baby's head. This usually necessitates a diaphragm that is an average of 5 mm larger in size than your previous one for each baby that you have had. If you have used a 75 mm diaphragm before your first child, you will probably need an 80 mm diaphragm after a vaginal delivery.

780. Is there any danger in forgetting to remove a diaphragm and leaving it in for an extra day or two?

Most, but not all women, will get an irritating, odorous discharge if they leave their diaphragms in longer than twenty-four hours. This probably depends on the bacteria that are in your vagina to begin with. The discharge will clear up just by removing the diaphragm. A rare complication can be toxic shock syndrome. Just as with tampon use, the occurrence of toxic shock syndrome depends upon what bacteria you have in your vagina to start with, and how long you leave something in there.

781. What percentage of women get pregnant using the diaphragm?

About 5 percent of women using a diaphragm get pregnant, even if they insert it and follow directions with every coitus. But many more women who use the diaphragm get pregnant because they leave it out once, either because they were half asleep and didn't think of it, or they just forgot it. Even more women get pregnant because they think they are in a "safe" period, such as during menstruation, and do not use their diaphragms at all.

BIRTH CONTROL: THE DIAPHRAGM (Continued)

782. Why do some women get pregnant even though they were using the diaphragm exactly right?

There are several reasons for this. As arousal occurs, the back of the vagina balloons out and gets larger, so the diaphragm is no longer tight, but slips around. This can allow sperm to pass and reach the cervix. Another well-documented situation involves a second coitus later the same night. After the first coitus, the diaphragm can slip so far down or forward that the penis can be inserted between the diaphragm and the cervix. Sperm are then quite free to enter the cervix. The advice for this situation is to check the rim of the diaphragm and be sure it is behind the pubic bone before the second entry, rather than just inserting more cream. Although this may help, too, inserting the cream below the diaphragm and the penis above the diaphragm is no help at all. Perhaps the safest way is to insert more cream after checking the rim of the diaphragm first. Women with a tipped or retroverted uterus, or pelvic relaxation are more likely to have problems with their diaphragms slipping. Unfortunately, such women usually have had several children already and really don't want any more.

783. Is it possible to put a diaphragm in "the wrong way"?

Of course, even pills can be taken the wrong way, mostly by misreading instructions or forgetting them. If the diaphragm is placed so that it is in front of the cervix, instead of covering it, the cervix is then exposed to the sperm. A diaphragm that is properly fitted will be large enough to make this position uncomfortable, but you should also check, by touching your cervix with your finger, to be sure that the rubber is over it before you have coitus. Arcing diaphragms are designed to avoid missing the cervix, but they can be inserted the "wrong way," too. The worst position, however, is to leave your diaphragm in the dresser drawer.

784. How long before having intercourse, can I insert my diaphragm and cream for it still to be effective?

A short time is best, but the effectiveness of the cream or jelly is generally one to four hours at the most. Of course, a diaphragm, even without any cream or jelly, is better than nothing at all.

785. Can I use any spermicide, or must it be especially made for a diaphragm?

Any spermicide, with the exception of suppositories and foams which are not adaptable, can be used with the diaphragm.

786. Which is better, cream or jelly?

Some creams and jellies are more spermicidal than others, but the final choice depends upon whether you like the additional lubrication of the jelly

BIRTH CONTROL: THE DIAPHRAGM (Continued)

or the heavier consistency of the cream. The cream is more like a normal vaginal discharge.

787. Are there any differences between the spermicidal creams and jellies that are used with a diaphragm?

Yes, they contain different materials, and they differ in their ability to trap and kill sperm, depending upon the amount and nature of the spermicide. The jellies are also more lubricating and slick. Some women feel burning with one type but not with the other type.

788. What are the ingredients used in foams and jellies that kill the sperm?

The most commonly used spermicidal ingredient is nonylphenoxy-polyethoxyethanol. This is poisonous to sperm, but not to other tissues around the vagina.

BIRTH CONTROL: THE DIAPHRAGM AND ITS SIDE EFFECTS

789. Does the diaphragm, used in combination with spermicidal creams or jellies, have any side effects?

Discomfort for the woman can occur if the diaphragm is too large or out of place. This discomfort is similar to the way you feel when you need to urinate. Discomfort for the male can occur if the diaphragm falls down into the entrance of the vagina. In its proper place, the male cannot usually detect its presence. Burning from a particular brand of cream or jelly may bother the male or female. Toxic shock syndrome has been associated with the use of the diaphragm, but there have not been many cases of this. If the diaphragm is too large, it can cause pressure on the urethra, which can lead to bladder infections.

790. I am susceptible to bladder infections. Should I use a diaphragm?

Probably not. The rim of the diaphragm presses slightly on the urethra, the tube leading from the bladder to the outside of the body. If your technique of coitus already presses against the urethra, this will lead to cystitis, and the diaphragm pressure would make it worse. Of course, if you want to use a diaphragm you could, and should, change your coital technique so that this won't happen. The first thing you should do is check to see that your diaphragm is not too large. If it is, you will have an urge to void, even without any coitus.

791. Can I get toxic shock from a diaphragm? If so, must I be in my menstrual period?

There have been a few recorded cases of toxic shock syndrome associated with diaphragm use. Women are advised not to wear tampons all

BIRTH CONTROL: THE DIAPHRAGM AND ITS SIDE EFFECTS
(Continued)

night to avoid toxic shock; yet they are told to keep diaphragms in eight hours or longer to be effective. Perhaps the spermicidal creams and jellies help prevent the toxic shock by being antiseptic, killing bacteria as well as sperm. This has not been fully investigated. You do not have to be having your period to get toxic shock with a diaphragm or tampon, but it makes it more likely.

792. Do diaphragms cause cervical cancer?
No, there is no relationship between cervical cancer and the use of a diaphragm or any other contraceptive method. There is more cervical cancer in sexually active women than in virgins, but it is not more frequent in those who use contraceptives than in those who do not.

793. Jelly burns me. Why?
Some women find that some of the creams or jellies are irritating to them. This isn't necessarily due to the spermicide; it may be the cream or even the perfume in them. There are many different kinds available, so try several before you give up. Also, be sure you don't really have a vaginal infection, such as yeast, that burns with intercourse, even without a jelly. If you burn with the use of a diaphragm moistened only with water, then it is not the fault of the cream or jelly.

BIRTH CONTROL: THE CERVICAL CAP

794. What is a cervical cap?
It is a soft plastic cup shaped to fit over the cervix itself. It acts as a barrier to the entry of the sperm into the cervical canal.

795. How does the cervical cap differ from a diaphragm?
It is different from a diaphragm in that it is much smaller in diameter and is designed to cover only the cervix. A diaphragm fits from the pubic bone to the end of the vagina and is a much wider cup.

796. How do I insert the cervical cap?
Like the diaphragm, the cervical cap is folded to insert it, and then placed over the cervix. It is easy to insert it behind the cervix, instead of in front of it, so the cap should be checked after insertion to see that it is in the proper place.

797. How long must a cervical cap be left in place after intercourse?
It must be left in place until all the sperm in the vagina are dead—at least six hours. Some people allow it to remain in much longer, sometimes for several days. It has not yet been proven that this is safe or that it promotes toxic shock syndrome. It is being tested.

BIRTH CONTROL: THE CERVICAL CAP (Continued)

798. What is the effectiveness of the cervical cap?

The cervical cap has been shown to be about 90 percent effective.

799. When will the cervical cap be available in the United States?

Very soon. It is now being tested by the Planned Parenthood clinics in the United States and is also being used by feminist clinics across the country.

800. Is the cervical cap more likely to cause infections? Odors?

Experience has shown that anything left in the vagina for over a day can cause obnoxious discharge with an odor. If staphylococcus is already present in the vagina, then toxic shock syndrome can occur. Therefore, the new rule is that tampons, diaphragms, and cervical caps should not be left in the vagina for more than eight hours; otherwise they can cause infections.

BIRTH CONTROL: THE INTRAUTERINE DEVICE (IUD)

801. What is the difference between the different IUDs on the market today? Is one better than the other?

One is not considered best over all. Each one has its advantages and disadvantages, and will suit some people better than others. One of the advantages of the older IUDs, like Lippe's Loop and Saf-T-Coil, is that they do not have to be removed at any particular interval if they are not causing any trouble. The disadvantages are that they are expelled more frequently, especially in women who have never had a pregnancy, and they seem to cause more bleeding and cramping with menses. The Cu-7 and Cu-T types must be replaced every three years, but have less bleeding and cramping and are seldom expelled, even with no previous pregnancies. The Progestasert must be replaced every year to keep the progestin in the stem working, but it seems better tolerated by some women who bleed and cramp more with all the others.

802. How do the IUDs that do not contain copper work?

The plastic inert IUDs depend on a foreign body reaction to prevent implantation of the fertilized egg.

803. Why do some IUDs contain copper?

Copper helps the IUD to be more toxic to the sperm and, therefore, makes it work better. IUDs that contain copper are smaller in overall area than some of the others, so they produce less adverse reaction and less expulsion. As a consequence, they need the additional copper or progesterone.

804. What effect does an IUD have on my body chemistry?

The copper in some IUDs helps immobilize the sperm that may enter

BIRTH CONTROL: THE INTRAUTERINE DEVICE (IUD)
(Continued)

the body of the uterus. The IUD itself produces a foreign body reaction that interferes with implantation. The IUD containing progesterone also prevents sperm passage and reduces spotting. The rest of your body has no change in its chemistry.

805. What was wrong with the Dalkon Shield? Why did it have so many problems? Have these problems been solved in the new IUDs on the market today?

Lawsuits regarding these questions are still in the courts today. One explanation is that the Dalkon Shield happened to be a popular IUD when it first came on the market, because it was not as easily expelled as those previously used. It was being used in large numbers when the problem of infection associated with IUD use were just being discovered, so it got most of the blame. Another problem was that the string used on the Dalkon Shield was formed by many filaments so that it made a ladder for the bacteria of an infection in the vagina, usually a venereal disease, to climb into the uterus and then into the tubes to produce much damage. In the case of a pregnant uterus, it resulted in a fatal infection. The rest of the strings of other IUDs were not so constructed since they were single filaments, and special care has been taken not to construct them that way since then. The Dalkon Shield is no longer being made or sold because of all the lawsuits.

806. How long can I retain the same IUD before getting a new one?

The Copper-7 (Cu-7) and Copper-T (Cu-T) have been approved by the Food and Drug Administration (FDA) for use for three years before changing them for a new one. The copper wears out and becomes less effective after that time. The Progestasert has a stem impregnated with a progestogen to help prevent cramps and spotting and wears out in one year, so it must be removed and replaced annually. The older IUDs, such as Lippe's Loop, Saf-T-Coil, and others, never went through FDA approval and have no time limit placed on them. They have been known to work well for as long as thirteen years, but they are to be removed whenever trouble develops. It is possibly a good idea to remove an IUD after a few years to prevent trouble. When they are removed years later, they have gritty calcium deposits on them, which must be irritating to the uterus.

807. What is the effectiveness of the IUD?

The IUD is about 97 percent effective; that is, three pregnancies occur per one hundred women per year. This percentage can be improved by using a barrier foam during the fertile time.

808. What percentage of teenagers are using the IUD?

Two percent of teenagers use the IUD, but these generally are teenagers

BIRTH CONTROL: THE INTRAUTERINE DEVICE (IUD)
(Continued)

who have already experienced a pregnancy.

809. What percentage of women use an IUD?

A recent survey showed that 6 percent of women between the ages of fifteen and forty-four use the IUD for contraception.

810. Is it easier to be fitted for an IUD if you've already had a baby?

Yes, the cervix is more open after you have had a baby, and the IUD is easier to insert and less painful. It is even easier if inserted shortly after the baby is born, such as six weeks or so later.

811. Does it hurt to be fitted for an IUD?

Yes, it does. It is usually not so painful that you need an anesthetic, but it feels like a severe menstrual cramp. It is not the fitting that is painful, it is the inserting of the IUD into the uterine cavity. It is a little less painful if it is inserted at the time of menstruation when the cervix seems to be a little more open.

812. Is there anything I can take to ease the pain of inserting the IUD?

A paracervical block anesthetic can be given to reduce the pain at the time of insertion, if it is known to be intolerable.

813. Is it also painful to have an IUD removed?

Yes, it is also painful to remove an IUD, but not as bad as insertion.

814. Does the effectiveness of an IUD decrease over time? For instance, I'm told that my Cu-7 will last for three years. Would I be smart to replace it in two years in order to increase its effectiveness?

No, apparently the effectiveness of the Cu-7 is the same for all three years and only begins to decrease after three years. The FDA originally advised using it for two years before replacing it, but changed it to three years after it was proven to be just as effective for that length of time.

815. Is it common for women to feel depressed or even inadequate from having something foreign, like an IUD, inside of them?

It is not really common, but it does occur with some frequency. It may occur more in women when it was not really their choice to use any contraceptive. Since they cannot forget the IUD or remove it themselves, they may feel trapped. It is especially true of women who are not enjoying sex anyway. They may feel that they are just being used and not even for their reproductive abilities, or they may feel rejected because no one wants their babies. If a woman has this reaction, she should reconsider her whole sexual life and relationships. Women who want to have sex without getting pregnant, on the other hand, usually do not feel inadequate with an IUD, but in-

BIRTH CONTROL: THE INTRAUTERINE DEVICE (IUD)
(Continued)

stead feel that they are in charge of their bodies. Some women do not want to have "something foreign" in them. An IUD has enough complications to cause this fear to be somewhat justified.

816. Why can some women use an IUD successfully and others can't?

The major reason is that women who have experienced a pregnancy, preferably a full-term delivery, are less likely to expel the IUD and less likely to have cramps and excessive bleeding from their reactions to the IUD, because the cavity of their uterus is larger from the pregnancy. Also, women who have a monogamous relationship with their partners are not very likely to have a pelvic infection, which would react badly with an IUD. Some women already have light, painless periods, and even if they become twice as bad, they are still quite tolerable. Some women have a larger uterus than others, even without pregnancy, and would tolerate an IUD better. If women have cramps and heavy menses before they insert an IUD, they will get worse afterwards.

817. How often should I check to see if my IUD is still in place?

It is sometimes advised to check your IUD for proper placement before each coitus for the first month and then after each menstrual period for several months.

818. My mother couldn't use an IUD; she expelled it. Will I have the same problem?

You are less likely to have this problem, because the newer IUDs are not as easily expelled as the older ones. Your mother may have tried one of the larger, older types, which were frequently expelled.

819. Is it safe to douche while using an IUD?

It is probably as safe to douche with an IUD as without one. Douching makes a diaphragm fail, but it does not make an IUD fail. Most gynecologists do not think anyone should douche, as it is usually unnecessary and a poor way to treat an infection if one is present. Douching can induce some yeast vaginitis by removing the normal bacteria that belong in your vagina to keep it healthy.

820. Should I stop using an IUD as a method of birth control after a certain time, in order to give my body a rest?

No, there is no known reason to stop using an IUD in order to "give your body a rest." If the IUD is giving you problems, such as severe cramps, heavy menses with clots, intermenstrual bleeding, or signs of infection, it should be removed. After the problems have cleared up, it can then be tried again. If you have been in a monogamous marriage and then get divorced

BIRTH CONTROL: THE INTRAUTERINE DEVICE (IUD)
(Continued)

and are going to have many partner changes and be exposed to venereal disease, it would be a good idea to change from the IUD to a contraceptive that helps prevent a VD infection from getting into your tubes, such as contraceptive pills.

821. I am now on my second IUD and have never had any problems. Should I assume that I won't have any problems in the future?

You are less likely than others to have problems with your IUD in the future; however, if you were to contract a venereal disease and a pelvic infection, you could have as much trouble with it as anyone else.

822. Is spontaneous expulsion of an IUD with no discomfort or even an awareness that it has happened a common occurrence?

Loss of the IUD, especially with the more modern ones, is not a common occurrence in the first place. Most women know when it comes out and they bring it into the doctor's office to show their doctors. Often it happens with a heavy menstrual flow, in which there is much cramping. Rarely, it seems to disappear without the awareness of the wearer. In that case, an X-ray or an ultrasound is done to see if it has gone inside the body. If it can't be found, then it must be assumed that it has just slipped out. This is a good reason to check the string periodically to see that it is still there, especially after heavy menses.

823. Do some men object to an IUD, because they can feel it during intercourse?

Yes, but they do not feel the IUD itself. They feel the synthetic string coming out of the cervix. This is especially noticeable if it is short and pointed toward them, and they can feel the end of it.

824. Could a man avoid feeling the synthetic string of an IUD?

They could avoid feeling the string if they would penetrate deeply in a downward direction and avoid hitting the cervix altogether. By downward, this means away from the bladder wall, going deeply under the uterus. This is the best way to have intercourse anyway, since hitting the cervix produces a cramping, uncomfortable feeling in the pelvis of the woman, and it should be avoided. Cutting the string shorter makes it worse, not better.

825. Could pressure caused by the male penis during intercourse force an IUD into the uterus?

It is not thought that this is possible. The IUD is entirely within the cavity of the uterus, and nothing is sticking out to put pressure on, except a little nylon thread. It is considered that if the IUD goes through the wall of the uterus, it happens at the time of insertion, but it is not detected until later

BIRTH CONTROL: THE INTRAUTERINE DEVICE (IUD)
(Continued)

when it travels further and the string disappears from the cervix. Sometimes, if it is in the wall only part of the way, the string can still be visible through the cervix. An exception to this would be if the stem of the Cu-7 perforated through the lower segment of the uterus or the back wall of the cervix after insertion. Intercourse has not been blamed as a cause of this.

826. Is the IUD essentially a form of abortion?

The answer to this question depends upon your definition of an abortion. The modern definition of abortion is the interruption of an implanted pregnancy. In that case, the IUD does not produce an abortion. What it does do is prevent a fertilized egg from implanting in the uterus. This is shown by the fact that an IUD does not prevent an ectopic pregnancy, in which the fertilized egg plants itself in the tube, on the ovary, or elsewhere. This is one of the dangers of the IUD; it does not prevent ectopic pregnancies. If, on the other hand, you believe that life begins when the sperm enters the egg, then you would feel that an IUD produces an abortion.

BIRTH CONTROL: PROBLEMS ASSOCIATED WITH THE INTRAUTERINE DEVICE (IUD)

827. Can I use an IUD if I have never been pregnant?

The newer IUDs will stay in your uterus if you have not had a pregnancy, but whether you should use them is open to question. If you can guarantee that you will not get VD, it would probably be all right, but few young women can guarantee that. Since the complications may involve a loss of your ability to have a baby and most young women may want a baby in the future, it is usually advisable for you to use something else.

828. As a teenager, should I use an IUD?

The intrauterine device is not as advisable for teenagers, because it makes VD worse if you get it, producing such damage to your tubes that you may never be able to become pregnant. This may not matter as much to a woman who has just completed her family as it would to you.

829. Does the IUD cause problems in females who have different sex partners?

Yes, but this is just another way of saying it causes problems in women who get VD. You do not really have to have two or more sex partners to get VD. Your partner may have two or more sex partners, and you may not know it. If you had five partners who only slept with you, you would not be liable to get VD, but then, this situation is also not liable to happen.

BIRTH CONTROL: PROBLEMS ASSOCIATED WITH THE INTRAUTERINE DEVICE (IUD) (Continued)

830. After my IUD was inserted, I began to spot before and after my periods. My doctor advised me that taking vitamin C regularly would correct this, and it worked. Why?

Vitamin C deficiency makes it easier for small blood vessels to bleed, and this can cause spotting. If you have a deficiency, you should certainly correct it by taking more vitamin C or drinking orange juice. But time probably corrected the spotting, because your uterus adjusted to the IUD. Spotting occurs mostly in the first month or two.

831. Is spotting common after the insertion of an IUD?

It is generally true that in the first two cycles after insertion of the IUD there may frequently be some spotting. This usually clears up by the third cycle, but if it does not, most doctors remove the IUD until the spotting clears up, and then they try again.

832. Can an IUD be damaging to surrounding tissues?

Yes, it can. In the uterus, the IUD is expected to be irritating enough to prevent implantation and perhaps increase menstrual flow and cramps. If any of these conditions are severe, the surrounding tissues are too irritated. If the IUD, particularly a copper one, travels outside of the uterus into the abdominal cavity somewhere, it seems to arouse a reaction in surrounding tissues, and unless it is removed fairly soon, it can become so damaged by the tissue reaction that removal is difficult. Such reactions can cause adhesions and even bowel obstruction.

833. What are the most common complications requiring surgery that are known to occur in women using an IUD?

Perforation of the uterus, where the IUD becomes misplaced in the abdomen, occurs in about one out of every six hundred insertions. Surgery may be required to remove the IUD from the abdomen. Infections that go up into the tubes and form abscesses are increased in women with the IUD, compared to women using the pill or diaphragm. Surgery can be required to remove the abscessed tubes and perhaps all the female organs involved, making the woman both sterile and menopausal. Estimates are that this occurs once in every five hundred women, depending upon the type of women being studied. However, these infections do not occur without the presence of venereal disease; therefore, they are much less frequent in stable partner relationships and much more likely where there is a frequent change in partners, making VD more likely to occur. Even then, the patient still survives.

BIRTH CONTROL: PROBLEMS ASSOCIATED WITH THE INTRAUTERINE DEVICE (IUD) (Continued)

834. Aren't IUDs incredibly dangerous?

An article in the *Wall Street Journal* once said that the IUD was the most dangerous contraceptive on the market. This may be true, but it is still not "incredibly" dangerous. The present day evaluation is that it can have more severe complications involving surgery than the pill, but it does not really have a higher death rate than the pill or any of the sterilization procedures. It is more dangerous to your fertility than the pill, because it can cause a venereal disease to go up into your tubes and damage them. This venereal disease is called pelvic inflammatory disease.

835. If I can feel the IUD itself, does this mean that it is about to fall out?

If you can feel the actual plastic portion of the IUD stem, then it is not properly placed in your uterine cavity. It could be expelled or else cause cramping and bleeding by being in the cervix. Worst of all, it might not prevent pregnancy. You should have a doctor, or preferably the same person who inserted it, check it and remove and replace it with a new one if necessary. Until you can do this, use another contraceptive, such as foam.

836. Could I expel my IUD at any time after it's inserted?

Possibly, but after an IUD has been in place for one year, it is much less likely to be expelled.

837. How does a doctor find out where a lost IUD has gone?

An X-ray or an ultrasound will usually show where it is.

838. If an IUD slips outside the womb, will it need to be surgically removed?

Usually, it is wise to surgically remove the IUD, whatever kind it is, from the abdomen by laparoscopy (a small incision under the navel) or by an incision in the vagina or lower abdomen, depending upon where the IUD is. The copper types must be removed, because they cause more tissue reaction.

839. What are the chances of an IUD slipping up into the womb?

The IUD belongs in the womb in the first place; that is where it is supposed to be inserted. Only if it perforates the wall of the womb, or uterus, does it become a problem, and this occurs in about one in every six hundred women using an IUD.

840. How great is the risk of suffering a perforated uterus as the result of using an IUD?

Depending upon the ability and experience of the person doing the insertion, about one out of six hundred women who have an IUD will suffer from a perforated uterus.

BIRTH CONTROL: PROBLEMS ASSOCIATED WITH THE INTRAUTERINE DEVICE (IUD) (Continued)

841. Is suffering a perforated uterus an extremely severe injury?

No, usually it is not if the IUD is found in your abdomen and removed before it makes any trouble there. If the IUD is not located and removed fairly soon, it can damage surrounding tissues, which can result in an adhesion or even bowel obstruction. Usually an IUD that has perforated your uterus can be found and removed by laparoscopy. Since this does not require opening the abdomen through a large surgical incision, the risk is not so great. However, sometimes a surgical incision is necessary. Of course, if you do not know that your IUD has perforated and wandered out of your uterus, you could get pregnant, since the IUD is not in place to protect you from this. Often it is not until you discover that you are pregnant that you find out you have suffered a perforated uterus. This does not bother the pregnancy, as the perforation quickly heals over.

842. What if pregnancy occurs while an IUD is in place; can it safely be removed without injuring the fetus?

No, it is not completely safe to remove the IUD, since the removal may dislodge the entire pregnancy and cause a miscarriage, but if you leave it in place, you are even more likely to have a miscarriage. So the medical advice is to remove the IUD if you want to continue the pregnancy. A more important reason for removing the IUD is that if it is left in place, it can contribute to a fatal infection of the pregnant uterus midway in pregnancy, in the fourth to seventh month, which can cause the death of the mother and baby. If you refuse to remove it, you are taking your life into your own hands.

843. What are the chances of never being able to have children as the result of using an IUD?

The estimates are that about one in five hundred women with an IUD will develop such a severe infection with VD that her tubes will be damaged beyond repair, so that she can never get pregnant. Of course, any woman who gets PID (pelvic inflammatory disease) with VD may suffer such severe damage that she also cannot get pregnant even without an IUD. The chances of this happening are estimated to be about 10 percent each time she gets PID.

844. Will the IUD prevent VD?

No. The IUD seems to make the VD germ go up into the tubes worse than if you were using nothing at all. You will not always get VD if you have coitus with someone who has it, but you usually will. With an IUD, the infection will go further; on the pill, the infection is less likely to involve the tubes and ovaries.

BIRTH CONTROL: PROBLEMS ASSOCIATED WITH THE INTRAUTERINE DEVICE (IUD) (Continued)

845. Does an IUD increase the risk of uterine cancer?

No, it does not. Any contraceptive, except birth control pills, may be associated with an increase in uterine cancer, when compared to the incidence of uterine cancer in women who had many children. This is because uterine cancer occurs more frequently in women who have never had children or have just had a very few as opposed to women who have had a lot of children. Uterine cancer occurs less frequently in women who have used the birth control pills for at least eight to ten years because of the effect of the extra progestogen they have taken all those years. But women who use an IUD do not have more uterine cancer than women who never had children and never took any contraceptive pills. The IUD is certainly not a direct cause of any cancer.

BIRTH CONTROL: OVER-THE-COUNTER METHODS— SPERMICIDES, FOAMS, SUPPOSITORIES, CREAMS, SPONGES

846. What are over-the-counter contraceptives?

They are contraceptives that do not require a doctor's prescription. You can buy them in drug stores.

847. What is the most reliable of all the over-the-counter contraceptives?

The best is a combination of condom for the male and foam for the female, used together at all times, or the sponge.

848. Which over-the-counter method is the least reliable birth control method?

The vaginal suppositories are probably the least effective. Douching is also not very reliable, nor is it a valid contraceptive method.

849. Where can I find over-the-counter contraceptives?

Over-the-counter contraceptives are available in pharmacies, drugstores, and sometimes in physicians' offices. Most of the female contraceptives are in the area of the store displaying "female hygiene" articles. They are also available at Planned Parenthood clinics and other family-planning centers. In Sweden, you can find them at bus stops and located in restrooms in coin-operated machines.

850. Do I have to be a certain age to buy over-the-counter contraceptives?

No, there is no law forbidding the sale of over-the-counter contraceptives to minors. It is only recently that advertisements for the sale of over-the-counter contraceptives have been on display in pharmacies or drugstores; previously, you had to ask the druggist for them. In California, in the last few years, a handbook for teachers was prevented from being

BIRTH CONTROL: OVER-THE-COUNTER METHODS— SPERMICIDES, FOAMS, SUPPOSITORIES, CREAMS, SPONGES

(Continued)

distributed, because it suggested that the teachers discussing contraception actually instruct the students how to go into the drugstore and purchase the contraceptives. There are still people who want to prohibit the use of over-the-counter contraception, because they feel it will lead to sex. Instead, it simply prevents pregnancies in those already having sex. There are heated arguments on both sides of the issue.

851. Are suppositories a popular method of birth control?

There recently has been a resurgence in the use of vaginal suppositories, primarily because women prefer to insert a suppository instead of using an applicator. Filling an applicator with cream or foam and depositing this into the vagina is considered to be messy. There has also been more advertising of suppositories, often making claims that they are far more effective than the 80 percent they are.

852. Must I use foam or jelly again, if I have intercourse a second time on the same night?

If four or more hours have passed, it is best to renew the foam or jelly by inserting more.

853. Is it true that certain herbs can prevent pregnancy?

The Chinese have made claims that there are several herbs that can prevent pregnancy, but when used by women's groups in the United States, the pregnancy rate was high.

854. What is the sponge?

The sponge first came on the market July 1, 1983. It is a vaginal contraceptive that is sold over the counter without a prescription. The advantage of the sponge over the diaphragm is that it does not have to be fitted to the individual. The disadvantage is that it does not have quite the effectiveness of a fitted diaphragm.

855. Can using a sponge keep me from becoming pregnant?

Ancient women added salt water or vinegar to real sponges from the sea and prevented pregnancy. The Food and Drug Administration (FDA) recently has approved an artificial sponge that is made of polyurethane, measures about two inches in diameter, and contains the spermicide nonoxynol-9 for contraceptive use. Called "Today," it can be used once, and costs $1.00.

856. How effective is the sponge?

The sponge with the spermicide is about 85-90 percent effective. This is in the same range as foams and jellies.

**BIRTH CONTROL: OVER-THE-COUNTER METHODS—
SPERMICIDES, FOAMS, SUPPOSITORIES, CREAMS, SPONGES**
(Continued)

857. Has the sponge been tested to be safe?

Three thousand women used it for five years, and only 2 percent were allergic to the spermicide. It will take more use to find out if a reaction similar to toxic shock syndrome will develop from leaving it in for twenty-four hours.

858. Is the sponge difficult to use?

It must be inserted before intercourse but remains effective for twenty-four hours. However, failures are attributed to not using it properly, so perhaps it isn't easy to insert it correctly.

859. How can I get a sponge?

They are sold over the counter in drugstores. It is not recommended that you make your own, because the spermicide used in the ones approved by the FDA is better than what women once added to sea sponges.

BIRTH CONTROL: DEPO-PROVERA

860. What is Depo-Provera?

It is a long-acting hormone contraceptive. You can receive the hormone by an injection every three months. The high dose of Depo-Provera (medroxyprogesterone acetate) blocks ovulation, changes your cervical mucus, depresses the endometrium, and changes the motility of your tube.

861. What happens to my menstrual period when I use Depo-Provera?

With Depo-Provera, menses usually disappear after about a year of shots.

862. Are Depo-Provera shots presently being used by women in other parts of the world?

Yes, they are quite commonly used in Mexico, Europe, and in seventy-eight other countries, although their use abroad decreased when the FDA withheld its approval of the drug in the United States. The United States cannot fund foreign contraception that is not approved here.

863. How thoroughly will new methods of birth control, such as the cervical cap and Depo-Provera shots, be tested before they are made available to the public?

They are first tested on animals for safety and effectiveness, then on humans for safety, and finally on larger numbers of people for effectiveness. Tests are now in progress on the cervical caps and have already been completed on Depo-Provera.

BIRTH CONTROL: DEPO-PROVERA (Continued)

864. When will Depo-Provera shots be available in the United States?

They will be available when the officials of the Food and Drug Administration (FDA) listen to the decisions of their own scientific committees, instead of listening to nonscientific groups who claim Depo-Provera is a dangerous drug, and bring about political pressure. Of course, Depo-Provera shots are really available now, because physicians are not required to limit drug use to that recommended in the PDR (Physicians Desk Reference) or by the FDA. Any drug on the market can be used for any purpose if the physician has a good reason for doing so and if it has been used elsewhere, so that it is not experimental.

865. What kind of special problem might be solved with Depo-Provera shots?

One such problem occurs in women in their forties who smoke and have irregular menstrual cycles with heavy bleeding. Birth control pills are usually taken away from women with these symptoms, but Depo-Provera solves both their bleeding problem and their contraceptive problem. Of course, they must first make sure that the bleeding is not due to cancer.

BIRTH CONTROL: THE RHYTHM METHOD

866. What is the rhythm method?

The rhythm method depends upon abstaining from intercourse at the time in your cycle when depositing sperm in the vagina can result in a pregnancy. Since sperm can live in the tubes for six days, it means avoiding coitus for six days prior to ovulation.

867. Is birth control necessary every time I have intercourse if I don't want to become pregnant, or is the rhythm method a good birth control method?

Birth control is necessary every time you have intercourse if you do not want to become pregnant. Given the biologic variability of the menstrual cycle and the time of ovulation, there is no absolutely safe time in which to have intercourse without contraception, unless you have been taking birth control pills for two months. Then it is safe to have intercourse in the week you are off the pill, provided that you take the pill properly during the next cycle. You must use all barrier methods of contraception, such as the diaphragm, every time you have intercourse.

868. What is the main problem associated with the rhythm method?

The problem, of course, is trying to determine when you are going to ovulate. If you have a very regular rhythm to your cycle, this is not so difficult, but if the rhythm of your cycle changes once in awhile, then the method frequently fails. For some people, the problem is abstaining from sex during the fertile period.

BIRTH CONTROL: THE RHYTHM METHOD (Continued)

869. Dr. Carson, when would you recommend that a woman use the rhythm method?

I would never recommend that a woman use the rhythm method, although if a woman wants to follow this method, I would certainly help her to make it work.

870. Why do most of the women who use the rhythm method select this form of contraception?

Most of the women who use the rhythm method do so because of their religion. The rhythm method is the only method of contraception available to Catholics who wish to strictly adhere to the tenets of their religion. Some women use it because they like to avoid sex, and they cannot say "no" without an excuse. Other women use it because they consider it to be "natural," and they can avoid pills, creams, and other methods.

871. When in a woman's life is the rhythm method best suited?

The rhythm method is best suited for women who are rhythmic. This almost limits it to women between the ages of twenty and forty, as women in this age group are most likely to have menses at the same time every cycle, and they predict with some accuracy when they will ovulate. It is also best suited for women who have a regular life, that is, a life without too many upsets or illnesses, as these might delay their ovulation and, therefore, make the rhythm method impossible.

872. Are more women today going back to the rhythm method because they want a natural form of birth control?

Yes, many women state that this is their motive. This is reinforced by attacks by the media on all forms of contraception as being very dangerous to your health and full of side effects. It is not certain how "natural" refusing to have sex really is, although it is natural to refuse sex when you don't want it. Some women like the rhythm method because they feel entitled to refuse sex at least part of the time. They would like to refuse it all the time, because they have never worked out their sexual technique to be pleasurable for them. I think the only natural state is to be pregnant or breast-feeding, but the world will deteriorate due to overcrowding if everyone continued to be that natural.

873 . Does backing up the rhythm method with creams, foams, jellies, or suppositories substantially increase effectiveness?

Yes, but only if these methods are used to protect the otherwise "safe" period, since it is not really so safe that you can use nothing.

BIRTH CONTROL: THE RHYTHM METHOD (Continued)

874. How effective would it be if I use other methods, such as creams, foams, jellies, or suppositories, in addition to rhythm during my fertile period?

It would be less than 80 percent effective to use these methods during your fertile period.

875. How can I determine the times during the month when I can or cannot get pregnant?

You can determine the times during the month when you can or cannot get pregnant by using the calendar method, the temperature method, or by analyzing your cervical mucus to find out when ovulation occurs.

BIRTH CONTROL: HOW TO DETERMINE WHEN I CAN AND CANNOT GET PREGNANT USING THE CALENDAR METHOD

876. How can I determine the times during the month when I can get pregnant using the calendar method?

You must first determine the length of your menstrual cycle over several cycles. Whatever this number is, subtract twenty-one and you will have the day of your cycle on which you should stop having intercourse (or start using another barrier method, if you are combining methods). If your cycle is twenty eight days, then your result will be seven, so it is after the seventh day that you can become pregnant. The first day of menses is day one of your cycle, so from then through the seventh day, you are safe and probably won't get pregnant. Then, since sperm live in the tubes for as long as six days, you count forward eight days (two extra days in case you ovulate a day or two late) to determine the time span in which pregnancy is most likely to occur. You do this because sperm placed in the vagina on the eighth day can still fertilize the egg on the fourteenth day when you ovulate. If your cycle is twenty-eight days, then after the fifteenth day of your cycle, your safe time (when you cannot get pregnant) has arrived. However, even then, your ovulation could be delayed and pregnancy could result after the fifteenth day.

877. Does the calendar method work for everyone?

If you are perfectly rhythmic and always have a twenty-eight-day cycle, the calendar method will work fairly well for you. However, even then, if you are upset or have an illness, ovulation could be delayed into the "safe" period, and pregnancy could result after the fifteenth day.

878. Is there any time in my cycle when I am absolutely immune to pregnancy?

There is no time that is easily detected. There is such a time theoretically, but practically speaking, you have no way of being absolutely sure when it is.

BIRTH CONTROL: HOW TO DETERMINE WHEN I CAN AND CANNOT GET PREGNANT USING THE TEMPERATURE METHOD

879. How can I determine when to abstain from intercourse to avoid pregnancy by taking my temperature?

You will need to buy an oral type of basal thermometer and prepare a chart on which you will keep track of your daily waking temperature. Each morning, beginning with the first day of menstruation, put the thermometer in your mouth as soon as you awake. Do this before you get out of bed or even talk. Wait three or four minutes, then record your temperature on the chart. You will find that for the first two weeks or so of your cycle, your waking temperature (basal temperature) will be quite low, even down to 96° and seldom above 98° F. It may vary a little since going to bed late or getting up late can change it. Then, immediately prior to ovulation, it will drop more than usual. Many women tend to miss this drop. However, after it occurs, in fact the next day, your temperature when you awake will be much higher, or at least a half degree higher. It may be over 98°, even above 98.6°, and it will remain this way, usually above 98°, until the onset of menses when it drops again. When charted on a graph, this pattern is called a biphasic curve. If your chart reveals such a curve, then you are ovulating. The specific time of ovulation is the time that your temperature rises and stays up, about fourteen to sixteen days before menses. Therefore, to be very careful, you should not have coitus without protection for at least eight days before the expected rise in temperature and certainly not again until after the rise confirms that you have ovulated by staying up for a day or two.

880. How does taking your basal temperature compare with the calendar method in determining my "safe" time for intercourse?

It is superior. The exact timing may turn out to be the same, but the basal temperature method allows you to know when you have really ovulated (by the rise in temperature), instead of just guessing by the calendar.

881. Are there any disadvantages to using the temperature method for determining which days during the month I am likely to get pregnant?

Yes. If you do not ovulate during a month, by using the temperature method, you will not have coitus at all that month, because you will spend the whole time waiting for ovulation to occur.

882. Can a cold affect the temperature method?

Yes. A cold can make the temperature rise, thus disguising itself as ovulation. As a result, you could be caught off guard, by mistakenly think-

BIRTH CONTROL: HOW TO DETERMINE WHEN I CAN AND CANNOT GET PREGNANT USING THE TEMPERATURE METHOD (Continued)

ing that you have ovulated when, in fact, you are experiencing cold symptoms. So, if you are sick, it is best that you do not trust the temperature method.

BIRTH CONTROL: HOW TO DETERMINE WHEN I CAN AND CANNOT GET PREGNANT USING THE CERVICAL MUCUS METHOD

883. How can I determine when to abstain from intercourse to avoid pregnancy using the cervical mucus method?

The cervical mucus method is based on the fact that the mucus from the cervix changes at the time of ovulation and, in fact, throughout the menstrual cycle. At the time of ovulation, it becomes transparent, clear, and stringy. It actually can be stretched a few inches, just like sugar syrup strings from a spoon as it cooks. This type of mucus is the best kind for letting sperm come through the cervix to reach the uterus and tubes. Therefore, the clear stringy mucus (called by the German word spinnbarkheit) is a sign that ovulation is about to take place. If you abstain from intercourse from the onset of menses until two days after this stringy mucus has disappeared, you will usually avoid pregnancy. You can then have intercourse after ovulation, which is the "safe time" for not getting pregnant. Of course, if you miss the stringy mucus altogether, you will not know when you ovulate or when your "safe time" is, so you have to check the mucus every day.

884. How do I check my mucus, if I am using the cervical mucus method?

To obtain a specimen, you must put your finger right against the mouth of your cervix. Using your finger is suggested, because it is difficult to insert an instrument there, since with the instrument you cannot feel exactly where you have placed it.

885. Is there a more scientific way to examine mucus to determine my "safe time" for intercourse?

A novel approach is to examine the mucus under a microscope. The clear, stringy mucus that signals ovulation will dry on a slide in a fern-like pattern. In fact, the mucus will appear this way from the end of menses until after ovulation; however, this is only visible when seen under a microscope. When the mucus no longer ferns, you are in your safe period.

886. Is there anything that might prevent mucus from forming a fern-like pattern, when viewed under a microscope?

Yes, an infection could keep it from ferning prior to ovulation.

BIRTH CONTROL: HOW TO DETERMINE WHEN I CAN AND CANNOT GET PREGNANT USING THE CERVICAL MUCUS METHOD (Continued)

887. Is it just an old wives' tale that I can determine the time of my ovulation from the type of mucus in my nose?

No, it is true. If you have a microscope, you don't even need mucus from your cervix. You can use the mucus from your nose. It will also fern until after ovulation, when it dries with no pattern at all. But, of course, a cold can interfere with displaying this pattern, too.

888. Which method of analyzing cervical mucus to determine the time of ovulation works the best?

If you don't have a cold or vaginal infections, the microscope or test tape methods work the best. They work even better if your cycle is regular and you can predict your approximate ovulation time. They also teach you a lot about your own body and how fluids change in your cycle.

889. Are there any other types of tests I can do on my mucus to determine the time of ovulation?

Yes. A sugar is produced in your cervical mucus just prior to ovulation, presumably to help the sperm along. This can be detected by inserting test tape against your cervix. When the test tape turns blue, you are about to ovulate. A day or two after that, you are safe from getting pregnant. Of course, you may miss the change, or a vaginal infection may obscure it. The tape can be purchased at the drugstore without a prescription.

BIRTH CONTROL: STERILIZATION—TUBAL LIGATIONS

890. Why would a woman want to have her tubes tied?

This seems more like an exclamation than a question. No matter what problems they may have with fertility control, some women would never want to permanently give up their reproductive ability by having their tubes tied. Others are at their wits' end trying to continue to have sex, yet not populate the earth all by themselves or cope with medical problems aggravated by pregnancy. Some women simply tire of their constant attention to contraception and are delighted to take all their risks in one day and never be bothered with contraception again as long as they live. This sounds delightful to some and abhorrent to others. Women who are very fertile and have many contraceptive failures are more likely to want sterilization than women who are not very fertile and even have a problem getting pregnant.

891. Is there any physical reason why I couldn't have my tubes tied before I'm twenty-one?

No, it is physically easy to tie tubes at age twenty-one, sixteen, or sixty-

BIRTH CONTROL: STERILIZATION—TUBAL LIGATIONS
(Continued)

one. It is a legal problem if the surgery is federally funded, because sterilization done before age twenty-one, regardless of the circumstances, is exempt from funding. State requirements in California demand that a girl be at least eighteen before she can be sterilized, regardless of the funding or who pays for it. Most doctors refuse to do it, unless they are convinced you know what you are doing.

892. I'm having trouble deciding if I should have a tubal ligation or my husband a vasectomy. Which one is more dangerous?

The tubal ligation has always carried more risk than a vasectomy. Of course, it is safer for the woman if the man has a vasectomy. The risk to him is much smaller, anyway, partly because a vasectomy only requires a local anesthetic. A vasectomy is much less expensive, and it is not a major operation. However, a vasectomy only sterilizes the couple, not the woman. If she were having sex with men other than her husband, she would obviously not be protected from becoming pregnant because her husband had a vasectomy.

893. What happens to my eggs after my tubes are tied?

After your tubes are tied, you still ovulate as before. The open, fringed end of the tube still catches the egg from the ovary, but it is trapped in the tube, which is now a blind alley. It does not get fertilized, of course, so after a few hours it dissolves and is absorbed. The egg is only as large as the smallest pencil dot visible on a piece of paper. It doesn't occupy much space.

894. What is "Band-Aid" surgery, and why is it called that?

It is a sterilization operation done through such a small incision that it can be covered by a small Band-Aid. Laparoscopic tubal ligation, postpartum tubal ligation, and minilaparotomy tubal ligation (minilap) all qualify as "Band- Aid" surgery.

895. What is the cost of sterilization by tubal ligation by the vaginal route, by laparoscopy, and by minilap?

The lowest cost would be around $350.00 in some clinics. Privately, it would be $1,500.00 or more. It is sometimes not covered by medical insurance, unless it is performed for a medical reason.

896. Which form of sterilization is more dangerous?

They are probably equally safe. The best method of sterilization is the one with which your surgeon is more familiar, because that is the one he or she will do best. The minilap requires less special training than the vaginal tubal ligation.

BIRTH CONTROL: STERILIZATION—TUBAL LIGATIONS
(Continued)

897. Which method of sterilization is preferred by most women?

The laparoscope method has become a popular method in recent years, primarily because it was the first method of sterilization that women could have done and go home the same day. Since then, the anesthesia used for the minilap and vaginal methods has been improved, so that the patients are also able to come in, have the operation, and go home the same day. The methods of laparoscopy and vaginal tubal ligation require special surgical skills, whereas the minilap can be done by most doctors who do any form of abdominal surgery. The actual frequencies of the methods are different in different communities and hospitals, depending upon which methods the individual physicians prefer.

898. What is the procedure involved in having tubes tied by minilap?

This surgery is done under general, spinal, or even local anesthesia. A small one-inch incision is made in the pubic area, just above the pubic hair in the midline of the abdomen. Tissues are separated and dissected until the abdominal cavity is entered, avoiding the bladder. A metal rod is placed in the cervix and uterus at the beginning of surgery so that the uterus can be moved around and brought up close to the incision. Instruments are then used to grasp the tube as it comes off the uterus. A portion is tied and cut in two places and a piece of the tube is taken out. This same procedure is then performed on the other tube. The remaining ends can be cauterized, and then the incision is sutured closed. The entire operation takes about twenty minutes.

899. What is the procedure involved in having my tubes tied by vaginal route?

This surgery is done under general or spinal anesthesia. A small 1½-inch incision is made in the upper part of the vagina, just behind the cervix, into the abdominal cavity. An instrument is used to grasp the tube on one side, it is tied in two places, and the portion of the tube between the sutures is cut out and sent to the pathologist to confirm that the tubal portion was removed. The ends can be cauterized, and the ovary is usually inspected. The same thing is then done on the other side. To be sure that there is no disease (pathology) in the uterus, a D & C also is usually done. The incision is then sutured closed. The entire operation lasts about twenty minutes.

900. What is the procedure involved in tubal ligation by laparoscopy, also known as "Band-Aid" surgery?

This is usually done under general or even regional anesthesia, but a few skilled surgeons have done it under a local one. A small nick is made in

BIRTH CONTROL: STERILIZATION—TUBAL LIGATIONS
(Continued)

the skin just under the navel (umbilicus), and a long needle is inserted through the abdominal wall into the abdominal cavity. Gas (carbon dioxide) is then put through the needle into the abdomen until the abdomen is swollen tight. A larger needle, called a trocar, is inserted into the same little incision, so that a long tubular lighted scope, the laparoscope, can be inserted through the trocar into the abdomen. The surgeon can look through this laparoscope and see the contents of the pelvic cavity (the uterus, tubes, and ovaries), because gas is holding the abdominal wall up and out of the way. A second probe is inserted through the abdominal wall lower down under the visual control of the laparoscope. An electric current goes through the second probe when it grasps the mid-portion of the tube, burning it for 1 or 2 centimeters. Some laparoscopes have an instrument that operates through the laparoscope itself, so the second probe is not used. Instead of cauterizing the tube, a clip may be placed on it by the instrument. After the laparoscope and probe are withdrawn, gas is pushed out of the abdomen, and the small incision is sutured closed. A Band-Aid is placed on the small incision. That is why it is called the Band-Aid surgery. If a woman is overweight or has had many surgeries resulting in adhesions, or infections producing adhesions, this surgery cannot be carried out. This operation only lasts for approximately ten minutes.

901. How large will the scar be if I have a tubal ligation by laparoscopy or minilap?

The scar will measure less than one-half inch just under the umbilicus with the laparoscopy, and about one inch just at the top of the pubic hair with the minilap. With a tubal ligation postpartum, performed just after delivery of the baby, it measures one inch just below the umbilicus.

902. What are the risks involved with tubal ligations?

The major risk of a tubal ligation is that due to the risk of anesthesia. Some people have unusual reactions even to the best anesthesia, and this is unpredictable. A cardiac arrest can occur, or something can go wrong with the surgery. The bowel can be cut by accident or perforated by the laparoscope. A large blood vessel can be injured and a hemorrhage occur. A bowel burn can occur when the tube is cauterized, or infection can be introduced, especially if the bowel is punctured. These complications do not happen often, and this is a relatively safe surgery. Still, it can be fatal as often as one in every ten thousand operations.

903. What sort of changes are likely to occur in my body as the result of having a tubal ligation?

The only change that usually occurs is that the tubes are closed to the

BIRTH CONTROL: STERILIZATION—TUBAL LIGATIONS
(Continued)

passage of the egg and the sperm. Such a closure should not affect the rest of your body at all, and some studies have confirmed this by showing that there are no subsequent differences in women with and without a tubal ligation. Other studies have asserted that when you cut or burn the tube, you interfere with the blood vessels in the area that supply the ovaries, and thus affect the function of the ovaries. Of course, any surgery can result in adhesions. Problems can develop from these adhesions, such as pain if they are on the ovaries or bowel obstruction if they are on the bowel. Having a tubal ligation does not insure that you will always have perfect menstruation thereafter. You are just as subject to problems in the female reproductive tract as someone who has not had a tubal ligation. The only difference is that you are just not subject to pregnancy, except in a very few cases.

904. What percentage of women who have a tubal ligation still get pregnant?

Approximately one in one thousand women still get pregnant, or 0.1 percent of tubal ligations fail and result in pregnancy.

905. Are there any emotional problems associated with women who undergo a tubal ligation?

Surveys show that most women are happy that they had the surgery and do not change their minds. Some, however, regret their decision to never have another child and often request reversal of the operation. This seems to occur more often in women who had the surgery when they were rather young, under thirty or thirty-five. It happens most often when the marriage dissolves and they remarry, which changes their decision to have no more children. Being younger, they have more time to change partners. There are no special emotional problems, other than regret that the surgery was done. Sometimes their husbands have the emotional problem; there have been men who have become impotent when their wives have had a tubal ligation. Fertility seems to have been important to their sexual lives. The sexual lives of women are more likely to increase in freedom and spontaneity when the fear of pregnancy is removed.

906. What percentage of tubal ligations have been successfully reversed?

About 60 percent of the attempts to reverse tubal ligations are successful. This percentage is based on using microsurgery, which is operating under a microscope. The success rate is higher for the tubal ligation if the tube is cut and tied instead of cauterized, because cauterization destroys so much of the tube. The clip is even more reversible, because it destroys such a small portion of the tube. The clip method, however, has a higher failure rate (occurrence of pregnancies), because it might not absolutely close the tube in the first place.

BIRTH CONTROL: STERILIZATION—TUBAL LIGATIONS
(Continued)

907. If it were possible to reverse my tubal ligation, what would be my chances of becoming pregnant?

Overall, the chances are about 60 percent that you could reverse the tubal ligation and become pregnant, but just opening the tube again doesn't make it work. The little cilia lining in the tube has to re-form and carry the egg down the tube. Microsurgery, operating under a microscope, has improved the chances of a successful reversal.

908. Can a tubal ligation affect sex drive or performance?

A tubal ligation has no direct effect on sex drive and performance. It does not change anything about the body that is involved with sex, although it can psychologically change a person's reactions. The usual effect is a release from fear of pregnancy and concern with contraception, thereby freeing the woman to enjoy sex as she never has before. If she regrets her decision, however, she may withdraw psychologically and feel she is being used against her desires, since she desires another child. As mentioned before, the husband may also react to sterility by becoming impotent, even though it was his wife who was sterilized.

909. Will I still menstruate after I have a tubal ligation?

Yes, the uterus will still react to the female hormones produced by the ovaries. It will grow and then shed a lining with each cycle, just as before. If you were on contraceptive pills right up to the time of the tubal ligation, you may be surprised at the character of your menstruation, since you probably will not have the same scant, painless flow that you had when you were on the pills. It may revert back to the heavy, painful flow that you had prior to taking the pills.

910. Will a tubal ligation decrease the problems associated with menopause?

A tubal ligation will probably not decrease any of the problems associated with menopause. It will only decrease the fear of a late, unplanned baby. The presence of and decrease in hormones will proceed just as they would have without a tubal ligation.

911. Do tubal ligations increase the chances of cancer?

No, there is no increase or decrease in cancer after tubal ligation.

912. When is the best time in life for me to have my tubes tied?

When you are sure that you don't want any more children and you find other effective contraception intolerable, then you are ready for a tubal ligation. If you do this before the age of thirty-five, you are more likely to want it reversed later.

BIRTH CONTROL: STERILIZATION—TUBAL LIGATIONS
(Continued)

913. Could a hormonal imbalance occur after having a tubal ligation?

Yes it could, but that does not mean that it is caused by the tubal ligation. Tubal ligation does not carry a guarantee that you will not have any hormone imbalance or any other problem. It just means you probably won't get pregnant.

BIRTH CONTROL: STERILIZATION—TUBAL INJECTION

914. What is tubal injection?

Tubal injection is a new method of sterilization, which is not yet in general use. By means of a hysteroscope, an instrument that allows the surgeon to look inside the uterus, a type of silicone is injected into the tube from the uterine opening. It then hardens into the shape of the tube. If this plug remains in place, it prevents sperm from entering the tube and fertilizing the egg. With the tubal injection, the hope is that if the plug is removed at a later date, the tube will not be so damaged, and it will still be able to work so that the woman can be fertile again.

915. What problems have developed with the tubal injection?

One problem is that the plug sometimes falls out, and the woman becomes pregnant. Another problem is that after the plug is removed from the tubes, the cilia of the lining have been so damaged that the tube does not work.

916. What are the advantages of the tubal injection?

One of the main advantages is that it does not require anesthesia or cutting in any form. It also can be done in a doctor's office.

BIRTH CONTROL: STERILIZATION—HYSTERECTOMIES

917. Are hysterectomies a chosen form of birth control among older women?

There have been several reported studies of women who had a simple vaginal hysterectomy for sterilization. It also is a preventive measure against cancer of the cervix, cancer of the uterus, and menstruation. But risk of hysterectomy is several times more than that of a tubal ligation, so most medical authorities do not approve of a hysterectomy for sterilization. Most insurance companies will not pay for a hysterectomy when it is only done for sterilization. However, the most frequent situation is that a woman has a reason for a hysterectomy, which exists for a long time, and when she finally decides she wants no more children, she then goes ahead with the needed

BIRTH CONTROL: STERILIZATION--HYSTERECTOMIES
(Continued)

hysterectomy. The sterilization is a side effect and added benefit but not the main reason.

918. Why are so many women in their forties being encouraged by their gynecologists to have a hysterectomy?

One of the reasons women in their forties seem to have more hysterectomies is because they have other conditions, which may have been present for many years before, that are getting worse. Heavy menstrual flow is a condition that may turn into a premalignant (precancerous) lining of the uterus, as determined by a D & C, when a woman reaches her forties; fibroids, which simply may be present when women are in their thirties, become larger and bleed more in the forties. Endometriosis, which caused pelvic pain when they were in their thirties, may be making large endometriomas in their forties. After having several children, the uterus may be falling down and dragging the bladder and rectum with it, so that women are unable to control their urine. Since most women don't want any more babies when they reach their forties, the repair that really required a hysterectomy long ago is carried out then. Birth control is an added benefit of a hysterectomy, but it is not the main reason. Childbearing is a reason for women not to have a hysterectomy until they are sure this stage of their lives is complete. Usually, when a woman reaches her forties, she has completed her childbearing years. She then takes care of the problem that has been bothering her for years, by having the hysterectomy she has probably put off for years.

919. What are the different procedures used to perform a hysterectomy?

Hysterectomies may be performed through an abdominal incision or through a vaginal entry.

920. How do I know which method of hysterectomy to choose?

The procedure used for a hysterectomy depends upon the reason the hysterectomy is being done. You can ask for the vaginal route, but it isn't always possible. Your physician will discuss your surgical needs with you.

921. When would a vaginal hysterectomy be advisable?

If you have a pelvic relaxation, a uterus that is falling out or a bladder and rectum that are bulging out (a cystocele or rectocele), then a vaginal approach is advisable. This would allow repair of the bladder and rectal walls to be carried out at the same time as the hysterectomy. If the hysterectomy is being done to eliminate bleeding that is not due to cancer and the uterus is a normal size, a vaginal hysterectomy is done because recovery is faster.

BIRTH CONTROL: STERILIZATION—HYSTERECTOMIES
(Continued)

922. When would a hysterectomy by the abdominal approach be advisable?

If the reason for the hysterectomy is to remove a large fibroid tumor or there are other problems involving the ovaries, such as an old pelvic inflammatory disease, then the abdominal approach must be used. With this approach, the surgeon will be able to handle the removal of the large tumor, such as fibroids, and still get around adhesions from disease. Diseased ovaries must be removed through the abdomen. Sometimes normal ones can be removed vaginally, but seldom can diseased ones be removed this way.

923. What is the cost of a hysterectomy?

A hysterectomy costs $3,000.00 to $10,000.00, depending upon the complications. It is not covered by medical insurance if it only is done for sterilization purposes.

924. Does hysterectomy affect sex drive or performance?

Most studies conducted on women who have had a hysterectomy have determined that sex drive and performance usually are not affected by hysterectomy. There is no reason that they should be affected, since nothing necessary for sex drive and performance is removed or changed. Only if the idea of sterilization makes you reject sex does hysterectomy have any effect, and the same problem could occur if your husband had a vasectomy. If the hysterectomy is combined with a repair of your vagina and the vagina is made too tight, then performance can be impaired until it has been dilated to the proper size. This occurs more often if the vagina is not used for a long time after the repair, and is allowed to shrink. It is especially common after menopause. If freedom from the worry of pregnancy is a plus, then sex drive and performance may be increased, due to the release from fear of pregnancy. Freedom from pain and bleeding can also improve sex drive.

BIRTH CONTROL: STERILIZATION—VASECTOMY

925. Is vasectomy new?

No, it is not new, but it has increased in frequency since the late 1960s when sterilization became a patient's right instead of a privilege conferred on a few. The first vasectomies were done in the early 1900s.

926. How were men sterilized before the 1900s?

In earlier times and for centuries, men were sterilized by cutting off their testicles, castrating them. This was usually done as a punishment or to make eunuchs (castrated men) for the harem. Castration stopped their hormones and made them impotent as well, especially if it was before puberty. Men today may think vasectomy is like this, and perhaps this explains their reluctance to have them performed.

BIRTH CONTROL: STERILIZATION—VASECTOMY (Continued)

927. At what age is vasectomy recommended?

Federal law requires that the patient be twenty-one years of age if federal funds are going to pay for his vasectomy. Actually, the physician must be convinced that the patient is sure he wants a vasectomy, regardless of age. Those men who request a reversal later were usually under thirty years of age when they had their vasectomies done.

928. Are vasectomies safe?

They are safe, and much safer than a tubal ligation in a female. Only 1-3 percent of the men who have a vasectomy have a medical complication, such as infection or hemorrhage, requiring further treatment. Most men may have a little pain, swelling, or a little bleeding under the skin, which soon clears up.

929. Are all vasectomies performed in the doctor's office?

Most vasectomies are done in an office or clinic, but they may be done in the hospital when combined with another operation that requires hospitalization.

930. Are vasectomies performed under a local anesthetic?

Yes, vasectomies are performed under a local anesthetic, unless they are being done in combination with other surgery that requires a stronger anesthesia.

931. How is a vasectomy performed?

A small amount of local anesthetic is injected in the skin high on each side of the scrotum, the sack that holds the testicles. A small slit is then made in each anesthetized area right over the vas, the tube that carries sperm from the testicles to the penis. These are then cut, tied, and/or cauterized (burned), so that they are blocked. Then sutures are used to close the slits.

932. How does a vasectomy work?

The cut and tie, or cauterization, of the vas block the transport of sperm from the factory where they are made, the testicle, to the dispenser, the penis. Sperm continue to be produced, but cannot be dispensed. Of course, sperm already past this point in the vas and stored in the seminal vesicle, a sac near the prostate gland, can still be ejaculated from the penis. Many women have become pregnant because they thought their husbands' vasectomy should work the next day. You must use other contraception until all the sperm are gone.

933. After a vasectomy, what happens to the sperm?

After a vasectomy, sperm are still produced in the testicles and continue to come down the vas, but they are stopped where it is blocked. The body

BIRTH CONTROL: STERILIZATION—VASECTOMY (Continued)

then reabsorbs the sperm, and in the process makes antibodies that inactivate them. These antibodies can be detected in men's blood, but they are not known to be harmful.

934. When is the man considered sterile after a vasectomy?

After a vasectomy, the man is considered sterile only after the ejaculate is found free of sperm.

935. Will it hurt?

After a man has a vasectomy, there is some discomfort for a few days. Inactivity and wearing a support, such as jockey shorts or an athletic support, help.

936. How long does it take to perform a vasectomy?

It takes approximately fifteen to twenty minutes to perform a vasectomy.

937. Is vasectomy reversible? If yes, what percentage are successfully reversed?

Vasectomies are sometimes reversible. Of those attempted, about 30-60 percent succeed in making a woman pregnant, which is the final test. Nearly all vasectomies can be reversed in that the vas can be reconnected and sperm can again be found in the ejaculate. According to many studies, 80-90 percent of vasectomies are reversible, but the pregnancy rate is much lower. Because of the man's antibody formation, the sperm are inactivated in many men and will not get anyone pregnant. Since some men make more antibodies than others, the rate varies from man to man, and this determines the man's ability to have children more than does the skill of the surgeon. The skill of the surgeon determines how many vas really will be open and transmitting sperm.

938. How long after a vasectomy can the operation be successfully reversed?

After five years, the chances of a successful reversal are definitely decreased, so the sooner the better.

939. Can a vasectomy reverse itself?

Yes, the vas can re-form, or recanalize, and again form an open duct to carry the sperm to the penis, but this seldom happens. It accounts for the small failure rate, less than 1 percent, of vasectomy.

940. How do vasectomies emotionally affect men?

There is no physical reason that men should be emotionally affected by vasectomy at all. Testosterone continues to be produced in their testicles and distributed at the same rate to their bodies after vasectomy. If men react emotionally, it can be because they really did not want to be sterilized, or else they changed their minds.

BIRTH CONTROL: STERILIZATION—VASECTOMY (Continued)

941. Do most men resist having a vasectomy? If yes, are they worried that it will affect their masculinity?

Most men are resistant to having a vasectomy. They may already lack confidence in their sexual performance, and they fear that something like surgery, especially with the possibility of hemorrhage or infection, could ruin their future. Some men just may not want to be sterile.

942. Does a vasectomy affect sex drive or performance?

Vasectomy does not reduce the body's supply of testosterone, made in the testicles, so there is no physical reason that sexual drive or performance should change. However, the freedom from worry about contraception, especially condom use or withdrawal, could enhance performance.

943. What are the chances of impotence occuring as the result of a vasectomy?

A vasectomy cannot physically cause impotence. However, impotence is usually psychological and can result from anything that makes a man lose confidence in his sexual performance, such as fear.

944. Have vasectomies been linked to an increased risk of cancer?

Not successfully. Everything is accused of causing cancer these days, even sex. But it has been shown that in many men there is an increase in the production of autoimmune antibodies (substances produced to inactivate protein) to sperm. This is predictable, since their bodies must do something to destroy or inactivate the sperm that they can no longer get rid of by ejaculation. Whether these antibodies do anything to men's bodies is, so far, conjecture.

945. Have vasectomies been linked to an increased risk of heart attacks in men?

Vasectomies have been claimed to cause an increase in heart attacks, but this is very difficult to prove, because men are very prone to heart attacks anyway, even without a vasectomy. The studies show an increase in certain lipids in the blood of monkeys, which might be related to heart attacks; however,this has not been shown to occur in men.

946. What is the cost of a vasectomy?

In a low-cost clinic vasectomies range from free to $50.00; in a private office, they are $150.00 to $300.00. Vasectomies are not always covered by medical insurance.

947. Would more women like to see their husbands have a vasectomy after they have a full family?

Yes, many women confide that they wish their husbands would have a vasectomy, but they are afraid to nag or push them into it. They are worried

BIRTH CONTROL: STERILIZATION—VASECTOMY (Continued)

that if they insist, then their husbands might blame them if anything ever went wrong with their sexual performance after the surgery.

948. Are there any other methods of sterilization for men, besides vasectomy?

No, there are no other voluntary methods of sterilization available to men. Involuntary sterilization can occur, however, if surgery for cancer of the prostate, penis, or testicle is done, because portions of the reproductive system are removed. Radiation can also cause sterilization.

949. With more men having vasectomies today, are fewer women undergoing tubal ligations?

No, the tubal ligations are steadily increasing. Since sterilization became a patient's right, instead of a privilege, around 1968, they have steadily increased for women.

BIRTH CONTROL: MEN'S ATTITUDES TOWARD THE USE OF CONTRACEPTION

950. Why do so many men object to using the birth control methods that are available to them?

The only birth control methods currently available to men interfere with their enjoyment of sex, so it is not really hard to understand why they object to using them. The condom requires application after erection and changes the sensation. Withdrawal requires that a man maintain enough control to remove his penis prior to orgasm.

951. Why do some men object to women using birth control?

The explanation for why men object to women using contraception is complicated and even mysterious. If women interrupt the love-making sequence to insert foam or a diaphragm, annoyance is inevitable. But when they have an IUD, are on the pill, or have previously inserted a contraceptive, then why do some men still object? Some men do this because they think contraceptives are dangerous for their loved ones. Other men really want to have children, so they don't want to use birth control. Others simply like the danger of possible fertility. These men sometimes refer to having intercourse with women who are using contraceptives as "shooting blanks." Unless women are willing to have a lot of abortions or unwanted babies, it is advisable to stay away from men such as these.

952. Are males more fertile at certain times in their lives than others?

Men are not fertile until they can produce prostatic fluid, sperm, and ejaculate. The onset of puberty is ten to fifteen, and the peak probably is eighteen. Men are then fertile and remain fertile throughout their lives if no

BIRTH CONTROL: MEN'S ATTITUDES TOWARD THE USE OF CONTRACEPTION (Continued)

disease process interferes and if they remain sexually active. Infection, radiation, injuries, and chemicals, even excessive heat, can reduce their fertility. Their sexual performance may make them infertile even though their sperm are fine. A spinal cord injury may paralyze them in their reproductive abilities, but the sperm go on being produced in the testicles. Once men are fertile, there is no natural rise or fall in fertility—only accidents. Their ability to perform sexually decreases in frequency from eighteen until old age.

953. Have condoms gone out of style?

Yes, condoms do seem to be going out of style. Even before birth control pills for women came into use, a survey done in 1955 showed that only 26 percent of the couples surveyed used the condom for contraception. Still, it was the most popular method at that time. Rhythm was used by 21 percent of the respondents, and 24 percent used a diaphragm. Withdrawal was the method used by only 7 percent of the couples surveyed. The condom used to be the primary method of birth control for unmarried sex; it also helped to reduce the spread of VD. Today, the use of the condom as the sole method of contraception is limited to 3 percent of couples. When used in combination with cream, suppository, or foam, it is 5 percent.

954. Will condoms prevent the spread of VD? Herpes?

Nothing will absolutely prevent the spread of VD, except eliminating intimate contact with a person who has VD. However, the barrier protection of the condom helps keep the infected material in the vagina away from the penis and infected material in the penis away from the vagina. Many people have coitus a little while before they put on the condom, in which case there is no protection. Condoms can protect the woman from herpes if the ulcers are on the penis, but since contact with the labia occurs even with the condom, it does not protect the male from the female at all. Herpes ulcers in the female usually are on the lips of the vulva.

955. Birth control pills for men have been under research for years. Why aren't they available today?

The most successful birth control pill for men (danazol) costs $1.00 per pill and requires a shot (testosterone) once a week. It does not work until it has been used for two to three months, and then it works only 80 percent of the time. It also takes several months for a man to return to a fertile sperm count after the use of the pill has stopped. Other less successful methods have stopped sperm production permanently.

BIRTH CONTROL: MEN'S ATTITUDES TOWARD THE USE OF CONTRACEPTION (Continued)

956. How far into the future can we expect chemical birth control pills for men?

A crystal ball for this is very cloudy. It may never happen, because sperm production (spermatogenesis) seems to be so delicate that once it is turned off, it is difficult to regenerate. At least fifteen years of research have not produced a satisfactory birth control pill for men.

957. In this day and age, what should a man's role in birth control be?

The ideal role for a man in regards to birth control really should be the same as for a female. Together, as a couple, they both should decide whether or not they want a pregnancy; together they should discuss their likes and dislikes and the merits of the many different methods of birth control; and then, together, they should choose one. After that, they should reinforce its use, whatever the method. Rhythm is most effective when calculated by the man, because he doesn't pursue sex at the wrong time, forcing the woman to do the refusing. Reminding her to take her pill can be a token of love, as can waiting for the diaphragm to be inserted. Tolerating the feel of the IUD string also may be his contribution.

BIRTH CONTROL: SOCIAL AND RELIGIOUS ATTITUDES TOWARD THE USE OF CONTRACEPTION

958. When in a relationship should I discuss birth control with my partner?

It preferably should be discussed prior to intercourse and certainly prior to marriage, as a difference of opinion could be disastrous. If the man thinks that you are taking care of it and you think that he is taking care of it, pregnancy could result. A real understanding of each other's attitudes about having babies and using contraception is an integral part of a deep relationship. This is why it is sad to see a woman using an IUD without her husband's knowledge, because he does not want her to use any kind of birth control. It would be even sadder for her to have many more children than she wants. Some men seem to want no responsibility for birth control, and yet they are illogical enough to become angry if their partner becomes pregnant. It is best that a woman find out early in the relationship how her partner feels about it. Many men know very little about contraceptives, especially their effectiveness.

959. What methods of contraception can I use without discussing them with my partner and which ones should be discussed prior to their use?

If you are taking birth control pills, discussion is not really necessary for a temporary relationship, but it is important for a permanent one. An

BIRTH CONTROL: SOCIAL AND RELIGIOUS ATTITUDES TOWARD THE USE OF CONTRACEPTION (Continued)

IUD also is not necessary to discuss if the relationship is temporary. However, barrier methods may depend upon cooperation and must be agreed to prior to their use, even on a temporary basis.

960. Does shared responsibility for birth control increase intimacy?

Yes, it does. Communication increases intimacy, and responsibility for birth control requires communication.

961. In our society it seems that women are burdened with the sole responsibility for birth control. Is it that way in other societies?

Yes, that is generally true. The birth control methods that women use seem to be more effective than withdrawal or the condom. Men actually take more responsibility in Europe and the United States than they do in some countries of Africa or the Middle East, where it is almost ridiculous to ask a man to use a condom. He would be insulted at the suggestion. It also may be that women are far more likely to be motivated to use contraception than men, since they have more to lose by not doing so. Before the pill, more men were willing to use the condom. However, even then there was a dispensing machine for condoms in Scandinavia that was installed in a women's restroom, with the motto, "He never will!"

962. Why do people fear birth control so much?

By publishing frightening articles that increase the fear of all contraception, the communications industry is partly to blame for this fear. For some women, whether they use birth control depends on what they fear more—pregnancy or the use of contraceptives. Women also rightfully fear that sex itself is dangerous, as they may get a venereal disease or be injured in some way. They also may know that sex is the cause of cervical cancer. However, you must not allow your fears to be out of proportion with the actual danger, for then your fears will control your life, and you will live in fear. Many parents have described birth control to young people as very dangerous. Their motivation really is to prevent them from having sex. Ministers and especially priests have given sermons about the danger of pills, saying they caused cancer, which is not true. They should have given the sermon on why you should not use contraception at all, since that is what they believe.

963. Why does the Catholic Church object to all forms of birth control, except the rhythm method?

Strict Catholic doctrine does not approve of the rhythm method, except in cases where there is a dire need to avoid pregnancy. The belief is that life should not be controlled. But the best way to find an answer to this question is to ask the Catholic Church itself, not medical science.

BIRTH CONTROL: ABORTION

964. How common is the use of abortion as a method of birth control?

Most women seeking an abortion have not used birth control, so most abortions are a form of birth control. There are over one million abortions a year, performed on over a half million women who used no contraception at all. Others really may be planning an abortion if they get pregnant, but they never get pregnant and therefore are not counted. A survey of the motivation for abortion would be difficult to carry out. Some people will only think about a problem when there is a crisis, and pregnancy produces a crisis. Often, women do not use contraception until after they have had an abortion.

965. How great are the emotional problems associated with using abortion as a method of birth control?

There are no emotional problems known to accompany the use of abortion as a method of birth control. More depressions develop from continuing a pregnancy than from abortion. If a woman does not adjust to the idea of an abortion easily, she should use another method of birth control.

966. Dr. Carson, as a doctor, how do you and other health workers feel about women who use abortion as a method of birth control?

I can attest to the emotional problems of physicians and health workers when they encounter someone using abortion as a birth control method. Most people in the medical field become angry and have bad things to say about a woman who is doing that, especially someone who is appearing for her fourth abortion in the same year. The feeling is that the medical system, as well as the economic system, are being abused, especially if the woman is on welfare. Even if she is using private insurance, the ones who are paying the premium are being abused.

967. What is the feeling in other countries about women who use abortion as a method of birth control?

The use of abortion as a birth control method has been discussed at the international level. Sweden, for instance, defends the right of a woman to an abortion if the circumstances justify it, regardless of how many she has had before. Abortion for Swedes, however, is still a committee decision. In Japan, elective abortion was legal long before birth control. The women of Italy fought for and won the right to abortions. In Latin America, they are still illegal, but frequently done.

968. What are the physiological damages, if any, to using abortion as a method of birth control?

If each abortion is performed prior to three months of pregnancy, no physiological damage can be detected, unless you have a hemorrhage, infec-

BIRTH CONTROL: ABORTION (Continued)

tion, perforation of the uterus, or anesthetic accident at the time of the abortion. But if each abortion is uncomplicated, it is no worse than having a spontaneous miscarriage with a D & C. If you have Rh negative blood, you should be given immune globulin (Rh antibodies) after each abortion so that you will not develop sensitization to Rh positive blood with these pregnancies, otherwise future babies could be affected. If you have to pay all the costs for each abortion, you will find it much more expensive than any other birth control method. This might be one of the reasons the public does not like to fund abortions; they feel women are using them for contraception instead of for an emergency or crisis.

969. Can any physiological damages occur if an abortion is performed while I am three to six months pregnant?

If the abortion is done in the mid-trimester, three to six months pregnant, then the procedures to dilate the cervix can damage it, and future babies literally fall out so prematurely that they cannot live at all. This occurs only in a small percentage of women, but it is still a good reason to have the abortion in the first three months rather than later.

970. Is an abortion easier if it is done early?

Yes, very much so. If you can detect that you are pregnant early, such as with a home pregnancy test, and then decide by the eighth week after the beginning of your last menstrual period that you want an abortion, it can be done outside of a hospital in an office or a clinic. A small plastic curette (a loop-shaped instrument with a sharp edge) can be used so that you will not have to have your cervix dilated. Therefore, the pain is so minimal that you can manage with a local anesthetic, such as a paracervical block. This takes five or ten minutes and has the lowest danger to your health, primarily because no general anesthesia is required. The cost is also low, $150.00 being the average cost throughout the United States for this procedure.

971. Is there any danger to my health if I get an abortion later?

Yes. An early abortion, under eight to twelve weeks, has a death rate of only 1 in 100,000 abortions. If an abortion is performed later, the complications increase, and the death rate rises to 4 in 100,000 abortions. Of course, this is still not as high as the total death rate for pregnancy including full-term deliveries, which is around 16 per 100,000 pregnancies.

972. How is an early abortion performed?

First, blood typing must be done, because if the woman is Rh negative, an immune globulin must be given so that she will not develop antibodies to Rh positive blood. Then she is placed on an examining table just as for a pelvic examination. After some cleansing, a paracervical block (local

BIRTH CONTROL: ABORTION (Continued)

anesthetic) is injected into the cervix. The top lip of the cervix is grasped with a hooklike instrument called a tenaculum, and a soft plastic curette is inserted into the cavity. Suction is then applied, either by a vacuum machine or by a large syringe with a stop on it so air cannot be injected. The curette is moved about until all of the material can be obtained, and then it is removed. All equipment inserted in the cervix must be sterile or infection could occur. Total time for the procedure is about five or ten minutes.

973. What is a "menstrual extraction"?

It is another name for an abortion done before you have missed your second period, or before the eighth week after the beginning of your last menstrual period. The procedure is the same as that in the previous question. Even though the pain is minimal, women would not like to endure it every month to "extract" their menses.

974. If I wait until after my eighth week to decide I want an abortion, how is it done?

Because the uterus and its contents are larger, it requires some dilation of the cervix. This also can require a more powerful suction machine than that used for the early abortion, so some form of general sedation or anesthesia is usually needed. Therefore, the abortion frequently is done in a hospital under general anesthesia, which becomes more expensive. By law, it can still be done in a clinic or office, but more equipment and anesthesia is required. It will usually cost more there, too.

975. If I wait until the fourth or fifth month of my pregnancy to decide to have an abortion, how is it done?

The most frequent and least expensive procedure would be a D & E (a dilatation and evacuation). It would also have the least complications. It requires general or regional anesthesia, and therefore is usually done in a hospital. The day before surgery a "laminaria" is placed in the cervix to dilate it slowly. This is a dried seaweed that takes up water in the cervix and swells, dilating the cervix. The next day you are anesthetized, and the contents of your uterus are removed by forceps as well by a large suction curette in order to remove all of the placenta. Blood loss is greater at this stage of pregnancy, as are complications, such as hemorrhage, infection, perforation of the uterus by the instruments, and something called DIC, disseminated intravascular coagulation, which is a severe bleeding disorder.

976. Are there any other methods of abortion that are available in the mid-trimester, after the third month?

Yes. The oldest method was hysterotomy, in which a little cesarean section was done. Of course, this was a major surgery, very expensive, and re-

BIRTH CONTROL: ABORTION (Continued)

quired the mother to have any future babies by cesarean section because of the scar on the uterus. The next oldest method was saline injection. Very saturated saline (salt solution) was injected through the woman's abdomen into the cavity of the uterus where the amniotic fluid is located. The salt would draw fluid into the uterus and cause labor; after eighteen hours or so of labor, the fetus and placenta would deliver. If the fetus but not the placenta delivered, a curettage was needed. With this method, the woman was given pain medication, but the experience was still more dreadful for her than a D & C given under general anesthesia. Another method consisted of a similar injection of a solution of prostaglandins (substances locally produced in the tissues that can cause cramps) into the amniotic cavity, the water around the fetus. It also started labor, sometimes more efficiently than the saline. A newer way is to put a suppository of prostaglandins into the vagina every four to six hours until labor starts and delivers the fetus, but it still takes several hours. Prostaglandins also are a problem because they not only cause contractions (that's how they cause menstrual cramps), but also cause nausea, vomiting, and diarrhea (like some women get with menstrual cramps). These methods are still used in mid-trimester abortions when the abortion is being done because of the likelihood of a congenital abnormality. They leave the fetus intact so the doctors can tell if it really had the abnormality.

977. How long does it take to have an abortion?

That depends upon how far along you are in your pregnancy, and what method is used. An office abortion takes about five minutes from the time the local anesthetic is given to completion. If you have a hospital abortion, it is perhaps fifteen minutes from the time of induction of anesthesia to the completion of the surgery, but it may take you an hour or so to wake up. A mid-trimester abortion, performed in the fourth or fifth month, can be by D & E (dilatation and evacuation), saline, or prostaglandins. A D & E requires a laminaria insertion into the cervix on one day, and anesthesia and surgery, which takes about fifteen minutes including anesthesia, the next day. Waking up may take an hour or two. Saline requires an injection that induces labor, which may take six, twelve, eighteen, or even thirty-six hours to complete. Prostaglandins are a little faster, and the suppositories usually work within about twelve hours.

978. Are abortions that occur in abortion clinics performed by certified doctors?

If you mean licensed doctors, yes. No state has yet allowed any licensed health workers, other than physicians, to do abortions, but these are not necessarily board certified obstetrician-gynecologists.

BIRTH CONTROL: ABORTION (Continued)

979. Who can legally perform an abortion?

Any licensed physician can perform an abortion.

980. Is there a limit to the number of abortions a woman can safely have?

No. There have been women who have had fifteen abortions, who were fine and able to have full-term babies afterwards.

981. What percentage of women who have an abortion were using birth control at the time they became pregnant?

Less than 10 percent were using birth control.

982. What is a therapeutic abortion?

A therapeutic abortion is an abortion that is done to improve the patient's physical or mental health because it is threatened by the continuation of the pregnancy. Elective abortion is an abortion that is done because you want one.

983. What kinds of tests are done before an abortion?

First, tests are performed to determine if you are pregnant. Then you have a blood test to be sure you are not too anemic and to determine if your blood type is Rh negative. A urinalysis is done to be sure that you do not have diabetes that is not under control. A physical examination with emphasis on the pelvic structures is also necessary.

984. Do some women have special problems that make it impossible for them to have an abortion?

Some women could have acute illnesses that would delay the abortion surgery, but there is no medical problem that would make delivering a baby safer than having an abortion. All women are able to have abortions, although it might be more difficult for some.

985. How and when are most abortions performed?

Today in the United States, most abortions are performed in the first three months of pregnancy in physicians' offices. A small plastic curette is inserted into the cervix and suction is applied by a vacuum machine or a large syringe especially made for this purpose. A local or general anesthesia, or just sedation, may or may not be used.

986. What is the difference between a D & C and an abortion?

An abortion is one purpose of a D & C. Other purposes of a D & C could be to stop heavy menstruation, diagnose cancer of the uterus, or to stop intermenstrual bleeding. The technique is a little different in that suction is more often used on the abortion type of D & C.

987. What were the earliest forms of abortion?

For centuries women have inserted long slender objects into their cer-

BIRTH CONTROL: ABORTION (Continued)

vixes to attempt to induce abortions. Coat hangers frequently were used, and catheters were also popular. "Slippery elm" was a stick that would swell and dilate the cervix after insertion and sometimes cause it to empty. Potassium permanganate tablets were also inserted in the vagina. These were so irritating that sometimes the uterus would empty, but sometimes it would just get burned. Women have drunk various poisons to try to get sick enough to abort. Of course, all of these were quite dangerous.

988. How are most illegal abortions done?

In this country, there almost aren't any more illegal abortions. In the past, most illegal abortions were done by nonphysicians who used poor methods, such as catheters and other similar instruments. It is hoped that illegal abortionists in other countries will avail themselves of the new techniques and equipment that are now available.

989. Will I bleed after an abortion?

Usually you will bleed for a little bit that day, stop bleeding for three or four days, and then bleed again as in a menstrual period. Sometimes there is not very much bleeding. If there is more, it is abnormal and should be reported to your doctor.

990. What symptoms should I watch for after an abortion that would indicate something is wrong?

Watch for pain, bleeding, and fever. Mild menstrual cramps on the day of the abortion are normal, but persistent or severe cramping is not. Bleeding as much as a menstrual flow is normal, but more is not, especially soaking four or five pads an hour or passing large clots. Any temperature over 100° should be reported to your doctor and investigated in case you are developing an infection, even if it may be due to a cold. Continuing to feel pregnant is also abnormal, because sometimes the abortion doesn't work and must be done again.

991. Will my period resume immediately after I have an abortion?

After the bleeding of the abortion is over, your next menstrual period usually will not occur until nearly six weeks later, and in half of the women, it occurs later than that. The same is true after a full-term delivery if you do not breast-feed.

992. If I have an incomplete abortion, will I have to go back for a second abortion?

Sometimes the abortion can be completed by using a drug, such as ergotrate, that clamps down the uterus and expels any contents left in it. But if you still have a growing pregnancy, you should have a second abortion.

BIRTH CONTROL: ABORTION (Continued)

993. How do I know if I have had an incomplete abortion?

If you are bleeding abnormally, developing a fever, or having severe pain, these are signs of an incomplete abortion, and you should report them to your doctor and take any action he or she advises, including a second abortion if necessary. If you still feel pregnant and do not bleed at all, you may still have a growing pregnancy. The best thing to do is to have a follow-up examination, including a pelvic, in a week or two following the abortion to be sure everything has returned to normal.

994. What complications can arise from an incomplete abortion?

You can have bleeding, fever, infection, or even a continuing pregnancy.

995. Can an abortion make me sterile?

Yes, if something goes wrong, but so can a full-term delivery. If you hemorrhage and require a hysterectomy to stop the bleeding, you will be sterile. If you get an infection that damages your tubes, you can also become sterile. These are rare occurrences with abortion.

996. Do abortions cause infections?

Any surgery can cause an infection. If the equipment is sterile, if sterile technique is followed, if the woman does not already have an infection, like gonorrhea, in her vagina, and if the abortion is complete with no tissue left in, it is very unlikely to cause an infection. Illegal abortions, however, caused many infections.

997. How many abortions are performed on women who, due to an error in the pregnancy test, were not pregnant?

Very few. The decision that a woman is pregnant is based partly on a pelvic examination and partly on a pregnancy test. Only about 1 percent or less of positive pregnancy tests are false. Some are inevitable, but it is impossible to know just how many, because the tissue is not always sent to a pathologist to determine if the woman really is pregnant. Sometimes when a pelvic examination suggests that a woman is not pregnant, but a pregnancy test says she is, the situation in a woman's life is such that she cannot wait to be sure that she is pregnant. She may have to leave for college or a trip perhaps to Europe, and cannot wait two weeks to be sure. So she goes ahead with the desired abortion, pregnant or not. It then becomes just a D & C. When there is real doubt in the surgeon's mind, the tissue is sent to the pathologist for confirmation of pregnancy, but to do this routinely becomes too expensive.

BIRTH CONTROL: ABORTION (Continued)

998. How long is the recuperation period in a woman who has just had an abortion?

This depends a little on the procedure and the stage of pregnancy, but it is never more than one day. Most women feel better than they did before the procedure, because they are rid of the cramps and nausea of pregnancy. They usually can return to school or work; some even go back to work on the same day. However, the psychological adjustment may take longer.

999. What rights does the father of the fetus have?

None. The woman has a right to control her own body, and the father does not have the right to use her body to carry his baby unless she agrees to do so. That is the law in this land. She does not require his consent for an abortion. Unfortunately, the opposite occurrence is more frequent: the woman tells the father that she is pregnant, and although she wants a baby, he forces her to have an abortion either because he does not want a baby or he does not want to support it. This has been going on for many years, long before abortions were legal. It was an even worse situation when the man forced the woman to have an illegal abortion and risk her life. Now she does not risk her life, because abortions are so safe, death being 1 in 100,000 abortions in the first three months. How does he force her to abort his child? By threatening to leave her and to withdraw his financial support as well as his love, if she does not do so. His threats are effective and society does not protect her from them.

1000. Does an abortion hurt?

That depends upon the procedure. A D & C (dilatation and currettage) or a D & E (dilatation and evacuation) done in the hospital under general anesthesia does not involve pain, but there may be a few cramps afterwards. An office abortion performed under a local anesthetic still involves quite a bit of pain, similar to labor pains, but this is often aided by some sedation. The saline and prostaglandins mid-trimester abortions involve as much pain as labor, but there is no restriction on how much morphine is given during this process; morphine is limited in real labor for the sake of the baby. Nevertheless, these methods involve the most pain for the woman.

1001. Will an abortion affect my ability to have children later?

If the abortion is performed early in pregnancy, before eight or twelve weeks, there is no effect on later births or the ability to get pregnant. Abortions done in the fourth, fifth, or even sixth month, can damage the cervix, so that future children may be born prematurely because the cervix simply opens under pressure. This also can happen to your cervix in a normal

BIRTH CONTROL: ABORTION (Continued)

delivery and can damage it so much that the next child is born prematurely. This is called an incompetent cervix. Of course, if you have complications of the abortion, such as infection or hemorrhage, requiring a hysterectomy, there may be no future pregnancies, but these complications are quite rare. And they can happen after a full-term delivery, too. So once you embark on the course of a pregnancy, whether you have an abortion or a baby, it can affect your ability to get pregnant and have a baby in the future. The course with the least problems is not to get pregnant at all until you want a baby.

1002. My doctor doesn't perform abortions. How can I get one?

First, be sure you are right about your doctor. If you are, contact your nearest Planned Parenthood clinic, your nearest medical school hospital, your nearest health clinic, or even your counselor at school or college. Frequently there are hotlines listed in your phone book or even in ads in your newspaper that provide help for pregnant girls who do not know where to turn.

1003. What does an abortion cost?

The early abortion, performed on women who are less than eight weeks pregnant, can be done in a private physician's office under local anesthetic for as low as $150.00. If performed in a hospital under anesthesia, it can cost over $1,000.00. The mid-trimester abortion is less for a D & E with its short hospitalization and short surgery, costing $600.00. Spending several days in the hospital for a saline abortion can cost over $1,500.00. Most insurance plans still cover abortion, but federally funded programs, like Champus, do not. You have to find out about your state to know whether Medicaid programs cover abortion. If everyone had to pay for them out of their own pockets, they would certainly come in earlier to get the least expensive kind, which is also the safest for their health.

1004. After an abortion, is it difficult to have a normal pregnancy?

No, it is not difficult to have a normal pregnancy after having an abortion, unless complications occurred with the abortion or there was damage to the cervix. Some Japanese women have had fifteen documented abortions, and then had a normal baby. It is also said that the average number of abortions (though illegal) in some areas of South America is seven or eight per woman. It is not really known how many illegal abortions American women used to have, so it is impossible to compare this number with a control group that never had abortions to see if there is any difference in the number of women who went on to have a normal pregnancy. Also, there is no large control group of women who never had abortions.

BIRTH CONTROL: ABORTION (Continued)

1005. When is it too late to have an abortion?

It is too late to have an abortion when the fetus is advanced enough that it could live outside of the uterus, yet so premature that it would live a life of misery due to brain damage and other abnormalities caused by prematurity, such as blindness and deafness. This is why the Supreme Court has limited the right to elective abortion to the first six months of pregnancy. Babies born in the last three months may live, but they will be defective. Medically, it is quite possible to interrupt pregnancy at any time, and this is sometimes done to save the life of the mother, but only then.

1006. Is an abortion more dangerous after a certain age?

Age is not such a problem by itself, but if a women has become diabetic, hypertensive, smokes, has heart disease, is obese, or is otherwise very unhealthy, then any procedure, including abortion, is more dangerous for her than it would be for a healthy young woman. The dangers of contraception are not really greater than the dangers of abortion, even in the older age group, and abortion is always safer than continuing the pregnancy at any age.

1007. Is abortion available without parental approval?

Abortion is available without parental notification or approval in California and other states, if the minor seems capable of making her own decision. In some states, laws requiring parental approval are now being reviewed by the Supreme Court. Some individual doctors and clinics may require parental approval; others, of a particular religion, will not give an abortion to anyone. Also, some hospitals require parental signatures, and sometimes the parents are required to pay for an abortion. This is a land of diversity, so the minor has to find her way around. Counselors are a big help, and so are hotlines and the phone book.

BIRTH CONTROL: BREAST-FEEDING AS A CONTRACEPTIVE

1008. Is it true that I cannot become pregnant while breast-feeding, or it this just an old wives' tale?

This is partially true. It has been found that whether or not you can get pregnant while you are breast-feeding depends upon your total body fat and total nutrition. In the United States, where both body fat and good nutrition are plentiful, very few women have an absense of menstruation for more than three or four months while they are breast-feeding. Instead, their menses return and so does their fertility. Yet, in other countries around the world, women who breast-feed their children for two or three years tend not to have another baby more than every three or four years. These women do

BIRTH CONTROL: BREAST-FEEDING AS A CONTRACEPTIVE
(Continued)

not get pregnant and do have menses while they are breast-feeding, at least for a year. Generally, a very thin woman who loses weight while breast-feeding is less likely to have menses or become pregnant, while a heavier woman who eats well is much more likely to do so. The World Health Organization has advised that contraception becomes necessary even though you are breast-feeding when: 1) you replace one feeding with other food, 2) the baby sleeps as long as six hours, 3) menses return, or 4) six months have passed.

1009. If I am not menstruating while I am breast-feeding, is this an effective birth control method?

You could calculate it as 80 percent effective, for as long as you do not menstruate. The 20 percent failure rate is because you can get pregnant on the first ovulation before you ever menstruate, and you would not even realize it. Even if you do not have menses, it is better to supplement with a vaginal foam or some barrier birth control. The minipill (progesterone only) or the low-dose combination pill also can be used without harm to breast-feeding of the baby.

BIRTH CONTROL: MENOPAUSE AND CONTRACEPTION

1010. Is birth control necessary after the age of forty-five?

Forty-five is a dangerous age to stop contraception, since many women ovulate and can get pregnant through the age of forty-six. Statistically, forty-seven would be a safer age to eliminate contraception. Perhaps it would be better to continue some effort at contraception until after fifty or until after one year of menopause, whichever occurs sooner. "Menopausal babies" are usually born to women forty-six years of age and younger who thought they were in menopause when they got pregnant.

1011. Is birth control necessary after menopause?

If it is truly menopause, birth control is not necessary. However, not every pause in menses is true menopause.

1012. How old was the oldest woman to have a baby in the United States?

The oldest woman to have a baby in the United States was fifty-seven years old.

BIRTH CONTROL: TELLING YOUR CHILDREN ABOUT IT

1013. When should I discuss reproduction and birth control with my children?

This should occur when your children are most curious about all

BIRTH CONTROL: TELLING YOUR CHILDREN ABOUT IT
(Continued)

aspects of sex and reproduction, usually when they are around four years old. A discussion of birth control should be included whenever you first explain reproduction to your child, as it may be frightening to the child to know that she can get pregnant if she does not know how to prevent it. It is also better to discuss contraception with children before they have a need for it, otherwise it may sound like an accusation.

1014. What should I tell my daughter about birth control and reproduction?

When explaining reproduction to a daughter, mothers should explain that if you do not have coitus with a boy, pregnancy will not occur. They should also explain that it cannot happen until a girl is fully developed and menstruating, otherwise, some girls might become obsessed with the idea that they are pregnant. People may laugh at the child, but if she does not understand that pregnancy cannot happen until she is adolescent and until she has coitus, then in her mind it is real. Added to this, a mother should explain that if you have coitus, pregnancy can be prevented by certain means or devices, such as the rhythm method or birth control pills. If birth control is not included, the girl may grow up debating whether or not she wants to have sex and have babies. Many decide that they want babies and no sex!

1015. What is being taught in our schools about birth control?

This varies from state to state, and from school to school. In California, it is the custom to include a series on menstruation and reproduction at the sixth grade level, which is the year before most girls start to menstruate. Then at the eleventh or twelfth grade level there is a more comprehensive series, which parents can review in advance and decide if they will let their child attend. This series includes discussions of contraception. Many schools also invite Planned Parenthood to make a presentation on birth control, and some invite gynecologists to discuss the subject as part of the course on family life.

1016. Why is a clear understanding of birth control at a young age so important in girls?

For a girl to understand her role in the world and be able to plan an education, such as becoming a doctor for example, she also has to know that she can control her reproduction with some means other than complete abstinence. Ambition begins early in life, and maybe one reason some girls give up their goals early is that they did not learn at a young age that reproduction can be controlled for their own purposes. In the past, she was given the choice of giving up sex and men in order to have a career, or giving

BIRTH CONTROL: TELLING YOUR CHILDREN ABOUT IT
(Continued)

up the career, because sex and men lead to children. She does not have to make that choice today if she accepts birth control.

BIRTH CONTROL: PLANNED PARENTHOOD

1017. What is Planned Parenthood?

Planned Parenthood is a national organization of clinics that provide family planning information and sometimes treatment. Their information includes contraception, abortion, abortion referral, and sterilization. Anyone can go to these clinics for information and help.

1018. What types of birth control methods do the Planned Parenthood agencies offer?

All types of prescription birth control pills, IUDs, diaphragms, and over-the-counter barrier methods are discussed and available at these agencies. Some even have the cervical cap available on a trial basis.

1019. What other services, besides offering birth control, do the Planned Parenthood agencies offer?

They have discussion groups on sexuality that are both educational and therapeutic. Some also offer help for infertility problems and with prenatal care.

BIRTH CONTROL: NEWEST METHODS OF BIRTH CONTROL— ANTI-LRF, DEPO-PROVERA, ANTI-PROGESTERONE PILL

1020. What other methods of birth control for women are currently being researched? What is in store for women in the future?

One of the most promising new methods of birth control for women is a synthetic anti-LRF (luteinizing hormone releasing factor), which can be given just at the end of menses and, it is hoped, in pill form rather than by injection.

1021. How does this new synthetic anti-LRF work?

It affects the menstrual cycle so that the luteal phase (the part of your cycle that starts after ovulation and continues until menses) is shortened and is, therefore, infertile for implantation. This will be a once-a-month pill.

1022. Where is the new synthetic anti-LRF pill being developed?

It is being developed in southern California, particularly at the University of California, San Diego.

**BIRTH CONTROL: NEWEST METHODS OF BIRTH CONTROL—
ANTI-LRF, DEPO-PROVERA, ANTI-PROGESTERONE PILL**
(Continued)

1023. Are Depo-Provera shots presently being used anywhere in the United States?

Depo-Provera shots are used in the United States, particularly by some Planned Parenthood agencies and individual physicians, for certain special problems of contraception. It is only approved by the FDA to treat late uterine cancer, not for contraception.

1024. What sort of guidelines does the FDA require before a new birth control method is made available to the public?

Animal studies are first required to show that the drug or device is safe for the health of the patient. Studies then are done on volunteer human subjects for at least two or three years not only to show safety, but also to show that there are no changes, as well as that it is effective. If no unfavorable effects that would forbid use are shown, they are then released for prescription or over-the-counter use.

1025. Are there any other new methods being worked on?

In France, an anti-progesterone pill has been announced that can be taken just at the time of expected menses. It is so effective that even if the pregnancy has implanted, the loss of progesterone will make it slough off with menses. Some people object that this is abortion, but it is so early that it is an ethical, not a medical, problem.

Chapter 5

Sex

Love is
    being happy for the other person when they are happy
    being sad for the person when they are sad
    being together in good times
        and being together in bad times
Love is the source of strength

Love is
    being honest with yourself at all times
    being honest with the other person at all times
    telling, listening, respecting the truth,
        and never pretending
Love is the source of reality

Love is
    an understanding so complete that
    you feel as if you are a part of the other person
    accepting the other person just the way they are
    and not trying to change them to be something else
Love is the source of unity

Love is
    the freedom to pursue your own desires
    while sharing your experiences with the other person
    the growth of one individual alongside of
    and together with the growth of another individual
Love is the source of success

Love is
  the excitement of planning things together
  the excitement of doing things together
Love is the source of the future

Love is
  the fury of the storm
  the calm in the rainbow
Love is the source of passion

Love is
  giving and taking in a daily situation
  being patient with each other's needs and desires
Love is the source of sharing

Love is
  knowing that the other person
  will always be with you regardless of what happens
  missing the other person when they are away
  but remaining near in heart at all times
Love is the source of security

Love is
  the
source
  of
life

— Susan Polis Schutz

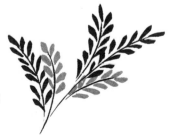

SEX

When women took charge of their bodies in matters of sex, it was first called a sexual revolution. Our sex lives were controlled by whatever our culture considered to be sexually moral. This was usually decided by our fathers, mothers, peers, schools, churches, city fathers, state legislatures, local police, and Congress. Unmarried women were not allowed to say "yes," and married women were not allowed to say "no." It was considered indecent for a woman to enjoy sexual activity of any kind, except holding hands.

Today some women really still feel more secure following all the old precepts governing sex, but they also may adopt the new attitude that they should enjoy sex as well. They will then wonder why they do not.

Most women now really want to learn—from others, from books, and from experience. They have assumed the right to sexual fulfillment, as well as the responsibility for control of their bodies. For human beings, sex is a learned behavior, not an instinct. Sex with a partner is always learned, and our culture does a poor job of teaching it, so many adults have problems, especially women. This chapter can help give information, dispel myths, and make you feel more sexually normal than you ever thought possible. "You shall know the truth, and the truth shall make you free." (John 8:32)

SEX: ATTITUDES TOWARD

1026. How have attitudes about sex changed through time in our society?

The biggest change is the attitude now that women have a capacity and a right to enjoy sex, and they are really learning to do so. Along with this has come a revolutionary change in the attitude about women having sex prior to marriage. There is more tolerance for couples openly living together without marriage. Openness and tolerance for homosexuality has also increased, and this is no longer classified as a disorder or disease in the medical world.

1027. How have the roles of men and women concerning sex changed in recent years?

The most significant changes in the role of women have been their increased awareness of sexual desire and their frequency of having sex. In the Kinsey Report on female sexual behavior, which was published in 1953, the frequency of sex among women was once every two weeks. Later, according to *The Hite Report* published in 1976, one-third of the women surveyed said that they have sex two or three times a week. A comparison of these two surveys also indicates that more women have learned to masturbate. As a result of this, they have become more aware of what will bring them to orgasm, and they have dared to ask men for it. More men, on the other hand, have become impotent in recent years trying to respond to this new sexual aggressiveness of women.

1028. How have changing attitudes toward sex affected sexual activity?

More premarital sex is occurring, to both the delight and chagrin of men. Couples are also using more varied positions and actions during sex, because they no longer think that it is intrinsically wrong or evil to do so.

1029. What is meant by "the double standard"? Do boys or men still abide by it?

Yes, most men and boys still abide by several double standards, and girls and women still hold on to them, too. Often women expect men to know more about the sex function than they do. They often wait for the male to be the aggressor in initiating sexual activity, and they pretend that they were not planning to cooperate. Many boys still feel it is their right to push for sexual activity and leave the responsibility of saying "no" to the girls. Boys leave the responsibility for contraception to girls as well. Many also still think that a girl means yes, even when she says no. Today, however, some of the double standards are changing, and many women are taking a much more aggressive role in sex.

SEX: ATTITUDES TOWARD (Continued)

1030. Is there a relationship between sex and the psychological need to be loved?

Yes, of course there is a connection between sex and the need to be loved. We obviously need to be loved more than we need sex. We also need to love ourselves. Women often, unfortunately, give sex in order to be loved. The ideal is to combine sex with the satisfaction of the need to love and be loved.

1031. How do I deal with guilt feelings resulting from sex?

If you are having sex with your best friend's husband, then you probably should feel guilty. However, if you feel guilty about having any sex at all, then you have been conditioned to think it is wrong under any circumstances. Group discussions with your peers, especially with a good leader, may change your attitude by peer pressure. Consultation with a psychologist or psychiatrist may help you trace the origin of your guilt and eliminate it. Reading books on sex or listening to programs and lectures by authorities who obviously don't think sex is a cause of guilt can help to dispel the feelings. Discussing your problem with your doctor, minister, or rabbi can help.

1032. What was the sexual revolution?

The sexual revolution was the declaration of the rights of women to have sex when and as they want to, without paying the price of pregnancy. This was made possible by the use of effective contraception, especially the pill, backed up by elective abortion.

1033. How does the way I feel about my body affect my attitude toward and enjoyment of sex?

If your self-esteem is based on the function of your body more than your appearance, you are more likely to enter into and enjoy sexual activity. Some of the most "beautiful" women derive no pleasure from sex, while some of the best long-term sex partners are possibly very obese. It may be that, in some cases, the "beautiful people" feel they do not need to be active in sex, and the less attractive bodies try harder.

SEX: EMERGING SEXUAL FEELINGS

1034. When does a female first begin experiencing sexual feelings?

Sexual arousal and response is present at birth. Little girls have vaginal lubrication in the first few hours of life in response to being touched, just as little boys respond to being touched by having erections as soon as they are born. Learning to recognize these feelings as being sexual comes later in the consciousness of the individual. Some women never recognize their sexual feelings for as long as they live.

SEX: EMERGING SEXUAL FEELINGS (Continued)

1035. To what extent is a person's sexuality determined in early childhood?

It has been shown that by the age of two, a child is very clear about his or her sexual designation and sex role. This awareness may precede speech. Sexual designation, feelings, and response, of course, are not related in this early stage.

1036. Do young children experience any sexual feelings before puberty?

Touch is a sexual feeling that babies and children respond to. Studies show that children who are not cuddled, fondled, and loved as babies and young children do not develop into normal adults. So touching is a vital part of human development. Some people might object to labeling this touch-response as "sexual," but then some people do not recognize the necessity of touch-response in sexual function as adults. Genital touching, more specifically, is seen in young children when they try to go to sleep. This is not labeled as sexual, although it is genitally directed, and some adults might call it masturbation. At school age, many of these activities are consciously suppressed and do not recur until puberty; some continue. The method by which parents and others socialize children by suppressing sexual activity will have a great effect on their sexual adjustment later.

SEX: SEX EDUCATION

1037. At what age is it best to begin sex education?

Sex education begins as soon as a child is born. Touch and response, pleasure with feeling and enjoying relationships, feeding at mother's breasts, enjoying the sensual part of life, and the child's observation of relationships, especially his or her parents, are all a part of sex education. More formal education comes when children ask questions about sex, as they do about everything else, and a discussion of the information often occurs when they reach three and four years old. Later, eight- to ten-year olds may become embarrassed by such subjects because their parents have been showing embarrassment and avoidance of these subjects. Children may even forget what they knew before. If education is attempted when they are embarrassed, the information is not retained. It is hard to teach children something they do not want to know. Greater interest occurs with the changes of puberty, and this is a good time for other education to occur, too.

1038. Is the sex education my children receive in school enough, or should I discuss sex with them at home, too?

Discussion of sex at home is far superior to the education your children receive at school, because you can include all your own values and attitudes in your home discussion.

SEX: SEX EDUCATION (Continued)

1039. Should sex be taught to daughters by their mothers and to sons by their fathers?

No! By tradition, sex has been taught that way in the home, if there was any sex education at all. However, the biggest problem we have in sex education is the lack of communication. If fathers would teach their daughters about men, and mothers would teach their sons about women, we might have very different results. It would break the ice about opposite sexes communicating with each other about sex. We might also know more about each other that way. Girls are no longer separated from boys when sex education is taught in high school. There is no longer an attempt to make one sex a mystery to the other, so there is no reason for it to be this way in the home.

1040. Dr. Carson, what did you tell your daughters about sex, and how old were they when you told them?

When my daughters were three and four years old, I made a point of giving information to them on how male and female bodies are constructed, and how the penis enters the vagina and places sperm there that can swim up and join an egg, when it is produced, to form a baby. I also made it clear that this could not happen until after they were twelve years old, at which time they could control it. I taught contraception along with conception information at the nursery school age. As each daughter reached that age, I talked about it again, the older and younger ones listening with interest. I have given lectures to nursery school parents about the advantages of educating their children regarding sex at this age. I think it is the only way to make contraception a part of their children's lives. I also think it is very necessary for little girls to know that their reproduction can be controlled; otherwise, how can they dream, even then, about being anything but a wife and mother? They forget much of what you tell them, of course, but you tell it over and over. That is teaching. Others teach them, too. One day my daughters came back from a neighborhood conference with their peers and informed me that I was wrong; they had found out from their friends that babies are purchased at the supermarket!

SEX: VIRGINITY

1041. When is a woman no longer a virgin?

When a woman has had sexual intercourse with a man, she is no longer a virgin. If something else tears her hymen, then she has a torn hymen, but she is still a virgin. If she has been so intimate with a man that he has ejaculated between her legs with no clothing interposed, but has not penetrated her vagina, she may become pregnant, but technically she is still a virgin.

SEX: VIRGINITY (Continued)

1042. Can a man tell if I am a virgin?

Most men cannot tell if you are a virgin. They try to judge this by your degree of tightness, pain, and bleeding, which, of course, can occur in a non-virgin. The only one who really knows if you are a virgin is you.

1043. Can my doctor tell if I've had sex?

Not always and not absolutely, but usually a doctor can tell if you've had sex. If your hymen has been broken into many pieces and/or is dilated to be quite large, then something bigger than a tampon has passed through the opening, and a penis is the most likely object. Some doctors, however, have not examined many virgins, other than children, and they are not familiar enough with the appearance of an intact hymen to know whether it has been stretched or torn.

1044. Is it unusual nowadays for a woman to still be a virgin when she marries?

Yes, it is unusual for a woman today to still be a virgin when she marries, but this is still the choice of many women.

1045. What percentage of women today are virgins when they marry?

According to the Alan Guttmacher Institute, which conducts national surveys on human sexuality and abortion activities, less than 10 percent of women today are virgins when they get married. Ten years ago, this figure was about 25 percent. These findings are based primarily on surveys taken in urban areas. Surveys in rural areas might turn out differently, but they are harder to carry out.

1046. What was the average age at which women lost their virginity in the 1950s?

In 1950, only 3 percent of women were sexually active by the age of sixteen and less than 10 percent of women had premarital intercourse. Therefore, the average woman lost her virginity when she married.

1047. What was the average age at which women lost their virginity in the 1960s?

In the 1960s, 20 percent of women were sexually active by the age of sixteen and half of all women had premarital intercourse. The other half lost their virginity when they married.

1048. What was the average age at which women lost their virginity in the 1970s?

In the 1970s, 30 percent of women were sexually active by the age of sixteen, and 75 percent of women had premarital intercourse. About 46 percent of women had sexual intercourse by the age of nineteen, so the average age for loss of virginity was about twenty.

SEX: VIRGINITY (Continued)

1049. What is the average age at which women become sexually active today?

According to the Alan Guttmacher Institute report for 1978, the average teenager begins sexual activity at about the age of sixteen. By other reports, 55 percent have been involved in sexual activity by the age of nineteen in the United States. In Sweden, 50 percent of teenagers are sexually active by the age of nineteen, and 61 percent by the age of twenty-six.

1050. Could a woman have sex and still be a virgin?

Since "sex" means having intercourse with the penis inserted in the vagina, the answer is no, a woman cannot have sex and still be a virgin. However, she could have intercrural intercourse, whereby the penis is inserted between her legs without any clothing interposed, and the male ejaculates in front of her vagina but not inside. That is certainly sex, but technically the woman's hymen is intact, and she could pass a medical examination as a virgin. I have seen a couple in their thirties who thought they had been having normal sex for years, and wondered why the woman wasn't pregnant. Her hymen was still intact, and their interpretation of intercourse was to put the penis between the legs. Although a woman can get pregnant this way, it is not very common.

SEX: WHEN AM I READY?

1051. When should I start having sex?

You should start having sex when you decide that your personal development and life situation make it possible for you to enter into a really good relationship with another person. You must also be capable of assuming responsibility for a pregnancy or its prevention, or for the treatment of a venereal disease or its prevention.

1052. Should I wait until I'm married before I start having sex?

You should start having sex when you decide that you are ready. Some women who are ready for marriage may not be ready for sex; others may be ready for sex and not ready for marriage.

1053. What is the average age for people to start having sex (coitus)?

This is variable for the culture and the individual. In some countries, it is common for marriage to occur in the mid-teens, so people begin having sex at that time. Long ago, this was also common in western civilization, but it is no longer. In the United States today, the age at which people start having sex with a partner is usually between fifteen and twenty-five, but marriage occurs later.

1054. At what age is a person mentally ready for sex?

Some people are never mentally ready for sex. Others are probably

SEX: WHEN AM I READY? (Continued)

mentally ready before they are physically mature enough to perform. In our culture, most people seem to be involved in sex between the ages of sixteen and eighteen. The ideal age of mental readiness is unknown.

1055. What is the ideal age for a woman to start having sex?

Most of the time, the onset of sexual activity is the result of a man initiating it. If the conditioning of women was such that they could choose the age that they begin having sex, we might find an ideal age for this. In the past, women were not really programmed to enjoy sex, but it was useful for reproduction. In this case, the ideal age, from a medical standpoint, would be between the ages of twenty-five and thirty-five. Before the ideal age for a woman to begin having sex can be determined, newer ideals for having sex will have to be set.

1056. Is there any relationship between the age a person first starts having sex and how much they enjoy it?

No, the actual age of the onset of sexual activity has nothing to do with its success or the satisfaction achieved.

SEX: HYMEN

1057. What is a hymen, and where is it located?

The hymen is a little rim of tissue that circles the opening of the vagina, which is located between the urethra (the opening tube to the bladder) and the rectum. The opening in the hymen is normally about as big as a finger. It is a pink-colored tissue that looks a little like a collar, and more like the diaphragm of a camera.

1058. What exactly happens to the hymen the first time I have sex?

The hymen can be dilated (stretched) to the size of the penis, or it can be torn. If it tears, it usually tears in two places, one on each side, but it may tear in even more places. It may or may not bleed when it tears. Sometimes the bleeding is hard to stop without medical help or suturing, but this is rare. Usually, it heals in a few days, but sometimes bleeds even the second time you have sex.

1059. Is it possible for the hymen not to be broken the first time I have sex?

Yes, it is possible to have sex and not break the hymen, especially if it is gradually dilated to the size of the penis prior to intercourse. Once it is dilated, it does not really shrink back to its original size.

1060. Once broken, does the hymen no longer exist?

Once it is broken, the hymen does continue to exist, but in pieces.

SEX: HYMEN (Continued)

These are the little bumps that can be felt or seen at the opening of the vagina that exist all through life. When the vulva and opening are infected and irritated, these bumps become red, and sometimes women think that they are abnormal. In fact, these bumps, which are remnants of the hymen, are normal structures; they may just be abnormally red and irritated. You can always see them with a mirror by spreading the lips of your vulva and straining down. Sometimes surgeons have been asked to sew them back up to make a girl a virgin again. This is more frequent in Middle Eastern or Latin American countries where it is very important to be a virgin.

1061. Can a tampon break my hymen?

A tampon is too small to really break a hymen, but it may dilate a small opening in the hymen. It could break a hymenal band, which is a thick string of tissue going across the circular opening of the hymen. It also makes the hymen less tender, which has its advantages later. When your gynecologist examines you with a small instrument, it will not break your hymen, but a larger, average-sized instrument, such as the one commonly used to examine most women, is large enough to tear your hymen. This is why virgins are examined with smaller instruments that fit them. You should be sure your doctor uses the smaller instruments if you are a virgin.

1062. Is there a way that I can see my hymen?

Yes. You can see your hymen by using a mirror. Lie on your back, then prop yourself up on one elbow with your knees up and your feet on the bed. Spread the lips of the vulva and bear down by holding your breath and pushing. You will see the hymen open a little bit in a circle, with an open space in the center. When you do not bear down, it appears closed and folded up.

SEX: THE FIRST TIME

1063. Is it important to have a pelvic exam before I have sex for the first time?

There are advantages to having a pelvic exam before having sex for the first time. It is possible that you have an obstruction in your vagina or an abnormality that would interfere with intercourse and could be surgically corrected before you try. A hymenal band, a vaginal septum (a wall dividing the vagina into two parts), a double vagina, and an annular hymen (hymen with a ring-shaped opening in the center) are examples of abnormalities. All of these are rare, but they do exist. Actually, if you can put your finger in your vagina without any obstruction or if you can insert a tampon without a problem, you probably do not have an obstruction, so it is not absolutely

SEX: THE FIRST TIME (Continued)

necessary to be examined prior to having sex for the first time. If you cannot insert a tampon, you should find out why you cannot.

1064. Is it normal to be scared the first time I have sex?

Yes. The fear of performance can certainly be interpreted as fright, both for the man and the woman. It can be eliminated with a gradual approach to the first time you have sex.

1065. How will I know if I am ready for my first sexual experience?

By "first sexual experience," you probably mean intercourse. Actually, the first sexual experience occurs when you look at, speak to, or touch your partner. If you follow your feelings and find pleasure in touching each other, then you can carry this further to genital touching and orgasm, modifying your actions according to the other's response. This way, you will learn to be lovers for each other. The process is gradual.

1066. How can a couple make their first sexual experience more comfortable and enjoyable?

If you are a virgin, inserting fingers into the opening in your hymen and dilating it gradually until two fingers can be easily inserted and spread apart will make it easier to insert your partner's penis without discomfort and, hopefully, with pleasure. It will also show your partner what the problem with the hymen is. Even if you are not a virgin and your hymen has been dilated or broken before, fear can make you tense the muscles around the vagina so that insertion is painful. By gradually inserting fingers prior to intercourse, you will learn to relax these muscles and put aside your fears. Kegel exercises, in which you learn to tighten and relax these muscles to get control, can also be done.

1067. Will putting the penis in gradually the first time I have sex help to reduce the discomfort?

Putting the penis in gradually does not help reduce pain because it is not a graduated cylinder that will gradually dilate the hymen.

1068. What can I do to mentally condition myself for the first time I have sex?

The first thing you should do is to stop thinking of sex as only meaning intercourse. Do you have to condition yourself to hold hands with someone of the opposite sex? This is the first of many steps that occurs before intercourse. It would be difficult to progress from holding hands directly to intercourse, but if you find that you like to hold hands with someone, then you have passed the first step. Progress from there can mean all kinds of love-making between two people, including heavy petting and stimulating each other to orgasm.

SEX: THE FIRST TIME (Continued)

1069. Is there anything a couple can do before their first sexual experience to eliminate the pain?

If a man uses his fingers to dilate a woman's hymen prior to intercourse in order to avoid pain, this demonstrates to the woman that he can handle her without hurting her. If he does hurt her, then she is obligated to tell him; otherwise, no learning will take place. The same would be true if he stepped on her toe; she should tell him that it hurts. If he hurts her breasts or clitoris or vulva, she must also stop him and tell him that it hurts. It is not at all necessary to be hurt physically during sex. Lovers are made, not born. If you are prepared by much love-making to arouse your passion prior to entry, especially to orgasm, and if you have permitted your partner to dilate your hymen with his fingers to the size of his penis (this process of dilating your hymen probably will take several attempts on several different days), then entry can be made without pain.

1070. Why does intercourse hurt the first time?

The opening in the virginal hymen is normally about the size of a finger, but not as large as a penis. If it is thin and filmy, it may tear or stretch without much pain or bleeding. If it is tight and thick or abnormally formed, the pain can be surprising, and the tear can be so bad that it produces bleeding. This bleeding will usually subside and the tear usually heals quickly. It is rarely so bad that the girl must go to an emergency room of a hospital for a suture to stop the heavy bleeding.

1071. Could I have my hymen surgically cut or removed prior to my first sexual experience in order to eliminate the possibility of pain?

Generally, if the hymen is normal, it is better to dilate it slowly with fingers than to cut it surgically, because the surgery takes a few weeks to heal and leaves a tender spot and scars.

1072. Do most women bleed the first time they have sex?

Probably more than half of all women bleed the first time they have sexual intercourse. Some women have a hymen that is thin and is not richly endowed with blood vessels, so it may not bleed when it is torn, but could still cause pain. Not all women dilate their hymen before their first sexual experience, a process which could prevent bleeding. Surveys on this subject are not complete.

1073. Can I get pregnant the first time I have sex?

Yes, and much to their surprise, many women have gotten pregnant the first time they had sex. If you have intercourse with a fertile man at the fertile time of your cycle, you have about a 25 percent chance of getting pregnant.

SEX: SEX BEFORE THE AGE OF THIRTEEN

1074. What percentage of girls who have not yet reached their teenage years have engaged in sex?

In a 1978 survey of six hundred teenagers, 7 percent of the girls who were interviewed had their first intercourse prior to the age of thirteen.

SEX: TEENAGERS AND SEX

1075. What percentage of teenagers today have had a sexual experience?

In the United States, approximately 55 percent of teenage girls today have had a sexual experience.

1076. What do I say to a teenager who is thinking about having sex for the first time?

Seldom does the opportunity arise for you to say anything to a teenager who is thinking about having sex for the first time. The best approach is to help the teenager analyze her motives, pressures, and her ability to handle peer and parental approval and disapproval. Subjects you should also discuss with her include contraception, the risks of venereal disease (VD), and her knowledge of sexual function. The most important approval she needs is her own.

1077. As a teenager, how should I say "no" to sex?

The main problem with saying "no" to sex is convincing your partner that you really mean it. So, if you don't think that you are ready for sex, you should be very honest with your partner, and tell him exactly how you feel. However, you might also tell him that sometime, when the time is right and you are ready, you could say "yes" to sex. Only when you are capable of saying "yes," will you be able to convincingly say "no."

1078. Could it affect my physical health if I start having sex at an early age?

Starting to have sex at an early age can only affect your health if you get pregnant, contract an infection, or if you are sexually abused.

1079. What are the harmful effects of teenage sex?

The most frequent effect of teenage sex is pregnancy. The second most common harmful effect is venereal disease and its possible damage. The third most common effect probably is a broken heart. Another harmful effect is the possible disruption of family relationships, which sometimes leads to teenagers leaving home, dropping out of school, and failing to develop to their full potential. Possible damage to their tubes from pelvic inflammatory disease may make them sterile so that later in life when they have a stable love relationship, they will be unable to have babies. According to sex therapists, another result of early sexual experience for girls is that they can begin to feel used and abused and later turn against sexual activity altogether.

SEX: TEENAGERS AND SEX (Continued)

1080. How common are teenage pregnancies?

In 1978, the Alan Guttmacher Institute report showed that of teenagers who were sexually active, 23 percent became pregnant. Eleven percent of all teenage girls in the United States that year became pregnant, for a total of 1,142,000 pregnancies.

1081. Can having sexual intercourse at an early age cause any physical problems later in life?

Sex at any time in life can cause physical problems related to venereal diseases and pregnancies, but there are problems that are especially related to early sexual activity. Studies show that a girl who gets genital herpes early in life is more likely to develop cancer of the cervix than if she starts sex and gets herpes later in life. The reason for this is unknown. The young girl may be more likely to get VD because she may not have an exclusive relationship. Having an early pregnancy increases her chances of later developing cancer of the cervix. Contrary to this, studies indicate that girls who experienced incest, which usually begins at a young age and generally stops by sixteen, do not have any of these physical problems later in life. Perhaps this is because incest is less associated with VD and herpes.

SEX: SEX BEFORE MARRIAGE

1082. Have most girls today had a sexual experience before they are married?

Most girls today have had a sexual experience before they have reached the age of twenty. In urban areas, 90 percent have had a sexual experience before they are married.

1083. Is peer pressure a reason why so many young girls engage in sex before they are married?

Sex is a natural function, and in our culture great value is placed on sex with a partner. There is a peer pressure, and parental and cultural pressure that conditions children not to participate in sexual activity with others. There is also parental pressure to stop masturbating. Counter to this type of peer pressure is another kind of peer pressure which advocates dating and forming a significant relationship (including sex). A great deal of literature exists that places value on having a relationship. Remember, Juliet was fourteen when she died for Romeo. In the past in our country, and even today in countries like Saudi Arabia and Indonesia, marriage and pregnancy in the early teens were normal and frequent. A girl of nineteen in Saudi Arabia is usually on her third or fourth child, and 80 percent of the teenage

SEX: SEX BEFORE MARRIAGE (Continued)

pregnancies in Indonesia are among married women. One of our cultural problems is that our teenagers receive mixed messages, both to participate in sexual activity and to avoid it.

1084. How many men does the average woman today have sex with before getting married?

A 1978 survey of teenagers showed that 41 percent of those girls who were sexually active had only one partner. Another 44 percent had two to five partners, and 7 percent had more than ten partners while still teenagers.

1085. Is premarital sex good or bad for a marriage?

Good or bad, premarital sex is probably here to stay. At least 75 percent of couples today engage in premarital sex, so there are few marriages with no premarital sex to study for comparison to see if it is good or bad. It has certainly not solved all the problems of selecting a mate for an enduring marriage, as marriages today are enduring less and less, but it should at least prevent some annulments that are grounded upon a lack of sexual performance.

1086. Is premarital sex the best way to find out if I am compatible with my prospective mate?

"Compatible" is an outdated term that became popular during divorce proceedings in which couples claimed to be "incompatible." The problem of selecting a mate based on premarital sex is that your premarital sex could be very fine and "compatible," but then when marriage takes place, you could become completely disillusioned. How you behave as lovers without marriage only shows how you behave as lovers without marriage; it does not show you how you will behave when you are married. Both parties can change their attitudes with marriage. The best way to find out if you are compatible with your prospective mate is to talk to each other about it.

1087. What are the advantages of having sex without marriage?

One of the main advantages of sex without marriage is that it is easier to break up and leave your partner if the sex is unsatisfactory to you. However, women tend to blame themselves if the sex is unpleasant, and they are not really quick to try another partner. Sometimes they even marry the sex partner even though the sex experience has been miserable. It is far more difficult to change the habits and educate the married partner than it is the unmarried one. Besides, a marriage is probably doomed if a woman is planning to educate her partner and change his habits.

1088. What are the disadvantages of having sex without marriage?

When you have sex without marriage, less responsibility is felt for making provisions for contraception. This is especially true of the unmarried

SEX: SEX BEFORE MARRIAGE (Continued)

man. He usually does not feel financially obligated to take care of any pregnancy, if it occurs. Without marriage, there is more likely to be a rapid change in partners or multiple partners, which exposes you to sexually transmitted diseases. There is also the disadvantage of having to deal with the disapproval of people who think that you should not have sex without marriage.

1089. Why did sex get better after my divorce?

This is certainly a common experience. Perhaps it is because you have learned what to look for and what to avoid in sex, from the experience in your marriage. Perhaps it is because divorce frees you from the expectations of performance that marriage gave you. You become free to be yourself; you learn to be demanding and discriminating. You stop trying to please someone else by depriving yourself. You are no longer inexperienced and shy, and you do not pretend to be a virgin. When sex in marriage has been unsatisfactory, the first reassuring thing you may want to do as a single woman is find satisfactory sex, so you bravely seek it.

SEX: SEX AND MARRIAGE

1090. How important is sex to a happy and healthy marriage?

Sex is certainly not the whole of marriage. Some couples have a happy and healthy marriage with very little or no sexual function at all, and other couples with an excellent sexual relationship break apart over other things. It is everyone's ideal to have a satisfying and interesting sex relationship with the one they marry, but the percentage of times that this actually occurs is probably less than half. Someone said that if sex is good in marriage, it becomes hardly 1 percent of the marriage, but if it is bad, it amounts to 99 percent of it. In other words, sexual dysfunction in marriage seems to loom over marriage as a large problem, but when sex is happy and satisfying, it does not seem to be such a large part of it. Each couple and each person places a different value on sex in marriage, and marriage itself has changed through the years. At one time, women never expected to enjoy sex; they just did it for reproduction. In the same tradition, men did not expect sexual satisfaction or fun in marriage; this was only expected outside of marriage. Marriage was an economic and family, lifetime arrangement. Now the emphasis in marriage is on sex and companionship, not economics and reproduction. Sex has become far more important in marriage than it used to be.

1091. Can sex make or break a marriage?

Apparently sex difficulties can break a marriage, but good sex cannot make one. Sex is often blamed for problems in a relationship when the prob-

SEX: SEX AND MARRIAGE (Continued)

lem is really in the relationship itself. Other problems in a marriage will keep any sex problems from being solved.

1092. Why do many couples, after they are married for more than ten years, seem to lose sexual interest in each other?

The need for sexual expression and release of tension does not really die out. Chronic disappointment in one's own performance or that of a partner can certainly lead to loss of interest. Out of love, some people suppress their own desires and try only to serve their partners' desires and, finally, the desires cease to occur. If your interests and lifestyles are the same, this can lead to boredom. To retain sexual interest in a partner to whom you've been married for more than ten years involves the whole art of the long-term love bond.

1093. How do I plan sex around the busy schedule of a family so that it remains fun?

As parents, you should encourage your small children to have an early bedtime and sleep soundly in their own rooms. This will provide you with the private time you need to have your own relationship with your husband. If you are afraid of a child waking and entering your room, a lock on the door will give you time to recover before answering. Children should also be taught to knock. Older children can learn that parents sometimes want to be alone in the bedroom without interruption. It is certainly not harmful for children to know that their parents have sex. The most important thing you need to accept, however, is that it is not harmful if your love-making is occasionally interrupted. Telephones may ring, people may come to the front door, or a child may call out.

1094. Is it common for a couple who has been married for a while to tire of sex?

It is common to tire of tiresome sex. Sex that is effective in arousing both partners to orgasm is not tiresome, but the constant disappointment of one partner is. Sexual dysfunctions, such as impotence, premature ejaculation, vaginismus (contraction of the muscles surrounding the vagina), and failure to reach orgasm must be solved, as it is unsolved problems that really lead couples to tire of sex. Ill health and depression also decrease sexual desire. The problem is complex.

1095. Is it wrong to think of other men when I am with my husband?

Fortunately, there is no system of ethics or morals to prescribe what you should think or fantasize. Fantasy involves many things and is useful for sexual arousal. Morality is concerned with what you do, not what you think.

SEX: HEALTHY SEX LIFE

1096. Is sex good for my health?

Good sex is good for you, and bad sex is bad for you. Nuns live to a ripe old age without any sex. Sex is probably really helpful because of its ability to release tension after the age of puberty, since tension leads to many health disorders. Of course, sexual relations can lead to serious complications of pregnancy, venereal or sexually transmitted disease, heartbreak, and frustration. Sex while alone, called masturbation, is harmless to your health and can relieve sexual tensions, but it may not bring as much ecstasy and happiness that sex in a good relationship with a partner can bring.

1097. What part do the sex chromosomes and hormone levels play in determining my emotional attitude toward sex?

The awareness of developing sex organs, pubic hair, breasts, and an increase in the sensitivity of these areas accompanies the increase in emotions and sexual desire that occurs at puberty. Once these things have occurred, additional hormones make no difference. The sex chromosomes control which hormones and which sex characteristics will be produced, but scientists disagree as to whether they control emotional attitudes toward sex.

1098. How can too much or too little sex affect my health?

The effect of too little sex on your health depends upon how much sexual tension is aroused and how it is handled. If not released, sexual tension can make you nervous. Some writers have expressed belief in the myth that too much sex is harmful. As long as sex is desired and comfortable, the quantity of sex should have no direct effect on your health. Pregnancy and venereal disease affect health as a consequence of sex. Any sex that is more than you want and is forced on you can turn you against the whole process.

1099. Is sex sanitary?

Yes. Since "sanitary" describes something that tends to promote health and is especially free of dirt and agents of infection, then sex is sanitary. If both partners have had no sex with anyone else, there can be no infection.

1100. Is sex ever dangerous to women?

It may be that sex is always dangerous, since it can get women pregnant, infected, or just disappointed and heartbroken. But the dangers can be offset by the pleasure, indeed the ecstasy, that sex also provides.

1101. How long should I wait after having gynecological surgery to have sex again?

This depends upon the surgery, but generally for major surgery you should wait six weeks, or until your surgeon has examined you and finds you to be ready to have sex again. Ask your physician.

SEX: HEALTHY SEX LIFE (Continued)

1102. How would you describe a healthy sex life for a teenager?

Puberty turns thoughts more clearly to sex. Teenagers may learn to or continue to masturbate to orgasm to relieve their tensions and satisfy their bodies' needs. The more important goal is to develop the ability to relate to others in a tender and caring way, as a basis for future intimacy and long-term relationships. This can involve caressing, and it may progress to coitus. If coitus occurs, it is only healthy if both parties are responsible enough to provide for contraception, to avoid sexually transmitted diseases, and to cope with pregnancy if it results.

1103. How would you describe a healthy sex life for an adult woman?

As a young woman matures, her relationships can mature along with her, and ideally she develops her sexual knowledge and abilities as well. She can enjoy sexual arousal and satisfaction, both independently in the form of masturbation if she wants to, and joyously with a partner of her choosing. She is willing to instruct her partner in the art of making love to her, and she is willing to learn from him how to make love to him. Such give and take should permeate their whole relationship. Ideally, she avoids sexually transmitted diseases as well as unwanted pregnancies, and she retains her fertility until she completes her family. With such a basis, her sexual relationship will survive the rigors of pregnancy and child raising.

1104. How would you describe a healthy sex life for a senior citizen?

As a senior citizen, if life provides you with a partner who is in good health, then the enjoyment of sex will not fade and disappear, but will adapt to any changes that may occur with age. If no partner is available, the aged person need not frantically find a new one if she can be comfortable with her body and if she wants to enjoy her own masturbatory orgasms along with her memories.

SEX: SEX DURING MENSTRUATION

1105. If I have sex during menstruation, will the bleeding increase?

No, you will not bleed more if you have sex during menstruation, but any blood in the vagina will certainly be pushed out, so you may appear to bleed more. Contractions of the uterus during orgasm could reduce the flow, if there were any effect at all.

1106. Is it harmful to have sex during menstruation?

No, there is no harm in having sex during menstruation, although some people consider it messy. It is harmful to have sex while you are still bleeding for the first two weeks after having a baby, and this has been confused with menstruation. It is harmful then because infection could get into

SEX: SEX DURING MENSTRUATION (Continued)

the open uterus. According to the Talmud, sex during menstruation was forbidden in the ancient Jewish religion.

1107. Is it normal for me to lose my desire for sex just before my period?

No, it is not normal, but there is a great variation in how women react to their cycles. Most women report being more interested in sex the week before their menses. This is the time when your hormones are at their highest level. It is also in the "safe" period for not getting pregnant.

1108. Do most women desire sex while they are having their period?

Yes, most women do desire sex while they are having their period. During menstruation the uterus bleeds, but desire for sex is not affected by it. Activity may be affected if sex is carefully avoided during menses, but there is no real reason it should be avoided at all. Some men and women consider it messy; however, it is not dangerous. After a hysterectomy, women may desire sex at any time. They still have a hormone cycle, but they have no good way of knowing what part of their cycle they are in, so they don't lose their desire for sex for a week each month.

1109. Why do I want sex more and like it better when I'm having my period?

There are two explanations for why you want sex more and like it better when you're having your period. One is that you are more aware of your sex organs because of all the feelings produced by menstruation, and therefore the awareness becomes desire. The other is that you know that you are relatively infertile during menses and are, therefore, somewhat safe from pregnancy.

1110. Why is sex better after I finish my period than before?

Women vary, but the majority do not feel this way. One explanation could be that before menses you suffer from premenstrual syndrome, and you are so uncomfortable and emotionally upset that you cannot concentrate on intimacy and sexual pleasure. Discomfort during menses can also prevent sexual pleasure. After menses, you have neither of these problems, so sex is better for you then.

1111. Is there any time during the menstrual cycle that a woman is more likely to desire sex?

With most women, there is no correlation between the phases of their menstrual cycles and their desire for sex. However, when studies are made, there is a group of women who consistently say that they experience an increase in sexual activity during the week before their menses. There are others who have an increase in sexual desire during their mid-cycle, at about the time of ovulation. If most women were like this latter group, pregnancies

SEX: SEX DURING MENSTRUATION (Continued)
would occur more often, since that is the fertile time of women's cycles.

SEX: SEX DURING AND AFTER PREGNANCY

1112. How will my sex drive change during pregnancy?
Some women have an increased sex drive during pregnancy. The explanation for the increase is that women have a greater awareness of their sex organs during pregnancy, and they are free from the bother of contraception. They also need the reassurance of intimacy to feel secure. Many other women have a decreased sex drive during pregnancy because they feel nauseated, tired, or uncomfortable.

1113. Can I enjoy sex regularly during pregnancy?
Yes, and you should more than ever. Contraception is not necessary, menses are not involved, and there is greater freedom than before. Intimacy reassures you that you are loved, and you need this reassurance more than ever when faced with childbearing and rearing children. Also, the father of your baby needs to know that he is not forgotten. Positions may have to be modified when you are near term to ensure comfort, but you will still be able to enjoy sex.

1114. Is it safe to have sex during the last few months of pregnancy?
If your partner has no infections and you have no obstetrical complications, it is safe to have sex during the last few months of pregnancy. Complications that might prohibit sex during this time include placenta previa (placenta over the cervix), any bleeding disorder, incompetent cervix (cervix is too loose and the baby falls out early), threatened premature labor, or any other problem that your obstetrician warns you about and advises you to stop having sex because of. You should discontinue sex, however, if your water breaks or labor starts.

1115. Is it true that if I have sex during pregnancy, I could hurt my baby?
This is true only if you have abnormal bleeding due to a placenta over the cervix (a placenta previa) or even a bleeding edge of a placenta. If you have one of these conditions and have intercourse, it can cause further bleeding that can be fatal to your baby and even yourself. Fortunately, these conditions are rare. Women who are threatened with premature labor are often advised to avoid intercourse because it might induce labor and a premature birth. There are also recent studies which show that women who do not have sex during their pregnancy have better results with their babies than women who were sexually active. The primary reason for the bad results among sexually active women is due to infection. The studies usually fail to mention that the infections were sexually transmitted diseases, such as

SEX: SEX DURING AND AFTER PREGNANCY (Continued)

gonorrhea, herpes, syphilis, chlamydial infection, or even hepatitis B and streptococcus infection, all of which could affect the baby. With no intercourse, you are unlikely to get any of these infections, but you also risk losing the attention of your husband. Perhaps fathers-to-be should be more eduated about the effects of their infidelity on unborn children.

1116. Is oral sex safe during pregnancy, or could germs be transmitted to my baby?

As long as your partner has no contagious disease, oral sex is safe during pregnancy. The bacteria in the mouth are not normally harmful or contagious, unless you are bitten. Then they can be very infectious. The membranes around the baby, however, will keep these kinds of bacteria and germs out. Of course, after the water breaks, any sex is dangerous, since bacteria can travel up through the broken membranes.

1117. How long must I wait after having a baby before I can safely resume having sex?

After three weeks, the heavy bleeding will have stopped and the stitches from a tear or cut will have healed, so that most women can safely have sex again without injury or infection, although you still may be tender. However, you are not safe from getting pregnant, so you will need to use contraception. Otherwise, on your six weeks' postpartum visit, you may discover that you are pregnant again.

1118. Does sex get better after childbirth?

If you have had a problem with the opening of your vagina being too tight, then the enlargement of this area, which occurs with a vaginal delivery, may be beneficial to you. However, most women find no improvement.

1119. Will sex be painful for a while after childbirth?

Yes, your vagina will be tender for a while after childbirth, until your stitches have healed. Breast-feeding can make your vagina tender for a few months unless you use a lubricant or an estrogen cream in the vagina.

1120. After I had my baby, I seemed to lose interest in sex for a while. Is this common?

Yes, it is common, and it protects the mother and baby in two ways. For several days after childbirth, caring for your baby occupies your entire time, and this is necessary for your baby's own survival. Also, the cervix is still open and bleeding, so if you have sex then, infection can be severe. When the stitches from a tear or cut have healed and the bleeding has more or less stopped, sex will become safe for you. Still, you may be exhausted from caring for a difficult baby, as well as taking care of the house, meals, and other children. If you are breast-feeding, your vagina may be dry and

SEX: SEX DURING AND AFTER PREGNANCY (Continued)

tender for lack of estrogen. Both of these problems may last for a long while, unless they are solved by getting some household help and by using a little estrogen cream or sometimes just a lubricant in your vagina. Some mothers can't associate being a mother with having sex and they tend to withdraw from their husbands. This is called a Madonna Complex. In this case, counseling could help.

SEX: MASTURBATION

1121. What is masturbation?

Masturbation is self-induced sexual pleasure. This usually means handling the genitalia in a way that will achieve orgasm. Some women can reach a climax just by squeezing their thighs together or by fantasizing, and that is still considered masturbation.

1122. Is masturbation an act of self-appreciation?

It could be interpreted that way because masturbation involves self-esteem. Children do it without such conscious thoughts.

1123. How early do children begin masturbating?

Almost as soon as babies have learned to coordinate their hand movements in a purposeful fashion, they have been observed touching their genitalia and showing pleasure. With diapers on, however, they only have an opportunity to do this during their baths. When teenagers are asked when they first masturbated, they usually give an age of thirteen to fifteen. They probably have forgotten their early childhood experiences. Nursery school teachers are taught to socialize masturbation rather than forbid it; that is, they tell the child who is found masturbating to reserve that activity for when they are alone in their bedroom going to sleep, rather than doing it in nursery school.

1124. Does everyone masturbate?

A very small number of men never have masturbated. Some of these men are also primarily impotent; that is, they have never had an erection and ejaculated. A larger percentage of women have never masturbated. One of the explanations for this is that mothers may be too strict in forbidding little girls to touch their genitals, but they aren't sure that it isn't normal for little boys to do so. Another explanation is that little boys learn to handle their penises when they urinate and are, therefore, given permission to do so. There is no similar reason for little girls to handle their clitorises.

1125. Is it normal to masturbate?

Yes. Ninety-five percent of adult men and at least 60-70 percent of adult women have masturbated. Children discover the process without being

SEX: MASTURBATION (Continued)

taught; boys often teach each other the process. Sex is a normal function, and masturbation is a normal part of sexual function.

1126. How common is masturbation among singles?

At least 85 percent of single women and 95 percent of single men masturbate.

1127. Dr. Carson, what place do you think masturbation occupies throughout a woman's life?

There is a widespread belief in the romantic idea that a girl can grow and develop without any sexual activity until she develops a relationship with a lover who is perfect for her and who will awaken all of her sexual responses to full sexual fulfillment for both of them. This does, in fact, occasionally happen, but it is not the usual experience for women. If you avoid all sexual activity, including sexual arousal and self-stimulation to orgasm, until you develop a relationship with the one man with whom you want to spend your life, you may find that sexual intercourse is disappointing. You might not reach an orgasm no matter what you do, but because you love him, you may stay in the relationship all your life, without satisfaction or orgasm. Ten percent of women never experience orgasm throughout their lives. Men do not have such a problem; 95 percent of them learn to masturbate to orgasm before they have any sexual contact with women. When women accidentally learn to stimulate themselves to orgasm (masturbate) prior to any sexual contact with men, they are more likely to reach orgasm in their love-making later with their partners. Orgasm is really important if you want to have continued interest in sexual activity. Masturbation is valuable because it teaches women this reflex and the stimulation that produces it. It is also valuable to a teenager and a young adult for relieving sexual arousal and tensions when love-making with a partner is not practical or advisable. Leaving this arousal and tension without relief makes a woman nervous and leads to many symptoms of tension that could have been avoided. The liberation of women in the last thirty years is partly due to the dissemination of information on how to masturbate, the value of masturbation, and the right to masturbate, which men have been doing since time began. Masturbation also may serve as the only sexual outlet for the aging female in a world where her partner may not survive into old age as she does. According to the Hite Report on women, 85 percent of single women surveyed masturbate. It is considered normal and advisable.

1128. Does masturbating increase a woman's desire for sex?

No. Masturbating may increase a woman's ability to function in sex, but it does not increase her desire; it temporarily relieves it. Masturbating to orgasm relieves and disposes of physical and sexual tensions, thereby allow-

SEX: MASTURBATION (Continued)

ing you to go on to other activities in life.

1129. Does masturbation make a woman "nonorgasmic"?

No, masturbation is the main technique that women use to become orgasmic. It is also a common way in which women first achieve orgasm.

1130. Does masturbation relieve sexual tension?

Yes, masturbation is very effective in relieving sexual tension. It does not, however, satisfy the need to be loved or to have a relationship.

1131. At what age do women generally stop masturbating?

Normally, most women never stop masturbating. For the isolated, elderly woman, masturbation is the only outlet available for releasing sexual tension. Many women stop masturbating when they get married, mostly because they have no privacy in which to do so. They may also think that they should only have sex with their husbands, or their husbands may tell them so.

1132. What are the dangers of masturbation?

Masturbation does not cause any of the dangers you may have heard about, such as growing hair on your hands, making pimples, stunting your growth, or ruining your sex life. There is no known physical effect of masturbation that is considered bad. The worst effect might be the psychological guilt with which some people associate it, but that is the fault of the society that gives them the guilt, not the fault of masturbation. Why, then, have religions and cultures placed a taboo on the act of masturbation? The dictionary equates masturbation with onanism, which usually means having intercourse and then withdrawing and ejaculating on the outside. This is forbidden in the Bible because there is wastage. Perhaps in times gone by, when more people were needed, it was considered a waste to perform sex without a chance of reproduction. Today, there is so much overpopulation that it is not considered wrong to perform sex without reproduction. Masturbation is certainly not reproductive, and today it has become more acceptable as a form of sexual expression. The only criticism of masturbation to be found in current literature is that it satisfies sexual desire and therefore takes away some of the motivation to form a relationship with another person.

SEX: SEXUAL DESIRE

1133. What other parts of the body, besides the sexual and reproductive ones, have a role in sexual desire?

The entire body is involved in sexual desire. The largest sex organ is the skin, and the most important role in sexual desire is played by the brain. The sense of touch is also important. The eyes, an extension of the brain

SEX: SEXUAL DESIRE (Continued)

perhaps, are important because they usually are responsible for the first sexual encounter. The heart and all of the blood vessels pound with excitement during sexual activity, and in women, the whole pelvis becomes congested with blood during sexual arousal.

1134. How is sexual desire aroused in women?

There are as many ways to arouse sexual desire in women as there are women, but touch is probably the most indispensible method.

1135. Why do some women desire more sex than others?

Variations in sexual desire can be due to basic drive and energy, different values placed on sex, positive and negative sexual experiences, religious attitudes, knowledge about sex function, and even opportunities for having sex.

1136. At what age does sexual desire peak in women? In men?

A woman's sexual desire peaks when she is in her thirties and a man's desire peaks when he is in his late teens and early twenties.

1137. Do most women desire sex as often as men?

No, most women do not desire sex as often as men. One of the most frequent problems in sex therapy is the adjustment of the differences in frequency of desire between partners. Usually, men want to have sexual intercourse more often than women. This may be a cultural difference rather than a natural one; nevertheless, it exists today.

1138. How frequently does the average woman desire sex?

The Hite Report, which surveyed a large number of women, showed that 46 percent of the women surveyed wanted sex one to three times a week, 33 percent wanted sex one or more times a day, and the rest wanted sex less than once a week.

1139. Will my desire for sex increase the more I have sex?

Most women report an increase in desire for sex with an increase in frequency of sex. However, it is probable that each individual has a limit of frequency that still increases desire. If you are pushed beyond that limit for more sex than you desire, then your desire is likely to decrease.

1140. Is it true that once I have had sex, I will want it more and more?

Sex is a natural function, and the desire for repetition is as natural as eating or sleeping. It is also natural to want to repeat an activity that is pleasurable. The better the activity, the more you want it. Nevertheless, some people are quite successful in inhibiting sexual activity, especially masturbation, even though they find it pleasurable. Others, who find that sex with a partner is painful, are able to inhibit repetition more easily. A

SEX: SEXUAL DESIRE (Continued)

repeated desire for sex can also stem from the hope that the next performance will be better than the last one.

SEX: SEX DRIVE—WHAT IS IT; WHAT AFFECTS IT; HOW DOES IT CHANGE?

1141. What determines a person's sex drive?

Your individual sex drive is determined by your basic energy level and inherited factors, modified by experiences and value judgments provided by the culture in which you live.

1142. How can I have a healthy, active sex drive?

The best advice is to protect your sex drive from harm from childhood onward. Do not abuse and reject it. Nurture it with kind treatment. Do not use it for purposes other than sexual pleasure. It is not to be sold, exhibited, ridiculed, or used to keep a friendship alive. It should not be forced in order to please others. Masturbation should be respected and used as a response to desire whenever it is socially convenient. If you value sensual pleasure and relationships, your sex drive will thrive. If you treat sex like an accomplishment, act like a spectator at your own performance, strive for frequency, or just use it for something to brag about, then your sex drive will wither.

1143. At what age do girls first develop a sex drive?

Girls are born with a sex drive, but it is usually not recognized as such until puberty. At that time, their development increases the possibilities of sexual activity and interest.

1144. What is the sex drive of the average woman like?

As a teenager or in college, most women have discovered how to masturbate to orgasm, using it at varying frequencies. Over half of all women begin sexual activity with a partner before they are twenty years old, but frequency of orgasm in these years is not high. As they get married and have children, they are very busy but eventually develop enough communication with their partners to be orgasmic most of the time. Their interest in sex seems to increase when they are in their thirties, and it may stay this way for many years. Coital frequency at this time is two or three times a week on the average. Family, marital, and health problems may suppress their sex drive in later years, but it can usually be revived if it is desired.

1145. If boys and girls were raised "equally," would their sex drives be the same?

No one knows the answer to this. Since women are capable of a great deal more sexual activity per day than men, if the two were raised equally, a very unequal situation could result. But, as long as girls can get pregnant,

SEX: SEX DRIVE—WHAT IS IT; WHAT AFFECTS IT; HOW DOES IT CHANGE? (Continued)

there will always be some difference in their attitudes toward sex. An absolutely 100 percent effective contraceptive will have to be easily available to women before this difference can be overcome. The pill comes close and has, indeed, done a lot to free the sex drive of many women. It has been said to have been responsible for a sexual revolution.

1146. What factors in daily life affect sex drive?

Probably everything in life affects sex drive. Sex permeates all aspects of your life and all of your reactions. You cannot keep it in the one room of the house called the bedroom. Sex occurs throughout the house. If the way you lead your daily life increases your self-esteem and happiness, it will probably increase your sex drive, too.

1147. What do estrogen and testosterone have to do with sex drive?

Estrogen and testosterone are responsible for sexual development. In girls, estrogen brings about the growth and development of the breasts and vulva. These changes make a girl more aware of her body, and so her sensitivity increases. In boys, testosterone develops the penis, scrotum, and puts hair on the chest, and their sensitivity increases. Boys also begin having ejaculations and spontaneous erections. These changes can occur without the sex drive being present, or the sex drive can be present before they take place.

1148. How do hormones affect sex drive?

In four-legged animals, sex drive is hormonally controlled, and it is seasonal. This is not true of human beings or other primates. In human beings, hormones do not control sex drive; the brain does. However, estrogens can relieve dryness and tenderness in the vagina of women, thereby removing the discomfort that hinders sex drive.

1149. How does diet affect my sex drive?

Extreme dieting or overeating can leave you without enough energy to do anything, including having sex. Otherwise, diet has little to do with sex. Only as diet contributes to good health does it contribute to good sex.

1150. How will having a child affect my sex drive?

Unfortunately, many women become so engrossed in baby care, and so fatigued from this twenty-four-hour job, that they seem to have no energy left for a sex drive. If you are breast-feeding, you may have a lack of estrogen and a dry, tender vagina that discourages intercourse. A little estrogen cream in your vagina and a lot of rest and help with your baby will encourage your sex drive to return. Another effect some sex therapists find is that women often think of their mothers as being too pure to have sex, so when they become mothers, they feel removed from sex.

SEX: SEX DRIVE—WHAT IS IT; WHAT AFFECTS IT; HOW DOES IT CHANGE? (Continued)

1151. How will my sex drive change as I get older?

Positive sexual experiences improve your sexuality, and negative ones damage your sexuality. It is difficult to separate getting older from the experiences that occur along the way. There is no natural reduction in sex drive with aging, except as a reaction to problems in the environment, the disappearance of opportunities for sex, and a decrease in general health and energy. If you solve each problem, then your sex drive can continue well into old age.

1152. How does menopause affect sex drive?

Menopause does not have an established effect on sex drive. The lack of estrogen during late menopause makes the vagina tender and dry and can produce shrinkage. This makes intercourse painful and can lead to avoidance. Depression with a mid-life crisis, which sometimes occurs at the same time as menopause, is often blamed on menopause and certainly interferes with sex. Feelings of worthlessness associated with the loss of a youthful appearance at the same time as menopause decrease sex activity. On the other hand, the freedom from fear of pregnancy and more time with your partner, since the children are grown and out of the way, can bring about better sex than you ever had before.

1153. How can sex drive be increased after menopause?

Treatment of the estrogen deficiency of menopause can solve the problems of flushes and sweats, and it also reverses dryness and shrinkage of the vagina. A new role or a new job can raise your self-confidence, as well as your sex drive. If your partner can convince you of your worth and value as a sex partner, all will be well after menopause.

1154. How will a hysterectomy affect my sex drive?

A hysterectomy has no direct effect on sex drive at all, although it may have an indirect effect of relieving pain and improving overall health. If you are in pain and bleeding most of the time before surgery, then after it is completed, you are free to be sexually active. If you are afraid of pregnancy before surgery, then afterward, you no longer have this fear. But, if you think that you should only have sex in order to have babies, then you could be in trouble if you need a reason to have sex. If you do not value sex for pleasure, you may stop having sex after a hysterectomy. Your partner cannot tell if you have had the surgery, and neither can you. However, impotency may occur in some men when their wives have a hysterectomy, because they see no use in sex if their wives can't get pregnant. Some women also claim to miss a uterine component in orgasm, felt as contractions.

SEX: SEX DRIVE—WHAT IS IT; WHAT AFFECTS IT; HOW DOES IT CHANGE? (Continued)

1155. How do drugs affect my sex drive?

The answer to this question could fill a book. Sedatives and tranquilizers may release inhibitions, but in larger amounts they simply lead to inactivity. Stimulants and antidepressants increase activity, including sexual activity, but not selectively. Other drugs have specific effects on male erections. Blood pressure medications, for instance, can cause impotence while they are being taken. Their relationship to women's sexual activity has not been as well studied. If you have a sudden change in your sex drive while taking a medication, it would be wise to ask your prescribing physician about its possible effect.

1156. How does smoking affect my sex drive?

Tobacco does not really affect the psyche or sex drive, except when it has produced so much ill health that performance is not possible. Some people are repelled by tobacco smoke, socially and sexually. Others find it attractive, as it is depicted this way in movies and on television.

1157. How does alcohol affect my sex drive?

Alcohol is used to remove inhibitions against sexual activity and may cause you to enter into activities that are normally rejected when you are not intoxicated. Alcohol does not produce desire, but removes the inhibitions of desire. However, as Shakespeare pointed out long ago, it can remove the ability as well. Research confirms that alcohol tends to make men impotent. With enough alcohol, all drive disappears into a state of stupor. A small amount of alcohol can make you more social and talkative, whereas a large amount can make you completely unsociable. There is, of course, a great deal of individual variation in reactions to alcohol.

1158. What kinds of things could reduce my sex drive?

Depression is one of the most common causes of a reduction in sex drive. If you are depressed and have a reduction in sex drive with no other explanation, you should consider seeking help for your depression. Another common cause is being pushed and bullied into sexual activity, so that an aversion to sex is developed. Anything that makes sex painful, such as an infection, will cause avoidance of sex. Loss of self-confidence will also tend to reduce your sex drive. It is common for men's sexual activity to be reduced when they lose their jobs or suffer business losses. Similar failures in women's lives, especially the loss of a child or feelings of inadequacy, are reflected in reduced sexual activity. Of course, ill health will reduce your energy level and all of your drives, including your drive for sex.

SEX: SEX DRIVE—WHAT IS IT; WHAT AFFECTS IT; HOW DOES IT CHANGE? (Continued)

1159. Will being active in athletics help to curb my sex drive before marriage?

No. Fortunately for athletes, participation in athletics does not damage or reduce sex drive. It simply absorbs a lot of energy and time that might otherwise be spent on sexual pursuits. In the past, the sexes were also separated in most sports activities, but this does not happen so much anymore.

1160. What are some of the reasons that my sex drive might increase?

Improvement in your general health, an increase in your self-confidence, and a general energetic feeling are associated with an increased sex drive. Sometimes simple sex education and finding out that you are normal releases your energy for sex. Certainly, eliminating causes of painful sex will help to increase your sex drive as well.

1161. Is there any kind of medication available today that would help to increase my sex drive?

No, it is not that simple. Sex drive is a natural characteristic, and when it is inadequate, the problems that interfere with it have to be found and solved. There seems to be a natural variation in sex drive among individuals, so it is not always an easy problem to detect. Why should we all have the same sex drive? The important thing is that partners be somewhat matched in sex drive, not that everyone be highly driven.

SEX: DECREASING INTEREST IN SEX

1162. What causes a lack of interest in sex?

A lack of interest in sex can be the result of early childhood training that created an abhorrence and revulsion for sex. Being completely involved in a particular pursuit can make you consciously avoid all interest in sex in order to succeed and not be distracted. Severe depression, such as that which accompanies a severe illness or severe financial crisis, characteristically decreases your interest in sex. Aversion to sex can result from being pushed too far to perform sexually, until you turn against the whole process. This happens to women more often than men, because men are sexually more aggressive in our culture. They can demand sex too hard and too often, while women can't. With more women today being sexually aggressive, however, men are starting to suffer from sexual aversion more than before. Also, religious training with the substitute satisfactions it offers can divert all of your attention away from sex.

SEX: DECREASING INTEREST IN SEX (Continued)

1163. Will I lose interest in sex when I reach a certain age?

No, your interest in sex will not naturally decline as you get older.

1164. Sometimes I'm just not "in the mood" for sex. Why not?

There are other pleasures besides sex. It is unrealistic to expect to be in the mood for sex all of the time. No one is hungry for food at all times, unless they never have enough to eat. Then they may be hungry most of the time. If you almost never enter into sexual activity, you may be thinking about it most of the time. On the other hand, when you are sexually active, you may wonder why it is not on your mind so much anymore. Even though it is "macho" for a man to pretend he is always in the mood for sex, in reality, he does not always feel this way. The sexual appetite can be satisfied.

1165. Is there anything I can do to "get in the mood" for sex?

Yes, a lot of things, such as movies, books, fantasies, and music, can get you "in the mood" for sex, but your question implies that there is a great deal of pressure on you to have sex. Pressure to perform really can create an aversion to sex. It would be better for you to avoid people and situations that force this on you, because trying to force yourself to be in the mood for sex is damaging to your own sexuality. You can educate the one who is putting the pressure on you by turning the tables. Pick out a time when he is engrossed in some other activity, such as watching a ball game. Approach him for sex and when he ignores you, explain how similar the situation is in reverse. He may then understand what it feels like to be pushed into "getting in the mood" for sex.

1166. What should I do if I'm bored with sex?

Do something else for a while. Forcing yourself into sexual activity or letting someone else force you is a sure way to acquire an aversion to sex. Sex should always be voluntary. Review your relationship, change your sexual routine, and perhaps get some professional assistance.

1167. I've been with the same man for a while, and my desire for sex has steadily decreased. Is this common?

Yes, it is too common. Newness adds excitement to any activity. If problems in sex are not solved, they get worse. When desires are satisfied, the problems do not seem as urgent. But, sex with the same person for an extended period of time can grow better, too.

1168. What should I do if my sexual appetite with my partner has decreased?

You should take a close look at your relationship. Consider whether most of your encounters with your partner result in orgasm. You should make sure that they do. Consider whether you let sexual desire go unsatisfied day after day until you can arrange an encounter with your partner. If so,

SEX: DECREASING INTEREST IN SEX (Continued)

your body may go on strike and refuse to get aroused anymore if it isn't satisfied. Consider whether you are tolerating pain in love-making and trying to go on anyway. Consider your general health. Consider that you might be withdrawing sexually to punish your partner for some other behavior of which you don't approve. Look for signs of depression, such as insomnia, or general or social withdrawal. Then, try to share with your partner all of the things that turn you on. A change of environment might help, too. However, if a vacation together doesn't improve the situation, perhaps you have problems in your relationship and should consult a counselor.

1169. Why didn't I enjoy sex as much when I was on the pill? Is this typical?

The typical reaction to the pill is a greater enjoyment of sex because it gives you freedom from the fear of pregnancy and eliminates the problems of messy barrier contraceptives. However, if you do not feel well on the pill, and especially if you are continuously nauseated, then you will not enjoy anything as much. But some psychiatrists believe that the problem is really quite more complicated than that. They find that women who do not enjoy sex as much when they are taking the pill really secretly want to get pregnant. These women would feel the same way if they were using an IUD. Some men dislike any good contraceptive because they enjoy the thrill that the risk of pregnancy adds to love-making. Perhaps some women feel this way, too.

1170. What can a couple do to be sure that their interest in sex continues after they've been together for many years?

Communicating your desires, combining honesty with intimacy, incorporating change when you feel like it, and solving sexual problems can assure your continued interest in sex with your partner. Placing the opportunity for sexual intimacy high on your list of priorities can also keep sexual interest alive. Many couples who have been together for a while put sex at the bottom of their list, which starts with earning money, caring for children, having a social life, being with relatives, taking time for religious activities, and more. Only if some time is left at the end of the day, when they are exhausted, do they turn to sex. When your relationship was new, the opportunity to be together intimately controlled all your plans. If you continue to provide for these opportunities, you will have a better chance of retaining your sexual interest. This may involve planning a vacation or weekend together in a setting you like. It could also simply involve devoting an evening to each other, instead of to everyone else, and installing a lock on the bedroom door. You may also want to try new techniques.

1171. Is it possible for sex to get better after I've been with the same man for a while?

Definitely. If you have good communication, a good relationship, and

SEX: DECREASING INTEREST IN SEX (Continued)

you are honest about your desire with your partner, sex can get better and better, especially if you both want it to!

SEX: FREQUENCY OF SEX

1172. How often does the average married couple have sex?

According to most surveys, married couples have sex an average of two to three times each week. Of course, the variation is great, from no sex each week to several times each day. The frequency is generally greater when a couple first marries, and less when the marriage has lasted for many years.

1173. How many times each week does the average person have sex?

If you were to average the number of times different people have sex each week—from the very young to the very old, the single to the married— the average would be much less per person than two to three times a week, which is the average frequency for couples living together.

1174. Is it normal to have sex once a year and be satisfied?

It would be very unusual to have sex once a year and be satisfied. A more common occurrence would be not to want sex at all. Then you would not bother with it even once a year.

1175. Is there such a thing as too much sex?

Physically, exhaustion is the limit. Socially, you are limited by the tolerance of your partner and the opportunities you are given. Economically, you need to reserve enough time to make a living. For fertility, if the male ejaculates more than twice a day, the sperm count becomes too low to get a woman pregnant. Psychologically, sex can lose its desirability, and any sex that is more than you want is too much.

1176. Do people with an active sex life live longer than those without?

Surveys show that married people, who presumably have a regular, active sex life, live longer than unmarried people.

SEX: MULTIPLE PARTNERS

1177. What are the dangers of multiple partners?

One danger is that if you get pregnant, you may not know who the father of your child is. The primary danger is that you may contract a sexually transmitted disease. Of course, if all of your partners slept only with you, as in a harem, then you would not get a venereal or sexually transmitted disease. But the more partners you have, the more likely it is that one of them will have had sex with someone else who has a disease, and then they will give it to you. If you just have sex with one man, but he has many

SEX: MULTIPLE PARTNERS (Continued)

partners, you are still very likely to get a venereal disease. There is also the possibility that your partners will become jealous of each other and physical violence could occur.

1178. Does early sexual activity and/or multiple partners cause female problems later in life?

Only if you get a sexually transmitted or venereal disease will medical or physical problems occur later in life. If you have multiple partners, you are more likely to catch a disease because you have more chances of meeting a man who has such a disease. If you get herpes simplex type II (genital herpes) when you are young, you are more likely to get cervical cancer twenty years later. Vulvar warts are also thought to cause cancer of the cervix. Gonorrhea, if it gets into your tubes, can make you sterile in later life and also causes chronic pelvic pain. If you have a bad sexual experience, you may develop an aversion to sex, or even vaginismus, a clamping down of the muscles around the vagina when attempting intercourse. You could also develop a "broken heart."

SEX: SEXUAL PEAK IN WOMEN

1179. At what age does a woman reach her sexual peak?

Most women commonly reach their sexual peak between the ages of thirty and forty, although with some women this occurs after they reach the age of fifty. When a woman reaches her thirties, she has usually freed herself from the sexual suppression of her upbringing, so that she enjoys and is interested in sex. At this age, she is still young enough to be active and physically attractive.

1180. Women are portrayed in society as being glamorous and sexy when they are in their late teens and early twenties, and yet I didn't feel that way until I reached my thirties. Sex is far more exciting now. Is this typical?

Unfortunately, it is typical. "Sexy" is a word that is often used to describe an attractive appearance that stimulates the male. Yet the "sexy" twenty-year-old female may not enjoy sex at all. Our culture does not teach women to enjoy sex, but rather suppresses their enjoyment of it while teaching them to look sexy. After the age of thirty, women gradually find out how to enjoy their sexuality, and through the years they increase their sexual abilities.

SEX: A WOMAN'S ROLE AND BEHAVIOR IN SEX

1181. What is a woman's role in sex?

A woman's role in sex changes with each generation, each culture, and

SEX: A WOMAN'S ROLE AND BEHAVIOR IN SEX (Continued)

each woman. It is probably better not to stereotype the role of women, but hopefully it will always be to participate and enjoy.

1182. To what extent is the sexual behavior of women controlled by men?

Sexual behavior is controlled by men to the extent to which women allow it to be controlled. Frequency of intercourse seems to be the factor most controlled by men, although some men might say that women control this. Since most men falsely assume the role of knowing more about sex, they also may try to control the pattern that sexual activity takes.

1183. Who should be the aggressor during sex, the man or the woman?

Each couple decides this to suit themselves, but I would suggest taking turns. The aggressor has the advantage of choosing the time when he or she most desires sex and becomes stimulated just by the decision to have sex. Traditionally, this has been reserved for men, and women were supposed to "respond." Today women can enjoy sex more if they are the aggressors sometimes, and they can count upon the men to "respond."

1184. How does a woman know what to do during sex?

If you do not know what to do during sex, your partner will usually be glad to teach you according to what he knows. But since he only knows what satisfies him, he is really not a very good teacher. It is better for you to teach him what to do for you. You can always read books on sex, explore yourself, find out what feels good, and then teach him.

1185. How old do I have to be before I can function 100 percent sexually?

Trying to reach some goal of sexual performance really interferes with your ability to perform. Seeking sensual pleasure in a good relationship is a more effective motivation. Emotional maturity is a necessary ingredient for a sexual relationship that is 100 percent effective. It develops in different people at different ages. Some girls are apparently rather mature at fifteen and others are immature at fifty. The usual range is probably from eighteen to twenty-five.

1186. Should I have sex with a man to whom I am not emotionally attracted?

If you do, you may find out the hard way that it doesn't work. But what you should and should not do lies entirely within your own particular and unique value system. No one else can answer that for you. You must make your own rules.

SEX: ENJOYMENT OF SEX

1187. Why do some people enjoy sex more than others?

There are many genetic, cultural, religious, and general health reasons

SEX: ENJOYMENT OF SEX (Continued)

why some people enjoy sex more than others. It may relate to how they were handled as babies and whether they learned to enjoy sensual pleasure in being touched. If their only pleasure was in being fed, then they may become gourmets, instead of lovers.

1188. Is there a name for the pleasurable sensation short of orgasm which women achieve during sex?

Sexual arousal, intimacy, and the pleasure of giving and loving are all pleasurable sensations. Many women value these sensations much more than orgasm, even though they have orgasms, too.

1189. What do women enjoy the most about love-making?

In love-making with a partner, women enjoy the intimacy—the excitement of sharing, the physical sensation of the other person's body, the involvement, as well as orgasm.

1190. What happens inside my body to make me become "turned on?"

Nerve endings, primarily for touch and pressure, carry signals to the spinal cord as well as to brain centers which cause a reflex dilation of blood vessels in the pelvis, vulva, clitoris, breasts, and skin. Changes in the heart rate and the force of the heart beat also take place. The vaginal wall releases a lubricant, and the cavity of the vagina barrels out and becomes larger. At the same time congestion occurs at the opening. These are all reflexes. The mind cannot direct them to happen, but it can interfere and suppress their occurrence, just as it can interfere with almost any other reflex.

1191. Why do some women enjoy sex and others don't?

In our culture, very little effort is spent on teaching girls to enjoy sex. Some women have just never learned how to experience sexual arousal and orgasm. They perform during sex only to please their partner. For other women, pleasing their partner seems to be sufficient pleasure. Still other women have never learned to place a value on sensuous pleasure, theirs or their partner's.

1192. Is it true that the more relaxed I am during sex, the more pleasure I will experience?

No. Relaxation sets the stage for sex by preparing the mind for an awareness of sensual feelings, but it has no place during orgasm. If you will observe the state of someone who is sexually aroused or having an orgasm, you will see that they are anything but relaxed. A state of tension almost always precedes orgasm.

1193. Is sex as enjoyable when condoms are used?

Most men and women feel that sex is not as enjoyable when a condom

SEX: ENJOYMENT OF SEX (Continued)

is used. The surface can be irritating and uncomfortable to women, and most men report that it reduces sensation. It is also distracting to stop and put the condom on. However, some women really like the condom because it is less messy. With a condom, they do not feel the ejaculate in their vaginas or over their vulvas and the chances of becoming pregnant or contracting a venereal disease are less. It may also be sexually exciting to your partner if you apply the condom.

1194. How can I increase my own pleasure during love-making?

You can tell your partner what you would like him to do. You can stop him from doing things that you do not find pleasurable. You can use fantasy to increase your sensuality. You can do exercises that heighten your awareness of sensual feeling, especially touch. Kegel exercises which contract and relax your perineal muscles may help (see question 1345). Above all, you must rid yourself of the idea that it is your duty to have sex whether you want it or not. This idea can be devastating to your sexuality. You can seek counseling with a sex therapist if you feel that you have a problem.

1195. How can I add excitement to my sex life?

Learn more about sex. Read books on male as well as female sexuality. Take group courses in sexuality and be open to change. But most of all, keep your relationship exciting so that sex can be exciting.

SEX: SEXUAL FULFILLMENT

1196. How important is loving my partner to achieving total sexual fulfillment?

That depends upon your definition of total sexual fulfillment. If love is part of your definition, then it is important and you must meet that requirement, but it is not necessary in order to reach orgasm or have a sensual experience. Some partners love each other deeply, but never achieve sexual fulfillment; others achieve sexual fulfillment, but they do not love each other.

1197. Has the new sexual permissiveness increased or decreased sexual fulfillment?

Surveys convincingly indicate that the sexual fulfillment of women has increased in the last thirty years. Other studies show that male sexual fulfillment has decreased. This is because men have developed more impotence and other sexual problems in recent years due to the fear of performance failure.

1198. Do women get the same sense of sexual fulfillment as men?

No. A woman will never know what it feels like to have an erection or

I want to wake him
and say thank you
thank you for
knowing me

I want to wake him
and say thank you
thank you for
understanding me

I want to wake him
and say thank you
thank you for
making me so happy

I want to wake him
and say thank you
thank you for transforming me
into erotic delirium

But there he sleeps
so quiet and peaceful
I'll just kiss him softly
and thank him tomorrow

— Susan Polis Schutz

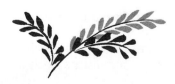

SEX: SEXUAL FULFILLMENT (Continued)

to ejaculate. A man will never know what it feels like to lubricate or to feel a penis thrusting in the vagina. A woman will never know what congestion in the scrotum feels like, and a man cannot know what the pelvic congestion in a woman feels like. Women are capable of multiple orgasms, and most men are not. Women can fantasize to orgasm, but there is no record of a man doing this. But how can we ever really know whether these different senses of sexual fulfillment are equivalent?

1199. How does the size of a man's penis affect a woman's sexual satisfaction?

All of a woman's sexual sensation is within the first two or three centimeters of the opening of her vagina, which even the smallest penis will reach. If a man's penis is large enough to project beyond his body and insert into the vagina, the size is adequate for a woman's sexual satisfaction. Some men are so fat and their penises are so small that this becomes impossible without weight loss. A larger, longer penis can become difficult for a woman to accommodate without pain caused by pressure, but comfort can usually be satisfactorily accomplished with lubricants and position changes. Contrary to the popular belief of men, a large penis does not create greater satisfaction, but rather it can create a problem.

SEX: THE FOUR STAGES OF INTERCOURSE

1200. What are the different stages that couples experience during the act of intercourse?

The four stages of intercourse are desire, arousal, orgasm, and resolution.

SEX: EROGENOUS ZONES, AROUSAL AND STIMULATION, FOREPLAY

1201. How do I discover what stimulates and pleases my partner?

This is the entire art of love-making. Ask, try, experiment. Above all, remember what works. Women often complain that they told their partner what to do once, but then he forgot and they never told him again. Tell him again. Don't be afraid to express yourself. In order to find out what pleases your partner, you must first of all have a good relationship, so you can communicate.

1202. Do most women find it difficult to communicate their sexual needs to their partners?

Yes. Our culture does not teach girls to communicate their sexual needs to their partners, but it does teach boys to communicate their needs by

SEX: EROGENOUS ZONES, AROUSAL AND STIMULATION, FOREPLAY (Continued)

"educating" girls about sex. Most girls grow up thinking that they do not need to know anything about sex, because their partners will teach them. Of course, the girl's partner needs the girl to teach him, but she may not be ready to do this. Women are better able to communicate their desires when they are in their thirties. But to avoid troubles in their relationships with men, women need to communicate their needs sooner.

1203. Where are the erogenous zones in a woman?

The erogenous zones in a woman are variable, and each woman is unique. However, they usually include the clitoris, vulva, breasts, mouth, lips, neck, buttocks, head, feet, G-spot (inside vagina), and even the anus.

1204. Why do some women enjoy having their breasts touched?

Breasts, as well as nipples, are erotic areas. There are genital corpuscles located in the nipples that are just like the genital corpuscles in the vulva. These respond as sexual organs. The nipples become erect with sexual excitement and change color. Orgasm has been known to occur with nipple stimulation. Male nipple stimulation is also sexually exciting to many men for the same reasons.

1205. What parts of the vagina are stimulated during sex?

Except for a feeling of swelling or fullness, the vagina itself does not have nerve endings for sensation. Organs surrounding the vagina, such as the urethra, bladder, rectum, and even the ovaries, the uterus, and the sacral bones can detect sensation, but this is mostly limited to pressure or pain. All of the really sensitive areas are at the opening of the vagina, such as the labia, the hood over the clitoris, the clitoris itself, and the G-spot, which is located just inside the vagina.

1206. There has been a lot of talk about the G-spot. What is it?

The G-spot was named for Dr. Grafenburg who first wrote about it many years ago. It is the most sensitive spot within the vagina, and is the junction between the bladder and urethra.

1207. Where is the G-spot?

The Grafenburg, or G-spot, is located about one inch inside the vagina in the middle of the upper wall, just below the urethra near the bladder. The urethra is the tube that carries urine from the bladder to outside of the body.

1208. Are women more difficult to sexually arouse than men?

Most writings emphasize that men are aroused primarily by visual stimulation, and woman primarily by touch. It is easier to provide visual

SEX: EROGENOUS ZONES, AROUSAL AND STIMULATION, FOREPLAY (Continued)

stimulation than physical stimulation. Our culture also teaches women to deny and suppress their sexual arousal. So in our culture the answer is yes, women are more difficult to arouse than men, but maybe it doesn't have to be that way.

1209. Why is it that I can sometimes be less or more stimulated than at other times, given the same situation?

The situation is never exactly the same. Your psyche and your whole state of physical sensation may be quite different, regardless of the similar mechanical aspects of the situation.

1210. Does my Adrenalin flow faster when I become sexually stimulated?

Yes, Adrenalin (epinephrine hormone) does flow faster when you are sexually stimulated. This is one cause of the increase in heart rate and cardiac output (heart pounding).

1211. How much foreplay is normal before sexual intercourse?

Normal is a difficult word to define when sex is being discussed, but foreplay should continue as long as either or both parties want it to last. If you are initiating the sexual encounter, foreplay is required at least until your partner has an erection. If he initiates it, he must continue until you are well lubricated. You may prefer an orgasm or two before his penis enters your vagina, and he may prefer lots of stimulation before he thrusts to orgasm.

1212. How long do most couples practice foreplay?

Most couples practice foreplay from five to twenty minutes, but some take much longer.

1213. Do most women like a lot of foreplay before sex?

Yes, they do like a lot of foreplay. Most women do not reach orgasm through intercourse, so they prefer enough foreplay to reach orgasm.

1214. How important is foreplay prior to intercourse in helping women to achieve sexual satisfaction?

It is very important. Even if you can reach orgasm with intercourse, you still need enough foreplay to lubricate. If you can only reach orgasm during foreplay, it is important for your sexual satisfaction.

1215. What causes a women to lubricate during sex? How does this occur?

Sensual arousal causes blood to flow in greater quantities around the pelvis and especially in the vaginal walls. Fluids and mucus come through the walls to produce the lubricating fluid. The normal vaginal discharge present in women who are producing estrogen contributes some of this fluid, and secretions from glands, like the Bartholin's glands located at each side of the entrance of the vagina, contribute the rest.

SEX: EROGENOUS ZONES, AROUSAL AND STIMULATION, FOREPLAY (Continued)

1216. What is the wetness I feel when I am stimulated sexually?

It is the lubrication which comes from the walls of the vagina. This substance consists mostly of mucus and water.

SEX: INTERCOURSE

1217. What part does my brain play in sexual intercourse?

Your brain is the most important sex organ, although it is not all powerful. It cannot experience orgasm without the spinal cord, but the spinal cord cannot function without the brain. In man and in other primates, the brain plays a larger role in sexual activity than it does in other animals.

1218. What role does concentration play in the sex act?

Concentration is very important in the sex act. Focusing upon sensation requires the concentration of the entire body. The world should seem very far away when you are concentrating on your lover. Concentration prevents distraction caused by the environment. Music may help, but television does not. Planning the grocery list at the same time as you are making love would be most insulting to your partner.

1219. What is the role of the cervix during intercourse?

The cervix is there to admit the sperm into the uterus in order to produce pregnancy. It has no role in sexual pleasure. Women who have had their cervix removed, as in a hysterectomy, feel no different during intercourse than women who have not. However, hitting the cervix with the penis can produce pain felt on each side of the pelvis. This can usually be avoided by shifting positions or by directing the thrust of the penis.

1220. Can a man's penis extend beyond my cervix during sex?

Certainly. The cervix is the roof, not the end of the vagina. There is less discomfort during intercourse if the penis goes below the cervix or beyond it, rather then directly into it.

1221. How long does sexual intercourse take?

The actual amount of time that the penis is in the vagina, not including foreplay and other stages of love-making, is usually five to twenty minutes.

1222. How long can the average male continue to engage in intercourse before ejaculating?

The average range is from five to twenty minutes, but there is wide variation among individuals. Some men ejaculate before intercourse even

SEX: INTERCOURSE (Continued)

starts. Others can continue to engage in intercourse for forty-five minutes or more before ejaculating. Some men are unable to ejaculate while their penis is in the woman's vagina, so they could continue to exhaustion without ejaculation.

1223. Sometimes I need to rest in the middle of sex. Am I out of shape, or is this typical?

Contrary to general opinion, sex does not have to progress steadily through a sequence of events to the ultimate end, orgasm. Orgasm has to be preceded by a plateau phase which is reached by stimulation, but a stop, hesitation, or rest can occur at any stage. It is monotonous always to follow the same pattern. Interruptions are not fatal to either party. Sex is not an athletic event for which you must be in shape. It is the psyche or the nervous system that dictates the pace, not the muscles or the cardiovascular system.

1224. Why is deep penetration so often painful?

Your pelvis is filled with tender organs. If pounding pressure is applied to them, they will hurt. If you assume the position of being on the bottom, pressure is more easily applied, because you can't move. If you are on top or on your side, you can't be hurt as much, because you are free to move a little if there is pressure. Pain may also indicate that something is wrong, so you should have a pelvic examination to find out.

1225. What organs can be tender during penetration?

The following organs can be tender during deep penetration: the cervix; the base of the uterus, if it is tipped back; the ovaries, especially if they are located toward the middle of the body; the rectum, especially if it is filled with hard feces, as in constipation; ligaments, if you have endometriosis nodules (small cysts); the coccyx (tailbone) and sacrum, especially if they are inflamed.

1226. Is it okay to have sex several times in a row?

As long as you both want to, there is no harm in having sex several times in a row. It is beneficial to the male who has premature ejaculation. When he has sex more often, he can delay ejaculation longer.

SEX: ORGASM

1227. What is an orgasm?

An orgasm is a reflex that is produced by erotic stimulation. The result is generalized tension and then relaxation of most of the body's muscles, rhythmic contractions of the pelvis, increased pounding of the heart, sometimes sweating, and flushing of the skin. You lose some control of your body and experience involuntary contractions, movements, and sounds. Orgasm is an ecstatic feeling.

SEX: ORGASM (Continued)

1228. How do I know if I've had an orgasm?

If you feel some or all of the reactions mentioned earlier, you have had an orgasm. You will know absolutely if you are having one, so if you are in doubt, you probably have not had an orgasm. In the Masters and Johnson research laboratory, women can be monitored to record all of these reactions.

1229. How long does an orgasm last?

A single orgasm lasts from five to ten seconds, according to the laboratory research of Dr. William Masters. Multiple orgasms, usually four or five, can last as long as a minute when fused together, or they can occur at intervals of one every few minutes.

1230. Is an orgasm biological or psychological?

It is both. Biologically, the spinal cord has to be in one piece, and psychologically, the brain has to cooperate.

1231. How does my mental state affect my ability to have an orgasm?

Like any reflex, a poor mental state can inhibit orgasm and stop the whole sequence of events. Your mind must be receptive to sensual pleasure in order to release the orgasm.

1232. How important is a healthy body to achieving orgasm?

General good health is not a requirement, but the spinal cord must be complete, as an injury to it can interfere with orgasm. Pain, weakness, and disease can interfere, but do not absolutely prohibit orgasm. Sensation must also be present, so that any injury to the nerves that would numb certain areas could certainly interfere with orgasm.

1233. How important is orgasm for a fulfilled sex life?

Orgasm is a necessity for a fulfilled sex life. No matter how loving and generous you feel, your body and nervous system cannot serve forever without the reward of orgasm. Sexual arousal without release is uncomfortable, so as a defensive mechanism, the body deprived of orgasm will stop being aroused by anything. From there, you'll progress to aversion and avoidance of anything sexual. It may take many years, but sex can wither away without orgasm.

1234. Why do we have orgasm?

This is a very philosophical question. A common answer is that orgasm serves the purpose of luring us into sexual activity so that we will reproduce, but this is only true if the sexual activity is with a partner and it is heterosexual. Orgasms relieve tension, reduce nervousness, and make life

SEX: ORGASM (Continued)

tolerable. So, we have orgasms to relieve tension, to have fun, and occasionally, to reproduce.

1235. Does orgasm vary from woman to woman?

Orgasm varies a great deal from woman to woman, more so than it does from man to man. The length, intensity, amount of pelvic thrusting, heart pounding, and sweating all vary, as well as flushing, which is not always present in all women. Some women have multiple orgasms, while others do not.

1236. What are the differences between a male and a female orgasm?

Except for minor differences, the physical sensations are essentially the same. There is tension and excitement, heavy breathing, flushing, heart pounding, muscle contractions, perspiration, release, and relaxation. The differences are that a man feels the ejaculation of semen from his penis and a loss of erection, while a woman has uterine contractions which she may or may not feel. The female can also have multiple orgasms, if the stimulation is continued.

1237. What makes a man have an orgasm?

Most people think that if you rub a man's penis, he will have an orgasm. Actually, he must be psychologically and sensually aroused to have an erection of the penis, and he must reach a plateau stage of sexual arousal. Then the stimulation goes from the penis to the spinal cord and produces a reflex of muscle tension and release, ejaculation of prostatic fluid, increased cardiac output (heart pounding), increased skin temperature, sweating, and then relaxation. Without the spinal cord, a man cannot have an orgasm, which is why men with spinal cord injuries have a problem with sexual fulfillment.

1238. What occurs during an orgasm?

Orgasm in women is similar to orgasm in men. While men are stimulated by rubbing the penis, women are stimulated by rubbing the area around the clitoris or the G-spot (located just inside the vagina). Instead of an erection, a liquid forms in the vagina, the upper part of the vagina enlarges and barrels out, and the lower part swells and thickens. The nipples darken and become erect; the vulva and chest flush, and all of this stimulation is transmitted to the spinal cord. There it produces the reflex of muscle tension and relaxation, often with pelvic thrusting motions, contractions of the uterus and other muscles, increased cardiac output, warm skin, and possibly sweating. This is followed by relaxation, if the stimulus is stopped.

1239. Does intercourse alone cause an orgasm?

The thrusting motion of the penis in the vagina is the form of stimula-

SEX: ORGASM (Continued)

tion that people most often expect creates an orgasm, but it is actually the least effective. According to Masters and Johnson, this works if the penis pulls on the labia minora (the little lips of the vulva which have no hair) and on the hood of the clitoris so that the clitoris is stimulated. This produces orgasm in approximately 30 percent of women.

1240. What is a clitoral orgasm?

It is an orgasm triggered by clitoral stimulation. The stimulation which produces orgasm may be limited to the clitoris, but the sensation of orgasm involves the entire body. Stimulation may also be limited to the breasts or just to the mind, as in an orgasm produced by fantasy.

1241. What is the difference between an orgasm produced by clitoral stimulation and one produced by vaginal stimulation?

According to Masters and Johnson laboratory research, there is no difference between an orgasm produced by clitoral stimulation and one produced by vaginal stimulation. However, the intensity or strength seems to be greater in orgasms produced by stimulation of the clitoris during masturbation. Some women have a "G-spot orgasm," which has a vaginally stimulated origin.

1242. Is it easier to reach an orgasm through clitoral or vaginal stimulation?

A clitorally stimulated orgasm is easier to reach than one which is vaginally stimulated. Vaginal stimulation reaches the clitoris, but it is less direct.

1243. What does the G-spot do? How do I achieve a G-spot orgasm?

The G-spot is the area in the vagina with the most sensation. When it is rubbed with the finger or penis, it swells. This is probably due to the enlargement of the periurethral glands and blood vessels which surround the urethra. Some women find this stimulating, and they reach orgasm as a result. At orgasm, the glands empty, and women feel that they have ejaculated. Some medical investigators have found that urine is mixed in with the secretions of the urethral glands. The danger in rubbing the urethra for sensation leading to orgasm is that it can lead to bladder infections following sex. The urethral glands contain many bacteria, and rubbing them introduces bacteria into the urine and perhaps back up into the bladder. This explains why many women frequently develop bladder infections, such as cystitis and urethritis. They depend upon the sensation of rubbing their urethra and bladder base in order to enjoy coitus and perhaps reach orgasm. It would seem better to use stimulation which does not lead to infections.

1244. What is the "myth of the vaginal orgasm"?

Sigmund Freud insisted that girls had clitoral orgasms, but when they matured into well-adjusted women, they changed to orgasms emanating

SEX: ORGASM (Continued)

from the vagina alone. This is the "myth of the vaginal orgasm." If it were true, only 30 percent of all women have ever matured. However, Dr. William Masters showed that when a man's penis is inserted into a woman's vagina, the labia are pulled over the hood of the clitoris, and it is stimulated. So it is still, indirectly, a clitorally stimulated orgasm. In the laboratory, Masters was unable to produce an orgasm by only using an instrument (with a camera in it) in the vagina. He found that a partner with a penis was required to produce an orgasm from vaginal stimulation alone. The term "vaginal orgasm" is falling into disuse.

1245. How long does it take the average woman to reach orgasm?

The time that it takes for the average woman to reach orgasm varies from one to twenty minutes, although most sex researchers agree on an average time of five minutes. Of course, the time involved depends upon the adequacy of the stimulation. Most women will not reach orgasm through intercourse alone, so even if it goes on for hours, they will not experience a climax.

1246. How often do most women experience orgasm?

Surveys show that most orgasmic women have an orgasm in 50 percent of their sexual encounters and 95 percent of their masturbation efforts.

1247. Are there women who never achieve orgasm?

According to most surveys, about 10 percent of all women never achieve orgasm by any means.

1248. Are some women incapable of achieving an orgasm?

It may be that a small percentage of women will be unable to achieve orgasm because emotional blocks to sexual response are so deeply ingrained. It is the experience of sex therapists that few women have this problem. Sex therapists consider nonorgasmic women to be preorgasmic, suggesting that any woman can eventually learn to be orgasmic.

1249. Am I considered frigid if I cannot achieve orgasm?

Frigidity is regarded as an obsolete term. In the old medical books, women who could not achieve orgasm were considered frigid. Today, however, this term is not used as much. The new term is "sex aversion," which means not wanting to have anything to do with sex or sexual arousal. It can occur in women who are very good at reaching orgasm, if they allow sex to occur at all, and it can occur in women who do not reach orgasm. Whether orgasm is achieved is not of primary importance in defining the problem.

1250. Can every woman reach orgasm if she and her partner try hard enough?

Trying hard to reach orgasm makes its achievement very unlikely.

SEX: ORGASM (Continued)

Changing the focus to feeling pleasure in sensuality would be more effective. Most women are capable of orgasm, but probably will not achieve their first one by trying hard, especially with a partner. Orgasm is more likely to occur after you have learned to feel more sensual in many ways. This is usually accomplished alone, through self-stimulation.

1251. Is there anything my partner can do to increase my chances of having an orgasm?

Yes, he can do what you have taught him to be the most effective for you.

1252. What can I do if I never get close to orgasm until after my partner has already climaxed?

You can have your orgasm before intercourse. Those people who think they are "close to orgasm" during intercourse are probably not close at all. They are just blaming their lack of orgasm on their partner. You should first find out how to have orgasms without intercourse, and then you will know how to reach them during intercourse. If your partner's ejaculation is very fast, less than five minutes, you can also help him make it last longer with the squeeze technique, as taught by Masters and Johnson (see question 1344).

1253. Should I expect to have an orgasm every time I have sex?

You should at least hope to have an orgasm, or else sexual arousal won't readily occur.

1254. What can I do to help myself have an orgasm?

Prepare your mind to receive and enjoy sensual pleasure, but concentrate on the pleasure, not the orgasm. When orgasm does occur, remember which stimulation worked, and repeat it.

1255. Why must some women be manually stimulated in order to reach orgasm?

That "some" is about 70 percent of all women, so it is normal. Why do some 30 percent of all women not require manual stimulation? Because, according to Dr. William Masters, during intercourse the penis pulls on the small lips of the vulva (labia minora) which pulls the hood back and forth over the clitoris and thus stimulates it. It is not known why this works for some women but not for most others.

1256. Why isn't the clitoris in the vagina, where it will be rubbed by the penis?

Women are built to have babies. When babies are born, tears occur

SEX: ORGASM (Continued)

around the opening of the vagina, sometimes tearing in every direction. This could destroy the clitoris if it were not safely placed under the pubic bone where it is protected and out of the way. In this location it is preserved for a sex life after the baby is born.

1257. Is it common only to achieve orgasm through foreplay?

Yes, most women reach orgasm through the sensual pleasure of stimulating the vulva and clitoris prior to intercourse. This is called foreplay because it is play before intercourse. If women instead of men controlled the language, intercourse would be called "afterplay," because it takes place after most women achieve orgasm.

1258. Why is it much easier for me to reach orgasm during my fertile times? Is there a correlation between hormone levels in the body and orgasm?

There is no correlation between hormone levels in the body and orgasm. Postmenopausal women with reduced hormones reach orgasm. How easily they do this depends upon their own experiences and sexuality. However, there is a correlation between feeling well and energetic, physically and psychologically, and the ability to have orgasm easily. So, if you feel particularly well at one portion of your cycle, you will respond better sexually at that time. According to surveys, most women record more interest in sex during the week before their menses, despite the fact that this is the time for the premenstrual syndrome. Perhaps orgasm is also influenced by whether or not you want to get pregnant and your impression of the fertile or safe time of your cycle.

1259. Is it possible to have an orgasm by just imagining sexy things?

Yes, it is possible for some women to have an orgasm through the use of their imaginations. For a long time, Dr. Masters could not find a woman who could fantasize to orgasm in his laboratory so that he could record it. Now women have been found who can do this, and it has been proven. Of course, many women already knew that it was possible.

1260. Can anal stimulation cause orgasm?

Yes, and some women prefer anal stimulation for achieving orgasm.

1261. Do women have any kind of ejaculation when they have an orgasm?

Most women do not have any kind of ejaculation during orgasm. A few women who emphasize stimulation of the base of the bladder and urethra (the Grafenburg or G-spot) release secretions from the urethral glands along with a little urine. They need not be embarrassed by this.

1262. Is there a sexual position which would increase the strength of my orgasm?

Yes. The position in which you are most likely to reach orgasm is the

SEX: ORGASM (Continued)

side position. In this position, the woman mounts on top of the man, slides one leg straight down, and turns to lie across the thigh of her partner, who has brought his thigh up for her to lie across. You can then move your pelvis at will to help you reach orgasm, and he has a free hand to add stimulation near the clitoris as you need it. This position certainly adds to the strength of your orgasm.

1263. How can I train myself to achieve orgasm?

Books have been written on various methods that women have used to stimulate orgasms. You can read and try them all.

1264. Is there a spot on a woman's body that a man can touch which will keep her in orgasm for a long time?

No, sex is not a push-button process. Life would be too simple if it were. If a woman is capable of multiple orgasms, she can tell her partner which process produced the first orgasm, and it can be used to produce more. Sex is a process, not a spot.

1265. Can I have more than one orgasm during the same episode of sex?

Certainly. You are capable of having multiple or repeated orgasms. The greatest number of orgasms that a woman has been known to have experienced is four hundred, and this occurred in a research laboratory.

1266. What is a multiple orgasm?

Multiple orgasm is arousal to the height at which orgasm occurs again and again through continued stimulation, without relaxing and then being aroused again.

1267. Am I having multiple orgasms when I have one orgasm, rest for an interval, and then resume sex and have another orgasm?

No, you are not. Men can do this too, although not as many times per day as women can. The woman who can achieve multiple orgasms remains at the plateau phase of excitement as long as stimulation continues and can have a second, third, and fourth orgasm without a resting interval.

1268. Can all women have multiple orgasms?

Possibly. Although it would be nice to think that they could, this has not yet been proven.

1269. Are multiple orgasms common?

Yes, multiple orgasms are common in women.

1270. Why do some women experience multiple orgasms while others do not?

Some women have never tried to have multiple orgasms. They stop

SEX: ORGASM (Continued)

the stimulation as soon as orgasm occurs and never think of going on or trying again. Others simply have one grand orgasm, feel completely satisfied, relax, and must be aroused again to have another. The reason for this is not clear. Perhaps it is a conditioned response.

1271. What causes me to make loud sounds while having an orgasm?

Involuntary contractions of nearly all of the muscles in the body are involved in an orgasm, including the ones that make sounds. But not all people make loud sounds when having an orgasm. Individual reactions have different patterns.

1272. What causes the total ecstacy and trance-like state during orgasm?

You are in a trance-like state when your attention is focused on one thing, to the exclusion of all outside distractions. During orgasm, the whole nervous system is discharged. Attention is focused entirely upon the sensation of the orgasm, so that outside stimuli, even painful ones, are ignored.

1273. Why am I so exhausted after an orgasm?

Such "exhaustion" is really relaxation and release of all tensions. Energy is expended during orgasm, but not enough to really exhaust you with only a few orgasms. In the laboratory of Masters and Johnson, a woman had four hundred orgasms in one day before she was exhausted. The result of relaxation just looks like exhaustion; both produce a collapsed body.

1274. What should I do if I cannot achieve orgasm?

Try to achieve orgasm alone. Read *For Yourself,* by Lonnie Barbach (published by Signet) or *The Hite Report* on women, by Shere Hite, and get some ideas on how others manage. If you still cannot achieve orgasm, consult a sex therapist in your community or a group for women about your problem. You can ask your doctor or call your nearest medical school for a referral.

1275. Are there any relaxation techniques that I could practice to help me achieve orgasms?

You cannot achieve orgasm by being relaxed, but relaxation can clear other problems and tensions out of your mind so you can concentrate on sex and sensuality. Good relaxation techniques are taught by many self-hypnosis tapes, Lamaze childbirth classes, motivational groups, and meditation groups. You simply relax one part of your body at a time until you have covered the whole body. By focusing upon relaxation alone, you clear your mind of other considerations.

1276. Will I continue to experience orgasms as I get older?

Yes. If you continue to experience the stimulation that produces

SEX: ORGASM (Continued)

orgasms, and if you do not have an injury to your spinal cord or a psychological depression that deters you from all sexual activity, then orgasms will continue as you grow older.

1277. Will the orgasms I have when I am older be the same as those that I experience when I'm young?

Yes, but it may take longer to reach them, and they may be less intense. Some women have their first orgasm at an older age than others. I know of a patient who was seventy-two years old when she accidentally learned, while in the bathtub, to stimulate her clitoris and only then reached her first orgasm. After that, she did it every week or two and felt more relaxed. She had been married many years and had six children.

1278. Can a woman still achieve orgasm at the age of seventy or beyond?

Yes. There is no age limit placed on orgasm. It may take a little longer to achieve, but it still occurs.

1279. Is it easier for me to delay my orgasm than for a man to delay his?

Yes, it is. All you have to do is stop the stimulation, and your orgasm will not come. With a man it is different. He reaches a point at which orgasm is inevitable, even if he stops the stimulation. There is usually no reason for a woman to delay her orgasm because she can always have another one later. But a man tries to delay his orgasm because with it he loses his erection, and it is difficult to regain it afterward.

1280. Why do I have an orgasm during one sexual encounter and not the next (even though my partner is the same)?

Sex and orgasm really do not work by pure mechanics. If you choose the time of the sexual encounter, you do so because you are already psychologically in the mood to be aroused, and orgasm is more likely. With coitus, the average woman reaches orgasm about 60 percent of the time.

1281. Does having an orgasm increase my chances of pregnancy?

No. Having an orgasm does not increase your chances of pregnancy, but it may make you desire sex more often, which increases your chances of becoming pregnant. Some women actually avoid orgasm because they think they will prevent pregnancy that way, but this is a mistake. After childbirth, some women have such a relaxed opening of the vagina that orgasm makes the semen empty out and interferes with becoming pregnant.

1282. Is it important for both partners to reach a climax at the same time?

No, it is actually important that you do not reach a climax at the same time. The joy of simultaneous orgasm is one of the biggest fallacies and myths of sex. The tension of trying to time the orgasms ruins the spontane-

SEX: ORGASM (Continued)

ity. When you are having your orgasm, you can't even notice his, and vice versa. You miss enjoying the pleasure of the other person's climax. Just the movements of orgasm that each one makes can disturb the reaction of the other. Dr. William Masters, of Masters and Johnson, lectures against simultaneous orgasm.

1283. Is it common for women to fake orgasm?

Unfortunately, it is quite common, but it is never too late to take charge of your body and tell your partner the truth. You will probably never have an orgasm if you keep pretending.

SEX: AFTER ORGASM

1284. What is the usual emotional state of a woman immediately after intercourse?

After intercourse and orgasm, most women are still aroused but go into resolution when stimulation stops. They still feel close to their partners and are open to emotional intimacy. Some may feel exhausted from their orgasms and be ready to rest and relax. Other women may still be aroused after intercourse and are still waiting for climax. Some may be angered by the cessation of sex prior to their climax, and still others may be glad that it is over because they were bored or in pain. It would be easier to describe the emotional state of men after intercourse, which usually ends when they ejaculate with orgasm, enter their resolution stage, become refractory to stimulation, and turn over and go to sleep.

1285. Why do women stay excited for a while after sex, while men cool off right away?

It is not known why this happens. It is a characteristic of the male that, following orgasm, he goes into a refractory state during resolution. At this time nothing can sexually stimulate him. Most women do not experience this, although some claim to have a refractory period after orgasm, just like men. This is a problem because some women who have not reached orgasm become angry when their male partners cool off before they have been satisfied. Of course, if you don't have an orgasm, you will certainly stay excited and only cool off gradually.

SEX: SEXUAL PERFORMANCE

1286. Does stress have any bearing on a person's sexual performance?

Sometimes stress produces such worry in people that they can't get their minds off of their problems long enough to concentrate upon sensuality. In this case, stress inhibits sexual performance. At other times, stress

SEX: SEXUAL PERFORMANCE (Continued)

simply increases a person's tensions, including sexual tensions, and sexual performance is more important than ever for release.

1287. Do women usually outlast men in sex?

Not always. Sometimes the man takes so long thrusting to orgasm that the woman loses interest and lubrication, so that her vagina becomes dry and uncomfortable. On the other hand, because she can have multiple and repeated orgasms, she can continue sex after orgasm longer than a man can.

1288. Can low levels of sex hormones affect a woman's sexual performance?

In general, low levels of sex hormones do not lower the sex drive in human beings. In women, however, it can make the vagina thin, tender, and dry, and thus it can make intercourse uncomfortable. This can happen during breast-feeding and after menopause. A little bit of hormone cream can restore the vagina to normal.

SEX: SEXUAL POSITIONS

1289. What are the most common positions used by couples during intercourse?

The most common position is with the woman on her back with her knees up and the man on top, but it is not necessarily the best. The next most common position is the woman on top, astride the man. The side position is probably the best for the woman because she is able to move. Rear entry, with the woman in the knee-chest position, is adopted in late pregnancy. There are many variations in positions; these are depicted in many books and on the walls of the ruins of Pompeii.

1290. What is the most popular position for sexual intercourse?

Probably the most popular position is the man on top of the woman, who is lying on her back with her knees up. But this is popular only because the man is more aggressive about initiating sex. If women initiated sex, they would probably choose another position.

1291. What sexual positions produce the most enjoyment for women?

Positions that allow the woman the greatest freedom of movement, such as the woman astride the man or the side positions, lead to more enjoyment. In the side position, her partner can use his hand to manipulate her vulva and clitoris to bring her to orgasm.

1292. What are the best positions for me to reach an orgasm vaginally, clitorally, and by the G-spot?

There really are not any best positions for these. Vaginally, orgasm is promoted if you are in a position to move your pelvis, such as the woman

SEX: SEXUAL POSITIONS (Continued)

astride the man, or better yet, the side position. Pressing downward with the penis, away from the bladder, pulls the lips and hood over the clitoris to stimulate orgasm. This is called a vaginally stimulated orgasm. Clitorally, any position that enables the hand or tongue to reach your clitoral area will work. If the man is bearing his weight on his arms, he cannot use his hands to stimulate your clitoris. The G-spot requires that the penis be inserted shallowly and pressed upward, toward the bladder, to rub the urethral area. This is usually achieved with the woman in the astride position. Since there is no need for simultaneous orgasm, position does not have to provide for stimulation of both of you at once. A position which is used to stimulate you can be changed when your partner is ready for his orgasm.

1293. Are there any sexual positions which would be harmful to my body?
Any position that is uncomfortable for you can be harmful to you. Painful positions indicate that joints and tissues are being pressured or stretched too much.

1294. Does the risk of pregnancy vary with the positions I use during intercourse?
As long as the ejaculate enters the vagina, the risk of pregnancy is high, regardless of the position.

1295. Are there any sexual positions that would be unsafe if I have an IUD?
No. The IUD cannot be touched or dislodged by sex in any position because it is positioned securely in the uterus.

1296. Are there any sexual positions that would change the placement of my diaphragm and thereby decrease its effectiveness?
No sexual position will change the placement of your diaphragm. However, sexual arousal enlarges the vagina, and the diaphragm becomes looser, which may allow sperm to pass through. A second intercourse after a period of rest may also allow the penis to enter over the diaphragm instead of under it. A quick check with a finger can prevent this from happening.

1297. How many different positions for sex are there?
The number of different positions for sex must reach infinity.

1298. Is it really possible to have sex while standing up?
Men can have sex in a standing position, but it would be very difficult for a woman to do so with her legs completely straight. However, if you were to squat a little, you could accommodate your partner's penis.

SEX: SEXUAL ACTIVITY AND BEHAVIOR

1299. What is the difference between sex and heavy petting?
In our language today, "sex" means intercourse, coitus, or the act of

SEX: SEXUAL ACTIVITY AND BEHAVIOR (Continued)

the penis thrusting into the vagina. Heavy petting is everything intimate except coitus, including manual or oral stimulation to orgasm.

1300. Is having sex the same thing as making love?

Yes, today "having sex" and "making love" share a common meaning. Both phrases refer to the act of having intercourse.

1301. What does it mean to be sexually active?

To be sexually active means to experience sexual intercourse on a continuing basis. The frequency of intercourse has not been defined, but being sexually active is different from having had intercourse only once in your life or only once each year.

1302. How do hormone levels change with sexual activity?

There has been research conducted which demonstrates that in men, sexual activity with ejaculation raises the testosterone level, while lack of activity lowers it. However, there is no similar change in women. Studies of hormone levels at the time of sexual intercourse do not show any changes.

1303. Are girls today more sexually active than they used to be?

If sexual activity means sexual intercourse, the answer is yes. The percentage of girls who have had intercourse before marriage and the percentage of teenagers who have had intercourse have increased greatly in the last twenty years. But that does not mean that there was no sexual activity before; it simply means that there was not as much intercourse. Sexual activity twenty years ago was limited to touching, talking, and fantasizing. The sexual revolution marked the inclusion of intercourse.

1304. What is promiscuity?

Generally, promiscuity means having sex with many different partners. It is a term that is most often applied to women, and it usually means having sex with several men during the same time period, or else rapidly changing partners one at a time. Men are seldom called promiscuous. This is part of the double standard; men are permitted to have many partners and to change partners frequently, but women are not. So, promiscuity refers to a woman who changes sex partners more frequently than is socially acceptable.

1305. Does nymphomania occur only in women?

By definition, nymphomania occurs only in women. The Don Juan syndrome occurs in men, and it is sometimes greatly admired. It seems to be more acceptable for men to desire sexual activity with many different women than for women to desire many different men.

SEX: SEXUAL ACTIVITY AND BEHAVIOR (Continued)

1306. What was the Hite report?
The Hite Report, conducted by Shere Hite (Macmillan, 1976), was a survey on the sexuality and sexual activities of women. It was first conducted on small groups of women and later on larger groups.

1307. What was the Kinsey report?
The Kinsey report was published in two volumes by Saunders. The first was *Sexual Behavior in the Human Male* (1948), and the second was *Sexual Behavior in the Human Female* (1953). Surveys directed by Alfred C. Kinsey through the University of Indiana were the first, and remain the largest, surveys ever conducted on human sexual behavior.

1308. What kinds of sexual activity are considered normal?
Any kind of sexual activity that is pleasing and acceptable to both partners is normal, no matter how unusual or odd. Anything that is painful or disgusting to either partner is not normal.

1309. What kinds of sexual activity are considered to be abnormal?
Almost every kind of sexual activity would be considered abnormal by somebody. What matters is whether you and/or your partner think it is abnormal.

1310. What is cunnilingus?
Cunnilingus is the stimulation of the clitoris and vulva of the female by her partner's tongue. It is an effective way to reach orgasm.

1311. Is oral sex new?
No, oral sex is not new. It is depicted in ancient drawings.

1312. During oral sex, is it unhealthy for a woman to swallow semen?
It is not unhealthy for a woman to swallow semen. It has no particular benefit to her health, nor does it cause any harm.

1313. What percentage of people engage in anal sex?
Kinsey's study, published in 1950, found that the number of women who had tried anal sex was neglible. A recent study, conducted in the 1970s, found that one-sixth of women surveyed under twenty-five had tried anal sex, and 6 percent used it occasionally.

1314. Does anal sex cause hemorrhoids?
No, anal sex does not cause hemorrhoids, but hemorrhoids can make anal sex uncomfortable.

1315. Why do some people engage in anal sex?
Sometimes it is used because the couple wants to avoid pregnancy. Other times, it is a sexual outlet when infection makes the vagina too tender

SEX: SEXUAL ACTIVITY AND BEHAVIOR (Continued)
for vaginal intercourse. Also, it is used because people enjoy it.

SEX: EFFECTS OF AGING AND MEDICAL PROBLEMS

1316. Will sex get better as I get older?

No, sex will not get better in a steady progression. For most women, sex improves between the ages of fifteen and thirty. During this time, you gradually learn to function in a way that is rewarding to yourself. Thereafter, any improvement may depend upon improving your relationships. An increase in frequency has been noted after menopause. This is attributed to freedom from the fear of pregnancy, but as methods of contraception improve, no such change should be noted. Postmenopausal problems of dryness, untreated with estrogen, can cause your sexual experiences to deteriorate, and general health problems can certainly interfere. On the other hand, freedom from raising children after menopause allows time for self-exploration and improvement in the sexual aspects of your life. Of course, if your partner's sexual performance has deteriorated, then it is hard for you to improve yours.

1317. Does sexual desire and drive continue for most people through their older years?

Yes, sexual desire and drive continue even if the opportunities for sex do not. As some older men say, "You can still look, even if you can do nothing about it!"

1318. What can women in the age bracket of sixty and older expect sexually?

Great variation exists in this age group just as in any other age bracket. Ideally, these women have solved their hormonal problems so that they have no vaginal difficulty with intercourse. They have solved their sexual difficulties in the past, so they are now capable of and interested in giving and receiving sexual pleasure and orgasms. They have worked out relationships with their partners so that they can communicate about sex better than ever before. Frequency will depend upon their partners, their lifelong pattern of energy, and their need to release tension.

1319. Why do some women continue to desire, enjoy, and pursue sex as they get older, while others push it out of their lives?

There are several important factors which have a bearing on how a woman will relate to sex as she gets older. First of all, menopause occurs between the ages of fifty and fifty-four. When a woman's estrogen is gone, her vagina becomes dry, tender, and sometimes shrinks. As a result, intercourse can become painful. Some women take estrogen; others continue to produce

SEX: EFFECTS OF AGING AND MEDICAL PROBLEMS
(Continued)

estrogen, so they do not have this problem. Others avoid intercourse. Second, aging in our culture is hard on the feminine ego. If a woman has a loving, adoring husband and family who keep her thinking well of herself or if she has a career that feeds her ego, she is more likely to retain her desire for sex and have a healthy outlook on life. If she loses interest in sex because she has no partner, and she has things to do that interest and excite her, she can still remain healthy and active despite her lack of sexual activity. If her ego is deflated every day and her self-image is very drab, her sex drive will decrease as a result of her depression. Thirdly, if her beloved sex partner has become impotent and can no longer perform, and he makes no substitution for her sake, she may suppress all of her sexual desires so that she can remain true to him. Many women do this consciously, but unnecessarily, since their impotent husbands could satisfy them in many ways. Many husbands do not even recognize the sexual needs of middle-aged women.

1320. Is there a trend toward being more open regarding sexual awareness and desire among women in their sixties, seventies, and over?

Yes, there is. The sexual revolution began some time ago, when these women were young, so they bring to this age a different attitude than that which their mothers had. They may have taken advantage of counseling offered for sex problems, and they probably have read modern books. They are not completely dominated by a religious or church-sponsored attitude toward sex, or they may belong to churches that take a modern view of sexuality in the human community. They are also physically healthier and more energetic for their age, due to the elevation of general standards of health in this country over those of their forebears.

1321. What happens sexually to a woman in her sixties? Does she still desire and pursue sex as much as she did in her thirties?

Very few women in their sixties enjoy and pursue sex as much as they did when they were in their thirties, although a few enjoy it even more. For some, the reason for this is atrophic vaginitis, a condition in which a deficiency of estrogen makes the vagina dry, tender, and sometimes shrunken. Estrogen cream or pills can be used to help this condition. For other women, this is not a problem. They still seem to have their own natural supply of estrogen after menopause. Even more important at this age is the state of a woman's health, which determines whether or not she has energy for any activity, including sex. If she is healthy and has a partner who is interested in sex, then she can be as sexually active as she was at any other time in her life. There are couples in their sixties who have time to be interested in sex for the first time in their lives because the children are finally raised and gone. Some

SEX: EFFECTS OF AGING AND MEDICAL PROBLEMS
(Continued)

couples who have had sexual dysfunctions get help from sex therapists at this age because it may be that it is the first time in their lives that they can afford it. At this point in their lives they know that they are going to stay together, so they decide to remedy any sexual difficulties. If the woman has no partner but still lives an interesting, active life, the lack of sex will not be so important.

1322. What happens sexually to a woman over seventy? Does she still desire and pursue sex?

Many women who are in their seventies still desire and pursue sex. There is no reason for them not to if their health is still good and if they have a healthy partner. Estrogen may be needed for comfort, but sex is still enjoyable. Many more women at this age are either disabled by their own illnesses or their husbands are so weak and feeble that they are afraid to attempt sex. Many women have misconceptions about the dangers of sexual activity at this age, and they avoid it without even asking their physicians if it is okay.

1323. How many times per week does the average senior citizen have sex?

The answer to this question is as elusive as that concerning the frequency of sex in teenagers. Many senior citizens have no sexual intercourse at all, due to ill health or the lack of a partner or an opportunity. Of those who are still active, some maintain a frequency of two or three times per week, which was the frequency most commonly found in earlier years, but most have a frequency of two or three times per month.

1324. Are there any precautions which senior citizens should take when engaging in sex?

The main thing that senior citizens worry about is having a heart attack. If you have a problem with your heart, then you should consult your doctor. If your doctor tells you that sex is safe for you to enjoy, believe it. Another problem which can occur in women is vaginal infections. Since pregnancy is no longer a consideration, precautions against becoming pregnant are no longer needed.

1325. Will my clitoris lose its sensitivity as I get older?

No, aging does not make the clitoris lose its sensitivity. Misuse and disuse cause this. If the clitoris is neglected for fifty years, it is not likely to remain sensitive. Care and attention might bring it back after such a long period of disuse, but only if your brain permits it.

1326. After a certain age, do women lose their attraction for men?

No. Although they may lose some attraction for some men, they may be attracted to others.

SEX: EFFECTS OF AGING AND MEDICAL PROBLEMS
(Continued)

1327. Is sexual stimulation a threat to a weak heart?

Yes, but only if the heart is so weak that it cannot tolerate climbing a flight of stairs. Your heart doctor can predict, from a stress test, whether your heart is strong enough for sex or any other form of exercise. Your doctor can also put you on a program of graduated exercise which can strengthen your heart.

1328. Can adult diabetes affect sexual activity in women? If so, how?

There are conflicting medical surveys concerning the effect of adult diabetes on sexual activity in women. Some studies demonstrate no effect and certainly nothing as devastating as the impotence it produces in men. Another study shows a reduction in the ability to lubricate. Theoretically, this would result from decreased circulation in blood vessels in the pelvis, as well as a reduction in nervous activity, which has been demonstrated in men.

1329. Does a very active sex life promote cancer of the cervix in women?

It is not the amount of activity which is so important; it is the presence of multiple partners, or a partner with multiple partners, that increases the chances of getting herpes simplex, warts, or any of the other sexually transmitted diseases that are found to be most often associated with cancer of the cervix. Even sperm is associated with cancer of the cervix, since it has been found to enter the cervical cells and transform the nucleus in a malignant manner. Virgins do not develop cancer of the cervix.

SEX: SEXUAL FANTASIES

1330. Are sexual fantasies more common among married or single persons?

There seems to be no difference. Sexual fantasies are present in the sexually active as well as the sexually inactive.

1331. Who fantasizes the most, men or women?

Women fantasize more than men. This is probably because they frequently find themselves in the situation of trying to reach orgasm without adequate stimulation, so they supplement stimulation with fantasy. A man is not expected to reach orgasm without adequate stimulation of his penis, so he does not need to fantasize as much.

SEX: INJURY AND PAIN DURING SEX

1332. Is it possible for me to be hurt by overly vigorous sex?

Yes, it is possible, but before you experience any physical damage you

SEX: INJURY AND PAIN DURING SEX (Continued)

will feel pain, and you should stop anything that is painful. Pain itself will damage your whole attitude toward sex. Intercourse that is forced upon you (rape) can be very damaging because the vagina and rectum can be torn.

1333. Is pain during intercourse more likely to occur in women with small bone structures than those with larger frames?

No. Pain in labor is more likely to occur in women with small bone structures, but not in coitus. If your vagina is shallow, the man's penis reaches the end sooner, but only force makes it painful.

1334. Can I suffer physical injury by having sex with a man whose penis is very large?

If the man's penis is longer than what you are accustomed to and if he uses force during intercourse, he can rupture your vagina. However, long before physical injury takes place, pain occurs, and you should not continue to have intercourse if it is painful. A man with a very large penis does not always present a problem during sex, as a vagina can adjust slowly to any size, even to that of a baby's head.

SEX: CELIBACY AND ABSTINENCE

1335. Is it easier for a woman to abstain from sex than for a man?

The Kinsey Report emphasizes that women can abstain from sex for very long periods, even years, and then participate again with full pleasure. When men abstain, they experience problems with impotence or premature ejaculation when they start again. This may be due to the difference in the male function, the accumulation of sperm when they do not ejaculate, and the suppression of testosterone when no ejaculation occurs. It may also be due to the man's conviction of his right to sexual activity and his clear recognition of his needs. Many women have no idea of what their rights are, and their sexual desires are so suppressed that they do not recognize them.

1336. A lot of women become widows in their late fifties or early sixties. They don't date men, but they seem relatively peaceful and content. How do they adjust to not having sex?

Of all natural functions, sex is the most easily suppressed. Kinsey's studies found that women could function well sexually for a period of time, and then not function sexually at all for long periods of time with no apparent ill effect. Men were able to do this much less frequently.

1337. Is it okay to abstain from sex?

Yes, it is okay to abstain from sex, but if you experience sexual arousal and refuse to satisfy it in any way, you will find that you begin to experience less and less arousal. This is a protective mechanism for the body. By not

SEX: CELIBACY AND ABSTINENCE (Continued)

satisfying your arousal, you will damage your ability to experience sexual arousal and satisfaction in later life. However, a small percentage of people never experience sexual arousal and can apparently do quite nicely without it forever.

1338. Could practicing celibacy for a while improve my sex life later?

Possibly. Celibacy removes the demand for performance, and it is this requirement for sexual performance which is so destructive to many people. Celibacy gives you time to think about yourself and what you want in life, without focusing upon pleasing others. In their cotherapy treatment of couples with sex problems, Masters and Johnson forbid all sexual intercourse at the beginning of therapy. Of course, when something is forbidden, desire for it rises. But if celibacy continues for a long time, sexual response may be suppressed. Masturbation and fantasizing about sex will keep sexual arousal and response alive more than celibacy will.

1339. How much strain does celibacy place upon a person's emotional nature?

Of course, this depends on how much a person desires a sexual relationship with another person. Most celibates claim not to masturbate, and this removes the natural outlet for the build-up of sexual tensions. In some people, very little sex tension is built up.

SEX: SEXUAL PROBLEMS AND CURES

1340. What percentage of all couples have sex problems?

Estimates are that at least half of all couples have some kind of sexual dysfunction that becomes a problem in their relationship.

1341. What percentage of married couples have a sexual problem?

It is estimated that at least 60 percent of all couples have a problem of sexual dysfunction that they must cope with in their marriage.

1342. What percentage of your patients tell you that they have sexual problems?

About 10 percent of my patients actually bring up a sexual problem without being asked about it directly.

1343. Are a couple's sexual problems usually solved?

Not all of their problems are always solved. Some of my patients bring up a problem for discussion, but will take no further action toward its solution. Others solve the problem as soon as they are given a little information or some suggestions. Some are referred to full-time sex therapists, usually along with their partners, for further help with the problem. Some work on a

SEX: SEXUAL PROBLEMS AND CURES (Continued)

problem by themselves or with help from professionals, but their partners will not join in the therapy or assist them with any change. Some solve their problems by changing partners. Others try this without success because the same problem follows them from partner to partner. Many people want to know how to raise their children so that their children will not be beset with sexual difficulties, as they were.

1344. How can I help keep my partner from having premature ejaculations?

You can learn the squeeze technique, as taught by Masters and Johnson and other sex therapists. You stimulate your partner's penis until he indicates that he is about to ejaculate, and then squeeze it between your thumb and index finger at the base of the glans (the cone-shaped head of the penis). This stops the ejaculation. Then you stimulate and squeeze again, until he can maintain an erection without ejaculation for five minutes or longer. During love-making, you mount him from above, dismount when he is about to ejaculate and squeeze the glans with your fingers. Then mount again and repeat the procedure until he maintains an erection for five minutes. With training, he can go longer and longer without requiring the squeeze to deter his ejaculation.

1345. What exercises can I do that will make me more aware of my body and perhaps help me to enjoy sex more?

Kegel Exercises (named after Dr. Kegel, who wrote a book about them) are said to enhance the sexual experience by tightening the muscles around the opening of the vagina. These exercises can make you more aware of your pelvic sensations, increase the blood flow to your vagina, and make your vagina feel tighter to your partner.

1346. Can proper exercise keep my vagina tight or make it tighter?

Kegel Exercises, or levator muscle exercises, will tighten the muscles around the vagina and can help to keep the vagina tight, but they will not always work in completely repairing damaged muscles. Sometimes surgical repair is necessary. A simple exercise you might try to tighten your vagina is to squeeze the muscles that stop urination while you are urinating.

SEX: HOMOSEXUALITY

1347. What percentage of all people are homosexual?

A rough estimate is that 10 percent of the overall population is homosexual.

1348. What makes a person gay?

Homosexuality is a natural occurrence, even among animals, but no

SEX: HOMOSEXUALITY (Continued)

one knows what causes it. Dr. Kinsey believes that you cannot classify people as being "gay" or "not gay." A more accurate classification would be: always gay, usually gay, sometimes gay, rarely gay, or never gay.

1349. What predetermines a person's sexual preference?

Sexual preference is probably not predetermined. It depends upon the experiences and the environmental factors of infancy and childhood that are unknown. Sexual preference can also change.

1350. Is it abnormal for women to look at other women, even though they are not gay?

Few people are 100 percent gay or 100 percent heterosexual. Most women have at least thought of having a sexual experience with another woman, even if they have never acted upon it.

1351. Why are there suddenly so many homosexuals?

There are not nearly as many homosexuals today on a percentage basis as there were among the Greeks when Athens was the center of civilization. It just seems as if there are more homosexuals, because homosexuality is discussed more openly today than it was thirty years ago.

1352. Can parents tell at an early age if their children have homosexual tendencies?

Probably not. It is quite normal for children to become more attached to other children of the same sex at certain stages of their development, even including a sexual experience. This does not mean that they are destined to remain in that stage.

1353. Can parents prevent homosexuality in their children?

It is not known if it is possible for parents to prevent homosexuality in their children. However, it has been demonstrated that children who are raised by homosexuals do not necessarily become homosexuals themselves.

1354. Are there any problems that are peculiar to gay women?

Unless they are hiding within a heterosexual marriage, gay women who want children have trouble arranging a pregnancy, adopting a child, or gaining custody of a child. If they never become pregnant or never use contraceptive pills, they have a higher incidence of endometriosis, endometrial cancer, ovarian cancer, and breast cancer.

Chapter 6

How and When to Get Pregnant

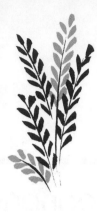

Today I woke up
feeling strange
but special
For the first time
in my life
I thought about the fact that I
could produce a baby
Out of me
from he
a little baby
Unbelievable

Sure all my friends
have had babies
but I never thought of myself
as a man's wife
or a child's mother
I am just me, leading
my own life
and in love with he

But today, I pictured
a little baby building sand castles
and it belonged to us

— Susan Polis Schutz

HOW AND WHEN TO GET PREGNANT

The opportunity to be able to decide when to have a baby is an opportunity that has only recently become available. In the past, the only decision women had was when to begin having sex, and that was equal to a decision to get pregnant. In today's world, it really takes courage to decide to have a child. For one person this is hard enough, but for two people to decide at the same time makes the decision to have a child even more difficult. Fortunately, many couples do decide to take the big step. Since you are probably only going to do this once or twice, you can put a lot of thought and effort into making it the best possible experience and getting the best possible result. Seek advice about the best time, age, and condition for becoming pregnant. Give up smoking, drinking, and even coffee. Some women find that they need to give up their jobs, professions, and/or education in order to create the time in which to have a baby or give early child care. Learn all you can about preparing for pregnancy and child care. After all this preparation, if you find that you cannot get pregnant, seek advice about your infertility. It is estimated that sixteen million couples in the United States find that they need help to get pregnant. That help can come from your gynecologist or an infertility specialist.

HOW AND WHEN TO GET PREGNANT: THE DESIRE TO HAVE A BABY

1355. Is it normal for a woman to feel strong urges to have a baby?

Having and raising a child is a fascinating, rewarding, and emotional experience that fulfills the need for close attachment like nothing else can. If this is denied, most people feel deprived, but women feel it more, because they grow up patterned to be mothers. Often there is not as much in their lives that is fulfilling, compared to the lives of most men. The desire for the joy of holding a small baby of your own may never leave you. It may even extend beyond all reasonable bounds of the number of children you can possibly raise or that the world wants. This is often a real conflict between a husband and wife, because the woman wants more children than the man wants to support. He also may not receive the gratification from the small baby that she does, because he has not been patterned for child care and its enjoyments. Counseling couples sometimes includes convincing the husband that having children is something his wife really wants out of life, whether he wants it or not.

1356. Do most women want to have children?

Yes, but not at all periods and all stages in their lives. In the past, most women have had more children than they wanted, because contraception was not available to them. When childbearing is their choice, women still want children, but not as many. Yet, some women do not want or need them at all. We must allow for variation in this respect. Just as it is accepted that all men will not be fathers, some women are not patterned to be mothers. Probably as many as 10 percent of women are not heterosexual, although many of them still want children.

1357. What is maternal instinct? Do all women have it?

An instinct is a patterned behavior that is hereditary. Instinct is very evident in other animals, particularly the female species' behavior toward caring for their young, although in some species, it is the male who does this. In the "higher" animals, like the monkey, and sometimes other primates, there seems to be no such maternal instinct. The mother will not take care of her offspring in captivity, because she has not seen this done by others. This has to be taught to her. Human beings are like primates in this respect; caretaking behavior toward the young must be taught to them. It is naturally taught by observation of others. Some women have had the opportunity to observe child care, and others have not. Studies have shown that children who play with dolls grow up wanting to have babies. If we want men to care for children, perhaps we should teach boys to play with dolls and to observe child care.

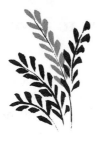

I had a
discussion
with a group
of women
They wanted to know
why I wanted
to have children
when the world
is so overpopulated
and since I couldn't
come up with
a great answer
they thought I
shouldn't have
any
But I asked
them why they
had children
and no one had
a good reason
I thought
about this
It would be
great to see
what kind of
person would
come from
the two of us
but that
seemed too
egotistical
It would be fun
to watch
and help someone
grow from a baby
to an adult
No, this wasn't
the reason either
And then all of a
sudden
I realized how
in this unstable
world
love is the only
important thing
and most of all
a baby would be
someone else to love

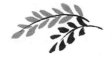

— Susan Polis Schutz

HOW AND WHEN TO GET PREGNANT: THE DESIRE TO HAVE A BABY (Continued)

1358. How can I mentally prepare myself for pregnancy?

Talking to friends who are pregnant and observing them is really very helpful. Reading books about pregnancy and preparation for childbirth is also a mental preparation. Taking childbirth classes is usually reserved for women who are already pregnant, but the books are available to everyone.

1359. How can I prepare my partner for pregnancy?

The most effective preparation for your partner is association with friends who are having babies. You must make clear in your partner's mind and in your own mind what your plans are regarding any change in activities that you expect to occur as a result of your pregnancy. Don't assume that he expects you to quit work and stay home. Discuss it in detail. Books written by psychologists about expectant fatherhood are also available. Apparently, our culture helps women a lot more than it does men in making the transition to parenthood, but this situation is improving.

HOW AND WHEN TO GET PREGNANT: THINGS TO CONSIDER BEFORE HAVING A BABY; IDEAL TIME TO BECOME PREGNANT

1360. What are some of the things my husband and I should consider before deciding to have a baby?

If you think about having a baby long enough, you may never have one. However, there are some problems that can be avoided by considering their solutions in advance. Both of you need to consider finances and your roles as parents. The prospective mother should ask herself the following questions: If I am going to stop earning money and take care of all the child care, will I be satisified in this role? Will there still be enough money? If I am going to work after the baby comes, what child care arrangements are available? If I become disabled by complications of pregnancy, how will the finances suffer? Will I become so maternal that I will lose my own identity? The prospective father should ask himself: Am I willing to give up the time and attention that my wife will be diverting to the baby? Both prospective parents should ask themselves: Do both of us agree on the methods and goals of child rearing? What are our reasons for wanting a child? How much will we have to change our lifestyles because of finances and child care? If both of you can answer all of these questions to your satisfaction, then you are ready to have a baby.

1361. How will a baby change my lifestyle?

The changes that a baby will make in your lifestyle depend upon the arrangements you make for child care. Responsibility for the child's care, by

HOW AND WHEN TO GET PREGNANT: THINGS TO CONSIDER BEFORE HAVING A BABY; IDEAL TIME TO BECOME PREGNANT
(Continued)

law, falls to the woman, while support falls to the man. But they can be traded and exchanged in individual arrangements. If you are to do all of the child care, your life will change greatly. If you share it with your husband, as many women now do, both of your lives will change somewhat. If you have had experience caring for younger siblings, you will know more of what to expect. However, even if you have help with your baby, you will always be aware of the responsibility.

1362. Are babies expensive?
Yes. Babies cost a lot in money, time, and effort.

1363. Where can I go for advice if I'm thinking about having a baby?
Discussing the subject with friends who have children can be very enlightening. Psychologists now hold group sessions on the subject of whether or not to have a baby. Your doctor can also answer many questions for you. However, only you and your husband can make the final decision.

1364. Is there a good or bad time to get pregnant?
The best time to get pregnant is when you want a baby. It helps if you are financially secure, in good health, and between the ages of twenty-five and thirty-five. It is also better when you are not smoking, drinking, or taking any drugs.

1365. I keep waiting for the perfect time in my life to get pregnant. Will there ever will be a perfect time?
Possibly not. If you are only going to have two children, you want to have them at the best possible times. However, if you wait too long, for finances to improve, for example, you may find that something has happened to your fertility.

1366. What are the ideal circumstances for becoming pregnant?
Ideally, this is when you are still fertile and financially able to enjoy pregnancy and child care without undue worry about money. You should also be joined in your desire by a participating father, and you should be completely healthy, with no genetic problems in your background or your partner's. You should be educated enough to be able to take care of yourself properly, and you should be aware of the available facilities for health care and delivery, as well as medical care for your child. If you are involved in other activities, ideally they are flexible enough for you to enjoy your pregnancy and your child without too much conflict with your other interests. If women were designing the world, there would be enough flexibility

HOW AND WHEN TO GET PREGNANT: THINGS TO CONSIDER BEFORE HAVING A BABY; IDEAL TIME TO BECOME PREGNANT
(Continued)

for fathers also to be able to enjoy the early childhood of their offspring. Part of the ideal situation is also having enough household help, so that you are not exhausted the first few weeks after delivery.

1367. Should I worry about getting pregnant if I've never had the measles?

Only German measles (rubella) causes birth defects. If you've never had German measles, you should have the vaccine to prevent it at least three months before you start trying to get pregnant. Getting rubella in pregnancy can be a disaster. However, there is a blood test to see if you are immune or not. Maybe you had them and didn't know it. You should find out.

1368. What are the ideal childbearing years for a woman?

Many obstetricians and gynecologists recommend that the ideal childbearing years are between the ages of twenty-five and thirty-five. In fact, they recommend having one child between twenty-five and thirty, and the second child between thirty and thirty-five. This allows the woman to become educated and mature before she has a child. Population experts say that the total population would be reduced more by women waiting until a later age to have children than it would be by reducing the number of children per person by one. The body is really not totally mature before the age of twenty-five, and a person is certainly not completely educated or financially independent until that time. However, this ideal is not what actually occurs in this country.

1369. What is the youngest age that a girl can get pregnant?

The youngest age on record, which is documented in the United States, is nine years old. Supposedly, there was also one girl in South America who became pregnant at the age of six; however, the documents concerning the girl's age were questionable.

1370. At what age do most women feel the urge to have a baby?

Most women have had a baby by the age of twenty-five. This may or may not be the result of an urge.

1371. Will my ability to have children decrease as I get older? If so, why?

Yes. Your fertility increases from the onset of menses to the age of twenty-five. After that, it stays about the same until you reach thirty-five, and then it begins to decrease. The decrease is due to the lack of ovulation (not releasing an egg every month). By forty-five, you will almost stop releasing eggs, and by fifty, ovulation would be extremely rare.

HOW AND WHEN TO GET PREGNANT: THINGS TO CONSIDER BEFORE HAVING A BABY; IDEAL TIME TO BECOME PREGNANT
(Continued)

1372. At what age is a woman too old to get pregnant?

Pregnancy becomes rare after the age of forty-six, and it is extremely rare after fifty. The oldest woman on record to have a baby was fifty-eight years old. Only sixteen women over the age of fifty had babies in the United States in a ten-year period. Statistically, that is one in many millions.

HOW AND WHEN TO GET PREGNANT: PLANNING FOR A FAMILY

1373. Do most couples today plan their families in advance?

Yes, they do, and if an unplanned pregnancy occurs, they might choose to terminate it. However, couples are usually better at contraception after they experience an abortion, so it usually only happens once.

1374. What percentage of births are not planned?

In the 1950s, surveys showed that seven out of ten babies were clearly unwanted, as well as unplanned. Today only about three out of ten pregnancies are unplanned. It is difficult to assess planning. Sometimes the woman plans the pregnancy but the man does not, so there is a conflict in the answer.

1375. How do I plan in advance for a baby?

You can obtain information about pregnancy, delivery, and child care so that you will be knowledgeable on these subjects. You should plan on including household help for the first few weeks after the baby is born. If possible, you should be able to provide financially for any possible disability or complication of pregnancy or delivery. You should investigate the cost of having a baby and your available assets, such as insurance coverage. Find out the policies of your employer concerning maternity leave. If your job is such that you will be disabled in pregnancy, this needs to be included in your planning.

1376. Should I tell my employer that I'm trying to get pregnant?

No, because there is always the chance that you may never get pregnant. However, you should inquire of your employer or the personnel department in the company where you work what the policies are toward women working late into pregnancy. You should also inquire about maternity leave, insurance coverage, and disability insurance, especially for your particular state. Most women find it is not wise to divulge their pregnant state until it becomes obvious, thus lessening the time of apprehension of employers and fellow employees.

HOW AND WHEN TO GET PREGNANT: WHEN TO HAVE MORE CHILDREN

1377. How soon after childbirth can I become pregnant again?

Some women are already pregnant again when they come in for their six-week checkup. For that reason, many doctors have women come in for a checkup three weeks after delivery as well as six weeks after, so they can start some form of contraception. If you breast-feed, you will usually not have menses or be able to get pregnant for at least three or four months after delivery. If you are slender and do not gain much weight, you may not have menses for as long as you breast-feed, even if that is two or three years. In that case, you may not be able to get pregnant until you stop breast-feeding. Most women who do not breast-feed ovulate and can get pregnant by six weeks after delivery.

1378. How long should I wait between children before getting pregnant again?

If you had a perfectly healthy pregnancy and an easy delivery, there is no real medical reason for you to wait at all. However, your baby might want some exclusive mothering for a year or two before it has to share you with another baby. If you have a baby every year, it is difficult to keep from becoming anemic, because each pregnancy is a drain on your supply of iron. Also, your abdominal muscles can certainly lose their tone if you have no time to exercise them back into shape between babies. There could be a financial drain if you are unable to work because you are constantly pregnant or nursing a baby. If they are all in college at once, your finances may be strained then, too. The advantage to having your children close together is that you can raise them all at once, and then you are done. When your deliveries are close together, the labor gets shorter and shorter. If you wait ten years, it is more like having a first baby again. Since breast-feeding is really best for most babies, it is natural to space children about three years apart. Then the older one can be in nursery school when the younger one is born. If you wait five years, the older one can be in kindergarten. There is more competition and sibling rivalry between children who are close in age, and more nurturing and care taking when they are spaced farther apart.

1379. Does having children close together affect their size or development?

If your nutrition is good and your finances are such that you can afford good medical care, there is no reason for the size of your babies to be affected. Physical development is not a problem of having children close together, but sometimes a child is emotionally and educationally deprived if its mother is caring for other children who are under the age of five. If you are free to spend time with each of your children and can get relief from housework, cooking, or other duties, this would not be so bad. A child

HOW AND WHEN TO GET PREGNANT: WHEN TO HAVE MORE CHILDREN (Continued)

raised alone is deprived of the companionship of other children. The financial drain from having many children may make it impossible to provide the education an only child would have.

1380. Do children who are born close together tend to suffer from vitamin deficiencies?

No. The mother's supply of iron decreases as a result of multiple pregnancies, but there is a mechanism in women's bodies that gives iron to their babies, even if they are anemic, so the babies do not become anemic, too. Vitamin needs change from day to day, and adequate diet will take care of that.

1381. If my first pregnancy was relatively easy, does that mean that my future pregnancies will be that way, too?

Yes, that is a good basis upon which to predict your future experiences. Generally, labor becomes easier and shorter with each subsequent baby. The only time this would not hold true would be if your general health changes, such as by getting hypertension, diabetes, or kidney disease. After five babies, however, certain dangers increase, such as placenta previa (placenta over the cervix), transverse lie (position of baby is crosswise), postpartum hemorrhage, and uterine rupture.

HOW AND WHEN TO GET PREGNANT: TAKING CARE OF YOURSELF BEFORE PREGNANCY

1382. What can I do before pregnancy that would help me have an easier pregnancy?

Solve any medical problems you have and get any dental care you need before you get pregnant. Get yourself within five pounds of your normal weight and in good physical condition through regular exercise. Stop smoking and drinking, preferably at least two or three months before you get pregnant. Take extra vitamin supplements, especially folic acid, to prepare your body. Stop using any medications that are not required. Stop taking birth control pills at least one cycle before you want to get pregnant, so that you will have one of your own menstrual periods. This way, it will be easier to calculate your delivery date. Get a medical checkup if you have not had one recently. Follow a diet that is nutritious and high in protein. Read all you can about pregnancy and childbirth.

1383. Is it true that the better my health is, the better my pregnancy will be?

Yes, that is generally true. However, there are some complications that are really accidents, on which good health would have no influence, so

HOW AND WHEN TO GET PREGNANT: TAKING CARE OF YOURSELF BEFORE PREGNANCY (Continued)

there are exceptions to this rule.

1384. How can what I do to my body before pregnancy affect it during pregnancy?

Many defects occur within the first two weeks of pregnancy, before you even know that you are pregnant. These defects can be caused by toxins and deficiencies that result from things you eat or don't eat, things you do, viral infections, radiation by X-rays, alcohol, drugs, and even having a fever of 103° or more. Taking care of yourself only after you find out you are pregnant is too late to prevent many defects.

1385. How important is good nutrition if I'm trying to get pregnant?

Your nutrition must at least be good enough to allow your body to ovulate, so you can get pregnant. It should be even better during the time when the new embryo is forming—before your first missed period, or before you know you are pregnant. The embryo is very sensitive to any drugs or alcohol you take at that time. If you are on a strict diet to lose weight, you will probably not ovulate anyway, but if you do and still diet, your embryo can be deprived. Taking vitamins, especially with folic acid, for two months before trying to get pregnant is recommended by many physicians to prevent birth defects.

1386. How long before pregnancy should I start improving my nutrition and conditioning my body?

Some studies suggest that what you do all your life will affect your pregnancy. Others suggest that improving your health for about two months before you try to get pregnant is helpful.

1387. If I watch my diet and take lots of vitamins and minerals, will I increase my chances of getting pregnant?

Yes. If your diet is nutritious and high in protein, you will increase your chances of getting pregnant.

1388. Should I start taking vitamin supplements before I try to get pregnant?

If you are going to take vitamin supplements at all, then this is the time to begin. Some studies have suggested that taking extra folic acid (or eating a lot of leafy green vegetables) could prevent neural tube defects. The embryo is most sensitive to any deficiencies that occur early in pregnancy. If your diet contains all of the needed vitamins, you do not need supplements.

1389. Should I be at a normal weight (not overweight or underweight) before I try to get pregnant?

That would be ideal, but sometimes the ideal is unattainable. If you

**HOW AND WHEN TO GET PREGNANT: TAKING CARE OF
YOURSELF BEFORE PREGNANCY** (Continued)

wait too long to try to get pregnant you will have the additional problem of
decreased fertility. Do the best you can.

**1390. Can being overweight or underweight affect my chances of getting
pregnant?**

Yes. Being extremely overweight or underweight is often associated
with not ovulating, and you need to release an egg to get pregnant. It does
not affect getting pregnant in any other way, unless it keeps you from being
sexually active as often as you need to.

1391. Is it dangerous to conceive if I am extremely overweight?

No, it is just unlikely. If you conceive and you are overweight, you are
not more likely to miscarry. You can have a perfectly normal pregnancy if
you continue to practice good nutrition and don't try to lose weight while
you are pregnant. In the past, overweight women who lost weight in
pregnancy fared badly. The poor outcome was blamed on their being
overweight, but it was really because they lost weight while they were pregnant. Overweight women should gain at least twenty-five pounds with
pregnancy, just like women of normal weight. Then their chances of getting
toxemia (a blood pressure disorder of late pregnancy) will not be increased.
Of course, it is a strain on your heart and back to carry the extra weight plus
the weight of pregnancy, but if you are young and strong, you can do it.

**1392. Are there any exercises I could do to tone up my body before preg-
nancy?**

All exercises would help. The ones that are most beneficial to help you
carry the baby nine months and then deliver it vaginally are those that tone
up the abdominal muscles. These include such things as sit-ups, leg raising,
swimming, and many forms of dancing.

1393. Do certain kinds of sports or activities make conception less likely?

Any long-term, strenuous activity that keeps all the fat off your body
and prevents menstruation altogether will certainly interfere with getting
pregnant. Running is the most frequent cause of this today, although it used
to be ballet dancing. However, if ovulation is still occuring, as can be shown
by a basal temperature chart, then the activity is not interfering at all, unless,
perhaps, it leaves no time or energy for sex.

1394. Could physical environment affect my chances of getting pregnant?

The only effect environment could have would be that it creates tensions that keep you from ovulating.

HOW AND WHEN TO GET PREGNANT: TAKING CARE OF YOURSELF BEFORE PREGNANCY (Continued)

1395. Should I look carefully into my family's past medical history before I consider having a child?

Yes, that would be a good idea. It is very frightening to find out bad news when you are already pregnant or have a child. You should look equally as well into the father's family. Then you should get good genetic counseling before you make any decision for or against having children. Your doctor or a hotline can refer you.

1396. What role does my husband's health play in conception?

If he is healthy enough to be able to have intercourse, ejaculate, and have a good, healthy sperm count, that is all that is required.

1397. Will my pregnancy be like my mother's?

We do inherit tendencies that affect pregnancies, so that mother's and daughter's pregnancies are more alike than those of unrelated persons, but it is not inevitable that they will be similar. If your mother had good pregnancies, have hope. If she had problem ones, try to analyze the problems and correct them, perhaps by being close to a normal weight and gaining at least twenty-five pounds with your pregnancy. Premature babies do keep occurring in families, but so does poor nutrition and smoking, and both contribute to prematurity.

1398. If my mother had a hard time getting pregnant, will I have a hard time, too?

If a pattern of poor ovulation or many chromosome defects were the reason that your mother had a hard time getting pregnant, the difficulty may be repeated. It depends upon whether or not you inherited those characteristics. You may be entirely different and take after your father instead.

1399. Should my husband and I have a medical examination before I try to get pregnant?

It is probably more important that you get a medical examination than it is for your husband to have one. All you need from him is healthy sperm, although he should also be free of any sexually transmitted diseases. A sperm analysis would provide as much help in this case as a medical examination would.

HOW AND WHEN TO GET PREGNANT: THINGS TO AVOID BEFORE PREGNANCY

1400. What foods, drugs, and other things should I stay away from when I am trying to get pregnant?

It is best that you not take drugs at all, but if you have a condition that

HOW AND WHEN TO GET PREGNANT: THINGS TO AVOID BEFORE PREGNANCY (Continued)

makes them necessary, consult with your doctor about their use in pregnancy. Thyroid medication and drugs for diabetes control and heart disease must continue. The medications needed for these conditions have been found to be safe to babies. Drugs to prevent convulsions, as with epilepsy, are sometimes a problem and may have to be changed before you get pregnant in order to have a healthy baby. One such drug, Dilantin, is a definite problem; phenobarbital is much safer for the baby, provided it will prevent convulsions with the same effectiveness as Dilantin. Aspirin, excessive caffeine, cigarettes, and alcohol should be avoided, because all of these have been implicated in birth defects. Any fever of 103° or more can produce nervous system defects in the fetus, even if it is produced by a sauna bath. If you have a fever, use cooling measures to reduce it. Avoid X-rays, especially of the abdomen. Shield the abdomen if you have dental X-rays. Stay away from children who have any childhood diseases, such as rubella (German measles), especially if you have not had them.

1401. Should I avoid X-rays if I'm trying to get pregnant?

You should avoid X-rays to your ovaries throughout your life. But if you are pregnant, you should not X-ray the small embryo. Unless the X-ray has to be of your pelvis, a lead apron over your pelvis will protect the ovaries and the new embryo if you are pregnant. If you must have an X-ray of the abdomen and pelvis, schedule it during or just after your menstrual period, when you are sure you are not pregnant. After ovulation at mid-cycle, you can't be sure of this.

1402. Are there any drugs (prescription, over-the-counter, or illegal) that might interfere with my chances of getting pregnant?

Any medication that contains estrogens or progesterones, including but not limited to birth control pills, can interfere with conception. Danazol, which is used in the treatment of endometriosis (small cysts), stops ovulation and prevents pregnancy. Some tranquilizers, such as Mellaril, interfere with ovulation and therefore with pregnancy. The agents used to kill cancer are usually violent enough to stop ovulation. Some of them can even produce abortions, if you are already pregnant when you start using them. Women between the ages of fifteen and forty-five should always discuss the effect of medication upon a possible pregnancy with their regular physician or obstetrician, unless they are abstinent or have been sterilized.

1403. What types of medication are safe if I'm planning to get pregnant?

The very safest thing for you to do is not to use drugs at all, so long as they are not necessary for your health. Some health conditions, such as

HOW AND WHEN TO GET PREGNANT: THINGS TO AVOID BEFORE PREGNANCY (Continued)

diabetes, hypothyroidism, and heart disease, are worse for the baby if you do not use medication. In other cases, such as epilepsy, some medications are much safer than others. Your regular doctor and your obstetrician can get together to discuss which medications are safe for you when you are pregnant, or are trying to get pregnant.

1404. Should I stop smoking before I get pregnant?

Yes! The answer to "Should I stop smoking?" will always be yes, no matter what the circumstances. Many women wait until the nausea associated with pregnancy makes it easier for them to quit smoking. If they have not stopped before that time, they certainly should then. Stopping at least two months before pregnancy assures that there will be no smoking in pregnancy. It also assures better nutrition for the first week or two of pregnancy when the fetal environment is so crucial.

1405. Does smoking affect my chances of getting pregnant?

Smoking can affect your chances of getting pregnant if it keeps your weight so low that you do not ovulate or menstruate. Some women have a severe loss of appetite, even nausea, with smoking.

1406. Can alcoholism decrease my ability to conceive?

Alcoholism can interfere with your ability to conceive only if it is so severe that you are malnourished and, therefore, are not ovulating. As long as you eat well, it seems to have no effect on fertility. However, if your partner drinks, it will affect his ability to have an erection.

1407. Does caffeine affect a woman's chances of getting pregnant?

No.

1408. I have been using drugs heavily for a while. How long should I be off of them before I attempt to get pregnant?

You should be off of them long enough to know that you are going to stay free of them for at least nine months and perhaps for twenty years, or long enough to raise a child. It may take as long as six months to regain your total health.

1409. Will smoking marijuana before pregnancy cause any problems?

No problems have been found in the research that has been done so far.

1410. Can early drug experiences endanger future pregnancies?

No. At first it was thought that using marijuana or LSD caused chromosome breakage in young people, but this turned out to be due to the laboratory methods that were used in the early research. Now it is known

HOW AND WHEN TO GET PREGNANT: THINGS TO AVOID BEFORE PREGNANCY (Continued)

that these drugs have no residual affect on the person who uses them.

1411. If my partner used drugs heavily in the past, what effect can this have on our children?

There is no known effect on the newborn baby, nor is there any future effect on the child. The only problem would be that of living with a partner who may return to heavy drug use.

1412. Is the quality of a man's sperm affected by improper diet, use of drugs, or excessive drinking?

No. Heat is more likely to affect the quality of a man's sperm. Wearing clothing that keeps the testicles close to the body warms them unduly. They function best at lower temperatures. This is why boxer shorts are better than jockey shorts for men who wish to father a child. Hot baths are supposed to reduce men's fertility, but they haven't done this very well in Japan. Extreme obesity, in which fat is all around the testicles, also reduces the sperm count. Some researchers believe that going nude would be the best way to prepare a man's sperm for reproduction.

HOW AND WHEN TO GET PREGNANT: PREGNANCY FOR A SINGLE MOTHER

1413. How many babies are born today to single mothers?

Since birth certificates do not specify whether or not the mother is married, records are not really kept on this subject. With the availability of contraception and abortion, the number of single mothers is less than it used to be, but 95 percent of single women today who become pregnant and have their babies keep them rather than have them adopted. This is because if a woman really does not want a baby, she usually has an abortion. Therefore, very few babies are available for adoption. Most single parents are teenagers, and 20 percent of babies born today are born to teenagers. Teenagers also have about 30 percent of the abortions.

1414. Is it normal for a single woman to want to have a baby?

It is quite normal. Some women decide to get married simply because they want to have babies and raise children.

1415. What are the disadvantages of being single and having a baby?

The primary disadvantage is the lack of emotional and financial support from the father during pregnancy, delivery, and early child care. Condemnation from family and friends may also be difficult to handle. If you have a child and then become widowed or divorced you may have more ap-

HOW AND WHEN TO GET PREGNANT: PREGNANCY FOR A SINGLE MOTHER (Continued)

proval from society than a single woman having a child, but you may still be at a financial disadvantage or be just as unprepared as a single parent.

1416. What are my legal rights as a single mother?

You have the right to obtain medical care without parental knowledge or consent if you are a teenager. Welfare programs will assist you financially with your medical care. Aid to mothers with dependent children is a category of welfare in all states that will help you financially as long as your child is young. All that does not make life exactly easy, but possible. You also have a responsibility to care for your child and not neglect it. If you are declared an unfit mother, your child can be legally taken away from you and cared for in a foster home. However, it cannot be adopted without your consent. Recent changes in adoption laws require the consent of the father as well.

1417. If I am single and get pregnant, do I have to tell the father?

No, and many women do not. The birth certificate has a place for the name of the baby's father, but some women just make one up. Even if you identify the real father, he may never know it, as he is not notified. If you put the baby up for adoption, then there must be an attempt made to obtain his consent. If you seek financial aid, you are required to give his name so that the welfare agency can seek financial support from him, which he is liable to provide. Some people feel that you should tell the father, especially if he does not deny parenthood, so that the child can have the possibility of financial support.

HOW AND WHEN TO GET PREGNANT: PREGNANCY AFTER THE AGE OF THIRTY-FIVE

1418. Will I have a harder time with childbirth if I have my first child after the age of thirty-five than I would if I had my first child at a younger age?

If you are in good health, with no blood pressure problems, diabetes, or kidney disease, then you probably will not have a hard time with pregnancy. However, many women who are over the age of thirty-five are not in good health. The first baby is always the hardest to have, even if you are young, so you will have a more difficult labor than someone of the same age who is having her fourth child.

1419. Is it unusual for a woman over thirty-five years of age to have children?

In 1980, 4.2 percent of the babies born were to women over thirty-five years of age; in the early 1960s, 7.5 percent of the babies born were to women over thirty-five. In the distant past it was not unusual for a woman to

At thirty-nine
I realized that
my career is just
what I always
dreamed that it might be
my love for my husband
is stronger and more exciting
than ever
my children are
more beautiful and fun
than I ever hoped they could be
At thirty-nine
I felt it was exactly
the ideal time
to have
another
child

— Susan Polis Schutz

HOW AND WHEN TO GET PREGNANT: PREGNANCY AFTER THE AGE OF THIRTY-FIVE (Continued)

have babies when she was over thirty-five, because contraception was not available to her and she was still fertile. When contraception became available, women chose to stop having babies when they had had enough. Usually they had had enough by the age of twenty-six. Now that contraception and even abortion are available to all women, including young teenagers, many women delay having a family at all until their other pursuits have been accomplished. They are frequently over thirty-five when this occurs. The figures also show that the average age that women are having their first baby is rising, because women under twenty are having fewer babies. However, it is still relatively new for women to have their first baby after thirty-five.

1420. If I am healthy and in good physical shape, can I safely wait until my late thirties or early forties to have a child?

This could never be called safe. At that age, there is always the chance that you are not fertile at all, but most women are still fertile, so you may be, too. On the other hand, you could be quite healthy and still get gonorrhea that destroys your tubes and makes normal pregnancy impossible. Your partner could also have something happen to lessen his sperm count. So if having a baby is a primary goal in your life, do it while you are young. If it is a secondary goal, you can take a chance on doing it later. You also never know if you are fertile until you become pregnant. It could be that you are not fertile while you are young, but you just won't know until you try to get pregnant.

1421. I am over thirty-five years old. Is there anything I can do to increase my chances of having a healthy child?

You can choose a man with a good genetic background, and you can do all the same things that young women do to have healthy babies. In addition, you can have a test called amniocentesis, in which amniotic fluid is taken from around the baby in order to obtain cells to study for chromosome abnormalities. You may also have other tests, such as an ultrasound. If a defect is found, you will be offered the option of having an abortion to avoid delivering a severely mentally retarded child. However, you may also choose to go ahead with your pregnancy. By eliminating defective babies, you increase your chances of actually delivering a healthy baby later, but your chances never reach 100 percent, because there are defects that cannot be detected before the baby is born.

1422. Dr. Carson, why did you wait until your late thirties to have children? Do you recommend this?

I began medical school late, due to finances, and could not afford to

HOW AND WHEN TO GET PREGNANT: PREGNANCY AFTER THE AGE OF THIRTY-FIVE (Continued)

complete my specialty training and finance child care, too. In addition, I had been responsible for much of the care of a younger brother and sister, and I did not want to do that again so soon. I was thirty-five before that feeling wore off. This can be a problem among some girls who have too much responsibility for child care placed upon them when they are quite young. I recommend that women have babies when they want them, whether they are fifteen or forty-five. Many professional women find it preferable to make their way in the world before starting a family, but if your whole life is designed around having children, you had better start when you are young and fertile, because later on that option may not be available to you. If you delay childbearing until you are thirty-five, you should prepare yourself for the possibility that it may not happen.

1423. Is there anything that I should do if I am over thirty-five before trying to get pregnant?

It is very important for you to be sure that you do not have high blood pressure, kidney disease, or diabetes, since the older you get, the more likely these become. Younger women seldom have these disorders. A prepregnancy visit to a physician to see if you have any major problems is a good idea. Otherwise, you should follow the same advice given to younger women. Normalize your weight, stop smoking and drinking, and eat a good, nutritious diet. Also, try to arrange to avoid all medications during this time, or else check to see which ones are necessary.

HOW AND WHEN TO GET PREGNANT: MENOPAUSAL PREGNANCY

1424. How common are menopausal pregnancies?

They are really not very common. Menopause in the United States occurs between the ages of fifty and fifty-four. Few babies are born to women of that age. A few more pregnancies occur than the number of babies born, but these end in miscarriages. Most so-called menopausal babies were born to much younger women who were skipping periods and just thought they were menopausal, without any medical or scientific testing or proof.

HOW AND WHEN TO GET PREGNANT: GENETIC COUNSELING

1425. What is genetic counseling?

Genetic counseling consists of analyzing your genetic history: the characteristics of defects known to occur in your family, in which relatives

HOW AND WHEN TO GET PREGNANT: GENETIC COUNSELING
(Continued)

they occur, and with what frequency. A genetics counselor is educated so that he or she knows what to ask and how to determine your chances of having a defective or normal child. None of us has a 100 percent chance of having a normal child. You will be given a percentage chance that is based on your family history. Counseling also includes the tests that can be done on you or your husband to determine whether you carry a certain gene, and also on the unborn baby to see if it has received that gene. Many things can be tested for, but many more cannot. At least with genetic counseling, you know what kind of a chance you are taking.

1426. When should a couple seek genetic counseling?

If there is a defective child in your family, especially if the child is mentally retarded, you should find out all you can from your relatives about your family history. Then you should seek counseling long before you get pregnant, in order to find out what your chances are of having a defective child. The counselor may find the defect is not inherited at all, and this will relieve your fears. If you are a woman thirty-five years old and are having a baby, this is another time to seek counseling, so that you might have an amniocentesis to look for a Down's syndrome, which occurs more frequently after thirty-five. You also can discuss other family defects during counseling when you are pregnant, but unless there is testing beforehand, it is a little late to decide not to have children.

HOW AND WHEN TO GET PREGNANT: POSSIBILITY OF BIRTH DEFECTS

1427. If there is a history of birth defects in my family, will my child be born with birth defects, too?

That is a question that only geneticists are trained to answer. Some defects are purely accidental and are not likely to recur at all. Some very bad defects can be prenatally detected in your unborn baby. With others, you just take your chances, but genetic counseling can tell you what chances you are taking. Some defects that are likely to occur are not bad enough to refrain from having a baby. Nearsightedness is a good example. It is dominant in familes, but it does not mean that life is not worthwhile. However, if both parents are nearsighted, they might as well plan on eyeglasses of some kind for their child.

1428. What are the chances of having a child born with birth defects?

Generally, there is a 2 or 3 percent risk of having a child born with serious defects. If both partners know their family history of inherited con-

HOW AND WHEN TO GET PREGNANT: POSSIBILITY OF BIRTH DEFECTS (Continued)

genital defects, a genetics counselor can calculate your chances of these repeating. This may be much higher than the general 2 or 3 percent.

1429. Does the likelihood of birth defects increase as a woman gets older? If so, why?

Yes, it does increase, but the birth defects that increase with age are limited to the chromosomal defects, not to other kinds of defects. The most frequent defect is a Down's syndrome baby, who has forty-seven chromosomes instead of the normal forty-six. With this syndrome, there is an extra twenty-first chromosome, called trisomy-21. There are also some other types of chromosomally defective babies, but they are still more frequent among older women than they are among younger women. Various estimates have been made of this incidence. One is that at the age of thirty, the incidence of Down's syndrome is 1 in 1,500, but at thirty-five it is 1 in 500. By forty, it is 1 in 100, and at forty-five, 1 in 50. Some tables show twice this many defects in the same kind of progression. The reason given is that all eggs are present when the baby girl is born, and the longer she lives in this world, the more radiation she gets. Background radiation is unavoidable, but routine chest X-rays and pelvimetry X-rays are now avoided in order to decrease the amount of lifetime radiation. This also is the reason that a lead apron is put over your ovaries when you have dental or other X-rays of the upper part of your body. Another theory is that defective eggs are difficult to ovulate, but when you run out of good ones, the bad ones then come to the surface and respond to the stimulation of the pituitary hormones. This seems to increase with age and with defective ovulation.

HOW AND WHEN TO GET PREGNANT: POTENTIAL PROBLEMS

1430. Is it possible for my doctor to tell me, before I get pregnant, if I will have any problems during pregnancy?

Certain health conditions, habits, and physical findings, such as high blood pressure, kidney disease, diabetes, or very small bone structure, can help your doctor to predict trouble, but the doctor can never guarantee that you will not have trouble. It happens to perfectly normal women.

1431. Does a tipped uterus cause problems in women who want to get pregnant?

No. One-third of women have a tipped uterus, and their fertility is not affected at all.

1432. Can I have children if I am epileptic?

Yes, of course. If you are taking Dilantin and certain other anti-

HOW AND WHEN TO GET PREGNANT: POTENTIAL PROBLEMS
(Continued)

epileptic drugs while you are pregnant, you will have a higher incidence of birth defects; however, if you take phenobarbital, you will not. Of course, you may pass your epilepsy on to your children, if you have the kind that is inherited. Sometimes it would be unwise to do this. You need counseling with a neurologist and a geneticist.

HOW AND WHEN TO GET PREGNANT: FEARS OF PREGNANCY

1433. Is it normal for a woman to fear pregnancy and childbirth?

Yes, it is. All women have heard of things that went wrong during someone's pregnancy, so they know this is possible. It is abnormal to have no fear at all and to feel perfectly safe about having a baby. You should have just enough fear, at least for your baby's sake, to deliver in a hospital where there is medical help.

1434. How can I alleviate my fears of pregnancy and childbirth?

Most fears can be calmed with knowledge. Reading books is one way to gain knowledge, but many people do not learn well from reading. A more effective way is to take a class in natural childbirth, even if you are not pregnant, so you can become familiar with the routines of pregnancy. Talking to friends who have been through it can also calm your fears. Sometimes the fears get worse, however, depending upon the attitudes and experiences of your friends.

HOW AND WHEN TO GET PREGNANT: DANGERS OF PREGNANCY; WHEN NOT TO GET PREGNANT

1435. What are some of the dangers of pregnancy?

One danger of pregnancy is the possibility of suffering an injury or disability that will keep you from your usual work. Discomforts of pregnancy are real, but they are not normally disabling, except from certain jobs, like ballet dancing. Some complications, like bleeding, threatened premature labor, or toxemia (a blood pressure disorder of late pregnancy), can make it necessary to be away from work and at relative rest until the baby is mature enough to be born. This may take weeks or months, and can interfere with the progress you make in your job or career. It is hard to plan for this. About 20 percent of deliveries result in cesarean sections, which means some disability after delivery, but this usually does not last longer than six weeks. Death is a very rare possibility. Only five hundred women die per year in the United States from pregnancy. Of those, nearly one hundred die from an ectopic pregnancy, a pregnancy in the tube that ruptures and bleeds inside

HOW AND WHEN TO GET PREGNANT: DANGERS OF PREGNANCY; WHEN NOT TO GET PREGNANT (Continued)

the abdomen when the woman is about six weeks pregnant. Books on pregnancy seldom list all of the dangers; however, you could find them all in a textbook on obstetrics.

1436. What are the dangers of pregnancy if I am not mentally prepared for it?

It is mentally and emotionally disturbing to be forced into an activity that you do not want and did not plan for. That is one reason why abortion is available. It may not reduce the number of births, but it allows women to stop a pregnancy that they do not want so they can get pregnant later when they feel more prepared. The dangers of an unprepared pregnancy are increased only because you are unlikely to take really good care of yourself while you are pregnant. Therefore, you could have more complications and worse results than someone who is ready for and wants pregnancy.

1437. Should I consider the dangers of childbirth before deciding to get pregnant?

Yes, of course, but the dangers should not be exaggerated or belittled. It is more dangerous to drive a car than it is to be pregnant. In fact, one of the greatest causes of maternal death is car accidents. If your desire for a child does not overcome your informed fear of the dangers of pregnancy, then you are not ready for a baby. To consider the dangers, you must seek advice, counsel, hospital care, and medical help. You should also learn all you can about pregnancy and childbirth. It is a good motive for obtaining knowledge.

1438. What percentage of women today die as a result of childbirth?

Only sixteen women per 100,000 live births actually die from childbirth. This amounts to about five hundred women per year in the United States. In underdeveloped countries, this figure is much higher. In 1900, it was about five hundred deaths per 100,000 births in the United States. Women in underdeveloped countries and those from long ago had a lot more to fear from pregnancy. If we were to abandon all medical progress and knowledge about how to make pregnancy safe, we would return to those kinds of percentages.

1439. When would you advise a woman not to get pregnant?

If you do not want a child, you should not get pregnant. Many women do not want a child, but they leave the decision up to fate. Even if you want a child, it is not advisable to get pregnant if that pregnancy is likely to damage your health so much that you will not live to enjoy your child. Such conditions exist with severe health problems, such as terminal cancer, extremely

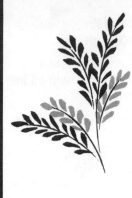

Many women
I have talked to lately
tell me that they are
extremely unfulfilled being housewives
that their work all day
is so unimportant
that they are not using
their minds —
These women must
do something that
interests them
but they must also
be reassured that
being a good mother is a
very important job
and that just because society
seems to say that raising children
  is a menial task
there is no reason to believe this
In fact many beliefs that society
imposes on the individual
are wrong
Women must realize
that whatever they do
is important
as long as they do it well

— Susan Polis Schutz

HOW AND WHEN TO GET PREGNANT: DANGERS OF PREGNANCY; WHEN NOT TO GET PREGNANT (Continued)

severe diabetes, severe kidney disease, severe hypertension, or congestive heart failure. Some pulmonary diseases are in this category, too. Other conditions are temporary, and it is best just to delay pregnancy until the necessary treatment for the disease is over, especially if that treatment would be harmful for the child, such as is chemotherapy. There are so many factors involved and each patient is a different case. The decision not to have a child must be made in a special way for each person separately. As medical care improves, women with special problems will be more able to have children.

HOW AND WHEN TO GET PREGNANT: WHEN TO STOP BIRTH CONTROL

1440. If I want my child to be born at a certain time, how far in advance should I start trying to get pregnant?

If you want your child to be born before a certain date, you should start trying to get pregnant thirteen months before that date. This will give you at least four months to get pregnant. You have only a 20 percent chance of having a child born in a particular month, no matter how hard you try nine months before.

1441. How soon before the time that I want to become pregnant should I stop using birth control?

You should stop using contraceptive pills one month before you start trying to get pregnant. With all other methods of birth control, you can stop the day you want to try to get pregnant.

1442. What is the probability of conception without using birth control each month?

If you are trying to get pregnant (intercourse every other day, lying down thirty minutes afterwards, and using no birth control), the probability of pregnancy is about 20 percent. In four months this adds up to 80 percent. If you have not gotten pregnant by then, it may take up to a year, and 10 percent of women never get pregnant.

1443. How long do I have to be off the pill before trying to get pregnant?

It is recommended that you stay off the pill for at least one menstrual cycle before trying to get pregnant, so that your expected due date can be calculated from your own natural menstrual period, rather than a pill period. Dates from a pill period are very inaccurate, and sometimes it is important to know a correct due date. However, even if you get pregnant while you are on the pill, it does not cause birth defects in the baby.

HOW AND WHEN TO GET PREGNANT: WHEN TO STOP BIRTH CONTROL (Continued)

1444. How long will it take for me to get pregnant after I stop taking the pill?

It takes four months, or four menstrual cycles, to get 80 percent of women pregnant when they stop using the pill or any other contraceptive, including abstinence.

1445. Will I have a harder time getting pregnant if I've been on birth control pills for a long time?

Not unless you've grown old in the meantime. If you take the pills until you are forty, you will certainly be less fertile, but this is not because you took the pills. Many women are shocked because they get pregnant one week after they stop taking the pills, even though they have been on them for ten years. Women usually underestimate their fertility.

1446. How long will it take for me to get pregnant after I have my IUD removed?

The same as any other contraceptive method: four months after it is removed, 80 percent of women will be pregnant.

HOW AND WHEN TO GET PREGNANT: EFFECTS OF USING AN IUD OR CONTRACEPTIVE FOAM

1447. What is the danger of finding out I am pregnant when I still have an IUD in place?

There are three dangers: removing the IUD can cause a miscarriage; leaving it in place can cause a miscarriage; and leaving it in throughout the pregnancy can cause a fatal infection of the uterus in both the mother and fetus.

1448. Does using an IUD affect my chances of getting pregnant later?

No, unless you get a pelvic infection or pelvic inflammatory disease. This is made worse by having the IUD in place and can lead to tube damage and blocked tubes. Then you cannot get pregnant at all. For this reason, IUDs are discouraged, except for women who are no longer interested in having another baby.

1449. Will foam contraceptives cause any abnormalities in the fetus if I become pregnant while using them?

No. There is a 2 to 3 percent chance of having a baby born with major defects in the general population. Using foam does not guarantee you will not have an abnormality, nor does it increase the chances of this happening.

HOW AND WHEN TO GET PREGNANT: EFFECTS OF A PREVIOUS MISCARRIAGE

1450. Does having a miscarriage decrease my chances of getting pregnant again?

No, not unless you had a complication of the surgery that completed your miscarriage, such as an injury from the D & C (dilatation and curettage) or an infection afterward. Normally a miscarriage does not decrease fertility.

1451. How long should I wait after a miscarriage before trying to get pregnant again?

It is recommended that you wait until you have stopped bleeding before you have intercourse, in order to avoid a possible infection through your dilated cervix. After that, you are free to try to get pregnant again. You probably cannot get pregnant for about six weeks, because it often takes that long to ovulate again, but there is no harm in getting pregnant sooner if you can.

HOW AND WHEN TO GET PREGNANT: EFFECTS OF AN IRREGULAR MENSTRUAL PERIOD

1452. If my period is irregular, does that mean I'll have a hard time getting pregnant?

If the irregularity consists of a longer time between cycles, it may take you a little longer to get pregnant. If your period is irregular because you do not ovulate, you will really have a hard time. You can find out if you are ovulating by keeping a basal temperature chart.

HOW AND WHEN TO GET PREGNANT: WHEN GENITAL HERPES IS PRESENT

1453. Should I get pregnant if I have genital herpes?

Of course, otherwise the population would dwindle rapidly. It is better to have genital herpes before you ever get pregnant, so that you will not get a primary or first attack during pregnancy. A primary case during pregnancy can spread to the baby before it is born, and a cesarean section will not save it. The only other problem with having herpes while you are pregnant is that if you have an open sore or active infection in your vagina when you start labor, you will have to have a cesarean section, so the baby will not be delivered through the infection. If you have an open cold sore on your lips, you should not kiss your baby, as it can be severely infected that way, too.

HOW AND WHEN TO GET PREGNANT: WHEN AND HOW AM I MOST LIKELY TO GET PREGNANT?

1454. At what point in my cycle am I most likely to get pregnant?

Pregnancy occurs when a sperm penetrates the egg you have released, which occurs about fourteen days before your usual menstrual period. If you have a twenty-eight-day cycle, this is about the middle of your cycle, or fourteenth day. If your cycle is thirty days, it is the sixteenth day. However, intercourse must occur in the day or two (sometimes more) prior to ovulation to give the sperm time to swim up through the uterus into the tube and wait there for the egg to come by. Usually, you are most likely to get pregnant in the ten days right after your period ends.

1455. How do I determine when my most fertile days are?

If you have intercourse every day you don't need to determine when your fertile days occur. If you are trying to get pregnant by having sex only once a month, you need some luck. How to determine this is covered in detail in the chapter on contraception. In general, you can use the sympto-thermal method to figure out the day you ovulate and consider that the two days before that are the most fertile. Symptothermal means noticing the symptoms in your body that indicate ovulation, such as a clear discharge, mucus that strings or turns test tape blue, or sensations of ovulation. More accurately, you can use a basal temperature chart that shows the curve of your ovulatory menstrual cycle. This is all so complicated that it is easier just to have sex all the time.

1456. It is true that I am fertile for only forty-eight hours each month?

The time when intercourse is most likely to get you pregnant is forty-eight hours before ovulation. However, some sperm live much longer than that. Therefore, intercourse can occur as much as six days before ovulation and still get you pregnant. The egg is probably only fertile for a few hours, but the sperm live in the tubes for two to six days.

1457. Are there certain times in a man's life when he is more likely to get a woman pregnant?

A man's sperm are just as good when he is sixty as they are when he is sixteen. Whether he is able to get a woman pregnant depends on his sexual activity, erections and ejaculations, and even his sexual preferences.

1458. How many times a week should I have sex if I want to get pregnant?

Since most men's sperm live in your tubes for forty-eight hours, you should have sex at least every other day, or three to four times a week if you want to get pregnant.

HOW AND WHEN TO GET PREGNANT: WHEN AND HOW AM I MOST LIKELY TO GET PREGNANT? (Continued)

1459. Can I have sex too often for the sperm to be fertile?

Yes, you can. Sperm are manufactured in the testicles at a constant rate, and they are collected in the seminal vesicles, little sacs at the base of the penis. These are emptied with ejaculation. If a man doesn't ejaculate for three days, a lot of sperm are stored so the count looks abnormally high, but some of them are rather old and not so fertile or active. If a man ejaculates three or four times a day, the actual count goes down and becomes too thin to be efficient. Ejaculation once a day does not present any problems.

1460. What is the best position to use during intercourse in order to get pregnant?

If you lie down shortly after ejaculation, it doesn't really matter which position you are in when you receive the sperm. The vagina is a closed place, as soon as the penis is withdrawn. If you stand in a vertical position, or especially if you get into a squatting position, the semen will leak out of your vagina. If you feel messy, just use a tissue or a towel, but do not jump up and go to the bathroom to wash.

1461. How can I be sure to keep the sperm inside of me?

If you are really trying to get pregnant, it is better not to get up for at least a half-hour after intercourse and not to douche at all.

1462. How can I increase my chances of getting pregnant?

You probably cannot increase your chances of getting pregnant above 20 percent per month, but having coitus at least every forty-eight hours, lying still for a half-hour afterwards, and using no lubricants or douches certainly helps. This is especially helpful from the end of menstruation until you are past your fertile time. Good general health, normal weight, and relaxation also increase your chances of ovulating.

HOW AND WHEN TO GET PREGNANT: GETTING PREGNANT WITHOUT INTERCOURSE

1463. Can I get pregnant if I just engage in heavy petting, but not intercourse?

Yes. If a man ejaculates between your thighs in front of your vagina, with no clothing interposed, it is possible for you to become pregnant. This is called intercrural coitus. Many couples think that if they do not penetrate the vagina with the penis, the woman will not get pregnant. They are wrong. It is possible for a girl who has never had intercourse to become a pregnant virgin with an intact hymen.

HOW AND WHEN TO GET PREGNANT: HOW LONG WILL IT TAKE?

1464. What is the average time span that it takes most couples to get pregnant? Is it the same for all ages?

A very fertile couple, usually between twenty-five and thirty-five years of age, will generally achieve a pregnancy within three to four months. The average couple in the United States is very fertile. Younger women, especially teenagers, usually take a little longer, up to eight months, because as many as 50 percent of their cycles release no egg at all. This is fortunate, or there would be more teenage pregnancies. Women over thirty-five also ovulate less often, but this becomes more prominent after forty when ovulation is much less secure. At these ages it may take twice as long, or eight months, to achieve pregnancy. Another factor is the frequency of sex. If it is rare, then the chances of it occurring at the right time for pregnancy are less. Teenagers have rather rare sex, averaging about seven times a year. Newly married couples have more frequent sex than couples who have been married for a while, regardless of their age.

HOW AND WHEN TO GET PREGNANT: PLANNING FOR THE SEX OF THE BABY

1465. How can I increase my chances of having a male child? A female child?

Most of what you hear on this subject is purely folklore. Some factors are real, however, based on the knowledge that the sperm containing the female X chromosome are hardier and live a bit longer, especially under adverse circumstances, than the sperm containing the male Y chromosome. Therefore, if coitus occurs several days before ovulation, and not again until after ovulation, more female X sperm will be surviving, and you have a greater than 50 percent chance of having a girl. If you have intercourse frequently, such as every day, you supply more Y sperm to increase the chances of a boy, but of course, there are X sperm there, too. Sperm that swim around in vinegar or soda don't get anybody pregnant, so douching is useless. If you really care about the sex of your child, there are techniques for controlling this. Some obstetricians take the male ejaculate, filter out the male sperm, and inject it by artificial insemination into the female vagina. Their success rate is 80 percent male.

HOW AND WHEN TO GET PREGNANT: SIGNS OF PREGNANCY

1466. What are some of the signs that I could look for that would tell me I'm pregnant?

The classic sign, and still the most reliable one, is missing a menstrual

HOW AND WHEN TO GET PREGNANT: SIGNS OF PREGNANCY
(Continued)

period. If you are usually regular and find that your period is a week late, it is a good idea to have a pregnancy test. If your period comes, but it is short and unusually light, you may still be suspicious. Urinary frequency is the most common symptom of pregnancy, but it can, of course, have other causes. Breast tenderness that continues longer than it usually does before menstruation is a significant sign. Fatigue without a clear cause is another general sign. Nausea and vomiting, without any diarrhea, is another classic sign of pregnancy, but only occurs in about one-third of women. Sometimes a lack of appetite or an increased appetite is significant. If you can see your cervix, you might be able to tell that it has turned blue. It also will feel softer. Your nipples become darker, and the little bumps toward the outside, called glands of Montgomery, become more prominent. Your stomach may be bloated with gas. You may have cramps that make you feel like you are going to have a period, but you don't have the period. However, none of these are proof of pregnancy.

HOW AND WHEN TO GET PREGNANT: WHEN TO GET A PREGNANCY TEST AND SEE A DOCTOR

1467. If I think that I might be pregnant, how long should I wait before having a pregnancy test?

Under normal circumstances, you should wait one week after you have missed a menstrual period. At that time, you could have a urine test, which is about 95 percent accurate in diagnosing pregnancy.

1468. What is the earliest that pregnancy can be detected?

A blood test, called an RIA (ratio-immune assay), can detect pregnancy as soon as six days after you ovulate and become pregnant, which is over a week before you even miss a period.

1469. Do I have to wait until I've missed a period before I go in for a pregnancy test?

Normally, if you are not having any problems, you should wait until you have missed your period by at least a week, so that the urine test will be accurate. If there is an emergency situation, such as needing X-rays after an auto accident, and you might be pregnant, the more sensitive RIA blood test can be done even before you have missed your period, but it is much more expensive.

1470. Where can I go for a pregnancy test?

You can buy one at a drugstore and perform it on your urine yourself,

HOW AND WHEN TO GET PREGNANT: WHEN TO GET A PREGNANCY TEST AND SEE A DOCTOR (Continued)

following the directions carefully, or you can ask your doctor to run one at his or her office or laboratory. Many clinics, especially family-planning clinics, can also run a pregnancy test for you.

1471. How soon should I go to the doctor if I think I'm pregnant?

A test to find out if you are pregnant can be done without scheduling an appointment with your doctor. This is usually accurate if you are a week overdue for your period. If you have odd symptoms, the doctor may want to do a blood test, even if the urine test is negative. The blood test is more sensitive, but it is also more expensive. A physical examination is usually a good idea by the time you have missed two periods, to be sure all is well and to diagnose twins or any other abnormalities that can be detected. If you have severe symptoms, such as uncontrolled vomiting, you will need help sooner.

1472. What is the most accurate test for finding out if I'm pregnant?

The RIA (ratio-immune assay) blood test is the most accurate test for pregnancy because it is the most sensitive. However, if the less accurate, less expensive urine test is positive, then you do not need any other test. The one-minute urine tests are not as accurate as the two-hour tube tests for urine. The test that is available in the drugstore for you to use at home is the two-hour tube test. Many clinics run the one-minute test on a drop of urine as a screening test, to be confirmed by some other method later.

1473. How accurate are blood tests in determining pregnancy?

At six days after ovulation, the RIA beta-subunit tests are 99 percent correct in diagnosing pregnancy; at fifteen days after ovulation, they are 99.9 percent correct. The errors usually come from HCG (human chorionic gonadotropin) shots that women sometimes take to lose weight. This can be detected in the blood, and pregnancy is incorrectly diagnosed.

1474. How is pregnancy determined from a urine sample?

When you are pregnant, your urine contains HCG (human chorionic gonadotropin), a hormone produced by the placenta. If particles form in a ring at the bottom of the test tube when the urine is combined with another solution in a urine test, then there is HCG present in the urine. This test takes two hours, although a similar one-minute test also can be done on a slide. In this case, the separation occurs quickly and only if you are not pregnant. These one-minute tests are, however, less accurate. The pregnancy tests you buy at your drugstore are very simple to perform.

1475. How was the rabbit used in determining pregnancy?

The woman's urine was injected into the rabbit. If she was pregnant, the urine's affect on the rabbit's ovaries was to make them swell. The rabbit

HOW AND WHEN TO GET PREGNANT: WHEN TO GET A PREGNANCY TEST AND SEE A DOCTOR (Continued)

was sacrificed (cut open after it was killed) and the ovaries examined. If they had reacted, she was pregnant. Sometimes, however, rabbits seemed to do whatever they wanted to, so the test was not always reliable.

1476. How reliable is taking basal body temperature in determining pregnancy?

If there is no illness or change in your habits of rising and retiring to change your body temperature, then this method is fairly reliable. A rise in temperature above the base line that stays up longer than sixteen days is considered to indicate pregnancy, until proven otherwise. This method is at least 95 percent accurate, but sometimes the temperature falls and yet you are really pregnant. This is especially common with an ectopic pregnancy (a pregnancy in the tube). It is best to confirm the results with a pregnancy test.

1477. How accurate are the pregnancy tests that I can do at home?

If you follow the directions, they are as accurate as the urine tests you have done in your doctor's office or laboratory. If the result is not clear, as when the ring is fuzzy and not clear cut, you should repeat the test.

1478. What are the tests for pregnancy that I can do at home?

Home pregnancy tests have many names, such as E.P.T., Fact, Daisy, and Answer. They are all similar. Some of your urine is combined with a test solution in a tube. If this forms a dark ring, you have a positive test for pregnancy. If it does not, the test is negative. If an irregular, fuzzy ring forms, pregnancy is doubtful, but the test should be repeated. Any urine will work, but morning urine is more concentrated. The cost of these tests in the drugstore is about the same as it would be at your doctor's lab.

HOW AND WHEN TO GET PREGNANT: WHO CAN GET PREGNANT?

1479. Why do some women get pregnant more easily than others?

Some women are fertile because they have excellent chromosomes with no abnormalities, a receptive, well-nourished cervix with clear estrogen mucus, open tubes, and perfect ovulation every cycle. They are also willing to have intercourse often. Other women seem very fertile, but this is really because their partners' sperm have a long life and lots of energy. They live in the tubes for a long time before the egg comes by. In other words, some men are more fertile than others. So far, fertility in men has not been correlated with their general health, but all the factors that make men's sperm better are not yet known.

HOW AND WHEN TO GET PREGNANT: WHO CAN GET PREGNANT? (Continued)

1480. What percentage of women who try to get pregnant will never get pregnant?

That is hard to estimate, because not all infertile couples are trying to get pregnant. Eighty percent of women will get pregnant in four to eight months, another 10 percent in about a year or so, and 5 percent more will become pregnant after they seek medical help for their problems of infertility. About 5 percent will never get pregnant. This figure could change if they all attempted test tube babies.

HOW AND WHEN TO GET PREGNANT: CAUSES OF INFERTILITY

1481. What are some of the reasons that so many couples have trouble conceiving?

Almost 40 percent of the time, it is because the man has a low sperm count. He has no way of knowing this without a semen analysis to count his sperm. When the woman is the cause of the problem, 40 percent of the time it is because she has blocked tubes, usually caused by a previous infection, such as gonorrhea or chlamydial infection. The next most frequent cause of infertility in women is not ovulating, or at least not ovulating very often. This problem usually can be corrected by study and fertility drugs. Fibroids also interfere with the implantation of the fertilized egg if they are numerous and large.

1482. What other causes are there for infertility?

After thirty-five, your ovulation will be less frequent, and you will become relatively infertile, usually completely infertile by the age of forty-six. Fibroids frequently occur in women who are in their thirties and can interfere with implantation of the fertilized egg if they are numerous and large. This may or may not be aggravated by birth control pills, although present day opinion is that the pills do not cause or make fibroids grow. In time, women may acquire other diseases, such as high blood pressure, diabetes, or severe kidney disease, that make it hard to complete a full-term pregnancy and have a healthy baby. They also may be quite fertile, but their male partners become infertile through disease, tumors, or surgery. If you consider having babies as a very important goal in your lifetime, then you probably should have them while you are young and fertile. Endometriosis (small cycts) acts in two ways to interfere with getting pregnant: by adhesions that prevent the egg from reaching the tube, and by endometriomas on the ovary that distort it. Hormones and surgery can help this, too. Sexual dysfunction may be the basic problem if there is no intercourse. After these causes are

HOW AND WHEN TO GET PREGNANT: CAUSES OF INFERTILITY
(Continued)

ruled out, the rest of the reasons for infertility become more complicated, such as antibodies produced by the woman against the man's sperm, cervical mucus that is hostile to sperm, or an inadequate corpus luteum phase in which she ovulates, but not well enough. Running and being underweight can also interfere with ovulation. Sometimes it is a simple problem of vaginitis or cervicitis that interferes with the sperm entering the cervix.

1483. Why haven't two healthy people, who have gone to many doctors and passed every test, been able to conceive a child after nine years of trying?

Sometimes the answer to this question cannot be found. One theory is that your genes and chromosomes are just not compatible and will not form a living fetus together. Your chromosomes can be studied, but only rarely can the actual cause of the incompatibility be determined. It may be there, but it cannot be seen. Perhaps sperm studies are not good enough to reveal when there is something wrong with the sperm.

1484. Is it true that wearing brief-style undershorts causes sterility in men?

Wearing brief-style undershorts does not cause absolute sterility, but it can reduce the sperm count, because restrictive shorts hold the testicles close to the body and keeps them too warm. The testicles naturally hang outside the body because sperm are produced better in a slightly cooler temperature. Testicles that stay inside the body, undescended, will not produce sperm; however, they still produce testosterone just as well.

1485. Can emotional problems hinder my chances of getting pregnant?

Yes, if the problems are severe enough to interfere with ovulation, then they could interfere with your chances of getting pregnant. Ovulation can be very sensitive to tensions and emotional upsets. If the problems require medication, such as tranquilizers, that can also interfere with ovulation.

1486. Could a severe blow to my abdomen (possibly the result of a fall or accident) cause me not to be able to have children?

No, not unless it destroyed both of your ovaries and you never menstruated again.

1487. Is it possible to "try too hard" to get pregnant?

If the attempt to get pregnant is harmful to the relationship of the couple and if the strain actually keeps the woman from ovulating, then it can interfere with conception. If trying too hard means having sex more than once a day, this reduces the sperm count.

HOW AND WHEN TO GET PREGNANT: CAUSES OF INFERTILITY
(Continued)

1488. Can worrying too much about getting pregnant be a reason why pregnancy does not occur?

If you are ovulating and having sex, then worrying does not really interfere with conception. If you worry so much that you do not ovulate, this will show up on your temperature chart. Pushing your partner to have sex in order to get pregnant can ruin the sex pattern of any couple. When no cause for infertility is found, it is easy to blame the woman by saying that she is worrying too much. That is not fair.

1489. I have frequently heard of couples who finally adopted a child after trying for years to have one of their own, and then shortly after that they were able to conceive a child. Why does this happen?

Usually, these are couples who, before adopting a child, had tests that showed no reason for their inability to have children. Most couples who adopt never have children of their own afterward. If pregnancy does occur, it may be that the woman ovulates better when the pressure to get pregnant is lifted.

1490. What are the chances of getting pregnant if one of my fallopian tubes has been damaged?

If one of your fallopian tubes has been damaged, there is a good chance that the other one is damaged in its interior as well, even though it looks all right on the outside. If both are blocked, your chances of getting pregnant are zero. If they are not blocked, but one is severely damaged, your chances depend upon the extent of the damage. You may need an X-ray (hysterosalpingogram) to find out. With this procedure, an injection of dye is put into your tubes so that their shape can be detected.

HOW AND WHEN TO GET PREGNANT: WHEN TO SEEK HELP FOR INFERTILITY; FERTILITY TESTS

1491. How long is too long for a couple to spend trying to have a child? Is it different with age?

Since trying to have a child means having frequent intercourse, there is no problem with doing that for the rest of your life! But if you mean how long should you try unsuccessfully before getting a medical examination to find out if something is wrong, the answer is four months for someone who is under thirty-five, and eight months for someone who is over thirty-five.

1492. In cases in which couples are having trouble getting pregnant, is it usually the man or the woman who is infertile?

A little more than half of the time, it is the female who has the problem. This is fortunate, because there are more solutions for women's infer-

HOW AND WHEN TO GET PREGNANT: WHEN TO SEEK HELP FOR INFERTILITY; FERTILITY TESTS (Continued)

tility problems than there are for a low sperm count.

1493. What kinds of infertility problems are easily treated?

If you are not ovulating because you run and are underweight, it is easy for you to change your habits and become fertile. If the problem is cervicitis and vaginitis due to infection, treatment of the infection and the cervix can result in pregnancy, even before the treatment is complete. Sometimes this happens inadvertently. If you are using inadequate contraception when the cervicitis is treated, you could become pregnant when you don't want to be. Correcting ovulation problems can be as simple as taking five birth control pills in one cycle. However, if you are not ovulating because you are in poor health, correcting ovulation becomes both a medical and an ethical problem because then you are an unhealthy woman who is pregnant, too. Encouraging sex at the right time of the cycle or stopping habits that interfere with fertility, such as standing up after intercourse or douching, can make a dramatic change. Correcting sexual dysfunction problems is not exactly easy, but it can be simpler than surgery.

1494. Where can I go for a fertility test?

Most family practice physicians, general practitioners, and obstetrician/gynecologists can perform the first simple tests and evaluations of fertility. Some gynecologists specialize in this field and offer more elaborate testing, including laparoscopy and tubal reconstructive surgery. Some clinics are devoted to this purpose. Ask your doctor for a referral, if he or she does not do this.

1495. What kinds of tests can my doctor do to find out if I am fertile?

Actually, the only way to prove you are fertile is for you to become pregnant. However, it is possible to prove that you are infertile. The first test is a physical examination, with a thorough pelvic examination. Examination of your cervical mucus containing sperm is done shortly after intercourse with your partner. Temperature charts or endometrial biopsies are done to determine ovulation and its quality. A semen analysis should be performed on the man. If needed, a hysterosalpingogram can be done to see if your tubes are open. This is an injection given on an X-ray table. Laparoscopy is a surgical examination of the abdomen performed under anesthesia with a small incision. Dyes can be injected at this time to see if they come through the tubes, thus avoiding the X-ray. Tests on your blood and urine for hormones, such as estrogen, progesterone, FSH (follicle-stimulating hormone), prolactin, thyroid, and others, can be essential. Your general health may require other testing, not directly related to fertility; if you are too thin, that could be your problem. Learn everything you can about the tests. Be sure you know about any risks that are involved.

1496. What kinds of tests can a doctor do to find out if a man is fertile?

A semen analysis is done first. The man ejaculates into a clean con-

HOW AND WHEN TO GET PREGNANT: WHEN TO SEEK HELP FOR INFERTILITY; FERTILITY TESTS (Continued)

tainer and brings it into the laboratory within an hour. The ejaculate is watched for six hours to see how long and what percentage of the sperm continue to swim. A count is done, and the shape and form of the sperm are studied. Any pus suggesting infection is noted, along with the quantity, acidity, and other symptoms. If this analysis is normal, the man is seldom tested anymore. If not, a urologist can examine his testicles, prostate, and urethra. Some men have a collection of varicose veins in their scrotums (varicocele); in that case, a biopsy of their testicles can be taken or surgery performed. This is the most successful treatment for any male infertility. For an unknown reason, sperm counts in men have been decreasing for the last thirty years. In 1950, the average count was 100,000,000 sperm per cc of semen; in 1980, the average was as low as 60,000,000 per cc of semen.

1497. Getting a sperm count is embarrassing for my husband. How can we avoid using his real name?

All medical tests are confidential, and no one will discuss the test with anyone, except you. If your husband is embarrassed, he can ejaculate into a clean container, and you can bring it into the laboratory to be tested. If you don't use your real name, there may be a mix-up in the reports. I should think you would be more embarrassed telling your doctor that you are going to use a false name, but, of course, there is nothing to stop you from doing this. Some men aren't embarrassed; they simply think it is wrong to ejaculate anywhere except into a woman's vagina. They will not even use a condom to catch the semen, because they think it is wrong to use contraception. Using a condom is a poor method anyway, because it is treated to immobilize sperm and makes them look abnormal. Sometimes the only way to find out if a man has any sperm is to examine the woman as soon as possible after she has had intercourse with him, to see if live sperm are in her cervix. This is called a Huhner test. However, it does not provide an accurate sperm count; it just lets you know if sperm are present.

1498. How accurate are fertility tests?

After a sperm count is taken, a man is told the percentage chance he has of getting a fertile woman pregnant. The results are not absolute, unless he has no sperm at all. Also, his sperm count can change with his environment and living habits, so that his sperm count last year may be different from one today. Similarly, the woman can change her ovulation pattern from month to month, so her diagnosis one month can be different the next month. Blocked tubes seem to only rarely change, so that they become unblocked, but even this can happen. Fertility tests result in possible causes of infertility, but they are not absolutely accurate about predicting the future.

HOW AND WHEN TO GET PREGNANT: WHEN TO SEEK HELP FOR INFERTILITY; FERTILITY TESTS (Continued)

1499. What are the dangers of fertility tests?

A hysterosalpingogram involves X-rays to the pelvis. In general, it is better to avoid X-rays to the ovaries, in order not to change chromosomes any more than background radiation already does. Also, you could be allergic to the dye that is injected, though this is very rare. A laparoscopy is performed under anesthesia, which always involves a risk. This procedure has its own risks, too, such as bleeding, infection, or puncture of an organ. It is, however, less dangerous than the previously used laparotomy, in which the woman's abdomen was cut open with a large surgical incision in order to look around for a reason why she was not able to get pregnant. Other tests have no dangers.

HOW AND WHEN TO GET PREGNANT: FERTILITY DRUGS

1500. What are the most common fertility drugs prescribed by doctors?

Clomiphene (brand name Clomid) is a pill that can be taken shortly after menstruation ceases to produce ovulation in women who ordinarily don't ovulate. It is effective for most women; however, some women who have a pituitary problem will not respond. These women require more powerful injections of another brand of fertility drugs called Pergonal (urinary gonadotropins extracted from the urine of menopausal women), perhaps combined with estrogen or HCG (human chorionic gonadotropin) from placentas. The art of inducing ovulation has been perfected in recent years, and there are many ways to do it.

1501. When should a doctor prescribe fertility drugs?

Fertility drugs are only useful for women who are not ovulating or not ovulating very well. Women who are infertile for any other reason will not benefit from these drugs. They are also used in the test tube baby program (in vitro fertilization) to make women ovulate several eggs at the same time. These eggs are then recovered by laparoscopy, fertilized in a dish, and returned to the uterus to improve the chances of a pregnancy. This, of course, can lead to twinning if more than one fertilized egg implants. Twinning, or even triplets, is always a problem with fertility drugs. If you can ovulate without them, you are usually better off.

1502. What percentage of women who take fertility drugs have multiple births?

About 10 percent of those women using clomiphene (Clomid) will have twins, and much fewer will have triplets. The percentage goes up when the dosage is increased or if other stronger drugs, like Pergonal, are used.

HOW AND WHEN TO GET PREGNANT: FERTILITY DRUGS

1503. How do fertility drugs promote pregnancy?

Fertility drugs only promote pregnancy by inducing ovulation. They do not do anything else.

1504. How soon after I start taking fertility drugs will I get pregnant?

If the fertility drugs produce ovulation, then you are like any normal fertile woman, and it will take an average of four menstrual cycles for you to get pregnant.

1505. What percentage of women who use fertility drugs get pregnant?

About 80 percent of women using fertility pills will ovulate. The remaining 20 percent will require more powerful drugs. Of those who ovulate, about 60 percent will end up with a baby. The others often have multiple problems, including partner sperm problems.

1506. Are fertility drugs safe?

The side effects of fertility drugs are few. These include hot flushes and headaches, especially when high dosages are taken. They also can produce large cysts on the woman's ovary that can rupture under pressure, but usually these will go away if the drug is stopped. Fertility drugs do not produce more abnormal babies than normal ovulation does, but they can produce multiple eggs and, therefore, a multiple pregnancy. Twins are not such a hazard, but triplets are. Often, women carrying triplets deliver prematurely and the babies die.

1507. Do fertility drugs have any long-term effects on the mother or child?

No, except that having twins affects both the mother's and children's lifestyles.

1508. Are there any risks involved in taking fertility drugs over a long period of time?

The risk of large cysts forming on the ovary is actually greater when you first start taking fertility drugs than it is after you have used them for a while. It is also more likely if the dosage is raised to a high level. You must have a pelvic examination at intervals to be sure that this is not happening.

HOW AND WHEN TO GET PREGNANT: ARTIFICIAL INSEMINATION, IN VITRO FERTILIZATION, MICROSURGERY

1509. What is artificial insemination?

Artificial insemination is the placement of semen into the vagina by artificial means, rather than by intercourse. It is sometimes performed with the husband's sperm to overcome the deficiencies of a low count or to place a high concentration of sperm over the cervix, avoiding the vaginal environ-

HOW AND WHEN TO GET PREGNANT: ARTIFICIAL INSEMINATION, IN VITRO FERTILIZATION, MICROSURGERY
(Continued)

ment. It is also performed in women who are unable to have intercourse with their husbands because of ejaculatory incompetence or impotence. Usually donor sperm, the sperm of a fertile male unknown to the woman, is used instead of the husband's sperm.

1510. How is artificial insemination done?

Artificial insemination is done by first obtaining either fresh semen from the woman's husband or usually frozen, stored semen from a donor who is known to be fertile, without disease, and who is paid for his ejaculate of semen. The family history of the donor is investigated in order to eliminate the possibility of defective babies. The woman must keep a temperature chart to know when she is going to ovulate. Within forty-eight hours of ovulation, the semen is placed in a small cup that fits over the cervix. This is usually done in the doctor's office. It is left in place for one-half hour, and then removed. If the woman ovulates, but menstruates two weeks later, the procedure is tried again before the next ovulation. Frequently when women are having aritifical insemination with donor sperm (AID), they fail to ovulate, apparently because knowing they are receiving sperm from another man is upsetting to them. It usually takes four such inseminations at the right time to get most women pregnant.

1511. Is artificial insemination dangerous?

No, the donor semen is carefully screened. The donor is also screened and examined to be sure he does not have a contagious disease and does have a good family history for having babies, preferably one that matches the charactertistics of the legal father. This is more protection than you have when you have intercourse with your husband. Legally, the child born from this method is in limbo; it is presumed to be the legal offspring of the husband, unless he denies it. Most husbands are advised to adopt the child, so there will be no legal loopholes concerning the child's inheritance.

1512. When would artificial insemination be advised?

The most common situation in which artifical insemination is advised is when the husband has such a low sperm count that his wife has very little chance of becoming pregnant. Occasionally, the count is high enough that placing it in the cup over the cervix will improve the efficiency enough to get her pregnant. But most of the time, a donor specimen of semen, carefully screened to match the husband's racial and other characteristics, is used. Of course, only very fertile sperm are used, to reduce the number of inseminations that are necessary. Once in a while, artificial insemination is carried out

HOW AND WHEN TO GET PREGNANT: ARTIFICIAL INSEMINATION, IN VITRO FERTILIZATION, MICROSURGERY
(Continued)

because there is a sexual difficulty that cannot be overcome, such as ejaculatory incompetence or impotence in a man who can still masturbate and ejaculate. Rarely is it used when the husband has a hereditary disease that has a high chance of recurrence and no chance of prenatal detection. Lesbian women ask for this service when they want to have children without having sex with a man, but they usually are refused. Artificial insemination with donor sperm (AID), is reserved for stable, married couples who want children. Doctors who provide this treatment are stricter than adoption agencies.

1513. Where can I go to have an artifical insemination?
Your doctor or, especially, your gynecologist will be able to refer you to a gynecologist who specializes in artificial insemination. This doctor will also handle obtaining and storing donor sperm for you to use, or else you can use your husband's. Sometimes the sperm are mixed so that you can't be sure who the father is. Clinics that specialize in infertility problems also usually offer this service. Artificial insemination is such a standard procedure today and has been used for such a long time that insurance companies usually pay for it.

1514. What other new treatments are available for infertility problems?
The newest treatment is in vitro fertilization. Women who have blocked tubes can have the eggs removed from their ovaries by laparoscopy. Semen is added to the egg in a Petri dish in a laboratory under perfect conditions of temperature, solutions, cleanliness, and timing. When the fertilized egg has divided into eight cells, it is carefully placed into the woman's uterus. Usually several eggs are used at once, to increase the chances of success. One hundred and fifty babies have been born from this method. The success rate of in vitro fertilization will increase the more it is studied and performed. Clinics for this purpose are springing up across the nation and around the world. It is an expensive treatment, costing about $5,000 per attempt, and four attempts may be needed for a pregnancy. This method also can be used when the husband's sperm count is low, since it takes much fewer sperm to fertilize an egg in a Petri dish than it does when the sperm are placed in the vagina. In vitro fertilization is recommended for couples who do not want artificial insemination with donor sperm. Another new treatment is microsurgery to repair damaged tubes. This also can be performed to reverse a sterilization surgery that was done previously. These operations have been 60 percent successful in reversing sterilization surgery, but less successful in repairing damaged tubes.

HOW AND WHEN TO GET PREGNANT: FEELINGS ASSOCIATED WITH INFERTILITY

1515. Do most women who have a difficult time getting pregnant become depressed?

If raising a family is their main goal in life, women who have difficulty getting pregnant do become quite frustrated and depressed, and sometimes desperate. However, this is not a frequent cause of suicide. There is always hope. Some men know they have a low sperm count and will not tell their wives. Men also feel depressed if they know that they have a low sperm count, and some women try to keep this information away from their husbands to protect their egos. Our fertility seems to be tied up with our egos, even if having children is not our goal. However, if men and women would seek help from their doctors for their fertility problems, perhaps their problems could be reversed and they could have children.

1516. Do some women who cannot have children feel that they are less of a woman than those with children?

Yes. Even though our culture says women are liberated and able to do almost anything they want in life, most people expect women to have and raise children, instead of or in addition to any other work. People show sorrow and sympathy for those women who do not have children, even if it is by choice. More astoundingly, when the fertility problem is entirely the males', many women still feel they have somehow been cheated in life and have not reached their full potential, because they have not experienced pregnancy and childbirth. In the not too distant past, it was really considered tragic to be a woman without children. It was even grounds for divorce or annulment, especially by royalty. Today, this is true in some undeveloped countries. The opportunities for women in the United States are too great for infertility to be a tragic problem.

1517. How can I get over the depression I feel from knowing that I cannot have children?

You can turn to other solutions, such as adoption. You can apply to be on the waiting list for in vitro fertilization, if that is appropriate for your problem. You can use your maternal yearnings in other directions, such as teaching children, working in day care centers or child development programs, or giving special attention to nieces and nephews. There are groups in every city that can help you to cope with your infertility. Your doctor can refer you to one, and so can a hotline referral number. But the most important thing to do is to regain your self-esteem and proceed with other goals in your life.

HOW AND WHEN TO GET PREGNANT: NOT HAVING CHILDREN

1518. What percentage of women never have children?

In the past, about 15 percent of women never had children, but today this percentage is increasing as more and more women find that they can live a full and happy life without having babies.

1519. What are some of the reasons why a woman might not want to have children?

Some women have a full, creative, and productive life that leaves them no room and no desire to have children. Others choose to avoid pregnancy with some pain, because they believe childbearing would end their careers. Still others feel that their lifestyles are not suitable for raising a child, even though they might want children. A few women have an inheritable disease in their families that cannot be prevented, and they do not want to pass on this inheritance. Others have responsibilities, such as caring for younger brothers and sisters or aging parents, and they feel they do not have the right or the time to care for children, too.

Chapter 7

Normal Pregnancy and Choices in Childbirth

NORMAL PREGNANCY AND CHOICES IN CHILDBIRTH

The hallmark of freedom for women is their range of choices in childbirth. In the distant past, women were in no way in charge of their bodies or their lives. Childbirth and child care controlled their existence, and only those who were sterile or who could avoid all sexual activity could devote their energies to anything else. Today knowledge, technology, culture, and the law give women freedom of choice in all aspects of childbirth and child care. A woman's first choice is that of a sex partner, a far cry from an arranged marriage. Then she is faced with contraceptive choices. This is sometimes a dilemma because of the many forces affecting her decision. Even after she is pregnant, she can legally back out of the process, with medical safety, up to the point at which the baby would survive.

Even if a woman has never before thought about how her body works, pregnancy makes her conscious of its mechanisms, from the first nauseous moment or breast tenderness to the climax of delivery of the baby. As she acquires knowledge, she realizes that she has many choices in every aspect. She can become disabled by vomiting and fatigue, or control it with frequent eating, vitamins, medication, or all three. She can perform her own pregnancy test or seek immediate confirmation of pregnancy from her doctor. She can deny pregnancy and its need for care, or she can decide to seek early medical care that suits her approach to childbearing. Her finances or insurance may control her choice of medical care, or she may interview or start care with several sources before she finds the right place. As she gains information, her choice may change. She has legal support for her choice to work or stay home. Exercise is now open to her, with many physical fitness centers promoting classes for pregnant women. She is recommended to gain at least twenty-five pounds, but there is no set limit on her weight gain; fear of her baby being premature may keep her from staying thin. If she fears defects that occur in her family or because she is over thirty-five, testing is available to determine if the fetus has defects. Ultrasound is a test that can show the normal contours of her fetus, and maybe even the sex. If a gross defect is found, she can choose to terminate the pregnancy, and become pregnant again. She also may choose to avoid all testing. If she can tolerate artificial insemination, she may even choose the sex of her child. Classes to prepare her for labor, delivery, and baby care abound, with the many differing styles including Lamaze, Leboyer, and Bradley. Her choice of anesthesia used to be either to use drugs and gas to put her and the baby to sleep, or to stay awake and feel everything, including pain. Medical care now provides local and regional anesthesia that safely lets her stay awake and comfortable enough to enjoy it all. Hopefully, she has a free choice of hospitals with their different approaches to childbirth. Most hospitals now have a special room called an ABC room (Alternative Birth Center) where she can experience delivery just as if she were having her baby at home with family and friends around her, without the inherent dangers of home delivery. A first cesarean section is not really a choice for her, but a repeat one may be, as she can, under some conditions, choose to try again for a vaginal delivery. The form of anesthesia for a cesarean section is a choice to be made by the woman and her doctor. In the United States, the decision to breast-feed is equally as popular as choosing to bottle feed. Child care choices are now astounding in their variety, with fathers and children playing a greater role than ever before. With regard to pregnancy and choices in childbirth and child care, there are no more set patterns in this aspect of life; therefore, knowledge is needed to choose the paths that are best.

This chapter does not attempt to include everything about pregnancy. (There are complete reference books on pregnancy in your local bookstores and libraries that you might want to read.) It does, however, provide a lot of information so that you can make choices that affect you in this most important event. We hope that after reading it you will feel more at ease with your pregnancy. You will be reassured that what you feel is probably normal, and if it is not, you will be knowledgeable enough to call your doctor.

Make the most of this miraculous experience.

NORMAL PREGNANCY AND CHOICES IN CHILDBIRTH: TAKING CHARGE DURING PREGNANCY; EMOTIONS AND STRESS

1520. When I am pregnant, I am happy one minute and sad the next. Why am I like that?

In early pregnancy, your emotions are on a roller coaster ride due to blood sugar changes. This is caused by the rapid removal of glucose from the bloodstream by pregnancy. When the level of glucose is high, you feel energetic and happy; if you let it drop, you feel faint, nauseated, and definitely unhappy. You can eat frequent, small meals of carbohydrates and some protein without fat to try to stabilize yourself. If you are very active, you have to balance this activity with food to an even greater extent. If you are relatively inactive, it is less of a problem. Another factor in rapid mood swings is your emotional adjustment to your pregnancy and to the prospect of having a baby. If pregnancy is unplanned, this can produce a crisis in your life situation, and you might have severe depressions until you solve all of your problems. Solving your problems even may include abortion, especially if the pregnancy is really going to ruin your mental health. Prior to ten years ago, when abortion became a personal choice, psychiatrists had to certify that the continuation of pregnancy would be hazardous to a woman's mental health. Today you do not have to ask them, although sometimes it is wise to do so.

1521. How can I take charge during pregnancy when I am irritable much of the time?

If your irritability is due to low levels of sugar in your blood, an injection of sugar into your blood could stop this from happening. An easier solution for controlling your emotions would be to eat enough carbohydrates to satisfy your need for sugar. It also is better for your baby not to experience extremely low blood sugars.

1522. How can I take charge of my body when my pregnancy symptoms have me completely disabled?

Instead of accepting that all the symptoms and discomforts of pregnancy are the price you pay for a baby, you need to gain as much knowledge as you can about each symptom and how you can reduce it or even make it disappear. Read books. Ask your doctor.

1523. Can my emotional state affect my unborn baby?

If your heart beats faster than normal, then your baby's heart also beats faster. The baby can respond with activity to the emotional state you are in. This does not really change the way in which the baby develops, nor does it cause any defects. However, if you are so depressed that you do not take in proper nourishment, then the baby can be severely affected.

Whenever anyone sees me now
they treat me as a pregnant woman
no longer a career woman
no longer sexy or attractive
just another pregnant wife
Whenever anyone speaks to me now
they speak to me as their own mothers
no longer about world affairs,
          or business,
or careers, or goals,
but strictly about diapers and babies
and family life
Why can't people treat me
as the person I have always been

— Susan Polis Schutz

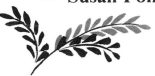

NORMAL PREGNANCY AND CHOICES IN CHILDBIRTH: TAKING CHARGE DURING PREGNANCY; EMOTIONS AND STRESS
(Continued)

1524. Should I avoid stressful situations while I am pregnant?

Situations only are stressful if you interpret them as such. There is no study or scientific evidence to indicate that stress to the mother is harmful to her baby. However, if your response to stress is to stop eating and not take care of yourself in any other way, then there will be some harm to your pregnancy. But if you just have emotional responses, these are not known to be harmful to your baby. There also is no evidence to indicate that stress causes the onset of premature labor. If you had to avoid stress during pregnancy, you would have to avoid all important jobs and positions. You also would have to avoid staying home and taking care of your other children. No one ever worries about the stress you experience taking care of your difficult children, just the stress from high-paying jobs.

NORMAL PREGNANCY AND CHOICES IN CHILDBIRTH: PRENATAL CARE

1525. What is prenatal care and where can I get it?

It is medical care starting with the first confirmation of pregnancy and ending with labor and delivery. Postnatal care is given for the six weeks following delivery or until you have recovered. There are many sources from which you may obtain prenatal care. Most prenatal care in the United States is given by private doctors in their private offices, and delivery is done in a private hospital. Organized clinics, such as the Kaiser Clinic, provide extensive prenatal care in which a group of doctors see the patients in rotation. Delivery is done by whichever doctor is on call when you go into labor. The large service hospitals for the Army and Navy give care in this same manner. Medical schools, church hospitals, county hospitals, and charity hospitals for the poor also give care in this manner, frequently by doctors in some stage of their training, at a reduced cost or even free. Care like this is provided on Indian reservations by our government for the Indian Service. Some community clinics and even Planned Parenthood groups also give prenatal care, even if they do not provide the final labor and delivery care.

1526. How important is prenatal care?

Even if you go to the best doctor and the best hospital in the world, if you only go when you are in labor and about to have your baby, the results will not be very good. Without prenatal care, the number of babies and mothers who die from childbirth will be high, and there will be more defective babies born. But if you seek medical care as soon as you suspect

NORMAL PREGNANCY AND CHOICES IN CHILDBIRTH: PRENATAL CARE (Continued)

pregnancy and follow the advice regarding testing and caring for yourself, the chances of this happening will be significantly reduced. Modern statistics reveal extremely low death rates for mothers and very low rates for babies. Rates for this country would be much better if all women got prenatal care, but they do not. Of course, seeking prenatal care and then ignoring all the information you receive does not produce a good outcome, either. If you choose to eat a strange and inadequate diet, drink alcohol excessively, smoke heavily, take drugs that are forbidden, expose yourself to diseases, and fail to treat problems, the outcome will not be much better, even though you visit a doctor. Even if you obtain good nutrition, exercise regularly, avoid bad habits, stay free of infection, and, in general, care for yourself, you still should seek medical care early in your pregnancy. A good standard of living and good health habits certainly improve the outcome for babies, but do not solve or prevent all problems. Prenatal care is the care you give yourself and the medical care you seek while you are pregnant.

1527. Do you advise women to attend prenatal classes?

Yes, indeed. They are an important supplement to prenatal medical care and provide you with information. They also teach you exercises in relaxation and body control, which will assist you in carrying your baby, as well as during labor and delivery. You can learn enough so that you can make choices in your childbirth experience. Child care is also taught for newborns. Fathers are expected to attend classes as well, because they will become the labor coaches. Some hospitals even have classes in sibling preparation, so that the other children can learn about what their mothers are going through and what to expect. Classes are available at hospitals, schools, churches, and many community centers. To find one, you can call your local hotline, ask your doctor, write the International Childbirth Education Association at P.O. Box 20048, Minneapolis, MN 55420, or ask your friends. This is a time to learn, and you will never be more interested.

1528. Do I have to have an obstetrician, or can I rely on my family doctor for prenatal care?

That may depend on your family doctor. Many of them do not want to deliver babies because they do not feel adequately trained, they do not like the restrictions it puts on their lives, or they do not want to pay the large price for liability insurance. There are not enough obstetricians in the United States to deliver all the babies. Family and general practitioners who are interested in obstetrics do an excellent job of caring for pregnant women who are neither high risks nor have complications. They know the whole family and, therefore, have special insight into their problems. If complications

NORMAL PREGNANCY AND CHOICES IN CHILDBIRTH:
PRENATAL CARE (Continued)

arise, they are trained to call in specialists for consultation, and the hospital where they practice makes sure that they do so. Many communities do not have an obstetrician located nearby, so care from the local family doctor is superior because of availability. It is also better than having to travel to a distant and sometimes unavailable obstetrician, except when complications arise. The same discussion applies to the choice of pediatrician or family doctor for your baby.

1529. How often will I need to go to the doctor while I'm pregnant?

Most doctors ask you to come in for regular checkups at least every three or four weeks until the last two months when they will want to see you more often. Of course, you must call whenever a problem arises, and extra visits may be necessary, both to the office or to the hospital. Your knowledge about pregnancy and your body will assist you in determining when to seek extra help. It also may prevent you from skipping visits for unimportant reasons.

1530. Why do I have to go to the doctor so often when I'm pregnant?

The reasons change in the different stages of pregnancy. In the first three months, you go to the doctor to diagnose pregnancy, to make sure the baby is in the uterus and nowhere else, and that it is growing normally. Tests are arranged as needed and an attempt is made to determine your due date. Care for your general health as well as the pregnancy and its symptoms are planned. This is a good time to discuss all the choices you want to consider in labor and delivery. During the second three months, or the middle of pregnancy, there are fewer problems and this allows even more time for education and discussion of exercise in pregnancy and planning for your recovery from delivery while caring for the baby. Proper growth of the baby is also observed. The last three months are more crucial and your visits generally are more frequent because the problems multiply. Diabetes can start during this time. High blood pressure and protein (albumin) in the urine may signal toxemia of pregnancy, a serious disorder occurring only in pregnancy that can cause convulsions and death of the baby and mother. Treatment and perhaps early delivery are crucial for survival. It can occur with no symptoms, although headache, vomiting, seeing white spots, and mental changes may occur. Toxemia was the original reason for starting prenatal care years ago. Signs of premature labor are monitored, and at term, signs of proper position of the baby and progress toward normal labor are checked. If you are overdue, special tests and actions may be needed. Rh blood-type problems have almost disappeared, but still require frequent blood tests and rechecks. Anemia has to be rechecked, too. If you skip even

A Doctor to Avoid
If You Are Busy

Last time I waited
two hours to see the doctor.
Today I thought I was smart.
I called the nurse right before
my appointment to see if he was
on schedule.
The nurse said, "Yes, you're next."
I rushed to the doctor's office
and checked in . . .
and waited
and waited
and waited.
I went to the desk and
told them that I was supposed
to have been next.
They said that they were sorry
and that there were five people
in front of me.
"Your doctor is very popular
and everyone waits for him,
and they feel that he is
worth it.
He's a very important man,
you know."
"I'M AS IMPORTANT
        AS THE DOCTOR, AND
I WON'T WAIT FOR HIM."

— Susan Polis Schutz

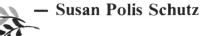

NORMAL PREGNANCY AND CHOICES IN CHILDBIRTH: PRENATAL CARE (Continued)

one visit, it may be at a crucial time when something should have been done in time for the baby's welfare or your own.

1531. Why does the doctor measure my stomach?

The doctor measures the height of your fundus, the top of your uterus or womb. This is done to be sure that the baby is developing at the normal rate, is not growth retarded or excessively large due to too much water (polyhydramnios), and to check for the presence of more than one fetus.

1532. What will the doctor do on each prenatal visit?

You are expected to bring an early morning urine specimen each visit, or give a specimen when you arrive, to be checked for sugar and protein, or diabetes and toxemia. You will be weighed, and your blood pressure checked. The doctor will observe the size of the uterus, or the baby, and listen to the fetal heartbeat if possible. Hopefully, you can discuss your symptoms, fears, plans, and choices. The first visit, of course, involves a complete history, physical examination, and blood tests. The extent of examination on subsequent visits depends upon the problems at hand.

1533. Every time I have a problem, I call my doctor and his nurse screens my calls. I never get to talk to him directly and he *never* returns my calls personally. He makes me feel like I'm making a big deal over nothing, or else he doesn't really care. What should I do?

The next time you see your doctor for a checkup, ask him under what circumstances he wants you to call him. If you do call him during the day, be sure that you leave a number where he can call you back later. If that doesn't work, why not try to call him in the evening? If he never wants to return your calls personally, you might consider going to another doctor who will.

NORMAL PREGNANCY AND CHOICES IN CHILDBIRTH: THE IMPORTANCE OF REST

1534. Will I need more rest when I'm pregnant?

Yes, in general. In early pregnancy many women feel very tired and sleepy, even when they are eating well. You can have a higher activity level without extra rest in the middle three months. In the last three months, quality of sleep becomes poorer, and fatigue may result unless there is additional rest in the daytime. Sleep studies have shown that there is no deep sleep after the seventh month. Frequent waking about every 1½ hours is characteristic, as if you are being conditioned to wake up and care for a baby! Swelling of the feet, legs, and hands occurs when not enough time is spent lying down.

NORMAL PREGNANCY AND CHOICES IN CHILDBIRTH: THE IMPORTANCE OF REST (Continued)

However, this is not dangerous and does not mean you are going to get tox-emia (a blood pressure disorder of late pregnancy), as doctors once thought fifteen years ago. Sixty percent of normal pregnant women swell during pregnancy. Lying down, especially at midday, gets rid of the swelling.

NORMAL PREGNANCY AND CHOICES IN CHILDBIRTH: WHEN WILL THE BABY BE BORN?

1535. How can I figure out when my baby will be born?

Count back 3 months from the first day of your last menstrual period and add 7 days to arrive at the due date. This only will be accurate if your periods are regular and about 28 days apart. If you know exactly when you got pregnant by an ovulation temperature chart, count forward 266 days. Human gestation is ten 28-day menstrual cycles, or about 9 months and 7 days from the beginning of the last regular period. Sometimes there is no period or ovulation record to count from and no idea when you got preg-nant. In that case, an estimate is made of the size of the uterus on the first visit and a due date is approximated. The fetal heart can usually be heard with an ultrasound doppler instrument at 10 to 12 weeks, and a due date can be estimated from the date it is heard. The baby usually kicks at about 4½ months, so a due date can be counted from that. The fetal heartbeat can be heard with a stethoscope at about the same time and that can be used to estimate a due date. A sonogram taken about the middle of pregnancy, when the top of the uterus (fundus) comes near the navel (umbilicus), can measure the diameter of the fetal head, and a rather accurate prediction of a due date can be made. X-rays were previously used near term to see if the baby was due, but now these are avoided. If it is really crucial to know if a baby is near enough to term to be delivered without getting premature lung disease, then an amniocentesis can be done to get a sample of amniotic fluid and test it for respiratory maturity by its content. This test involves some risk, as under the direction of a sonogram, a needle is inserted into the fluid around the baby. But if it prevents a premature delivery, it is worth it. Calculating the baby's due date is not always simple.

NORMAL PREGNANCY AND CHOICES IN CHILDBIRTH: INVOLVING FAMILY MEMBERS

1536. How can my husband or partner become more involved in my pregnancy?

Share your excitement and happiness, as well as your nausea and fatigue with him. Let him read the books you read on the subject or visit the

NORMAL PREGNANCY AND CHOICES IN CHILDBIRTH: INVOLVING FAMILY MEMBERS (Continued)

doctor with you. All childbirth preparation classes are now open to fathers-to-be. These classes are designed to teach your partner to be your labor coach as well as your emotional support before, during, and after delivery. If his work does not allow his going to classes or going to the doctor with you, share the knowledge you obtain with him. His interest in child development will increase with his knowledge on the subject and by observing other interested men in the class. This is the meaning of family-centered childbirth. If you encourage his involvement, he will say, "**We** had a baby." The rewards for shared parenthood are great.

1537. How can I include my other children in my pregnancy?

Your pregnancy can be a very educational, as well as joyful and emotional experience for your other children if you are willing to share it with them. Teaching them about getting pregnant can be adapted to their level of understanding. Books are available with explanations for children of the growing baby and the changes it makes in you. You can take your children to visit the doctor with you and perhaps let them hear the baby's heartbeat. Movies of childbirth may be appropriate for them. Some hospitals have sibling preparation classes designed to prepare children for the event of birth and the new arrival in their home. If you like, and if your doctor and hospital provide an alternative birth room where they can be present at delivery, your children can watch the childbirth with another adult who is there to care for them. If this is not possible, they can see you right after the birth with the baby in your arms. Most hospitals now at least provide for "sibling visitation" by appointment a day or two after delivery, in which your other children, with an adult, visit you and your new baby—provided they have no contagious disesase! Letting them participate in the care of your baby, without allowing opportunity for harm to the baby, is a wonderful experience for your other children.

1538. Can my children be with me during or immediately after my delivery?

If you want your children to be present at the great event of birth, do not believe for a moment that this has to occur at home. Every community does, or can and should, have a birthing room in a hospital where you can deliver with family and friends of your choice, as long as you have a normal delivery with no high risk for problems. No one knows whether this experience is good or bad for children, so you are free to choose to include them if you wish. If you have a complication or need special anesthesia or forceps, you and your husband will leave the ABC room (Alternative Birth Center) and go to the delivery room without the children, so you will need someone with them who is old enough to care for them in that event. Even if

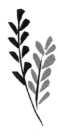

What more beautiful sight
is there than for
you to run along the beach
with our angelic little son following
and his little puppy following him
You run in and out of the waves
playing and laughing, chasing after each other

I sit in the sand
on the chair you both made for me
to make me more comfortable
seven more weeks before we have our new baby

I am so happy
to have such a beautiful family
so happy to be so much in love
I have dedicated my whole life
to being with you
every minute of the day and night
and to loving you and our son
every minute of the day and night

— Susan Polis Schutz

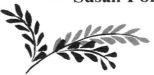

NORMAL PREGNANCY AND CHOICES IN CHILDBIRTH:
INVOLVING FAMILY MEMBERS (Continued)

you do not want them to see the delivery, you can invite them into an ABC
room after delivery to see the new baby in your arms. If you cannot deliver
this way, especially if you require a cesarean section, most hospitals today
allow for "sibling visitation" in the first day or two after delivery. You have
to be sure that they do not have a contagious disease, such as chickenpox or a
cold, so they will not infect others. They will need to wash their hands and
put on hospital gowns before they come see you and the new baby. This conditions them for the big change at home when you bring the new baby into
their world.

NORMAL PREGNANCY AND CHOICES IN CHILDBIRTH: THE
IMPORTANCE OF BEING COMFORTABLE

**1539. What can I do to be more comfortable during the "uncomfortable"
months of pregnancy?**
        You need to take care of all the minor complaints of pregnancy. In the
beginning you need to fight nausea with frequent eating. You can fight
headaches the same way. Backaches are common, but can be relieved with
good posture and exercise programs. The heaviness in late pregnancy can be
aided by good posture and exercise, but you also may require a maternity girdle in order to feel well. Heartburn can be relieved by harmless antacids,
which are available over the counter and are quite effective. Itching skin on
your abdomen and breasts, which are stretching, responds to cream lotions,
especially those containing lanolin. Any vaginitis can be treated after it is
diagnosed by your doctor and should not be ignored until after you deliver.
Any other illnesses that occur deserve treatment; do not just ignore them
because you are pregnant. Varicose veins can cause discomfort, but support
hose can provide relief. Don't give up on your body just because it is pregnant; make it as comfortable as possible.

**1540. When I sleep on my back, my chest hurts. It is hard to sleep on my big
stomach. Is there a comfortable position to sleep in when I am pregnant?**
        It is best not to sleep flat on your back after you reach the seventh
month of pregnancy, because the weight of your uterus actually cuts off circulation to your heart and lungs and you may become breathless. Sleeping
on your stomach is impossible because of the bulge. The only way to sleep is
on your side, preferably with one knee brought up and bent so that your
back will be straight, and one arm behind you so it will not be crushed under
your body. This is also a comfortable way to lie while you are in labor.

NORMAL PREGNANCY AND CHOICES IN CHILDBIRTH: THE IMPORTANCE OF BEING COMFORTABLE (Continued)

1541. Will wearing a maternity girdle support my muscles or make them weak? Will it help me to be more comfortable?

Wearing a maternity girdle can make you feel much better while you wear it by relieving backaches, fainting, low and high abdominal muscle pain, and even leg aches. It also can make you look better and less pregnant because it holds the baby up. Wearing a maternity girdle does not strengthen or weaken your muscles; only exercise, or lack of it, does that. It is not harmful to the baby, because it is designed without a constricting waist band like those in an ordinary girdle. The more pregnancies you have, which weaken and separate your abdominal muscles, the more you need a girdle for comfort.

NORMAL PREGNANCY AND CHOICES IN CHILDBIRTH: THE IMPORTANCE OF DIET AND VITAMINS

1542. Do I have a choice in the foods I eat, or do I have to follow a certain diet to have a good pregnancy?

All over the world women have good pregnancies and healthy babies, and they certainly do not eat the same foods. Both vegetarians (as long as they have some animal protein, milk protein, or vitamin B12) and meat eaters can have equally healthy babies. The basic requirements are: to consume enough calories per day to provide at least 200 calories above your normal diet, usually 2,300 calories; to consume enough protein for good fetal growth (especially after the fourth month), usually 75 gm per day; to consume enough vegetables and fruits to provide all the vitamins and minerals needed; and to consume enough fiber and roughage to avoid constipation (common in pregnancy). This can be done in any country with the foods that are available there. It is difficult to get enough iron in foods, so an iron supplement is a good idea. Most people do not eat enough leafy, green vegetables to get enough folic acid, so l mg may be taken, perhaps with other vitamins. If you are aware of the importance of these basic requirements, you do not have to follow a specific diet with certain listed foods. You can make your own selections and still nourish your baby.

1543. Are there any foods that an expectant mother should avoid?

In the first three months of pregnancy, foods high in fat will make the expectant mother more nauseated. The FDA (Food and Drug Administration) has issued a warning against excessive caffeine, because of its effects on pregnancy as shown in animal studies. This means eliminating coffee, tea, chocolate, and all soft drinks with caffeine added. Since women in late pregnancy have trouble sleeping, it is probably good to avoid caffeine anyway. Of course, the most important time that it would matter in forming

NORMAL PREGNANCY AND CHOICES IN CHILDBIRTH: THE IMPORTANCE OF DIET AND VITAMINS (Continued)

the baby would be in the first month or two. Alcohol can at least be considered in the diet, but should be quite limited. According to studies, excessive use of alcohol creates a particular kind of defect in babies, called the fetal alcohol syndrome. This syndrome occurs when more than one ounce of alcohol is consumed per day. This is equivalent to one cocktail, two small glasses of wine, or a large beer. No minimum that is really safe is known, however. Being aware of this is also especially important in the first few weeks, before you even know you are pregnant.

1544. Do I have a choice as to whether I take vitamins in pregnancy? Calcium? Iron? Fluoride?

A national council on nutrition in pregnancy advises taking supplemental iron. They found that in pregnancy there seems to be increased requirements for folic acid (a B vitamin) to prevent or treat a macrocytic (large red blood cell) anemia. All of the other vitamins, including calcium, can and should be obtained in your daily food. Many doctors prescribe a supplement with iron, folic acid, calcium, and all other vitamins as somewhat of a safety measure. However, these can upset your stomach, especially in early pregnancy, and they are difficult for some people to swallow. Iron pills are available in chewable form, and you can sample different types until you find one that won't cause diarrhea or constipation. Rechecking for anemia in the last few months of pregnancy ensures that you are taking enough iron. The reason you need extra iron is that the baby takes iron from you and you lose even more if you bleed at delivery. If you have pills left over, take them after delivery to build yourself up again. Many women report that vitamin B6 helps to relieve their morning sickness symptoms. Studies also have shown that fluoride taken in water during pregnancy prevents cavities in the baby's first set of teeth. Fluoridated water during childhood prevents cavities in adult teeth. Most major cities fluoridate their water supply for this reason.

NORMAL PREGNANCY AND CHOICES IN CHILDBIRTH: THE IMPORTANCE OF WEIGHT GAIN

1545. Do I have a choice in how much weight I gain in pregnancy, and when?

Yes, you do. Prior to 1970, women were advised to limit their weight gain to fourteen pounds, no matter how skinny they were. If they were overweight, they were encouraged to lose weight. Doctors used to think that gaining weight caused toxemia (a blood pressure disorder of late pregnancy). We still do not know a specific cause for toxemia, but we have found that it is definitely not due to weight gain, so doctors now are taught never to limit

NORMAL PREGNANCY AND CHOICES IN CHILDBIRTH: THE IMPORTANCE OF WEIGHT GAIN (Continued)

calories or weight gain in pregnant women and never to encourage weight loss. Research has also shown that being underweight at the beginning of pregnancy, along with poor weight gain, leads to premature delivery. That is why many teenagers have premature babies. Today a minimum weight gain of twenty-five pounds is advised and encouraged, even if you weigh three hundred pounds at the beginning of your pregnancy. Good nutrition may help prevent toxemia, but high or low weight gain does not guarantee it. Some women gain a lot of weight because their diets are too low in protein. Others have too few calories for their activities and for the growth of their babies, even if they eat enough protein. You should gain twenty-five pounds or more, and eat protein. Most of the weight gain occurs after the first three months and is best gained at a steady rate of one pound per week for the last twenty-five weeks. But if you gain a lot in the early months of your pregnancy, it is not safe to stop gaining altogether in the later months. You should gain at least one-half pound per week even if you are grossly overweight.

1546. How much is too much weight gain during pregnancy?

Medical authorities no longer set any limit on weight gain during pregnancy, because it is not a medical problem. However, it may be a problem to you or your husband if you are grossly overweight after delivery. Since our culture values slenderness, both of you may become depressed over it. You also may be more uncomfortable at the end of your pregnancy because you are heavy, but this will not affect the course of your pregnancy, labor, or delivery. It can, however, make it difficult for a cesarean section incision to heal.

1547. What percentage of the weight I gain during pregnancy is fat?

If you gain twenty-five pounds, about 20 percent of your weight gain is fat. Within three weeks from the time of delivery at term, you will lose twenty pounds without even trying. The five pounds of fat seem to be provided to help breast-feeding and should be lost over the following six months. You will not lose more than the twenty-five pounds without exerting great effort.

1548. Is it all right to try to lose weight during pregnancy?

The primary consequence of losing weight or inadequate weight gain during pregnancy is premature delivery. This can produce a damaged or even a dead child. When you lose weight, you burn fat and that produces ketones (a breakdown product of fat) in the blood; keto acidosis (breakdown of a lot of fat) is a bad environment for a developing fetus. Fasting is specifically ad-

NORMAL PREGNANCY AND CHOICES IN CHILDBIRTH: THE IMPORTANCE OF WEIGHT GAIN (Continued)

vised against. A restricted diet can be so poor that it may cause toxemia, high blood pressure, protein in the urine, and even convulsions in late pregnancy. Poor nutrition can interfere with the development of the baby, especially its size. In general, larger women have larger babies, and women who gain a lot of weight have larger babies. Small babies do not fare as well. Large women who lose weight can have small babies, although the chances of this happening are even greater in small women who lose weight.

1549. Will I gain weight after my baby is born?

In the first three weeks after your baby is born you will lose weight. Most women lose about twenty pounds, but not all in one day. After three weeks, some women gain and some lose, depending upon their activities and the calories they consume. If they eat very well, in order to breast-feed, they will lose less. If they don't breast-feed and don't diet, they will not lose the extra fat they gained during pregnancy.

NORMAL PREGNANCY AND CHOICES IN CHILDBIRTH: EXERCISE

1550. Do you encourage exercise during pregnancy?

Encouragement of exercise during pregnancy is a step toward liberation for pregnant women. In the past, because miscarriage and premature labor were not understood, they were blamed on the physical or sexual activity of women and both were forbidden. When miscarriages were found to be due to chromosomal abnormalities of the fetus, exercise was exonerated. Having a baby is an athletic activity; in a vaginal delivery, it requires muscles that are conditioned to carry the baby and to push it out. Ballet dancers make the best patients, and you cannot stop them from exercising. If exercise is carried so far that the woman loses weight and burns so much fat that she forms ketones (a breakdown product of fat) in her blood, then this is not a good environment for a growing baby. Frequent eating and rest are important. As in all things, moderation is the key word for success. The availability of exercise classes for pregnant women is increasing, and women are encouraged to participate. This also provides women with the energy and incentive to work in active jobs until their labor begins, without feeling that they must be harming their babies. Certain complications will always exist to prohibit some women from work or exercise, such as placenta previa (placenta covering the cervix), toxemia, threatened premature labor, twins and triplets. But people must learn not to treat all women as if they had complicated pregnancies. Most pregnant women are healthy and normal and should be encouraged to continue normal, healthy lives, which includes exer-

NORMAL PREGNANCY AND CHOICES IN CHILDBIRTH:
EXERCISE (Continued)

cise. When people grow accustomed to seeing pregnant women who are active, they no longer will assume a woman has to take nine months out of her life to have a baby. It changes the entire view of womanhood, especially for young girls.

1551. Do I have the choice of exercise during pregnancy? Is it good or bad for me?

Today it is recommended that you stay physically fit while you are pregnant. This is necessary so that your heart, as well as your back, will be able to carry the load of pregnancy. It also gives you the strength to deliver your baby vaginally without extra help, like forceps. Having a baby is an athletic activity. Exercise is good for you, and you may have to exercise, especially if you want natural childbirth without anesthesia. (Anesthesia is needed if forceps are used.) Ballet dancers and swimming instructors do very well during pregnancy and delivery, and they continue to work out during their pregnancy. Lack of activity or exercise makes you fat and weak, and it reduces cardiac efficiency. However, exercise can be harmful if you get an injury from it or if you carry it to such an extreme that you are burning your fat and filling your blood with ketones for a long period of time. It can also interfere with weight gain. Medical research is just beginning to study how much exercise is beneficial in pregnancy. So far, studies have been limited to mild and moderate exercises, and the studies show that these exercises have had positive results. For obvious reasons, human experiments that might injure the baby have been avoided, but reports from women who did this on their own supply some information. We need to learn what the limits on exercise are.

1552. What are some effective exercises I can do to stay in shape while I'm pregnant?

Any effective exercise you have been doing before pregnancy that cannot cause you an injury, as skiing might, is all right to continue unless you find it gives you too much discomfort. New sports are not recommended because of your lack of conditioning and possible awkwardness due to the bulge of pregnancy. If you have not been exercising before pregnancy, walking briskly is highly recommended. Stretching and relaxation exercises are taught in childbirth preparation classes, as well as by many fitness centers and athletic clubs that have programs designed for pregnant women. Manuals on pregnancy include these, too. Floor workouts (not on your stomach) are fine; tailor sits that spread your pelvis and even sit-ups are allowed until they become impossible. Leaning over to touch the floor with your hands is not recommended, because it strains your back in pregnancy and puts a lot of pressure on the baby.

NORMAL PREGNANCY AND CHOICES IN CHILDBIRTH:
EXERCISE (Continued)

1553. Are there any exercises that I could do that would make childbirth easier for me?

Yes. Relaxation exercises are taught in Lamaze and other classes to help you relax and focus on breathing for your first stage of labor, while your cervix is dilating. Tailor sits, which spread your pelvic area and help in bearing down, are also taught to help you in the second stage. These are all described in books, such as *Six Lessons for an Easier Childbirth,* by Elizabeth Bing. However, reading about them in books is still second best to attending classes.

1554. Are exercises that cause shortness of breath dangerous during pregnancy?

No, but your lungs may respond less in late pregnancy due to upward pressure from the uterus. Your heart also is taxed by the burden of circulating blood to the placenta and uterus and by the extra weight of pregnancy. You will experience shortness of breath with activity that previously did not bother you, but this is not harmful. If you are short of breath while at rest and not just during or after exercise, you should tell your doctor in order to be sure that your heart and lungs are not in trouble.

1555. Do women who are active in sports have easier deliveries?

Women who are active in sports do well in labor and vaginal delivery. Being active does not shorten the first stage of labor, but it may shorten the second stage. There was an old wives' tale that said such women became muscle bound and had a hard time having babies. That is not true. Exercise does not change the width of your bony pelvis. If it is too small, the baby will not come through, no matter what the exercise pattern.

1556. When should I discontinue strenuous exercise?

You should reduce strenuous exercise when you fail to gain weight or if you do not have a quick recovery from exhaustion. Such exercise also should be discontinued when the bouncing of the uterus or enlarged breasts makes it miserable, or when you become so awkward that you are liable to fall or become injured. Of course, with the onset of labor, all strenuous exercise should stop.

1557. Is it all right to jog or ride a bicycle during pregnancy?

Yes, especially if you are already accustomed to doing these things. Running long distances that exhausts you and burns fat into a state of ketones (a breakdown product of fat) or prevents weight gain has the danger

NORMAL PREGNANCY AND CHOICES IN CHILDBIRTH: EXERCISE (Continued)

of producing abnormalities in your baby. In the case of the lack of weight gain, it may also cause premature labor. This is especially dangerous if you were underweight when you began your pregnancy.

1558. Are active sports, such as bareback riding, water skiing, or racquetball, dangerous during pregnancy?

They are only dangerous because of the possibility of injuring yourself. When you are pregnant and do these things, you also risk injury to your baby. You could be hit in the abdomen by a racquet ball, thrown from a horse, or whacked with a water ski. If you can do these activities without an accident, they do not harm your baby. For instance, if you have a mild-tempered horse, horseback riding may be safer than riding in a car driven by an angry person.

1559. If I exercise before and during pregnancy, will my stomach go back into shape faster after my baby is born?

Yes, it will. The more tone and strength your muscles retain, the better they will work after delivery. However, you need to continue exercise then, too.

NORMAL PREGNANCY AND CHOICES IN CHILDBIRTH: MOST COMMON DISCOMFORTS

1560. What are the most common discomforts of pregnancy? Is there anything I can do to alleviate these discomforts?

Urinary frequency (voiding often) and breast tenderness are the two most common discomforts of pregnancy, and there is almost no relief available, except a convenient toilet and a good brassiere. Nausea and vomiting are next. Swelling and edema (fluid in the tissues) can occur in the early months, but 60 percent of women have these symptoms in the last three months. Brown spotting on the face, acne, and darker moles are annoying, but not uncomfortable. Pelvic cramps can occur throughout pregnancy, because the uterus contracts all the time. Heavier discharge is normal, but itching and burning discharge should be treated. Heartburn in late pregnancy is common and responds to antacids. Headaches in the first few months are commonly caused by low blood sugar and may respond to orange juice. In late pregnancy, headaches may be due to a rise in blood pressure and are abnormal. Backache during pregnancy is so common that it is almost normal. It can be relieved with special exercises and correct posture, especially when lifting. Pregnant women feel warmer, but that is not always bad. In the last few months, insomnia is usual. Sharp pelvic pain,

I am a prisoner
of my own body
My stomach is so huge
I cannot even put on my shoes
My thighs hurt so
I cannot walk
My legs cramp
I cannot stand still
The baby kicks my ribs
I cannot sit in a chair
I am so tired
I cannot finish most activities
I am so big and puffy
I hate to look at myself
My body is king
I am its helpless servant
But when the baby kicks
I forget about
being so uncomfortable
and I can't wait
for it to be
born

— Susan Polis Schutz

NORMAL PREGNANCY AND CHOICES IN CHILDBIRTH: MOST COMMON DISCOMFORTS (Continued)

when ligaments are pulled, can be relieved by kneeling in a knee-chest position. Leg cramps after four months can be relieved by taking extra calcium at bedtime, elevating the foot of the bed to help circulation, and antacids to help absorb calcium. Fainting can be quite common when there is standing, warmth, and lack of food. A maternity girdle helps prevent faint feelings in late pregnancy by preventing pooling of blood in the abdomen. Research shows pregnant women experience more nightmares as a response to crises. Feeling the baby kick can be more than distracting. Varicose veins are not really normal, but commonly cause increased leg aches. Discomfort with intercourse can be relieved by changing positions. Hemorrhoids with itching, pain, and bleeding are almost normal.

1561. Is it normal for my breasts to be tender during pregnancy?

Yes. Breast tenderness is almost the first sign of pregnancy, but it is confused with the breast tenderness that normally precedes menses. When your hormones are very high in the first three months of pregnancy, your nipples are particularly tender and your breasts enlarge and feel heavy. In late pregnancy this is felt again, although it may be less distracting during the middle months. The heaviness and the preparation for lactation (milk production) contribute to the discomfort.

1562. What is the substance that leaks out of my breasts that is not milk?

This is called colostrum. It is a watery substance that contains cells (lymphocytes), antibodies, and even protein, but it does not contain the fat globules that make it into milk. Colostrum looks clear or grey.

1563. Is it common for a woman's breasts to leak during pregnancy?

Yes, about 30 percent of women have spontaneous leakage from their nipples during pregnancy. You can wear little pads or even a tissue in your bra to catch it.

1564. Is there anything I could do to insure myself of firm breasts after pregnancy?

You could not gain much weight and not breast-feed, but eliminating both of these things is harmful to your baby. Wearing a brassiere does not help at all, it only makes your breasts look firm while it is worn. Exercises only improve posture; they do not change the breasts.

1565. What can I do about morning sickness, nausea, and vomiting?

If you consider that nausea of pregnancy is a condition due to a low blood sugar, instead of a mental state, you will be more successful in treating it. Eating small meals frequently, such as every two hours around the clock,

NORMAL PREGNANCY AND CHOICES IN CHILDBIRTH: MOST COMMON DISCOMFORTS (Continued)

can keep you from vomiting or even being nauseated. If what you eat contains enough carbohydrates to raise your blood sugar quickly, you get quick relief. If it has a little protein, too, the relief will last a little longer. But you cannot relieve the nausea with a high-protein diet, as you can when you are not pregnant. You must have some starch and sugar for your body to use quickly. You must avoid fats, because they are nauseating to the pregnant woman. Sweet drinks work very well, especially fruit juices, but avoid citrus drinks because they may irritate your stomach. If you cannot control vomiting with eating like this, ask your doctor for a medication to help control it. Bendectin was an approved treatment for nausea, but it is no longer being marketed as the result of a lawsuit that identified it as the cause of a baby being born with a deformed arm. Starvation and vomiting have affected babies and these are not better than taking a medication. If diet and medication do not work, it is better to be hospitalized than to lose more than ten pounds. Intravenous sugar-water will stop your nausea and your vomiting, but it is less expensive to stay at home and drink fruit juices. Many women also report that by taking vitamin B6 supplements daily they do not get nauseous.

1566. Why does vitamin B6 help to relieve morning sickness or nausea?

There seems to be a greater need for vitamin B6 during pregnancy. Perhaps taking a vitamin B6 supplement remedies the deficiency of B6 in the diet of pregnant women. It also probably helps to maintain the blood sugar level, which relieves the symptoms of nausea and morning sickness.

1567. How long does morning sickness usually last?

Usually morning sickness only lasts for about the first three months of pregnancy, although it is also fairly frequent in the fourth month. Sometimes it lasts until you correct your diet to control it. Morning sickness usually parallels the high levels of estrogen and progesterone seen in early pregnancy.

1568. What can I do about brown patches on my face during pregnancy?

You can prevent them by wearing a sunscreen or makeup with a sunscreen in it, if you know you are sun sensitive. If you already have brown patches on your face, you can fade them with fade creams, which are now sold over the counter. A constant application is necessary every night at bedtime, but this will not work unless you also apply a sunscreen during the daytime. This is especially important when you are in the water or on the beach in direct sun. A hat is also protective, and it is wise never to lie face-up in the sun.

NORMAL PREGNANCY AND CHOICES IN CHILDBIRTH: MOST COMMON DISCOMFORTS (Continued)

1569. What causes swelling of my hands and feet? How can I prevent it?

In early pregnancy, swelling is caused by a high estrogen level that retains water. In late pregnancy, the cause is the obstruction of the uterus, which interferes with circulation of blood returning from the legs. More water has to be retained to have enough pressure to circulate the blood upward. If you limit salt or take diuretics, you retain less water, but then the blood circulation to the baby is not as good. This is harmful to the baby, so today this practice is forbidden (although fifteen years ago it was recommended). Lying down helps circulation, and also the kidneys are able to get rid of water better when they are in a horizontal position. This works especially well if done at midday for an hour or so. Water retention is not harmful, does not lead to toxemia (a blood pressure disorder of late pregnancy), and does not have to be treated or prevented. You just can't get your shoes or rings on, so you are advised to remove rings before you have to cut them off.

1570. Why do I always feel hot when I am pregnant?

Your metabolic rate rises when you are pregnant, and you really do run a higher temperature, but not over 99°. Usually you have more dilated blood vessels at the surface of your skin, so it feels warm. The extra weight from fat and fluids acts as insulation against the cold. Thirty percent of pregnant women even have hot flushes, like women in menopause, but these are due to chorionic, instead of pituitary gonadotropins. These are hormones that come from the placenta, instead of from the pituitary gland.

1571. Do I have to be constipated and get hemorrhoids while I'm pregnant?

No, but these symptoms are quite common. Some people inherit a tendency for hemorrhoids and develop them no matter what they do. They frequently occur during and after the strain of pregnancy. Eating bran may help to avoid the hard stools that produce hemorrhoids during bowel movements. Some people have better results from eating fruit. Others need a stool softener, which is available over the counter. It has many brand names and comes in a capsule form, to be taken once per day. Sometimes this is included in your prenatal vitamins, because constipation is so common. Laxatives just make the situation worse.

1572. Will hemorrhoids go away?

No, but they will get better within six weeks after delivery. If they still bother you after that time, a hemorrhoidectomy (removal of hemorrhoids by surgery) can be performed.

NORMAL PREGNANCY AND CHOICES IN CHILDBIRTH: MOST COMMON DISCOMFORTS (Continued)

1573. Why did my belly button (umbilicus) enlarge and protrude when I was pregnant? Could I prevent that?

You could only prevent it by preventing pregnancy. You must have been born with an umbilical hernia that closed when you were a baby, but under the pressure of the enlarging uterus came open again. This allowed it to balloon out as the abdominal wall was stretched. You can have a surgical repair if it still bothers you, but it is not dangerous.

1574. Is there any truth to the old wives' tale that a woman's teeth "go bad" during or after pregnancy?

There is no reason for your teeth to go bad, unless you neglect them because you are so busy with other cares. The calcium in your teeth does not leave them during pregnancy, although it does leave the bones of your body. The condition of your gums can get rather bad in pregnancy, but they will recover afterwards. If you fail to get your teeth cleaned or see a dentist regularly, you may have trouble with your teeth. If you continue to take proper care of your teeth, they will not change during pregnancy.

NORMAL PREGNANCY AND CHOICES IN CHILDBIRTH: STRETCH MARKS (STRIAE)

1575. Can I avoid stretch marks by limiting weight gain during pregnancy?

No. You can only avoid stretch marks by not getting pregnant. Weight gain does not cause them and weight control does not diminish them. They are an inherited, defective elastic tissue layer in the skin that causes the skin to break instead of stretch. They should be called break marks; medically they are called striae. If you did not inherit them, nothing you do will give them to you; if you did, nothing stops them. They are red and purple during pregnancy, but fade to white later. Studies to find a prevention for stretch marks have been done on everything you can think of: oils, creams, vitamin E, cocoa butter, lanolin, olive oil, sunshine, and tanning. Regardless of the treatment, the percentage of women who get stretch marks remains the same, so don't bother trying to prevent them. If the stretching skin itches, lanolin creams will help reduce the itching, but that is all.

NORMAL PREGNANCY AND CHOICES IN CHILDBIRTH: VARICOSE VEINS

1576. How can I prevent varicose veins?

You really can't prevent varicose veins, but you probably won't develop any during pregnancy if you did not inherit the tendency to get them. With a strong family trait, even men get varicose veins. Pregnancy cer-

NORMAL PREGNANCY AND CHOICES IN CHILDBIRTH: VARICOSE VEINS (Continued)

tainly increases your chances of getting them, so avoiding pregnancy will help you avoid varicose veins. They will improve within six weeks following delivery, perhaps to the point at which you can forget about them. Wearing support hose or elastic hose brings comfort to aching legs, but does nothing to prevent the increase in varicose veins during pregnancy. Surgical removal of veins by stripping must not be done during pregnancy, because of the extra bleeding it causes. This procedure can be done between babies or after childbearing is over. However, it should not be done for cosmetic reasons, because the scars can look just as unsightly as the varicose veins do. It is done for comfort, to relieve aching legs, or because the veins are so bad that the skin is breaking down.

NORMAL PREGNANCY AND CHOICES IN CHILDBIRTH: THINGS TO AVOID DURING PREGNANCY

1577. What things should I avoid during pregnancy?
There is a general practice in our society of forbidding things to pregnant women, sometimes without reason. In the past, women could not work, appear in a classroom, exercise, go to the beach, or even appear in public when they were pregnant. Sex was forbidden and they weren't even supposed to experience excitement or emotions. Now all of these rights have been restored, but there is a new list of things to avoid. The list follows; you must decide if you will comply.

Cigarettes: Smoking is probably the worst thing you can do to your unborn baby. While you are smoking, the blood vessels to the placenta clamp down and interfere with your blood circulation; this can clearly be shown on a thermogram. Cigarette smoking interferes with the nutrition of the baby. Of those women who smoke ten or more cigarettes per day, there is an increase in the number of premature babies (some fatal) and small babies born at term, who are less able to cope with problems. There is an increase in abruption of placenta (the placenta separating from the uterine wall and bleeding), causing labor and sometimes loss of the baby. Since cigarettes are also harmful to you, leading to lung cancer, bronchitis, heart attacks, ulcers, high blood pressure, cardiac irregularities, bladder cancer, even osteoporosis (thinning of the bones), it is obvious that it would be best to stop smoking, whether you are pregnant or not. The nausea of early pregnancy is increased by smoking, so it makes it easier to stop smoking at that time.

Alcohol: Most people are considered alcoholics if they have five or more cocktails per day. Alcoholic women have babies who are born with fetal alcohol syndrome (small, mentally retarded babies, with malformed

NORMAL PREGNANCY AND CHOICES IN CHILDBIRTH: THINGS TO AVOID DURING PREGNANCY (Continued)

ears and wide set eyes who resemble people who are alcoholics). If heavy drinking does this, what would light drinking do? Probably a little alcohol is not harmful, if you can stop there. Drinking during pregnancy has had such publicity that your associates will frown if you look pregnant and drink, but the most important time to drink in moderation is before you even know you are pregnant. If you are trying to get pregnant, don't drink much, or you will feel guilty if there is a defect in your baby.

Medications: It is simple to say, "Avoid all medications, except those that your doctor prescribes," but if your head is splitting, your nose is running, or your heartburn or backache is killing you, you want relief. Aspirin is not recommended; first, because it has caused cleft palates in rats, and second, because it has caused bleeding disorders in babies. Acetaminophen (Tylenol and other nonaspirin pain killers) has not been found harmful, and it can provide pain relief. Pregnant women can become addicted to nasal sprays, but they are harmless to their babies, so they can be used for a short time with a cold. Antihistamines and decongestants are under suspicion, at least for the first three months of pregnancy. Antacids are harmless and can be used for heartburn. For all other medications, you must check with your doctor. When you have a serious disorder, it is better to use medication and to stay alive and well, almost regardless of the medication's effect on your baby, but the least harmful one will be chosen. If another doctor prescribes a medication for you, you can cross-check the medication with your obstetrician to be certain it is safe for your baby. There are books about medications for doctors to consult that state which drugs are harmful when used during pregnancy; you also could purchase one of these books in most local bookstores.

X-rays: Routine X-rays are not advised, in order to minimize all radiation, but if you need dental X-rays, a lead apron can protect your abdomen. If you need X-rays for a serious problem, such as a broken hip, you must take the X-ray and solve the problem, but use the least radiation possible. The damage from diagnostic X-rays to the baby is only theoretical. The known damage to unborn babies comes from treatment radiation, such as radium, which produces babies with small heads (microcephaly). At least ten rads (radiation absorbed doses) are required to do this; diagnostic X-rays don't reach this level.

Immunizations: If possible, you should avoid routine immunizations while you are pregnant. This is because it is thought best not to activate antibody reactions in general, since they might increase blood-type antibody

NORMAL PREGNANCY AND CHOICES IN CHILDBIRTH: THINGS TO AVOID DURING PREGNANCY (Continued)

reactions for the baby. Live vaccines could also pass the live virus to the baby, who cannot produce antibodies and might suffer. However, having a tetanus booster is better than having the tetanus, if you are in danger. Similarly, if you are traveling to a country where you will be exposed to cholera, it is better to be immunized against cholera than to contract the infection.

Infections: German measles (rubella) is a disaster to the baby if you contract it in the first eight weeks of pregnancy, affecting more than half of babies with blindness, deafness, and mental retardation. Up to the sixteenth week, the effect is still present, but affects less than half of babies. If you are not immune, stay away from children with rashes. Immunize your other children, since you can't stay away from them. Immunize yourself at least three months before you get pregnant, if you are not immune, especially if you are a teacher who is exposed to this epidemic every spring. Other infections are less disastrous, but any illness that gives you a fever of 103° or more can affect the formation of your baby's nervous system. Colds seldom do this, but flu can. If you have a fever, keep it down with acetaminophen (Tylenol or other nonaspirin pain killers) and cooling measures. Do not volunteer to care for sick people, other than your family members, while you are pregnant. Toxoplasmosis is a disease that can harm the baby without harming you. You can get it from your cat by handling kitty litter, so get a cat door or have someone else empty the litter. You also can get it through eating raw meat, such as in steak tartar.

Jacuzzis and saunas: Research has shown some defects in the nervous systems of babies born to women whose temperatures rose to 103° in a sauna, causing them to faint. Moderation is advised; you really should not use a sauna while you are pregnant. No cases of defective nervous systems have been found in babies born to women who use jacuzzis, but you will see a sign above public ones forbidding pregnant women to enter. If you do not allow your temperature to rise too high, it is not harmful. When pregnant, you faint more easily if you get too warm, so don't go alone, because if you faint, you could drown.

Using common sense will help you to decide many of the things you should avoid during pregnancy; many of them should be avoided even when you are not pregnant. You might be careless with yourself, but when you are pregnant you are responsible for another human being: your baby. You should want to do everything possible to insure that the baby is born healthy.

NORMAL PREGNANCY AND CHOICES IN CHILDBIRTH: INJURIES AND ACCIDENTS

1578. How dangerous are falls, injuries, and accidents during pregnancy?

Falls are not as likely to cause a miscarriage as fiction would have you believe. However, if you have a serious fall after the sixth month of pregnancy and your uterus absorbs much of the blow instead of your hands and knees, it can literally knock the placenta off the uterine wall. This causes bleeding behind the placenta, violent labor, and loss of the baby. If you just break a leg, there is potential danger in the anesthesia and medical treatment you may require to have it set. However, most of the accidental injuries to babies come from automobile accidents in which the pregnant woman goes through a windshield. If you use your seatbelt, it will prevent this, but sometimes the seatbelt is worn incorrectly and can itself cause pressure to the uterus. The seatbelt should be positioned in the fold of your legs (the groin), so that it does not lie over the baby. A shoulder strap is needed, too. There is no activity that is harmful to pregnancy, unless it leads to bodily injury, which can lead to the loss of the baby. For this reason, dangerous sports are frowned upon. Unfortunately, our most dangerous activity is automobile riding.

1579. How well protected from injury is my baby in my womb?

In the first three months of pregnancy, the fetus is within the body pelvis and cannot be damaged, even with a blow to the abdomen. For the next six months, after the baby rises into the abdomen, a blow directly to the abdomen can injure the baby or its placenta. However, your baby is in a water bag, which spreads the pressure out like a hydraulic suit, so the blow would have to be severe for the baby to be injured.

NORMAL PREGNANCY AND CHOICES IN CHILDBIRTH: SEX, DURING AND AFTER PREGNANCY; BIRTH CONTROL AFTER PREGNANCY

1580. Do I have to avoid sexual intercourse if I want my baby to be the best it can be?

No. If everything is normal in your pregnancy, you can enjoy intercourse right up to the time you start labor or your water breaks, whichever happens first. After that, infection can be introduced, so you should stop all sexual intercourse until after delivery when your doctor tells you it is all right. If you have an abnormal pregnancy, such as threatened premature labor or bleeding in the last few months of pregnancy from a placenta previa (placenta covering the cervix) or abruption of placenta (premature separation of the placenta), then you should be at rest and, particularly, should avoid sex. This applies to very few people. The vast majority of women need

NORMAL PREGNANCY AND CHOICES IN CHILDBIRTH: SEX, DURING AND AFTER PREGNANCY; BIRTH CONTROL AFTER PREGNANCY (Continued)

the reassurance of love provided by sexual intercourse, and they need to enjoy the release from tension that it brings. Positions may need to be changed for comfort and to prevent too much pressure on your abdomen. Studies are still being published that suggest women who have intercourse during pregnancy have more infections in their pregnancies, but these studies fail to mention that these infections are sexually transmitted. If your partner gives you a venereal disease during pregnancy, then it does become dangerous for your baby, but if he has sex only with you during this time, you will not have this danger. Sexual intercourse also is frequently accused of causing miscarriages, but this is not true. Chromosome abnormalities and other types of defective fetuses cause miscarriages. Of course, if you are nauseated, vomiting, tired, or uncomfortable, you may not want to participate in sex until you feel better. After delivery, the bleeding, stitches, and danger of infection make sexual intercourse not very safe until about three weeks have passed, and everything has healed.

1581. How long after childbirth must I wait before resuming sexual intercourse?

As long as you are bleeding, it is easy to become infected, so sexual intercourse is usually not advised. Until your stitches heal, it could be most uncomfortable as well. They could be torn open if you try this before ten days have passed, which is the length of time it usually takes for stitches to heal. Most women bleed very little three weeks after delivery, but it is best to have an examination to be certain everything is healed and normal before you have sex again. This way you also can obtain contraceptives. It is possible to conceive in the month after a baby is born, so don't leave out contraception even if you are breast-feeding. Sexual intercourse may cause the vagina to feel very tender if you are breast-feeding. This is due to having little or no estrogen during that time, so the vagina becomes thin, dry, and tender. A lubricant will not alleviate the tenderness, but a little estrogen cream used twice a week can return the vagina to proper condition for sexual activity. Ask your doctor for some, especially if your vagina is quite tender after your first resumption of sex. Do not blame all of your discomfort on your stitches; even women with cesarean sections, in which the stitches are on the abdomen, hurt after sexual intercourse while they are breast-feeding. If you take large amounts of estrogen, you can suppress your breast milk, but a little cream will not suppress it. Using the cream is something you can do for your husband, who has stood by you all these months. He does not want to hurt you, but it would reassure him if you could have sexual intercourse.

NORMAL PREGNANCY AND CHOICES IN CHILDBIRTH: SEX, DURING AND AFTER PREGNANCY; BIRTH CONTROL AFTER PREGNANCY (Continued)

1582. When should I start using birth control again?

You should start using birth control methods before you have sexual intercourse. All forms of birth control are available to you; even an IUD (intrauterine device) can be inserted six weeks after your delivery. The low-dose birth control pills (minipills) will not suppress your breast-milk or in any way be harmful to your baby. Diaphragms must be refitted, because your vagina may have been stretched. Breast-feeding may be contraceptive for a while, but ceases its protection when your menses return, your baby sleeps six hours, you replace one feeding with other food, or six months have passed.

NORMAL PREGNANCY AND CHOICES IN CHILDBIRTH: AMNIOTIC FLUID

1583. What is amniotic fluid made of?

Urine from the baby makes up most of the amniotic fluid. It also may contain some cells from the baby's skin, fetal saliva, secretions from its lungs, and, on some occasions, meconium (baby feces), which turns it green.

NORMAL PREGNANCY AND CHOICES IN CHILDBIRTH: FEELING THE BABY MOVE

1584. When should I feel the baby move?

At approximately the fourth month you can begin to feel flutters inside, but it will be about 4½ months (or twenty weeks) from the beginning of your last menses before you will be able to feel a kick on your abdomen with your hand.

1585. How much movement is normal?

Movement is detected more in the sixth, seventh, and eighth months of pregnancy and then less in the ninth month, when there is less amniotic fluid to give the baby room to move. On the average, if you are quiet for ten minutes, you can note six motions.

1586. Should I worry if I don't feel the baby move very much?

Worry is seldom helpful, but if you do not clearly feel the baby move for a day, you should let your doctor check to see that it is all right. This will either reassure you that the baby is all right, or it will make it possible to run tests to confirm fetal death, if movement has really stopped.

NORMAL PREGNANCY AND CHOICES IN CHILDBIRTH: FACTORS AFFECTING THE BABY'S WEIGHT

1587. What factors affect the weight of my baby?

The weight of your baby is something that really can be controlled by what you do, because to a great extent the size of your baby depends upon your weight gain while you are pregnant. It also depends upon your size when you became pregnant. To a much lesser extent, size is inherited from the baby's mother and father. In general, larger babies survive better and have a greater chance of achieving higher intelligence than smaller babies. Even though a smaller baby would seem easier to carry around for nine months and to deliver, smaller babies are usually more difficult after they are born, because they eat and sleep only a little. They also become ill more easily and are less resistant to heat and cold. Convenience during pregnancy and delivery is not worth the problems you may have for the next twenty years if the baby is so small that it does not develop well.

NORMAL PREGNANCY AND CHOICES IN CHILDBIRTH: DETERMINING THE SEX OF THE CHILD

1588. At what point in pregnancy is the sex of the fetus determined?

Sex is determined at fertilization when the sperm enters the egg, carrying either an X or Y sex chromosome. The egg has only an X chromosome. The fetus does not look like a male or female until the fourth month of pregnancy, when the scrotum closes and the penis enlarges in males, or the vagina opens and the vulvae form below a small clitoris in females.

1589. Is there any way to determine the sex of my child before it is born?

Yes. Sonograms taken in mid to late pregnancy can suggest the sex of the fetus if the shadow of the penis and scrotum is seen, but this is usually uncertain. Amniocentesis actually obtains a picture of the chromosomes, showing XX (a girl) or XY (a boy), so there is no doubt as to the sex of the child. It is the most accurate way of determining the sex of your child.

1590. Does the way I carry my baby (high or low) have anything to do with the baby's sex?

The way you carry your baby has very little to do with the baby's sex. It has more to do with how strong your abdominal muscles are. If they are weak, they sag even with a little baby. A big baby will make them sag more, and on the average, boy babies are one-half pound heavier than girls. If you guess that larger babies will be boys, you will be correct a little more than half of the time. Tossing a coin works almost as well.

NORMAL PREGNANCY AND CHOICES IN CHILDBIRTH: GENES

1591. What are genes?

Genes are small units of a specially formed chemical that, by their patterns, carry the information of inheritance that gives us our characteristics. There are thousands of genes on one chromosome.

1592. What role do genes play in how my child will look?

The size of your baby depends primarily on your nutrition and health, while the shape and features of the baby's appearance are controlled by the genes. All characteristics that are inherited, such as eye color, hair, shape of mouth, ears, skin color, and even emotional make-up, are controlled by genes.

NORMAL PREGNANCY AND CHOICES IN CHILDBIRTH: BIRTH DEFECTS, TRYING TO PREVENT THEM

1593. What causes birth defects in babies?

Many causes of birth defects are unknown. Genes that are inherited can cause birth defects, which are repeated within families, or they can form in a baby for the first time and cause a defect. This probably is due to the background radiation that we all experience, and which accumulates as we grow older. Infections, such as syphilis, gonorrhea, chlamydial infection, rubella (German measles), herpes, and toxoplasmosis can cause defects; each has its own special problem. Uncontrolled diabetes causes many more than the average number of defects, but the chances of this happening are reduced when your blood sugar is strictly controlled for two months before you get pregnant. Alcohol abuse, especially when it is excessive, can cause the fetal alcohol syndrome. Vitamin deficiencies and excesses cause defects in experimental animals and also may cause them in people. Certain drugs can cause defects; more knowledge is being gained about this all the time. High fevers of 103 ° or more, or even the high temperature of a sauna, have caused central nervous system defects. There are even studies that show a higher incidence of babies born with low I.Q.s following a particulary hot summer. Some researchers believe men's clothing keeps their testicles too warm, which produces defective sperm or sperm that cause defective genes. Obesity in men has the same effect on the testicles. Accidents can cause defects; an example is a traumatic rupture of the lining of the amniotic sac, forming strings that bind around a developing limb and stop its growth. Fetal position, such as a breech (buttocks first), can flatten the baby's head against the top of the uterus, or the legs can be held in a position that forms dislocated hips. All this does not even include defects such as deafness, cerebral palsy, and many others, that occur simply because the baby is born very premature.

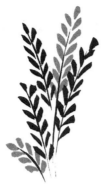

Will our baby
have sky-blue eyes
that examine
and understand
and that melt
with sensitivity
like his father
Will our baby
get lost in
his own genius
concentrating and
deciphering
new subjects
like his father
Will our baby
appreciate the solitude and beauty
of the outdoors
like his father
Will our baby
face and conquer
every challenge
becoming stronger and
wiser with each
like his father
Will our baby
be as
truthful and
good and
honest and
gentle and
unselfish and
loving and
beautiful
as his
father
— Susan Polis Schutz

NORMAL PREGNANCY AND CHOICES IN CHILDBIRTH: BIRTH DEFECTS, TRYING TO PREVENT THEM (Continued)

Lack of oxygen, at any time during pregnancy or after delivery, can also cause brain damage and cerebral palsy. Although not all of these defects occur at the time of delivery, this can be a traumatic time for the baby.

1594. What are the chances of having a child born with serious birth defects?

The general population has a 2-3 percent chance of having babies born with a major birth defect. If you or your husband have defects in your families, your chances may be much higher. You will need a genetic study and counseling to determine what your chances are.

1595. Can I control whether or not my child will be born with birth defects?

Yes, you can control it to some extent, but not absolutely or perfectly. Controlling birth defects requires knowledge and effort on your part, plus medical teamwork to accomplish it. Prevention of birth defects would be better than prenatal diagnosis and abortion, but it is not always possible.

1596. What percentage of babies that are aborted spontaneously would have been born with birth defects?

Through chromosome studies it has been proven that 60 percent of the babies that were aborted spontaneously would have been born with birth defects. If there were a way to study the balance of them, it probably could be proven that these babies also would have been born with defects. Miscarriage is a fairly good screening mechanism for eliminating birth defects from the population; however, 2-3 percent of babies are still born with a defect.

1597. What are the most common birth defects in children today?

The following are the most common birth defects, given in order of frequency and regardless of whether they are a major or minor problem (frequencies shown are the rate per 1,000):

13.50 Inguinal hernia	1.89 Pyloric stenosis (obstruction of small intestines)
8.04 Heart defects	
7.36 Extra fingers	1.83 Dislocated hip
3.80 Club foot	1.45 Hydrocephaly (water pressure in the head)
3.74 Hypospadias (urethra opens low on penis)	
	1.40 Ureteral obstruction (dilated ureter, kidney)
3.38 Cleft lip, gum, and/or palate	
	1.40 Pectus excavatum (chest depression)
2.74 Benign tumors	
2.49 Syndactylism (webbed fingers or toes)	1.01 Umbilical hernia
	1.01 Undersized limb
2.20 Urethral obstruction	.88 Cataract

NORMAL PREGNANCY AND CHOICES IN CHILDBIRTH: BIRTH DEFECTS, TRYING TO PREVENT THEM (Continued)

.80 Anencephaly (no brain)

.76 Skin tag on ear

.70 Meningomyelocele (spinal cord defect)

.66 Polycystic kidney

.64 Agenesis of lung (no lung)

.60 Absent limb

.60 Craniosynostosis (head bones closed)

.52 Malformed lung

.52 Adrenal atrophy

.52 Anal atresia (closed anus)

.52 Malignant tumor (cancer)

1598. What steps can I take to prevent birth defects and insure the good health and development of my baby?

You can select the father of your child from a family who has no known defects. You can ask your own family about defective children in your family history, so you can get proper genetic counseling. You should get proper tests for the defects known to exist in either of your families. Marry a young man, because those over forty-five years of age have more defective children, even if you are young. Make him wear boxer shorts and avoid hot baths and saunas, so that his sperm will not be defective. Seek prenatal care as early in pregnancy as possible and follow advice given to you by your doctor. Avoid radiation, at least until after you have had your children, except when necessary to maintain good health. Take care of your health and avoid infections, including herpes. Two months before you get pregnant, have a medical checkup and review any medication that you are using. Stop, or at least limit, smoking, drinking alcohol, and consuming caffeine. Good nutrition is important for at least two months before you become pregnant, and so is being near your normal weight. If you are diabetic, make certain this is under control. Take vitamins, expecially those with folic acid, for two months before pregnancy. Folic acid is thought to prevent neural tube defects (spinal column and brain). Avoid any fevers or excessive heat, especially in early pregnancy, and have all medications approved by your obstetrician. Do not allow vomiting or weight loss to continue for very long. Avoid injury and all infections during pregnancy. Exercise with moderation. Provide good nutrition. Arrange for good obstetrical care in a good hospital, and do all you can to make labor and delivery easy for your baby. Prepare for natural childbirth, so you can avoid medications, but if medication becomes necessary, accept regional anesthetic, for the sake of your baby, when it is recommended. If you and your husband are Jewish, get a blood test for Tay-Sachs disease (a degenerative disease in children causing blindness, mental retardation, and death by the age of three or four), preferably before you are pregnant. Plan an amniocentesis if genetic counseling suggests it or you are over thirty-five years old. This a test in

NORMAL PREGNANCY AND CHOICES IN CHILDBIRTH: BIRTH DEFECTS, TRYING TO PREVENT THEM (Continued)

which fluid is taken from around the baby to find out what kind of chromosomes it has, so you can have an abortion if the baby is defective. The fluid is also tested for alpha-fetoprotein, which can show spinal cord defects. The ultrasound, which is used during amniocentesis to control where the doctor places the needle to get the fluid, also can show a major defect in the formation of the baby. Even if you don't have an amniocentesis, you can have a blood test for alpha-fetoprotein or an ultrasound examination to look for visible defects at about the fifteenth week of pregnancy.

1599. What is the testing called that is available to pregnant women who have a disease to let them know if their child will be born with the same disease? How is it done?

This is called prenatal testing. When testing for sickle-cell anemia, this entails taking some blood or amniotic fluid from the baby, and performing a test to see if the baby has that form of anemia. Other diseases have special tests, too. Chromosomal disorders can be detected by amniocentesis and a culture of the cells that shed from the baby's skin.

NORMAL PREGNANCY AND CHOICES IN CHILDBIRTH: AMNIOCENTESIS

1600. What is amniocentesis?

Amniocentesis is a test performed on amniotic fluid to determine the chromosomes of the unborn baby.

1601. Who should have an amniocentesis performed?

If you will be over thirty-five years old at the time your baby is born or if genetic counseling about defects in your family suggests it would be a good idea, then you should plan an amniocentesis. If hemophilia (a blood disease) affects the men in your family, you could be a carrier and your sons may be born with it. In this situation, you can have an amniocentesis to find out if the baby is a girl or a boy. To prevent hemophilia, you could abort the baby if it is a boy. Without the test, you might be afraid of having children at all. Most amniocenteses are performed because the woman is over thirty-five.

1602. How is amniocentesis performed?

Usually in early pregnancy, a sonogram picture is taken, or some other method is used to determine the date that you will be fifteen weeks pregnant. At that time, under the guidance of an ultrasound machine, a needle is placed through your abdominal wall into an area of fluid in the uterus. The fluid is withdrawn and sent to the laboratory for study. A little

NORMAL PREGNANCY AND CHOICES IN CHILDBIRTH: AMNIOCENTESIS (Continued)

local anesthetic may be injected into the skin prior to the needle being inserted.

1603. When is it given?

The fluid needed for the test can be obtained at about the fifteenth or sixteenth week of pregnancy. Before that time, there is such a small amount of fluid that it would be too hard to find it with a needle. Amniocentesis can be done after the fifteenth week, of course, but since it takes two or three weeks to culture the cells, you could be more than twenty weeks pregnant when an abortion is decided upon. Generally, it is preferable to do an abortion by the twentieth week of pregnancy, because after that time, the fetus is possibly capable of surviving outside the uterus.

1604. Does amniocentesis hurt?

All needles hurt. Even the needle used to inject an anesthetic into the skin hurts a little. Sometimes the needle being inserted into the uterus hurts, too. But the main fear isn't pain, it is inserting a needle so near an unborn baby.

1605. What are the risks involved in amniocentesis? How many women have problems?

Even using ultrasound to see the baby with experienced doctors inserting the needle, about one in two hundred women nationwide lose their babies because of complications. The needle can hit a blood vessel in the cord of the placenta, and the baby bleeds right then. It can cause bleeding in the uterine wall or behind the placenta that causes labor or premature separation of the placenta. Infection can occur, even though sterile technique is used. Much more rarely, the needle will touch the baby itself and leave a mark that is visible at the time of birth. Sometimes the procedure simply can't be done because of technical difficulties, especially when the placenta is on the side of the uterus nearest to the abdominal wall.

NORMAL PREGNANCY AND CHOICES IN CHILDBIRTH: ULTRASOUND TESTING

1606. What is ultrasound testing?

An ultrasound machine gives you a sonogram, a picture of your baby, on a screen. Sound waves are bounced off the baby and all its tissues, and the results are projected on a screen, either as a still shot or as a moving image. The baby's head can be measured, the heart chambers and valves observed, and the brain, liver, kidneys, lungs, and all the major organs can be viewed. If the legs of the fetus are spread just right and if a penis and scrotum are visible or labia can be identified, the sex of the baby can also be determined.

**NORMAL PREGNANCY AND CHOICES IN CHILDBIRTH:
ULTRASOUND TESTING** (Continued)

1607. How accurate is ultrasound?

The picture on the screen is shadows, and these have to be interpreted cautiously. The experience of the machine's operator has a lot to do with the interpretation. Things can be missed and problems can be exaggerated, but the results are improving all the time, as the machine and experience with it improves.

1608. Is ultrasound testing good for my baby?

Ultrasound can benefit your baby in many ways. Ultrasound can indicate the extent of the baby's development, and thus prevent a decision to deliver the baby too prematurely. It is safer than using X-rays to determine if the position of the baby is breech. It can show problems of blocked kidneys, so that surgery to relieve the blockage can be performed, even before the baby is born. In that case, it can really save the life of your baby. This is called surgery in utero. Of course, if the ultrasound shows a serious defect, it can lead to abortion. Severely affected babies have been known to sue later in life for "wrongful life," because they were born with defects, which could have been detected and an abortion could have been performed.

1609. How safe is a sonogram for me and my unborn baby?

Sonograms have been in general use for ten or fifteen years, and no damage of any kind has been found in mothers or babies who have had them. They are much safer than X-rays, which were previously used for many of the same purposes. The total amount of ultrasound that can be given safely is not known. Therefore, ultrasound machines are used at the lowest dosage and smallest time interval necessary to accomplish the needed examination; a high dosage should never be reached. Safety studies in animals do not show damage from sonograms. One large study of pregnant women having sonograms seemed to show that they had smaller babies on the average, but this was due to the fact that the studies were made on women with medical and obstetrical problems, which usually do result in smaller, premature babies. The average would be expected to be lower in these women than in women who were without problems. In this country ultrasound is not routinely used on every pregnancy, but is frequently used to find and solve problems. In some countries, laws have been passed that require every woman to have at least two ultrasound examinations while they are pregnant.

1610. My doctor told me that because we don't know the risk of sonograms, he wasn't going to order one for me. He said, "We thought DES was safe, too." Do you agree?

The use of ultrasound in the clinical practice of medicine is generally

NORMAL PREGNANCY AND CHOICES IN CHILDBIRTH: ULTRASOUND TESTING (Continued)

considered not to inflict a hazard on the patient. Although no definite risk is known, the intensities of the sound waves are kept as low as practical to still receive a good image of the desired organs. Studies on the risks of sonograms have not yet been done, and it will be many years before they are available. The safety standards, therefore, are simply to minimize the acoustical (sound) exposure to the patient. If you wait for the safety reports on sonogram, you may be beyond the childbearing years, so you must weigh any possible unknown risks of the procedure against the present benefits to be obtained.

1611. I'm going to have my third sonogram. Have I hurt my baby?

No. There is no evidence at the present time to indicate that having several sonograms will hurt your baby. If you have had three of them, there must be a very good reason.

NORMAL PREGNANCY AND CHOICES IN CHILDBIRTH: TOXEMIA (ECLAMPSIA)

1612. What is toxemia?

Toxemia is a disorder of pregnancy that most often occurs in the last three months. The symptoms are high blood pressure that was not present previously; large quantities of protein (albumin) in the urine, often with severe edema (swelling); and, worst of all, convulsions. This condition can be so difficult for the baby that it does not grow well and sometimes dies before it is born. Maternal deaths have also occurred, although they occur less often than deaths of the baby, usually happening when the convulsions are not controlled or when there is a cerebral hemorrhage. Delivery is the best cure for toxemia, but the baby may be born prematurely.

1613. Is there anything I can do to keep from getting toxemia?

Since the specific cause of toxemia is not known, it is hard to say exactly what to do to prevent it. There is much less toxemia in women who receive good prenatal care and who have a good income with a high standard of living. This may be because these women are generally well nourished and well cared for. Some studies show that improvement in diet decreases toxemia of pregnancy. Doctors used to think that avoiding weight gain and going on a low-salt diet to avoid swelling would avoid toxemia. This is no longer held to be true, and now no limit is set on weight gain or salt intake.

NORMAL PREGNANCY AND CHOICES IN CHILDBIRTH: X-RAYS DURING PREGNANCY

1614. My doctor has scheduled me for an X-ray while I am pregnant. Isn't that dangerous for my baby?

If you have a problem that your doctor wants to diagnose with an X-ray, you should have it done, because the danger of the problem is probably far greater than any theoretical danger of an X-ray. It takes 10 rads (usually ten X-rays) to produce a known change in the fetus. One X-ray will not do that. In general, routine X-rays are no longer performed, because they radiate the reproductive organs of the baby and the mother. This is done in an attempt to keep the total life radiation down, not because there is recorded damage from diagnostic X-rays. The damage comes from treatment radiation, which uses 4,000 rads.

NORMAL PREGNANCY AND CHOICES IN CHILDBIRTH: ABNORMAL SYMPTOMS OF PREGNANCY

1615. What are some abnormal symptoms of pregnancy? Which ones require my calling a doctor?

Bleeding should always be reported to your doctor, even if it is not severe, because it may indicate other problems. Nosebleeds and bleeding hemorrhoids can be so severe that they produce anemia. Vaginal bleeding and cramps can mean a miscarriage in early months or a separation of the placenta in later months. Both situations need the immediate attention of a doctor. Severe vomiting with weight loss may require hospitalization for treatment. Spotting and severe pelvic or abdominal pain, especially if it is sudden, should be reported immediately, as it can indicate an ectopic pregnancy (fertilization of the egg outside the uterus) with internal bleeding requiring surgery. An average of eighty-two women per year die from ectopic pregnancies because they don't receive surgical help in time. Severe headaches and seeing bright stars, perhaps with vomiting, can lead to convulsions due to toxemia in late pregnancy. A rare occurrence in the fourth or fifth month is a molar pregnancy, where no fetus forms and grape-like cysts can be passed from the vagina, resulting in a miscarriage. Premature labor contractions are difficult to tell from normal contractions, but if they are strong and regular, they should be reported to your doctor within two hours. The bag of waters can break at any time after the third month, so if the water running down your leg is not urine, it should be reported immediately. On rare occasions, the entire bag of waters, which looks like a clear sac, balloons out of the vagina due to a damaged cervix opening up without labor, usually prematurely. If the water has broken, the cord can fall out, and you would see a blue rope hanging out in a loop. Fever, especially 102° or more, should

NORMAL PREGNANCY AND CHOICES IN CHILDBIRTH: ABNORMAL SYMPTOMS OF PREGNANCY (Continued)

be reported no matter what the cause. In childbirth education classes, you will learn all about the signs of labor and when to call your doctor. Usually when strong contractions occur every three to five minutes, or sometimes just closer than ten minutes, they must be reported to your doctor. Any other illness during pregnancy, such as diarrhea, deserves treatment, and you should at least inform your obstetrician of the problem. Unless you know you are immune, a red rash that might be rubella (German measles) must be reported to your doctor so tests can be done to diagnose it. Severe, persistent pain in the back of your legs could be phlebitis (blood clotting), and it also must be reported.

NORMAL PREGNANCY AND CHOICES IN CHILDBIRTH: PREMATURE DELIVERY

1616. How can I help to prevent a premature delivery?

Recent studies have shown that one of the best ways you can prevent premature delivery is to learn the signs of premature labor, report them immediately to your doctor, and go to the hospital so measures can be taken to stop the labor before it has gone past the point of no return. Another way you can help is to avoid the factors that tend to induce premature delivery. One of these is being underweight at the onset of pregnancy. Another is the lack of sufficient weight gain during pregnancy or the lack of good nutrition. Urine infections also have been blamed for premature labor, so signs of infection should be reported to your doctor and treated diligently. Even severe diarrhea and strong laxatives can cause labor, so treat diarrhea and avoid laxatives. Injuries to your abdomen that cause bruises on your uterus can dislodge the placenta and cause premature labor, so protect your abdomen from injuries. Wear your car seat belt correctly, at the fold of your thigh, not up over your uterus. If you have high-risk conditions that make you liable to have premature labor, such as a twin or triplet pregnancy or bleeding in the last three months of pregnancy, try to have more bedrest and avoid sexual activity to help prevent labor. Do not douche, because douching can dislodge the membranes and cause them to rupture too soon, also causing labor.

NORMAL PREGNANCY AND CHOICES IN CHILDBIRTH: MISCARRIAGE

1617. What are the warning signs that a miscarriage is likely to occur?

Usually a pregnancy that is going to result in miscarriage is not accom-

NORMAL PREGNANCY AND CHOICES IN CHILDBIRTH: MISCARRIAGE (Continued)

panied by nausea or vomiting, because the hormones being produced by a blighted pregnancy are not enough to produce all these symptoms. If you have no symptoms of pregnancy, except a skipped period and a positive pregnancy test, you should be checked closely to see if your uterus is enlarging properly. If it is not, the pregnancy test can be repeated. If you begin spotting and then bleed much more heavily, especially if the bleeding is associated with cramps, you are probably miscarrying. If you pass grey tissue, which is more solid than blood clots and it is determined to be fetal or placental tissue, then a miscarriage is certain.

1618. If I am pregnant and bleeding, does it always mean a miscarriage?

No, indeed. About 30 percent of women who go on to have healthy babies bleed in their first three months of pregnancy. So do not assume that you are having a miscarriage until there is more proof. If you are pregnant and bleeding a little, especially if you have pain on one side, you may have an ectopic pregnancy (a pregnancy developing in the tube or ovary), which cannot succeed. When it grows large enough, it causes bleeding inside the abdomen by rupturing the tube or ovary, which is very painful. If you have these symptoms, you need emergency care.

1619. When during pregnancy is a woman most likely to suffer a miscarriage?

A miscarriage is most likely to occur in the first twelve to fourteen weeks of pregnancy.

1620. What are the chances of having a miscarriage?

Most studies indicate that about 20 percent, or one in five pregnancies, result in miscarriage (called abortion in most medical circles). There actually may be many more than this, but they occur before the diagnosis of pregnancy has been made. The miscarriage just seems like an unusual menstrual period that is a few days late.

1621. What should I do if I think I am having a miscarriage?

Call your doctor, tell him or her your symptoms, and be able to estimate how much blood you have lost. Be willing to meet your doctor at an emergency room of a hospital. If you have no doctor, go to an emergency room for care. Do not eat anything if you are bleeding and cramping, in case a general anesthetic must be given for a D & C (dilatation and curettage). An empty stomach is better for taking anesthesia. You may have passed most of the tissue by the time you are examined. In that case, the doctor may do nothing more than examine the tissue. If you pass something besides just blood and clots, be brave: pick it up, place it into a plastic bag, and take it

NORMAL PREGNANCY AND CHOICES IN CHILDBIRTH: MISCARRIAGE (Continued)

with you to the hospital so that it can be examined to see if your miscarriage is complete. You also may be given Pitocin (contains the hormone oxytocin) to contract the uterus and control the bleeding, perhaps in an intravenous solution, or in ergotrate pills to be taken for a few days.

1622. How do I know if my miscarriage is complete?

When your miscarriage is complete, you will stop cramping and bleeding heavily. The tissue you passed will appear complete to someone who knows how to examine it.

1623. Will I have to have a D & C during or after a miscarriage?

Not always, and certainly not if your experience is so mild that you couldn't even tell you had a miscarriage. If you bleed heavily, such as soaking six pads in an hour, it is an emergency regardless of the cause, and you must seek emergency care to stop the bleeding. A D & C (dilatation and curettage) is the best way to do this. If you don't bleed too much, but the cramps are so severe that you can't stand them, you should seek emergency care. Removing the tissue that is lodged in your cervix can relieve the cramps, as well as stop the bleeding, and this is usually accomplished with a D & C. If you are not bleeding profusely and your cramps are not too painful, you may still choose to have a D & C in order to end the miscarriage quickly. You can bleed to death with a miscarriage, so do not decide to ignore it altogether.

1624. What are some of the causes of miscarriages?

The most frequent cause of miscarriages is a genetic abnormality—a combination of chromosomes that will not develop into a full-term baby. The most common abnormality is a set of chromosomes in which there is only one sex chromosome, one X instead of two, for instance. The next most common abnormality is a defective spinal cord or brain (a neural tube defect). Third is Down's syndrome, or Mongolism. Of babies who are miscarried, 60 percent have obvious defects or chromosome abnormalities. The others probably have them, too, but this can't always be determined. Some defects are so severe that the fetus doesn't form at all; there is just an empty sac with a placenta forming. Therefore, there is no great effort to prevent miscarriages.

1625. Can I control whether or not I have a miscarriage?

No, you are not in control of a spontaneous miscarriage; therefore, you are never responsible for it happening. You can suspect miscarriage if you are bleeding and cramping. Your doctor will suspect it, too, if your

NORMAL PREGNANCY AND CHOICES IN CHILDBIRTH:
MISCARRIAGE (Continued)

uterus does not grow larger and your pregnancy test turns out negative. You can be very sure that miscarriage is likely if you have an ultrasound examination (sonogram) that shows there is, indeed, a pregnancy sac in the uterus containing no fetus at all, or containing a dead one that does not move or have a heartbeat. This is called an inevitable abortion, and you can decide to have it aborted by a D & C whenever you like, or you can wait for it to happen naturally. That is about all the control you have over miscarriage in the present state of medical knowledge.

1626. Does taking hormone shots or pills work to prevent miscarriages?

No. This was attempted in the past, but it has been proven that hormones are not effective in preventing miscarriage, so they generally are no longer advised.

1627. If I have already had a miscarriage, does that mean my chances of having another miscarriage are greater?

No, not if you have had just one miscarriage. If you have had several, it may be that you and/or your partner have some abnormal chromosomes; therefore, you have more frequent abnormal chromosome pregnancies. You both can be checked for this by having the chromosomes in your blood analyzed.

1628. Is it possible to have a miscarriage and not know it?

Yes. If your menses are a little late and a little peculiar, you may suspect a miscarriage. You can only be certain of a miscarriage if you had a positive pregnancy test earlier or if you have a D & C to find out if the tissue looks like pregnancy tissue. Of course, it is not worth having a D & C just to know that, so there are many more miscarriages than women actually know about.

1629. Do most women find it hard to recover emotionally from a miscarriage?

Yes, for about a week. Part of the reason for this is grief over a lost baby, even if there was no baby at all. When women find out they are pregnant, most of them assume that they are carrying a fetus. When they miscarry, they also assume they lost something wonderful, not something defective. Miscarriage is a disappointment to a couple who is planning heavily on having a baby. Even women who didn't want a baby somehow feel they are imperfect as women if they miscarry, although it is through no fault of their own. Women who have a miscarriage need to know that it did not happen because of something they or anyone else did. Reassurance and an explanation of why miscarriages occur will help them.

NORMAL PREGNANCY AND CHOICES IN CHILDBIRTH: MULTIPLE BIRTHS

1630. How can I find out if I am having twins?

You can suspect the possibility of twins if you are much larger than normal for your length of pregnancy, especially if your doctor thinks so, too. You probably will have twins if the baby doesn't kick until it is far above your navel (umbilicus). To be certain, you need a sonogram to actually show the number of babies. This was previously checked by X-ray.

1631. Why is it important to know if I am carrying more than one baby before delivery?

There can be complications of position, such as twins being locked together, that make delivery impossible. If you delivered one baby and were given Pitocin (contains the hormone oxytocin) to control bleeding before you delivered the second baby, your uterus could clamp down around the second baby. Also, because you are more likely to go into premature labor with multiple babies, if you know you are carrying more than one, you can take precautions against premature labor, such as more bedrest. You could also take measures to stop premature labor as soon as it starts, instead of waiting until it is too late. Twin pregnancies can look as though they are at term when they are not, and sometimes labor is induced without realizing that the babies are premature. It is worth the cost and any vague theoretical risk of a sonogram to avoid these real dangers.

1632. In cases of multiple births, can the babies be delivered by natural childbirth, or is a cesarean section always necessary?

Depending upon the position of the babies and how premature they are, you can still have a natural birth. Very premature babies cannot tolerate a vaginal delivery as well as term babies, especially if one or more of them is in a breech position. The babies can even be locked together, especially if the first is breech and the second is head first. Even triplets can be successfully delivered vaginally when all three are head first.

1633. How can I control my chances of having a multiple birth?

You are less likely to have twins or triplets if you have babies while you are young, and you are more likely to have them as you become older. If you take fertility pills or injections, your likelihood of having twins and triplets is increased by at least 10 percent and sometimes even more. By choosing a partner who is a twin or who has many twins or triplets in his family, you only increase your chances if they are identical twins. Identical twins have exactly the same inheritance and are the same sex, since they come from the same egg. If they are fraternal twins (that is, two eggs ovulating at the same time), then your chances of a multiple birth are not increased.

NORMAL PREGNANCY AND CHOICES IN CHILDBIRTH: TAKING CHARGE OF LABOR AND DELIVERY

1634. Can I really control what happens to me in labor and delivery, or is that entirely up to my doctor and the hospital?

Your doctor and the hospital cannot absolutely control what happens to you. They cannot always predict a difficult or an easy labor, a cesarean section, a hemorrhage, or a perfect baby. They always have depended upon you to determine when you are in labor, to monitor your self-control while you are in labor, and to report when you need help. But today you have more opportunity to take charge of your birth experience than ever before. You can design it to meet the needs of you and your partner. Hopefully, you can select a physician and a hospital that support your choices, but also offer safety and emergency procedures if anything goes wrong or if your needs change. You cannot control the outcome so well that you can be certain of a safe home delivery. The best-trained obstetrician in the world cannot make home delivery a safe procedure. When a problem arises, there may be insufficient time to get to the hospital before there is damage, possibly fatal, to the baby and even the mother. But you do not need to make that choice today, because you can have a home-style delivery in the hospital. Hospital Alternative Birth Centers (ABC rooms) are approved and supported wholeheartedly by the American College of Obstetricians and Gynecologists to assist in family-centered childbirth. If you want anesthesia, such as an epidural, from the moment you reach the hospital in active labor, that can be done, too. But you have to find the doctor and hospital that will provide this service. Your demands are what control the delivery of medical care. If you cannot change to another doctor or hospital that better meet your needs, then change your doctor's and hospital's ways of thinking so they will better meet your needs. You do not have to retreat into a corner and give up all medical care to take charge of your birth experience.

1635. Can I ask for labor to be induced?

You can always ask. The last month of pregnancy is so uncomfortable, most women would like their labor induced at the end of the eighth month. But, of course, that would result in a premature baby who might not do well. Induction of labor for relief of discomfort is frowned upon for two reasons. One is that the baby might really be premature, since due dates are not especially reliable. The other reason is that it could cause a long and difficult labor. It also could fail entirely and require a cesarean section that might have been avoided if you had waited a little longer. If you have a medical problem, like toxemia (a blood pressure disorder of late pregnancy) or prolonged ruptured membranes, which really requires the induction of labor, that is a different matter. When delivery is required, an attempt to in-

NORMAL PREGNANCY AND CHOICES IN CHILDBIRTH: TAKING CHARGE OF LABOR AND DELIVERY (Continued)

duce labor is more desirable than immediately resorting to a cesarean section. Another situtation in which induction may be offered or insisted upon is when you are two or more weeks overdue, by the best calculations. If the cervix is soft, ready for delivery, slightly open, and the baby's head is in place, it may be easier to induce labor than to wait longer, even if tests show that the baby is in good condition and could wait. Tests also can show when the baby is not in good condition and labor must be induced or the baby delivered in some manner. This test is performed simply by applying a fetal monitor and watching the baby's heart rate after fetal motion, like kicking, or after uterine contractions, natural or induced. The placenta also can become old and provide poor nourishment for the baby when you are extremely overdue, so if your doctor is anxious to induce labor, don't fight it too long. Labor is easier to take when it starts naturally, but sometimes it is not safe to wait for that.

1636. Do I have a choice about whether I have an I.V. (intravenous fluid) during childbirth?

If you are going to have anesthesia, an I.V. is absolutely required so that fluid balance and blood pressure can be maintained, and medications can be given quickly to balance blood pressure, if it drops. Without any anesthesia, except a local, use of an I.V. is debatable, and you can discuss this with your obstetrician. In an emergency, it is sometimes lifesaving to have an intravenous line available to give medications that are needed suddenly to control hemorrhage or to stop convulsions, or even to give a blood transfusion. If you do not have one, your veins may be so collapsed in shock that a cut-down (an incision over a vein) may have to be made to find a way into a vein. These require sutures and leave a scar. But should everyone have an I.V., with its limitations of motion, for the one emergency in one hundred or so cases? If your doctor needs it for confidence, allow it. If you don't like it and your doctor does not care, avoid it, but complications may make it quite necessary.

1637. Do I have a choice as to whether my pubic hair is shaved?

Most delivery rooms no longer shave pubic hair. It was previously done in an attempt to prevent infections, but it seems infections were no greater when it was not shaved. It is certainly more comfortable in the few weeks following delivery without the stubble growing back in. You can ask your doctor about this in advance. You also can refuse it at the time of your admission to the hospital. If your doctor really wants it done, you will find that out soon enough. If you are going to have a cesarean section, the upper part of the pubic hair must be shaved, so that the hair will not contaminate

NORMAL PREGNANCY AND CHOICES IN CHILDBIRTH: TAKING CHARGE OF LABOR AND DELIVERY (Continued)

the abdominal incision or get tangled in the closing sutures. This step seems to be necessary, because there are more infections after a cesarean section than a vaginal delivery. More sterile technique (keeping germs out) is required for a cesarean section.

1638. Do I have a choice as to whether I have an enema?

Most delivery rooms have omitted the enema, which was previously given in early labor upon your arrival at the hospital. It was meant to speed up labor, but today delivery rooms are not so crowded that they have to speed up anyone. It was never intended to make room for the baby or to make delivery more clean. The watery return of feces at the time of delivery is harder to handle than solid feces. Enemas are still used to help induce labor or to speed up a slow labor. Do **not** give yourself one at home and do not take castor oil or any laxative, because you do not know how far along in labor you are, and speeding it up might be a disaster. If any procedure is offered during delivery that you do not want, refuse it and ask to talk with your doctor about it. If the doctor really wants it, you will learn all about it and perhaps be convinced.

1639. Do I have to have my arms strapped down when I have my baby?

As a rule, straps are not used anymore, except in some rare cases and during a cesarean section. Women who have gone to childbirth classes and learned about what is going to happen during delivery and who have not been given many drugs are not wild and do not wave their arms around in the air as women used to in times past. You probably cannot imagine what the delivery room was previously like. Women were so frightened that they screamed and struggled against everything, so straps were necessary for their own safety. Others had so many injections of drugs that they were out of their minds and had to be restrained so the baby could be delivered. Situations like that no longer exist, except in rare cases that involve immigrants who do not speak English and have had no preparation before coming to the hospital for delivery of their babies. With these women, you get a glimpse of how babies were delivered in the past. Of course, if you have a cesarean section, then it is important that your hands not enter the sterile field over your abdomen, so arm boards with small velcro straps will be used to remind you to keep your arms in place. This is especially true if you are under general anesthesia. The father's presence is also helpful in this regard, since he can hold your hand and keep you comforted.

NORMAL PREGNANCY AND CHOICES IN CHILDBIRTH: LABOR

1640. How can I decide if I am in labor?

If you have read about it or been to childbirth preparation classes, you are not likely to mistake labor. If you make up your mind exactly how it is going to be, you are more likely to mistake it, because it is liable to be different than what you expected, even if you have had labor before. If your doctor has examined you and told you that your baby has dropped into position and the cervix is ready, you are more likely to be correct when you diagnose labor. Usually the mucus plug, or bloody show, is seen sometime during the day before labor starts. It can be clear, pink, brown, or red mucus. If there is heavy bleeding, more than a menstrual flow, you have a problem and should report it to your doctor immediately. You will usually have a continual backache and intermittent contractions every half-hour or so. Then you will find that they are happening every ten minutes or even more closely. When the contractions are five minutes apart, you can be fairly certain that you are in labor. However, sometimes it is labor even when they are six and eight minutes apart, but very strong. Your uterus will become hard at the same time that you feel the labor contraction. You may feel it low in front, in the back, or even in your thighs, just like menstrual cramps. If it is your first baby, you can wait until the contractions have been five minutes apart for an hour or two before calling and going to the hospital. But if it is your second child or more, don't wait that long; an hour is enough. The safest place to be in labor, especially for the baby's sake, is in the hospital where nurses can listen to the baby's heart and know it is all right. If your water breaks and runs down your leg, you don't need any other sign. You should call or go to the hospital. But don't wait for the water to break, because the baby can be born without it breaking.

1641. How will I know if I am in premature labor?

This is one of the most difficult diagnoses to make, and obstetricians have a hard time with it. However, if there is to be any improvement in the prevention of premature labor, pregnant women need to be very alert for its signs. These signs need to be reported immediately, so premature labor can be treated and stopped before the labor has gone too far to be turned back. There are medications available now to stop the contractions of premature labor, provided it is wise to do so. If there is a severe hemorrhage, this may not be wise. If you have contractions at regular intervals of five minutes, even though you are only seven or eight months pregnant, you should call or go to the hospital to be examined to see if premature labor is threatening. The monitor for labor can sometimes diagnose this. If you are in premature labor, then steps can be taken to stop the labor, if that is the best choice. If

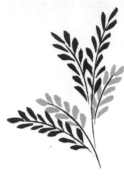

Oh my God
I think I'm in labor
20 minutes apart
15 minutes apart
10 minutes apart
It's not as bad as
I thought
except that I know
it will get worse
and I can't back
out now
No one can bail me out
Oh my God
I'm really scared
This is it
No one can help me
share the pain
Oh my God
I'm really scared

— Susan Polis Schutz

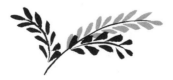

NORMAL PREGNANCY AND CHOICES IN CHILDBIRTH: LABOR
(Continued)

the cervix has dilated halfway, then it is too late to stop it. Sometimes even a strong pressure in the pelvis or a bloody show gives you a clue that something unusual is happening that might be an early labor. Do not be embarrassed to check on it. Premature labor is a difficult diagnosis for well-trained medical people to make, so how can you be certain? For the safety of your baby, or in an attempt to keep it inside your abdomen a little longer, report your symptoms to your doctor and seek help early. If it is not labor, just celebrate your good luck. It is not that much trouble to go in and be examined. Do not let anyone ridicule you for this.

1642. How will I know if I'm having false labor?

False labor is contractions that seem like labor at full-term pregnancy, but that stop before they dilate the cervix at all. It is a frequent occurrence and may necessitate several trips to the hospital or doctor to be examined to attempt to diagnose real labor. Many women act embarrassed if they go to the hospital on a false alarm and then go home because it is not real labor, even though they have followed the instructions of their doctors, waiting for two hours of contractions five minutes apart before going to the hospital. Sometimes husbands or relatives ridicule them for not knowing it was a false alarm. This is a dangerous cruelty to women, because their reaction may be to stay home until the baby is born the next time. This can be dangerous both to the baby and to the mother, since the baby may need help at birth and the mother could have an immediate hemorrhage. Do not be timid; demand to go to the hospital to be checked to determine if you are in labor. If you are not in labor, go back home with good cheer and with no apologies to anyone. You are doing this for the safety of your baby. There is no instinctive knowledge as to whether labor is real, until you have waited dangerously too long. When the head is showing, that is a little late.

1643. Can I walk around while I am in labor?

Recently there has been a resurgence of the idea that walking around helps promote labor. In some conditions, walking around is dangerous. If you want to walk around, ask your doctor if it's okay. If it is forbidden, ask why. There may be a very good reason for you not to walk around. You could have ruptured membranes or the baby's head may not be well applied to the cervix, which would allow a cord to prolapse. Both situations would be real disasters.

1644. Is it all right to sip an alcoholic beverage during labor to relax myself?

It is good to relax during labor, but alcohol can stop labor altogether. Intravenous alcohol used to be one of the methods of stopping premature

NORMAL PREGNANCY AND CHOICES IN CHILDBIRTH: LABOR
(Continued)

labor; drinking it worked well, too. An ounce of alcohol would usually stop labor within an hour. If you are trying to stop premature labor on the way to the hospital, it might be a good idea, but there are now better medications with fewer side effects than alcohol for premature labor.

NORMAL PREGNANCY AND CHOICES IN CHILDBIRTH: LAMAZE METHOD

1645. What is the Lamaze method of natural childbirth?

Lamaze is a method of pain relief, relaxation, and self-control accomplished by focusing on breathing techniques. It began in Russia and was patterned after the Pavlov conditioned reflex, but it was made popular in France and in the world by Pierre Vellay, who worked with Dr. Lamaze and then wrote books about it. You and your labor coach, usually your husband, learn to focus your attention on a certain point and to breathe in a specific pattern; frequency of breathing increases as the labor contraction increases in strength. The pattern changes as transition is reached, in order to keep you from bearing down too soon. You learn to pant and blow. After dilation of the cervix is complete, you learn to bear down in an effective manner to expel the baby. In the United States, the role of the father is emphasized, including his participation in the delivery room. He learns to rub your back, count while you push, remind you of the breathing pattern, and generally attend to your comfort. He is a useful member of the childbirth team. Lamaze has been called psychoprophylaxis, or self-hypnosis. It certainly can bring about relaxation, which reduces pain.

1646. Will Lamaze really make childbirth easier?

Yes. Control of fear helps to make childbirth easier, and all methods of childbirth preparation reduce fear through the knowledge that has been gained. Lamaze also adds a method of concentration on breathing patterns that distracts the mind from the sensations of labor. It is a little like self-hypnosis. For at least 30 percent of women, this provides enough relief for the entire process of labor and delivery. For others, additional relief is really necessary and should be provided. A woman who is out of control and hyperventilating in active labor is not providing the best environment for her baby. Anesthesia really can make conditions better for the baby, as well as for the mother. It also can be essential, if the baby's position is not ideal or if it is exceptionally large for the birth canal, in order for your doctor to perform the necessary procedures to help your delivery. Of course, Lamaze does not provide enough pain relief or control for a cesarean section. Childbirth preparation does not prevent cesarean sections.

NORMAL PREGNANCY AND CHOICES IN CHILDBIRTH: LEBOYER METHOD

1647. What is the Leboyer method?

The Leboyer method emphasizes how the baby feels during and immediately after delivery. An easy delivery (which is not possible for all women), low lights, pleasant sounds, and a warm bath immediately following birth make the world more pleasant to the baby, according to the French obstetrician, Leboyer. The expression on the child's face also seems to confirm this. Leboyer has little to say about labor, or even the father's presence in the delivery room. Fetal monitoring is also a form of being attentive to how the baby feels, with more accuracy than just using a stethoscope, but its use is not included in Leboyer's book, *Birth Without Violence*.

1648. Do most hospitals have the necessary facilities, such as the bath after birth, for using the Leboyer techniques?

Yes, of course. It just takes a tub of warm water.

1649. My sister and her husband had a "Leboyer birth," and it was great! How can I get that?

Ask your doctor if he is willing to use the Leboyer method. It is not a Leboyer birth if your husband is present, because Leboyer never had the husband present in France. Leboyer learned about that in the United States, but a modification of the Leboyer method allows husbands in the delivery room. So don't just ask for a Leboyer delivery, ask for the specific techniques that you want, such as holding the baby soon after birth, bathing it in a tub of warm water, and, after the delivery or the episiotomy is repaired, having the lights low so that the baby will open its eyes. The lights may also be lowered after the doctor has had sufficient light to see that the baby is in good condition. Be specific about what you want. Do not just use the word Leboyer; it can mean a lot of different things to different people.

1650. If my physician is strongly against using Leboyer techniques, would it be worthwhile for me to push for them?

There really are no special techniques used in the Leboyer delivery. The baby is not delivered any differently than in a normal delivery. Be specific about one or two things you would like to have done, instead of trying to change your doctor's entire manner of delivery to something that sounds new or foreign. If you want the tub of warm water, ask for it. If your doctor is against it, ask why. If you want the lights low, ask for them to be that way.

NORMAL PREGNANCY AND CHOICES IN CHILDBIRTH: BRADLEY METHOD

1651. What is the Bradley method?
Dr. Robert Bradley emphasizes the participation of the father during childbirth. He uses a different breathing pattern than Lamaze, but this is still the method of pain relief. Although his book, *Husband Coached Childbirth,* is moderate in its approach, some of his followers teach that you can only use the Bradley method at home. That would be giving up all medical safety just to try to control your childbirth experience.

NORMAL PREGNANCY AND CHOICES IN CHILDBIRTH: BIRTH UNDER WATER

1652. I have heard of women today giving birth under water. Is this true? Where did the idea originate?
It is true, and supposedly it started in Russia. I do not think we are really amphibious, and besides, the baby needs air to breathe when the cord stops pulsating. In the one such birth experience in San Diego County, both parents were in the water. Mother and baby were both later hospitalized for infection. It is hard to say what need this idea meets. It is novel and dangerous.

NORMAL PREGNANCY AND CHOICES IN CHILDBIRTH: HOME BIRTH

1653. Are more women today having home births?
Women are having more home births than they did fifteen years ago. This increase is among middle-class women who want to control their deliveries and provide the best emotional experience. It is partly a product of the women's movement that gave them the courage to exercise their rights, and partly the confidence they attained from attending childbirth preparation classes that dispelled all fear. Thirty years ago, home deliveries occurred only among the urban poor and the rural isolated. At the turn of the century, most deliveries were at home. The maternal death rate for women then was 500 per 100,000 live births. Now the death rate is 16 per 100,000. At the turn of the century, babies died at the rate of 3,000 per 10,000 births. In 1982, the rate was 112 per 10,000 births. The improvement has been accomplished through the use of antibiotics, blood banks, safe anesthesia, safe cesarean sections, fetal monitoring, neonatal intensive care units for babies, and advanced medical technology, as well as a better standard of living. The price paid for this momentous reduction in deaths of babies and women was the loss of the emotional side of the home delivery. Now an effort is being made

NORMAL PREGNANCY AND CHOICES IN CHILDBIRTH:
HOME BIRTH (Continued)

to bring that emotional side to the hospital by participation of the husband and even the entire family in childbirth. The emotional needs of women and their families should be met, but not by sacrificing the medical gains of the century. Women need to demand what they want in the hospital setting.

1654. What are the chances of having a successful home birth?

If you are properly screened to be sure that you are a low risk for any complications and if you are transferred to the hospital at the first sign of trouble, you have about an 80 percent chance of delivering successfully at home. There is a 5 percent chance that the baby will be distressed and need emergency care that it cannot get at home, or the mother will have trouble with delivering the placenta and need hospital care. Five percent is too high a price to pay for the satisfaction of home delivery, especially when the same satisfaction can be obtained at the hosptial.

1655. What are the dangers of home birth?

Home birth has all the dangers of obstetrics. Normally, things do not go wrong, but when they do, they do not give five minutes' notice. A hemorrhage can occur at any time during labor, delivery, or afterwards. The cord can prolapse, fall out of the vagina, and be shut off by the pressure of labor. There can be only minutes in which to perform a cesarean section to save the baby. Placental circulation and cord problems can cause the baby to have less oxygen and be distressed at any time. If the birth is not properly monitored, this may go undetected until after the baby is damaged or dead. High blood pressure and convulsions of the mother can occur at any time without much warning. The uterus can turn inside out when the placenta is delivered, causing hemorrhage and shock. Labor can be much too slow, but if drugs are used to speed it up, you need the safety of the hospital for control. You may need anesthesia, which is not available to you at home, so drugs are used instead, which make the baby sleepy. When the infant is born, you never know if it is going to breathe all right. It may need the most sophisticated resuscitation in the first five minutes of life. The baby may be born with a defect that needs immediate expert attention. The list is endless, and all of this can be treated in a hospital setting.

1656. Are home births legal everywhere?

There is no law against home births. Personally, I think they constitute child neglect. The American College of Obstetricians and Gynecologists does not approve of them because they are unsafe. The California Medical Association agrees. Most obstetricians will not participate in home births, because they are terrified of the dangers. The less

NORMAL PREGNANCY AND CHOICES IN CHILDBIRTH:
HOME BIRTH (Continued)

educated general practitioners do more home deliveries, but eventually stop when they run into enough trouble. Certified nurse midwives prefer a hospital setting but can't always get privileges, so they are doing home deliveries. Lay midwives, who are completely uneducated and untrained, do most of the home deliveries. It is interesting to note that the less birth attendants know, the more they do home deliveries; and the more they know, the more they avoid them. If you consider the whole world, only about 10 percent of women have a trained birth attendant of any kind. The death rate of mothers and babies is still high, except in developed countries.

1657. What are my rights if I wish to have a home birth?
You have the right to change your mind at any time, and if you do change your mind, no birth attendant should tell you it is too late. You cannot force anyone to attend you at home, but you can call an ambulance and go to a hospital where emergency care will be given to you and your baby. This is actually happening more and more often. You have the right to know the experience and training of your birth attendant, and whether he or she is connected with a doctor who has hospital privileges in obstetrics. There should always be at least two people with you during a home birth, one to stay with you while the other seeks help.

1658. What kind of training does a midwife receive?
A certified nurse midwife first receives the education required to become a Registered Nurse (R.N.). She then receives an additional eighteen to twenty-four months of special obstetrical training during which she delivers low-risk patients screened by doctors in a hospital setting under the supervision of an obstetrician. The American College of Obstetricians and Gynecologists approves of this setting for midwives to practice. At no time are midwives trained to do home deliveries. Many people who call themselves midwives have no training and very little experience. This was the way babies were delivered in the United States two hundred years ago. Two out of five babies died then, as did many, many mothers.

NORMAL PREGNANCY AND CHOICES IN CHILDBIRTH:
ALTERNATIVE BIRTH CENTERS

1659. Are birthing rooms in hospitals as safe as having a baby in a delivery room?
No, but they are far safer than having a baby at home. If you are not frightened by the appearance of a hospital delivery room and only require that your husband be present, you would be safer in the delivery room,

NORMAL PREGNANCY AND CHOICES IN CHILDBIRTH: ALTERNATIVE BIRTH CENTERS (Continued)

instead of an alternative birth room (ABC room). The sterile technique (keeping out germs) of the delivery room makes infection less likely and emergencies can be met more quickly. There is no attempt to get women to change from delivery rooms to ABC rooms, but there is an attempt to get women who want to deliver at home to change to the hospital. This is done by providing them with everything they could have at home.

1660. Why don't all doctors like to use the alternative birth rooms?

Some doctors feels that the sterile technique of the delivery room is very important. They would rather be in a room where they can handle an emergency, including a cesarean section, without having to move the patient after the problem arises. In the delivery room, anesthesia can be given quickly. There also are better facilities there for resuscitating the newborn if it is necessary.

1661. Am I taking any chances by using an ABC room?

You are taking some chances when you drop the sterile technique of the delivery room. There is almost no sterile technique in the ABC room; there cannot be. There is an effort to keep the rooms clean, but it is impossible to keep everything surrounding the birth of the baby sterile. Thus far, there has been no increase in infections in mothers or babies, but there could be. Long ago, childbed fever (parametritis) killed many women, but at that time doctors did not even wash their hands, much less put on gloves. The question of how much sterility is required during a perfectly normal delivery has not been settled. It is certainly required when the doctor has to rotate the baby by using forceps or deliver a breech birth. Of course, even more sterile technique is required with a cesarean section.

NORMAL PREGNANCY AND CHOICES IN CHILDBIRTH: OTHER PEOPLE IN THE DELIVERY ROOM

1662. Can I have anyone I want with me at the time of delivery?

If you deliver in a delivery room where sterile technique must be maintained, most hospitals limit your companion to one significant other person. This can be the father of the baby, your mother, a friend, or a labor coach. This certainly is true if you have a cesarean section. Sterile technique (keeping out germs) is very important with open abdominal surgery or with vaginal manipulations, such as rotating the baby's head using forceps or the vacuum extractor, at the time of delivery. If you deliver spontaneously without any intervention, sterile technique is not as important. You could deliver in an ABC room, an Alternative Birth Center, where the rules are

NORMAL PREGNANCY AND CHOICES IN CHILDBIRTH: OTHER PEOPLE IN THE DELIVERY ROOM (Continued)

relaxed and other people are allowed to be present. No one wears masks, and your other children can even be present. This makes your birth experience like a home delivery. You certainly can't have a sterile technique in a home delivery; but you could have friends over.

1663. Do most women want to have their husbands or partners in the delivery room?

Yes. In hospitals where it is allowed, about 95 percent of women have their husbands or partners present. However, no one should be forced to do this.

1664. Why won't my doctor let my husband in the delivery room for my cesarean section when I need him and he wants to be there?

Some hospitals require that persons who wish to be present during a cesarean birth attend a course on the subject. Your doctor may feel that the anesthesiologist is in charge of making you feel comfortable and relaxed. Your doctor also may not feel comfortable with an inexperienced person, like your husband, watching him do surgery. You should want your surgeon to be comfortable and relaxed, so he can do a good job for you. If your husband's presence makes him tense and anxious, you may not have the best results. He also may feel it is harmful for your husband to watch. Why don't you just ask your doctor what his reasons are?

NORMAL PREGNANCY AND CHOICES IN CHILDBIRTH: VAGINAL DELIVERY

1665. How can I know in advance if my birth canal is big enough to have a vaginal delivery?

You can't know this. You can know if it is of average size or even that it is large, but you do not know how large the baby will be. X-rays are no longer advised to measure the pelvis for this purpose. Instead, it is measured by the examiner's hand, placed inside the vagina, feeling the sacrum and other bones. Even if the pelvis seems small, it is best to attempt labor, because sometimes the joints spread so much with pregnancy that the pelvis is much larger at term. Perhaps the baby will be small, too.

1666. Will my vaginal canal be stretched and stay that way after I deliver?

This varies with different people who have different tissues and different sized babies. If an episiotomy is done before the tissues are badly stretched, you may not notice very much difference. However, if you are using a diaphragm for birth control, you will usually go to a larger size after delivery because of some stretching. If you have a large baby and no

NORMAL PREGNANCY AND CHOICES IN CHILDBIRTH:
VAGINAL DELIVERY (Continued)

episiotomy or tear, and tissues that are not very elastic, you may have quite a problem with stretched bladder supports (cystocele), rectal wall supports (rectocele), and even uterine supports (prolapse of the uterus). These conditions are collectively called pelvic relaxation. You can inherit the tendency to have pelvic relaxation, but it is brought out by having a baby. With a cesarean section, there is less stretch and damage to these tissues, but you have an abdominal scar.

1667. Can I have natural childbirth and vaginal delivery after previously having a cesarean section?

If the reason for the cesarean section is no longer present and there is no new reason for a section, today it is allowed to try a vaginal delivery, provided certain safeguards are present. First, the original section must have been made with a low transverse (crosswise) incision in the uterus, not a classical up and down incision, which is more likely to rupture. You cannot tell which type of incision you had from the scar on your skin, so you will have to get records to prove it. Then the labor must take place in a labor suite that has the ability to do a cesarean section quickly if it is needed because of an impending rupture of the uterus. Fetal monitors must be used, as well as contraction monitors, to be sure all is well. As more and more experience is gained with vaginal delivery after cesarean section, perhaps the rules will relax.

1668. If a vaginal delivery is possible after a cesarean, then why won't my doctor let me try it?

You should ask your doctor his or her reasons for not allowing this. Not all women who have had a cesarean delivery are good cases for trying a vaginal delivery; only about half of them would be relatively safe. If you had a vertical incision in your uterus when you had your C-section (cesarean delivery), vaginal delivery is too dangerous. If the original reason for your C-section was a pelvis that was too small, it probably has not grown, and the same reason is still present. Vaginal delivery after a cesarean section is also only allowed in a delivery suite with excellent monitoring facilities. Anesthesia and surgical teams for cesarean section must be available immediately in case of a rupture of the uterus. A vaginal delivery after a cesarean section is sometimes possible, but not routine.

1669. Is it dangerous for a child to be born vaginally to a woman who has genital herpes?

If the herpes is active (there is an open sore on the vulva or a positive herpes culture), then the virus can contaminate the baby as it is being born through the vagina. This can result in a very damaging or fatal infection to

NORMAL PREGNANCY AND CHOICES IN CHILDBIRTH: VAGINAL DELIVERY (Continued)

the child. Of course, it is also possible for the child to pass through the vagina and not get infected. To avoid the problem, a cesarean section can be done, so the child will not come in contact with the herpes. This is especially recommended before the membranes have ruptured. Sometimes, however, a child is born affected by herpes, and no one ever knew that the mother had it. She did not have any sores, and since there was no history of herpes, a culture was not taken. This happens in about half of the cases in which a baby is born with herpes. If the woman has had herpes in the past, but has not had an open sore for several weeks or has a negative herpes culture, she can deliver vaginally. This is usually the case.

NORMAL PREGNANCY AND CHOICES IN CHILDBIRTH: FETAL MONITORS

1670. What is a fetal monitor?

The fetal heart monitor is a machine that is usually wheeled to your bedside on a table. It will tell the doctor how your baby is doing during labor by measuring each of your uterine contractions and the baby's heart.

1671. Are fetal monitors really necessary?

In high-risk situations, such as premature labor, induction of labor, or even overdue labor, fetal monitors are a necessity for the safety of the baby. In low-risk pregnancies, where everything is quite normal, they are not as necessary, but they still provide a much better report on the condition of the baby than listening with a stethoscope every fifteen minutes. They also are probably more comfortable than being poked with a stethoscope. Fetal monitors are a little like seat belts on an airplane. You don't wear them when you walk up and down the aisle, but while you are sitting, you are encouraged to fasten the seat belt for safety. When the plane is really on a rocky course, everyone must sit down and put on their seat belts. Babies can get into trouble without any warning during labor; without listening to them, it would be impossible to know that they are in trouble. Fetal monitors have made labor much safer than it used to be. They prevent some cesarean sections by showing that the baby is in good condition, and they bring about other cesarean sections by showing that the baby is probably in great distress and must be delivered as soon as possible. Most of the monitors used today are external; they are placed on the abdomen and held on by soft belts. If these do not work, an internal one can be placed on the baby's scalp (or buttocks). It is something like the electrode on an EEG, a tiny wire inserted just 1/16th inch under the skin. Watching the monitor can be fascinating to you and others who are with you in the labor room. You can tell how the fetal

NORMAL PREGNANCY AND CHOICES IN CHILDBIRTH: FETAL MONITORS (Continued)

heart rate reacts to your contractions and just when your contractions start and end. You do not have to lie still; if you move and the belts get out of place, the nurse will adjust them. If you did not have the monitor on, the doctor would have to listen with the stethoscope instead. If you want it off, say so. If your doctor wants it on, ask why.

1672. How can I walk around if I have a fetal monitor on?

Of course, you cannot walk around, so when you do, it is removed. The nurse then comes in at intervals to listen with a stethoscope. Someday we will have little monitors that are worn in the vagina; then you could walk around **and** be monitored. These are still experimental at the present time.

NORMAL PREGNANCY AND CHOICES IN CHILDBIRTH: EPISIOTOMY

1673. Is an episiotomy necessary for all women?

No, but it usually is. If your vaginal opening was stretched by a previous baby, you probably can deliver your next baby without any more stretching, tearing, or cutting. On a first baby, however, only a few women will stretch without tearing and then be able to return to almost normal size. Most will tear and need stitches or have hidden tears so that the stretched tissue never goes back to normal size. Bladder and rectal walls can bulge out of the vagina, or the whole uterus can fall out for the rest of your life. You can lose control of your bladder, which may cause you to wet your pants whenever you laugh or sneeze, and this cannot be controlled no matter how much you exercise your perineal muscles. You may have to brace your vagina with your fingers to empty your feces. In desperation, you may even ask for a surgical repair after a few years. An episiotomy is a cut made with scissors (under at least a local anesthetic) in the tissue between the vagina and rectum. It opens up the area for delivery of the baby's head, without tearing or stretching too badly. It probably is better to have too many episiotomies than too few, because having an unnecessary one simply results in painful stitches for a few days, but not having a needed one can make trouble for the rest of your life.

1674. When I asked my doctor about needing an episiotomy, he replied, "We'll just wait and see if you need one." Why can't he tell me now?

The doctor cannot determine if you have an elastic opening that will not tear until the last minute before you actually deliver the baby. Most women who are having their first baby really do need an episiotomy to prevent a complicated tear through their rectums and to prevent damaging

NORMAL PREGNANCY AND CHOICES IN CHILDBIRTH: EPISIOTOMY (Continued)

stretching of the supports of the bladder and rectal walls. Some women have tissues that are very elastic and open easily, but most do not. The stretched opening hurts for as many days as the stitches of an episiotomy do. Of course, if you were stretched in a previous delivery, then this delivery will be painless afterwards, but you will remain stretched for the rest of your life.

1675. Isn't it true that doctors do episiotomies routinely, whether they are needed or not, because it makes things easier for them?

No, that is absolutely false. It is more difficult to repair an episiotomy than to stretch the perineum (tissue between the vagina and rectum) and deliver the baby without stitches. A tear also can be harder to repair, especially if it goes through the rectum. The talk against episiotomies sometimes comes from midwives who are not allowed to do them or repair them. If an episiotomy must be done or a tear repaired, midwives must call in a doctor. Since they often do not want to call the doctor, they praise having a baby without an episiotomy.

1676. What is perineal massage?

Perineal massage is done by the doctor or midwife to help the vaginal opening stretch around the baby's head.

1677. Why won't my doctor give me a perineal massage?

Perineal massage will not allow you to entirely avoid an episiotomy. Your doctor is trying to avoid your being stretched for the rest of your life and needing surgery in later years to tighten your vaginal opening. Let him tell you why he won't do a perineal massage.

NORMAL PREGNANCY AND CHOICES IN CHILDBIRTH: USE OF FORCEPS AND VACUUM EXTRACTORS

1678. Why are forceps used?

Forceps are used to help deliver the baby. Sometimes a woman simply cannot push hard enough to deliver her baby, and she needs help. Forceps are very uncomfortable, unless anesthesia is given before using them. If the baby is in a bad position, such as face up instead of face down, then the head needs to be rotated; this can be done with forceps and anesthesia, thus avoiding a cesarean section. If the baby shows signs of distress while the woman is bearing down in the second stage of labor and needs to be delivered quickly, forceps can accomplish this. If the woman chooses to have anesthesia, then forceps may be used to deliver the baby for two reasons. One is that she may not bear down as well when she is not in pain; forceps used for this reason do absolutely no harm or damage to the baby. The other

NORMAL PREGNANCY AND CHOICES IN CHILDBIRTH: USE OF FORCEPS AND VACUUM EXTRACTORS (Continued)

may be that if the baby is premature, anesthesia and forceps can be used to prevent damage to the baby's small, soft head. It is not easy for the baby's head to push the vagina open and come out. A hard head can take it, but a premature baby does not do as well. Forceps are used to protect the head during the delivery process, so they usually are used whenever the woman has anesthesia. Their use also shortens the second stage of labor, but this is not usually the reason they are used. Forceps can make slight red marks over the baby's cheeks, just from the pressure, but these disappear in a day. They are designed to give pressure only over the cheeks and not all over the head. No one should be afraid to use forceps, except perhaps if they are used without anesthesia, which would cause pain for the mother.

1679. What is a vacuum extractor?

It is a suction cup applied to the baby's head upon which traction is then applied.

NORMAL PREGNANCY AND CHOICES IN CHILDBIRTH: POSITIONS OF DELIVERY

1680. Do I have to have my legs in stirrups, or can I deliver in any position I like?

If your doctor only has experience with one position for delivery, and you have none at all, it would probably be best for you to use the position in which your doctor performs best. A new position can be so confusing to the doctor that he or she can't even tell what position your baby is in, face up or face down. If you both agree to try something new, then that is up to the two of you. Most deliveries in the United States take place on delivery tables with the woman's legs up in stirrups and the head of the table somewhat elevated. This forms a kind of chair with a back but no seat, except for the stirrups. Several delivery beds have been designed, mostly for use in the ABC rooms (Alternative Birth Centers), in which the bed breaks at the lower third and elevates so that it forms a kind of chair with a seat, a raised back, and a place for the feet to rest on the lower third portion. If needed, stirrups can also be added. These beds have different names, like Borning or Adel. The Delivery Chair looks even more like a chair, but some of them have a fixed angle for the back, and it is not always just the angle you would like. So all deliveries, except cesarean sections, are done in somewhat of a squatting position, as if you were sitting in a chair, but the appearance of the chair and the angle of tilt can be different. A flat surface is not best for delivery, because if the baby's shoulders are a tight fit, space below must be available to bring the head down to deliver or rotate the shoulders. Besides being adapted to the

NORMAL PREGNANCY AND CHOICES IN CHILDBIRTH: POSITIONS OF DELIVERY (Continued)

delivery of the baby, the table or chair also needs to provide the doctor with enough room to be able to put in any stitches that are needed after the delivery. Tables or chairs in the United States are not adapted for delivery in the sideways position, although the British use a curved bar with a sling to hold the upper leg to do this.

1681. What is the lithotomy position?

It is lying flat on your back with your knees up and feet down, also called the supine position.

1682. I read that the lithotomy position will increase my chances of needing an episiotomy. Why can't I sit at a 45° angle on the delivery table without using the stirrups?

You can read almost anything. There is also a study that discourages use of the birthing chair because fourth degree tears (through the rectum) are so frequent. Drawing the legs up, whether you hold them up with your hands or they are held up by stirrups, makes more room at the opening of the vagina. Stirrups were invented because women often stopped holding up their legs at a crucial point of delivery. In the ABC rooms (Alternative Birth Centers), stirrups are usually not used. They can also be eliminated in the delivery room, but it is very hard to maintain a sterile condition when the woman's legs are thrashing about. The 45° angle can be used with the stirrups as well.

1683. I've heard that squatting is the best position for giving birth. Can I squat in the delivery room?

Not everyone agrees that this is the best position for delivery. Does the baby's head then go into the floor? In the delivery room, sterile technique must be maintained to permit certain interventions by the doctor. If you want to squat, you should deliver in the ABC room (Alternate Birth Center) with a doctor who will permit that. Most doctors are not trained to help you in that position, so it would be new and experimental.

NORMAL PREGNANCY AND CHOICES IN CHILDBIRTH: ANESTHESIA

1684. Do most doctors today recommend natural childbirth or the use of an anesthetic?

There probably is no doctor who would refuse to give an analgesic (pain reliever) or anesthesia to anyone. But there are still doctors who refuse to allow natural childbirth to anyone! They have been trained only to deliver babies with anesthesia, and they do not want to change. The majority of

NORMAL PREGNANCY AND CHOICES IN CHILDBIRTH: ANESTHESIA (Continued)

doctors advise women to learn about natural childbirth and prepare for it, but recommend anesthesia if they do not cope well, if they change their minds and ask for relief, or if complications of delivery require it. This is more likely to happen with a first baby, rather than on repeat performances. You should discuss this question on your first visit with your doctor, so that you can know what to expect.

1685. What percentage of women today use an anesthetic during childbirth?

In some places, women do not use any anesthetic, because no one will give them any. When there is a choice, about 70 percent of women choose to have anesthesia during childbirth. Some doctors insist that all women have anesthesia, in which case this figure rises to 100 percent. If you count a local injection for the stitches needed after delivery as an anesthetic, then almost 99 percent of women use an anesthetic during childbirth.

1686. What are the different kinds of anesthesia for childbirth, and will I have a choice in the kind I have?

Your choice is definitely there, but it is limited by your ability to tolerate pain and by what is available at the hospital where you deliver. If you have been to childbirth preparation classes and have learned Lamaze or some other method of breathing to control your attention to pain, you may not need or want any other form of pain relief, except perhaps a local anesthetic for any stitches you may require. This can be a local, an injection of anesthetic directly into the place where the episiotomy or stitches will be, or it can be a pudendal block. A pudendal uses an anesthetic solution that is injected through the vagina into each side near the pudendal nerve. This serves to anesthetize most of the vulva and relieves some of the discomforts of the delivery and the stitches. A paracervical block is another form of local anesthesia that is injected into each side of the cervix during the first stage of labor, before you are completely dilated. It relieves some of the pain of labor, especially transition. However, some anesthetic from this occasionally reaches the baby and slows its heart rate, so the paracervical block has fallen into disuse in recent years. If you dislike labor intensely once it has started, you may choose to have a lumbar or caudal epidural. This is a long-lasting, regional anesthetic injected by a catheter outside the spine that can be continued for many hours to make you numb around the waist. Epidurals are not available in all hospitals, because they require a sophisticated anesthesiologist who is available at all times, and that is expensive. If you tolerate labor up to the second stage when you are bearing down to push the baby's head out but you can't quite do it or you can't stand the pain, a saddle block, which is a form of spinal, will get you through the last hour. A

NORMAL PREGNANCY AND CHOICES IN CHILDBIRTH:
ANESTHESIA (Continued)

spinal is an injection of a small amount of anesthetic into the spinal canal to numb the lower half of the body for an hour or so. The saddle block uses a heavy solution of anesthetic, so only the lower portion of the body, which is involved in delivery, is numb. Some places still give nitrous oxide gas or even Trilene gas for you to breathe at intervals between or during contractions just for some relief, but it does not completely knock you out. Some doctors may still use general anesthesia and put you completely to sleep, but this is usually only done for emergency cesarean sections. All anesthesiologists will discuss anesthesia with you before giving you anything, except in a life-threatening emergency, and even then they will try.

1687. Doesn't all medication and anesthesia carry some risks to the baby?

Nothing is absolutely safe, so you have to learn the relative risks of anesthesia to the baby. If it makes you go to sleep, it is more likely to make the baby sleep, too. An anesthesia solution that is injected to make you numb reaches the baby in such small quantities that it has no effect. Not having anesthesia also carries substantial risks to the baby. Hyperventilating and moving about because of the lack of anesthesia can be quite risky to your baby.

1688. Is there any harm in wanting to be completely knocked out during childbirth?

By being completely knocked out, you will miss one of the greatest experiences of life: birth. If you are knocked out too long before the baby is born, the baby will be knocked out, too. General anesthesia (where you are completely knocked out) makes your obstetrician have to hurry to deliver your baby vaginally or by cesarean section. Most babies can stand a lot of sedation, but if the baby is premature or already in trouble, the anesthesia can make a difference in how quickly and how well the baby breathes. If you have eaten recently and there is still food in your stomach, you may vomit while you are knocked out and get the food into your lungs, which can be fatal. Even if you ate only an hour or so before labor started ten hours ago, there may still be food in your stomach, because labor interferes with digestion. In this case, if a general anesthetic has to be given, a tube is put down your throat to protect your lungs from any such vomiting. This can make your throat a little sore the next day, but it is much safer than allowing vomiting when you are unconscious. Vomiting while under anesthesia used to be one of the major causes of maternal death, but no longer. Obstetrical anesthesiologists have specialized the way anesthesia is given for having a baby. It is now much safer, as well as a better pain relief.

NORMAL PREGNANCY AND CHOICES IN CHILDBIRTH:
ANESTHESIA (Continued)

1689. If I use an anesthesia during childbirth, will it harm my baby?

That depends upon the baby and the anesthesia. In the 1940s, when scopolamine, Demerol, and morphine were used in large quantities to make women groggy (called "twilight sleep"), most babies who were strong and at term had no problem. They just did not breast-feed as well for a day or two. But the premature baby or the one already having difficulty became overly sedated by the drugs, and sometimes had to be given an antidote so it would breathe. If the baby were severely depressed, this could make quite a difference in survival. Today, that kind of drug treatment just isn't used anymore, although a narcotic or tranquilizer may be given in mild doses. This would not be enough to keep the baby from breathing, but perhaps enough to keep it from breast-feeding well for a day or two. Again, if it is a very premature baby or in distress from some other cause, use of a narcotic or tranquilizer could make a big difference. General anesthesia, in which the mother is completely asleep, can make the baby sleepy, too, unless it is delivered quickly. Regional anesthesia, like epidurals, spinals, saddle blocks, and even paracervical blocks, do not make the baby sleepy at all. Paracervical blocks have fallen into disuse because the anesthetic injected around the cervix was absorbed by the baby and sometimes slowed the baby's heart rate alarmingly. Local anesthetic for the stitches, or episiotomy, actually contains a greater quantity of anesthetic than that injected with an epidural or spinal, but it still is not enough to reach the baby and have any detectable effect on it. Any blood pressure drop with a spinal or epidural would be harmful to the baby, but is prevented by giving lots of fluid intravenously before the anesthetic. Blood pressure elevators are also given if the pressure starts to drop. When the choice used to be between ether, which put you to sleep, or no pain relief at all, mothers wrestled with the problem of possible harm to their babies from being sedated. With regional anesthesia, there is no such problem to wrestle with. The only decision is whether you want to feel the entire process of delivery and do it yourself, or whether you dislike feeling it, or you really can't do it yourself without the intervention of the obstetrician's hands, forceps, or vacuum extractors. The cost of the anesthesia may also be a factor.

1690. What are the side effects of the different kinds of anesthesia?

Narcotics, which are injected, make you sleepy; scopolamine gives you amnesia and can make you a little wild; spinals can be followed by a postural (spinal) headache; and sometimes even epidurals can be followed by headache, but not as often. General anesthesia is frequently followed by nausea and vomiting. It can last for several days and spoil the fun you are

NORMAL PREGNANCY AND CHOICES IN CHILDBIRTH:
ANESTHESIA (Continued)

having with your baby. Wearing a tight abdominal binder, taking fluids, antihistamines, and analgesics (pain relievers), or just lying flat can help relieve nausea. If nausea is severe, a blood patch (some of your blood) injected over the site of the needle hole where the anesthesia was given can stop it altogether. Some women don't believe that childbirth is completely natural if they have anything at all for pain relief, including injections of narcotics or tranquilizers or even a local anesthetic for the stitches. Having a baby is not a game to see if you can go without analgesia (pain relief) or anesthesia (being completely numb). You should use whatever you need that is available. If you are one of the 30 percent of women who do well in childbirth without anything, except perhaps childbirth preparation training, such as Lamaze, you should not be bothered with anesthesia. Forceps are not harmful to the baby, so you should not try to suffer pain in order to avoid them.

1691. Is there anything I could take that would ease the pain but still allow me to have a natural delivery?
The definition of a natural delivery is difficult. If you mean that you still can push the baby out by your own strength, instead of having forceps used, this is sometimes possible under all anesthetics and pain relievers. On the other hand, sometimes it is impossible, even if there is no anesthesia. That is why anesthesia is needed, so that forceps or rotations can be used to deliver the baby.

1692. My doctor told me that he routinely delivers all babies with forceps, so I would need anesthesia. I really wanted to try to have a natural childbirth, but it's so late in my pregnancy that I'm afraid to change doctors now. What should I do?
You should have discussed this point during your first visit with your doctor. The use of forceps and anesthesia is a basic attitude that needs to be clarified right away. Late in pregnancy is not the time to discuss it. There is a good chance that you will need an anesthetic and forceps, even if you try for a natural birth, especially if this is your first birth experience. You would feel quite disappointed if you changed doctors so you could have a natural birth, and then found that you required the same things your first doctor was planning for you. If this is the best way your doctor delivers babies and he is not trained in natural delivery, you are better off to do it his way. With your next baby, you can look for a doctor who is willing to try natural birth.

1693. If I have an epidural, will I still be able to push the baby out?
Sometimes women cannot push their babies out, even if they do **not** have an epidural or any anesthetic. In fact, this occurs frequently. It is not

NORMAL PREGNANCY AND CHOICES IN CHILDBIRTH: ANESTHESIA (Continued)

guaranteed that with an epidural you will be able to push the baby out. It is, however, still possible for some women, especially if it is not their first baby. Since the pain is relieved, some women are less motivated to push it out, and they do not try as hard as when they are suffering. In this situation, forceps are used. Without an anesthetic, forceps are too painful to use, but with an epidural there is no problem in using them.

NORMAL PREGNANCY AND CHOICES IN CHILDBIRTH: CESAREAN SECTION

1694. When is a cesarean section necessary?

Fifty years ago a cesarean section was done only to save the life of the mother, never to save the life of the baby. This was because cesarean sections were considered too dangerous to risk the mother's life for the sake of the child. But with safe, modern anesthesia, better operating suites in the delivery area, antibiotics for infection, and probably healthier patients, they are now considered quite safe. Cesarean sections are now done for the benefit of the child, as well as for the mother. Prolonged labor, or failure to progress, has always been a good reason and still is one of the most frequent ones for having a C-section (cesarean section). If you had a previous C-section, this almost used to be an absolute indication for another one because of the danger of rupturing the old incision during labor and delivery. But with the newer type of incision that is made crosswise (transverse) in the lower segment of the uterus, rupture is much less likely, and under certain conditions a vaginal delivery can be done. It is successful in about half of the cases. Cephalo-pelvic disproportion, where the baby is too big for the mother's pelvis, is another common cause for cesarean section. This can be determined early in labor, but sometimes it is diagnosed only after forceps have failed to deliver the baby's head. Breech birth (buttocks first) has become an increased reason for cesarean section, to avoid all the injuries and damage that breeches cause with vaginal delivery, especially if the baby is very premature or very large. Some diseases, such as diabetes, Rh blood sensitization, toxemia, heart disease, and kidney disease, require that delivery be done before the cervix is ready for induction of labor. This can lead to a cesarean section to accomplish early delivery. If fresh herpes ulcers are present on the woman's vulva at the time labor starts, or if a herpes culture is positive, a C-section would be performed. Fetal distress, such as a declining heartbeat, passage of meconium (baby's feces), or a scalp blood sampling showing acidosis (a chemical state of the infant suggesting dire consequences if delivery is not immediate) would necessitate a cesarean section. Sometimes

Cesarean Section

My baby was
brought into this
world without
pain or suffering
He was born in ten minutes
My operation was completed
and shortly after
I held my little son
in my arms
What a miraculous way
to give birth
to a child

— Susan Polis Schutz

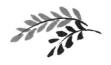

NORMAL PREGNANCY AND CHOICES IN CHILDBIRTH:
CESAREAN SECTION (Continued)

abnormalities of the infant, such as a tumor on the baby's neck or in the abdomen, can be discovered by sonogram, and it would be less susceptible to injury if delivery were made by C-section, rather than by the vagina. Hemorrhage of the mother can be caused by separation of the placenta or the placenta being located over the cervix. Both situations would probably require a cesarean section to save the mother, as well as the baby.

1695. What percentage of women have cesarean sections today?

In major hospitals, the rate of cesarean sections varies from about 15-20 percent of women having babies. Thirty years ago, 6-10 percent of women had them.

1696. When will I know if I need to have a cesarean section?

Sometimes you will only know five minutes beforehand, with the discovery of a prolapsed umbilical cord in your vagina, for instance, or there may be ten or fifteen minutes of fetal distress before a C-section (cesarean section) is decided upon. If you have had a previous cesarean section, you may even know before you get pregnant that you will need one again, especially if you had the first one because you have a small pelvis. Most of the time the decision for a cesarean section is reached gradually over a period of hours in labor.

1697. Can I decide whether I will have a cesarean section?

You cannot choose to have a cesarean section if your doctor does not recommend one simply because you want to avoid labor. That day has not yet come. However, if a cesarean is recommended by your doctor or his consultant, you will be asked to sign a consent form giving permission to do the surgery. If it is an extreme emergency and you are not capable of discussing it, a relative will be asked to sign for you. If you refuse the cesarean, you will be informed of the consequences of not having it, such as your own hemorrhage, prolonged labor, worsening toxemia or infection, or possible damage to the baby. Usually the decision to have a cesarean is made by you and your doctor. It is sometimes discussed for several hours before it is actually done. Sometimes you may know in advance of labor that a cesarean is likely; this would be the case if you have a very small pelvis, a very large baby, twins in a bad position, or a breech or other malposition of the baby. Most of the time the decision for a cesarean section is made after labor has started but has failed to progress, or a complication, such as fetal distress, has arisen. One situation in which you can choose to have a cesarean section is with subsequent pregnancies that follow a cesarean delivery. If conditions are right, you could also choose to try for a vaginal delivery. It is still somewhat new to

NORMAL PREGNANCY AND CHOICES IN CHILDBIRTH:
CESAREAN SECTION (Continued)

have a vaginal delivery after previously delivering by cesarean section, so no one is forced into that.

1698. Why do women "look down" on cesareans?

Some women feel that the primary role of a woman is to have a baby, and if she cannot deliver it in a completely natural way, without drugs, anesthesia, or assistance from anyone, then she has not properly fulfilled her role. It even is assumed that some women ask for the cesarean, so they can stop having labor; of course, that is not the case. Women can't really ask for cesareans. In the past and in other countries today, women who do not have large families are looked down upon. There also is the attitude that if you have a cesarean every time you have a baby, you can only have two or three babies, because it must be impossible to have more than two or three cesareans. This is really not true. As many as six, and sometimes as many as a dozen, cesarean sections have been performed on one woman. However, because it is so easy to have a tubal ligation at the time of surgery, many women do have this done after their second or third baby. There is an organization in the United States, called C-Section, Inc., that tries to combat these negative kinds of ideas. Their motto is that having a cesarean section is having a baby, too. They encourage family-centered childbirth, so that the father is present at the time of the cesarean section and bonding with the baby is provided for, rather than whisking it off to the nursery in the middle of the surgery. C-Section, Inc., is a group that voices concerns of women who have had cesarean sections; since 22 percent of women have them, this is a lot of people. Many women who have cesareans go through hours of labor, as well as surgery. They deserve more appreciation, instead of less. The father who stays with his wife through the surgery also has a more difficult experience and deserves admiration as well.

1699. Are cesarean sections dangerous?

A cesarean section is major surgery, involving more danger to the mother than an easy vaginal delivery. However, in certain situations, it may be far more dangerous for some women to deliver vaginally. The death rate for the safest of major surgeries is still about one in ten thousand operations.

1700. Exactly how is a cesarean section performed?

First the woman is anesthetized, her abdomen is scrubbed, and the drapes are put into place. Then an incision is made in her skin, either in the midline (up and down) or low across the top of the pubic hair, which has been shaved off. This latter method is called the bikini cut. Then the fat is cut, and bleeding vessels are tied or cauterized (burned) to stop bleeding. The

NORMAL PREGNANCY AND CHOICES IN CHILDBIRTH:
CESAREAN SECTION (Continued)

covering of the muscle, called fascia, is cut with scissors and pulled back. The muscles are separated in the midline, and the thin lining of the abdominal cavity (the peritoneum) is cut. After that, the lower half of the uterus is visible. Scissors are used to cut the attachment of the bladder from the uterus. A knife is used to cut into the lower part of the uterus, until membranes or amniotic fluid appears. This is extended with scissors across the uterus. At this point, the baby is visible. A hand is placed under the baby's head, and with the help of assistants, pressure is put on the top of the uterus, so that baby is pushed out. After it is breathing, the cord is clamped and cut, and the baby handed off to a nurse or doctor. The placenta is removed from the uterus by hand, and then the incision in the uterine muscle is closed by layers of stitches or sutures. The bladder flap is sutured back into place. Ovaries and tubes are inspected, and then the peritoneum layer is sutured. The fascia over the muscles is sutured back into place, the fat layer is sutured, and finally the skin is closed with clips, staples, or sutures.

1701. What different kinds of anesthesia are used with cesarean sections?

General anesthesia, in which the woman is completely and deeply asleep, and regional anesthesia, in which she is numb from the waist down, are the two major kinds of anesthesia used with a cesarean section. Various gases and drugs are used for the general anesthesia, with consideration given to the effect on the unborn baby. General anesthesia is often used when there is a hemorrhage, an immediate cesarean for an emergency, or hypertension. The side effects are mostly nausea afterwards and a possible sedated effect on the baby if it is not delivered quickly. Regional anesthetics used are either a spinal (saddle block) or an epidural (lumbar type). These are administered by an injection of anesthetic solution either into the spinal canal or just outside of it. Regional anesthetics are used when there is more time for the cesarean section, when the mother and father want to witness the delivery, or when there is an attempt to avoid sedation of the baby. Side effects are an occasional postural headache, which may last a few days; this occurs more often with the spinal than with the epidural. Rarely are cesarean sections done under local anesthesia.

1702. Will I have a choice in what anesthetic I will get?

Yes. If you have strong feelings about which anesthetic you want, you should make this known to the person who is giving you anesthesia. He may convince you that you should have something different, but your opinion is important to him in his selection. Unless there is a dire emergency, there is time to discuss the anesthesia before doing the cesarean section. If you are already under an epidural anesthetic for labor when the decision to do a

NORMAL PREGNANCY AND CHOICES IN CHILDBIRTH:
CESAREAN SECTION (Continued)

cesarean section is made, this anesthesia can just be continued with a little higher and more intense anesthetic solution to make you numb enough for surgery.

1703. How long does it take to perform a cesarean section?

A cesarean section takes forty-five minutes to an hour to perform. It takes only five or ten minutes to go in and get the baby out; the rest of the time is spent suturing the area closed.

1704. How long will the intravenous line (I.V.) be in my arm after the operation?

If you have regional anesthesia (spinal or epidural) and are not nauseated or vomiting, and if you are taking fluids, the intravenous line can be removed in a few hours. If you are so nauseated that you are vomiting for a day or so, as can happen with a general anesthetic, then the I.V. must stay in place so you can be given fluids to help reduce your vomiting. If you want to get the I.V. out sooner, try hard to take fluids as soon as they are offered. If you need it, ask for something to combat nausea.

1705. Will a cesarean section damage my stomach muscles?

No, but carrying a baby nine months will. The stomach muscles are not cut during the surgery, only their coverings are, and those are sewn back together. Because of the healing scar, the muscles may be a little slower to exercise and return to normal, but they will eventually operate as well as muscles do after a vaginal delivery.

1706. If I have a cesarean section, is there any harm to my baby?

Often a cesarean section is done to prevent harm to your baby. If the section is done to prevent harm to you, that also prevents harm to the baby, since harming you usually harms your baby. Comparisons have been made between repeat sections (where no problems exist) and vaginal deliveries. The main problem that arises from C-sections (cesarean sections) is premature babies that are delivered too soon.

1707. Will I still go through labor when I have a cesarean section?

Even if you know you are going to have a cesarean section, many times it is advisable for you to at least start labor, to be sure your baby is really at term. Scheduling the cesarean before you start labor might be delivering the baby early. But if the reason for the section is to deliver the baby early, this does not apply. When you don't know that you are going to have a cesarean section, labor may go on and on until either you or your unborn baby shows signs of exhaustion or distress that is enough to warrant ending the process. But there is always the hope that in just one more hour

NORMAL PREGNANCY AND CHOICES IN CHILDBIRTH: CESAREAN SECTION (Continued)

the baby will deliver vaginally. If you are in good condition and the monitor shows your baby is all right, it is fine to try a little longer. Your opinion can be influential either way.

1708. How will I feel after a cesarean section? Is there much pain?

There is more pain after a cesarean section than after a vaginal delivery. It is felt across the lower abdomen where the incision is. The pain after a vaginal delivery is felt in the tissue between the vagina and rectum, whether you stretched, tore, or were cut. After a vaginal delivery it is hard to sit down, but after a cesarean section it is hard to pull yourself up to a sitting position or to stand up. Sitting is all right, and so is lying down. More and stronger pain relief medication is offered after a cesarean section than after a vaginal delivery, at least for the first day or two. Gas in the abdomen is worse after a cesarean section, and it takes longer for the bowels to work again. Relief from gas can be obtained by suppositories, enemas, tubes, or other remedies. It is worse the second day after surgery, and eventually goes away.

1709. How long will I be in the hospital after a cesarean section?

On the West Coast, the average time spent in the hospital after a cesarean section is three or four days. It seems to be a bit longer elsewhere.

1710. How long will it take for me to heal after a cesarean section?

Six weeks is the usual time needed to recover from having a baby, whether it is by vaginal delivery or by cesarean section. The first few weeks after a cesarean section are more difficult than the first few weeks after a vaginal delivery with an episiotomy, but by six weeks there is not much difference. Bleeding after delivery occurs off and on for about six weeks. The uterus is a little slower to return to its normal size after a cesarean section, but accomplishes this within six weeks.

1711. Are infections more common after a cesarean section?

Yes, infections do occur more often after a C-section (cesarean section) than they do after a vaginal delivery. If an infection is expected, antibiotics may be given during surgery to avoid it.

1712. How big is the scar?

Usually the scar from a cesarean section is about six inches long, whether it is up and down or across the abdomen. If it is crosswise, when the pubic hair grows back, you won't see it as much.

1713. How long should I wait after having a cesarean section before doing any exercises?

Three weeks after a cesarean section, healing is usually sufficient to

"Cesarean Stigma"

Everyone: "Susan, I am so sorry
that you had to have a
cesarean."

Me: "Why are you sorry?"

Everyone: "Well, you didn't get the
chance to see Jared being born."

Me: "So what?"

Everyone: "Well, it's just so beautiful and
meaningful."

Me: "To me, the beautiful and
meaningful part is that a new life
has been born, and he is from us
and will be loved by us forever."

Everyone: "Sure, that's true, but it would
have meant that much more if you had
seen the actual birth of Jared."

Me: "Do you love your mother,
father, brother and husband?"

Everyone: "Yes."

Me: "Well, I'm sorry."

Everyone: "Why are you sorry?"

Me: "Because you didn't see
the actual birth of them."

— Susan Polis Schutz

NORMAL PREGNANCY AND CHOICES IN CHILDBIRTH:
CESAREAN SECTION (Continued)

begin doing exercises, such as those in which your legs are raised, and even sit-ups, swimming, or running. However, you should be examined by a doctor before you begin exercising. That is a good reason for a three-week checkup, as well as one at six weeks. For the first three weeks after the operation, it is enough exercise just to live, walk around, take care of your baby, and perhaps prepare some meals. You can drive a car when you no longer need pain pills and can turn and look for traffic without clutching your abdomen.

1714. Are cesarean sections used too much today?

Cesareans have definitely increased in both numbers and in percentages. There are several factors that account for the increase. The most frequent cause for a cesarean section is a previous cesarean section. The danger of rupturing the uterine scar from a previous section is thought to be too dangerous to deliver subsequent babies vaginally. Since cesareans are increasing, too, the repeat sections have a snowball effect in terms of increasing the numbers and percentages. There is a widespread attempt today to encourage vaginal delivery of subsequent children, if the original reason for the cesarean section is no longer present. In hospitals today, these attempts are made safer by the availability of fetal monitoring devices and the immediate availability of facilities and anesthesia to perform emergency cesarean sections. But only about half of such attempts succeed. These attempts will not greatly reduce the cesarean rate, and the procedure is not available in some delivery suites that cannot do rapid cesarean sections if the rupture starts to occur. Primary sections, those done for the first time, are also increasing.

The rise in cesarean sections has been accompanied by a reduction in deaths of babies, and with good reason. Another factor that increases the number of sections is the decision that a breech delivery, which used to damage many babies, is just too dangerous, especially for a first-time mother. This accounts for 10 percent of the increase. Fetal distress, that is, signs of trouble that may threaten the baby's survival, without any failure to progress in the labor, also accounts for about 10 percent of the increase in sections, and is credited to the new fetal monitoring machines that tell us how the baby is doing with greater accuracy than the old stethoscopes could. What mother would want to continue labor when she knows that her baby is about to die before it is born? Herpes accounts for a very small rise in cesarean sections; the section is done in an attempt to keep the baby from being infected by herpes on the vaginal area. A social cause of increased cesareans is the change in family size. Since most women now only have two

NORMAL PREGNANCY AND CHOICES IN CHILDBIRTH:
CESAREAN SECTION (Continued)

babies, instead of five or six, a much larger percentage of babies being born are to first-time mothers, called primagravidas. Twenty-five years ago these made up only 30 percent of the women in labor, but now it is closer to 45 to 50 percent. If families were ever reduced to one child per family, 100 percent of the women in labor would be in labor for the first time. Everyone knows that the first baby is the hardest one to deliver, taking a much longer time and running into many more problems than a third or fourth child. This factor alone accounts for about a 50 percent rise in the percentage of cesarean sections.

A recent consensus panel of the National Institutes of Health considered the question of whether obstetricians are simply doing more sections because they are too impatient, lazy, or because they want to make more money. They found that this was not the case. No woman or doctor would want a three-day labor and a damaged or dead child just to reduce the cesarean section rate.

NORMAL PREGNANCY AND CHOICES IN CHILDBIRTH:
CESAREAN STIGMA

1715. What is the cesarean stigma?

The cesarean stigma is the attitude that a woman who cannot deliver a baby vaginally is not a complete, feminine woman. Some people accuse women who have cesarean sections of not being brave enough or strong enough to go through labor and delivery, as if somehow they were inadequate. Of course, this is not true. The decision for a cesarean section comes from the women's obstetricians, and today they are done most frequently for the welfare of the babies. Women who have a cesarean section are really so maternal that they are willing to undergo the additional risk of major surgery and additional pain of recovery from the abdominal incision. A vaginal delivery is less risky for the mothers, and it is easier to recover from. Women should be admired for undergoing the cesarean section, instead of being put down for it. It is partly this stigma that makes women wonder if their cesarean section was really necessary. They also may feel that they did not really have a baby, that someone else had it for them. People feel sorry for women who have cesarean sections. A national organization called C-Section, Inc., is devoted to demonstrating that having a baby by cesarean section is having a baby, too, and can be just as exciting as natural birth. The father can be there, and the mother can be awake and alert if she is not under general anesthesia. After the baby is born, the father can hold the baby right next to the mother's face as the surgery is being completed. The pediatrician

NORMAL PREGNANCY AND CHOICES IN CHILDBIRTH: CESAREAN STIGMA (Continued)

does not usually need to whisk the baby off to the nursery. The baby can be left in the care of the surgical personnel as long as the parents are in the room. The parents can also visit together afterwards with the baby in the recovery room; this is called bonding time. By making the cesarean section a family-centered childbirth experience, it becomes much more acceptable to those who have it.

NORMAL PREGNANCY AND CHOICES IN CHILDBIRTH: BONDING

1716. Can I keep my baby with me all the time in the hospital after it is delivered? Can I go home right away with my baby?

If your baby is in good condition at birth, most hospitals allow some time for the two of you (or three with father) to be together and visit for a while after delivery. This is called bonding time. It can be a very special time for you to get acquainted and is a reward after your day of labor. State laws that require preventive treatment for the baby's eyes have been relaxed to allow a delay of up to two hours before this is done, so that your baby can look back at you for a while. Most modern hospitals also allow some form of rooming-in. If yours does not, you should request it. The reason the baby is taken away at all is to provide the treatment to the eyes, to measure and weigh it, and to perform a medical assessment of its condition. Of course, the doctor who delivered it evaluated it right away to see if it was safe to leave it with you for awhile, and then the nurse who is checking on your recovery also checks the temperature of the baby to see that it is not getting too cold. Newborns can get cold very easily. If you plan to go home soon, such as in six hours, after it is fairly certain you are not going to have a hemorrhage, then a pediatrician must examine the baby to see if it is all right to go home that soon. Early discharge also means you must bring the baby back to be examined and tested again in a day or two, or someone, such as a visiting nurse, must visit your home to see if all is well. If you are staying in the hospital for a few days, you will be moved to your postpartum room while the baby is taken to the nursery. In some hospitals, rooming-in is limited to daytime hours, although the baby is brought back for breast-feeding at night. Some other hospitals allow the baby to be with you at night as well, but with nursing care that carefully watches the baby and you. Some women would rather sleep without the baby for a night or two until they have recovered. Others cannot stand to be separated for a moment. A few women don't like rooming-in with the baby at all. This is really your choice, provided the hospital gives you the opportunity. Discuss rooming-in with your doctor, and try to bring pressure on the hospitals in your area to provide this

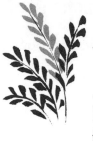

I can't believe it
I'm not pregnant anymore
it's over
it's really over
the operation is over
We have a healthy baby boy
I can't believe it
no more huge stomach
or bloated face
I'll be able to walk again
I'll be able to play again
The pain is so
unbearable
But I don't want pills
to put me to sleep
I want to be alert enough
to realize that it's really over
and that I have a beautiful baby
it's over
Thank God

— Susan Polis Schutz

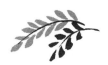

NORMAL PREGNANCY AND CHOICES IN CHILDBIRTH:
BONDING (Continued)

service. It certainly promotes breast-feeding, and it teaches the mother how to care for her newborn baby with confidence.

1717. I've read it's easier to develop close family relationships right after birth and that people who are separated from their newborns have a higher incidence of child abuse. We don't want to do anything that might minimize our loving relationship with our child. After all, it's our baby. Why should we have to be separated at all?

If you have a great desire to be with your child, you will bond with that child even if it does not occur immediately after delivery. There is no danger that you will be abusive parents. The bonding that you read about is an effort to make loving parents out of people who are not. Separation from your baby is eventually necessary to perform certain measurements and assessments of the child, to observe it for abnormalities, which you are not really capable of doing, to give it the eye treatment required by law within two hours of birth, and to have someone watch and take care of it while you are asleep. If your baby is with you while you are asleep in your room, no one is watching the baby, and it has just been born! It is fun to be with the baby right away, even for a few minutes, but the same bonding can take place later, too.

NORMAL PREGNANCY AND CHOICES IN CHILDBIRTH:
AFTER CHILDBIRTH

1718. Will I be weak after childbirth?

If your labor was long and hard or if you had a cesarean section, you will have some weakness for the day or so following your delivery. After that, if you get up and around, your strength will return, provided you get adequate rest during the daytime to make up for the time you spend with the baby at night. If you never sleep, you will be very tired and weak. If you stay in bed for ten days after you have your baby, you will be so weak that it may take a month for you to get up and around again. So you need a happy medium: some rest and some activity.

1719. Will my stomach go back into shape after my baby is born?

Not completely. It almost will return to its original shape if you exercise by doing sit-ups, leg raising, swimming, running, or dancing, but it may take six months for this to happen. If you have gained a lot of weight, this may interfere.

1720. How long will I bleed after childbirth?

It is normal to bleed a little, off and on, for as long as six weeks following childbirth.

Jared Polis Schutz
a whole little person
a miracle
from God
to Stephen, to me
to the world

Jared Polis Schutz
a beautiful little person
eight healthy pounds
delicate light skin
soft red cheeks
huge bubbly ocean-blue eyes

Jared Polis Schutz
a precious little person
who will share
our days
and nights
our life
our love

— Susan Polis Schutz

My Son

From the day you
were born
you were
so special
so smart
so sensitive
so good
It was so much fun
        to watch you
As you grew
you became your
own person
with your own
ideas
and your own way
of doing things
It was so exciting
        to watch you
As you grew more
you became more independent
still special
still smart
still sensitive
still good
I am so proud
of everything about you
and I want you to know
that I love
everything about you

— Susan Polis Schutz

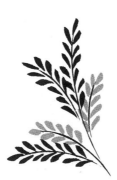

To My Daughter

When you were born
I held you in my arms
and just kept smiling at you
You always smiled back
your big eyes wide open
full of love
You were such a
beautiful
good
sweet baby
Now
as I watch you
grow up
and become your
own person
I look at you
your laughter
your happiness
your simplicity
your beauty
and I wonder
where you will be
in fifteen years
and I wonder
where the world will be
in fifteen years
I just hope
that you will
be able to enjoy a life
of sensitivity
goodness
accomplishment
and love
in a world that is at peace
But most of all
I want you to know that
I am very proud of you
and that I
love you dearly

— Susan Polis Schutz

We had a beautiful
little girl
I want to shout it
to the clouds
I want to yell it
across the ocean
It's all over

We had a beautiful little girl
Nine months of worry
and discomfort
and there she was
all pink and cuddly with
long almond-shaped eyes
perfect little hands and feet

We had a beautiful little girl
I want to shout it
across the mountains
I want to yell it
through the fields
It's all over

Jordanna is beautiful
Jordanna is healthy
Jordanna is perfect
Thank you Jordanna
Thank you God

— Susan Polis Schutz

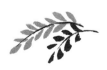

NORMAL PREGNANCY AND CHOICES IN CHILDBIRTH: AFTER CHILDBIRTH (Continued)

1721. When will I start my period again?

One-half of the women who do not breast-feed will have a menstrual flow by the sixth week after their delivery. Others may take three months before they have a period. If you breast-feed, you probably will not menstruate for three or four months after the six weeks of bleeding is over. Some women will not have a period for the entire time they breast-feed.

1722. Will it really take a year after childbirth before my body gets back to the way it was before pregnancy?

Your body never really gets back to the way it was before your pregnancy. Your abdominal muscles get tighter, but they are not as tight as they were. Your stretch marks fade, but are still there. Your varicose veins get smaller, but remain. The dark spots (chloasma) on your skin fade slowly, perhaps within six months. The cesarean section scar gets pale after a year. The scar of your episiotomy can always be seen by a doctor. Your vagina is never quite as tight as before, and your breasts sag.

1723. Where can I go for help and advice with my new baby?

The doctor who delivered your baby may want to take care of it, too. This could be a general practitioner or family-practice doctor. If you had an obstetrician deliver your baby, then you should also have a pediatrician who can advise you on the care of your infant. If you had a nurse midwife, she can refer you to a nurse practitioner who deals with newborn well-baby care. Most county and city health departments have well-baby clinics where you can go to see if your baby's progress is normal and to get advice on how to care for your baby. Visiting nurses are sometimes available to help you with newborn baby care. Be sure to ask about this when your baby is delivered. If you have moved, inquire about infant care at your nearest hospital, health department, or clinic.

NORMAL PREGNANCY AND CHOICES IN CHILDBIRTH: BREAST-FEEDING

1724. Should I breast-feed my child?

The majority of medical opinions agree that it is better to breast-feed your baby. It even is beneficial if you just do it for a little while, a week or two, and then stop after that. The human milk contains cells (lymphocytes) that contain antibodies to diseases. When the baby drinks it, they line the baby's intestinal tract and protect it from some diarrhea infections. Human milk is usually the most easily digested because of its protein and small curd.

NORMAL PREGNANCY AND CHOICES IN CHILDBIRTH: BREAST-FEEDING (Continued)

The act of breast-feeding provides the mother and child with a close body relationship that helps parenting and satisifies the child more than being held at arm's length and fed by a bottle. You can cuddle a child while feeding it from a bottle, but many parents don't do this because they don't have to. You can't breast-feed at arms length. At the breast, the baby takes only what it wants and no more. If you have an irregular lifestyle, that might make it very hard for you to be with your baby at the times it wants to breast-feed. When you are away from your baby, your breasts become painfully engorged, and the baby fusses at the bottle. Many women are able to combine bottle-feeding with breast-feeding, partially to adapt to their schedules. Others find the whole process of breast-feeding repulsive. In this case, it would be better to have a smiling mother behind a bottle than a disgusted mother behind a breast. Some men do not like to see their wives breast-feed. They feel jealous and replaced. Some women like to bottle-feed, so that the fathers can share equally in feeding the child. Each couple must decide for themselves.

1725. Can I choose whether or not I will breast-feed my baby?

You can decide whether you want to breast-feed before your baby is born by taking classes, reading, and talking with your pediatrician, obstetrician, family doctor, or friends. However, it takes two to breast-feed, so you must have a baby who is willing. Some babies will not breast-feed. Some are too little or too premature, and they cannot suckle well. Others simply fight and cannot be calmed down enough to learn how. They like bottles instead, where the hole is big and the milk pours out. Long ago, before baby bottles, babies who would not breast-feed probably just did not survive. Now we have bottles and baby formulas of many types to suit each baby. Some women also have inverted nipples that do not allow them to breast-feed, and even with breast shields, it can be difficult to obtain milk.

1726. Should I do anything during pregnancy to prepare my nipples for breast-feeding?

There are many opinions on this subject. In general, the only helpful thing you can do is to pull your nipples out, especially if they are slightly inverted, with your fingers. But if you stimulate your nipples too much, your breasts will produce milk, even during pregnancy, and then they will leak or cake. The best preparation for breast-feeding takes place in your mind. Attending a lecture on how to put the baby to your breast, how to hold it, how to get the whole nipple, and not just the end, into its mouth will do more good than any handling of the nipple. Toughening a nipple does not prevent

NORMAL PREGNANCY AND CHOICES IN CHILDBIRTH:
BREAST-FEEDING (Continued)

trouble; it makes trouble. A nipple that is hard to the touch will crack when it is being suckled on; a soft one will not. Rubbing your nipple with a towel, a toothbrush, or painting it with something does not make it soft. Lanolin softens, but there is time enough to use that after the baby is born, if you want to. You cannot avoid all pain when breast-feeding. The let-down reflex, when the milk shoots into the nipples, hurts for a moment, but it soon goes away. This usually happens when the baby first latches on, so you get set for it. If your nipples hurt more and more as the baby suckles, you are not putting them in the baby's mouth correctly. Try again to put more of the nipple into the baby's mouth. The baby's gums should clamp down at the edge of the areola, the brown part. Also, don't nurse for more than five or ten minutes at a time, at least not at first. The baby can empty the breast in that time, and after that you are acting as a human pacifier. If your nipples can stand it, it is all right, but if not, let the baby suckle on something else.

1727. How long should I breast-feed my child?

This certainly can be a matter of choice, and sometimes it is the baby's choice. When other foods are introduced, some babies switch to them entirely and refuse the breast. Also when a bottle is started, some babies turn away from the breast and only take the bottle. So the choice is not always absolutely yours. Only about one-half of the women in the United States breast-feed for as long as three or four months. About 10 percent breast-feed for as long as six months. A few women who really enjoy it feed the baby this way for two to three years. Of course, by that time breast-feeding is reserved for just the morning and evening, and most of the baby's food is obtained elsewhere. But it is soothing to the baby and still beneficial. A baby with teeth will not bite your nipples if it has always been breast-fed. If you are using breast-feeding to keep from being pregnant because your religion does not allow you to use any form of birth control, then breast-feed for as long as possible. In the developing countries, most babies are breast-fed for one or two years.

1728. How common is mastitis in breast-feeding mothers?

About 20 percent of women who breast-feed will have at least one episode of mastitis (an infection of the breast caused by bacteria). With mastitis, a hard, red tender area develops in the breast and there may be fever. Treatment is by the application of heat and perhaps antibiotics. A few cases go on to form a severe infection with high fever, and even an abscess that has to be opened and drained in order to heal. It is much better to treat the small spot quickly than to wait for this to happen. It is also better to continue breast-feeding the baby instead of letting your breasts become more engorged. It will not hurt the baby to breast-feed during this time.

NORMAL PREGNANCY AND CHOICES IN CHILDBIRTH:
BREAST-FEEDING (Continued)

1729. What is breast milk made of?

Breast milk consists of water, sugar (lactose), protein (mostly casein), fat (butterfat), some cells (lymphocytes) and antibodies, and a trace of almost anything that also is in the mother's system, such as vitamins A, B, and C, but not very much D.

1730. When will my breasts start producing milk?

Even if you do not let your baby stimulate your nipples by suckling, 80 percent of women will have the milk come anyway about forty-eight hours after delivery. If you let your baby suckle and stimulate your nipples, it can come in sooner; nearly 100 percent of women will have breast milk within forty-eight hours.

1731. Is my baby getting everything he/she needs from breast-feeding?

If you are not sure, ask your pediatrician. Most pediatricians believe that babies need extra vitamin D, especially if they are breast-fed, because there is not very much in breast milk. Vitamin D is added to cow's milk.

1732. My doctor told me I would have to introduce a bottle regularly, or I'd never be able to leave my baby. Is this true?

Some people hold this opinion, but others do not. When you leave and your child is very hungry, it may learn to take a bottle for the first time. If it doesn't catch on quickly, the babysitter and the baby may have a very tough time until you return. Find out if your baby will take a bottle at all. Your baby will probably take one from someone else better than it will take one from you, because with you it detects a better supply nearby.

NORMAL PREGNANCY AND CHOICES IN CHILDBIRTH:
POSTPARTUM DEPRESSION

1733. What is postpartum depression?

The degree of postpartum depression varies from woman to woman. One type is when women feel sad and bored because the excitement of childbirth is over, and the routine of baby care takes up their time twenty-four hours a day, with no relief in sight. Basically, they are exhausted because there is not enough help with the housework or the baby. Sometimes there are real psychotic depressions in which women hallucinate, deny their babies are theirs, and require major treatment or hospitalization for depression.

1734. What can I do to get over postpartum depression?

If your depression is severe, you need medical and psychiatric help. This type of depression usually occurs in women who have had similar prob-

NORMAL PREGNANCY AND CHOICES IN CHILDBIRTH: POSTPARTUM DEPRESSION (Continued)

lems before pregnancy, perhaps years before, but the strain of childbirth brings it all back. The postpartum depression caused by being tired because of the birth is easier to handle. This requires some planning for recreation time away from the baby, preferably with your husband. Babysitting relatives or hired babysitters can watch your baby while you go out and enjoy yourself. It would be best if this relief were planned along with everything else that is planned before having a baby. Postpartum depression is worse with a difficult baby when there is no relief during the day or night and no help from your husband. Help from your husband is important, especially if he lets you get out of the house for a while, but a housekeeper is very helpful for relieving depression, too. Basically, you will need to get an adequate or more than adequate amount of sleep every night so that you do not remain exhausted. Also, some relief from the many chores of motherhood will enable you to pursue other interests that make life exciting to you.

"Postpartum Blues"

"Postpartum blues"
Surely there is such a thing
but what a misnomer
it is exhaustion
it is physical weakness
How dare people reduce
this result of a very
traumatic experience
to just the "blues"

— Susan Polis Schutz

Chapter 8

Women's Diseases and Surgery

WOMEN'S DISEASES AND SURGERY

Many women are able to take charge of their bodies as long as they are healthy, but they completely panic when something goes wrong and turn their entire welfare over to their doctors, even letting their parents and husbands make any decisions that have to be made after that. It is normal to become dependent when you are sick, and it is a good idea to seek help. But if you can maintain some perspective on your problem, you still can exert influences on the choices, the outcome, and especially the disability produced by whatever is wrong. This does not mean that you should ignore all standard medical care and run to a friend or even a book for help. Discuss it with a friend and read a book, but if the problem is important, seek the best medical care you can find and afford. You deserve it.

How can you have choices when you have a disease? You can be cooperative and even influential in asking for tests that can help make the diagnosis, even in a small matter like an irritating discharge. By law, you must give an informed consent before any surgery or major medical treatment is done. To do this you must know what is going on, what your alternatives are, and what the medical treatments as well as surgical treatments could be. You can discuss and be influential in deciding what anesthesia you have for surgery. Hysterectomies may be done in several ways. Options, such as abdominal versus a vaginal approach, midline or bikini incision, keeping your ovaries or removing them, are for your selection. When there is a disease, you take charge of selecting a physician, but you are still in charge of your body; your doctor is your advisor and the instrument to carry out the decisions you both reach. This chapter covers the most common women's diseases and types of surgery. It does not cover every disease and it is not all inclusive, but it will give you a background so that you can discuss your problems with your doctor. Diseases of your breasts are covered in Chapter 3.

WOMEN'S DISEASES AND SURGERY: VAGINITIS—WHAT IT IS, SYMPTOMS

1735. What is vaginitis?

Vaginitis is an inflammation, infection, or irritation of the vagina and usually of the vulva, too.

1736. How common is vaginitis?

The waiting rooms of practitioners', nurses', and doctors' offices are filled with cases of "vulvovaginal disease." It is one of the ten problems most frequently encountered by gynecologists. Yet, the diagnosis and treatment of vulvovaginal disease does not get "prime time" in most medical schools, because it is considered an unimportant annoyance. The discomfort, the interference with the day-to-day routine of women, and the problems it creates in sexual relationships should make it Number One in importance as far as most women are concerned.

1737. What are the usual symptoms of vaginitis?

This depends upon the cause of the vaginitis. Some common symptoms are pain during intercourse; odorous discharge; severe or mild itching; burning; burning with urination; heavy, thick, or watery discharge; and skin changes, such as redness and perhaps cracks in the skin from scratching.

1738. How do I know when I have a vaginal infection?

If you have been avoiding intercourse and using simple measures, such as cortisone cream for itching, and the symptoms of itching and burning have not gone away within a few days, then you must have a vaginal infection. You also are more likely to have an infection if your discharge changes from its normal character to a very heavy discharge of a different color and odor.

1739. What causes vaginal itching?

What you refer to as vaginal itching is not really what it seems. There are no itch nerves in the vagina, but there are plenty on the vulva, the lips around the vagina. These nerves on the vulva are responsible for vaginal itching, and there are many causes. A little burning and itching is very common following dry intercourse; it occurs when you are not adequately aroused and lubricated. This type of vaginal itching will go away in a few days with no treatment, or you can get comfort by using cortisone cream. The most severe itching is caused by the fungus (yeast) infection of Candida albicans. Other infections, such as herpes genitalis or trichomonas vaginitis, also can be accompanied by some itching.

1740. How common is vaginal itching?

There is no woman alive who has not had vaginal itching at some time in her life. It is as common as the common cold.

WOMEN'S DISEASES AND SURGERY: VAGINITIS—WHAT IT IS, SYMPTOMS (Continued)

1741. How do I know if my vaginal discharge is normal or abnormal?

The abnormal vaginal discharges are associated with changes in odor, itching, burning, irritation, and pain during intercourse. If you do not have any of these symptoms, your discharge may be different in quantity, but it is probably normal. The final way to prove that your discharge is really normal would be to culture it for every possible infection. The negative results would tell you that your discharge is normal. A normal cervix and a normal Pap smear would also prove that you have a normal discharge.

1742. Is it abnormal to have a discharge that is extremely heavy, yet has no odor, change in color, or irritation?

No, it is not abnormal. The amount of discharge reflects the amount of hormones you have in your body. The quantity also reflects the amount of vaginal lubrication you produce in response to sexual arousal. Watching a sexually arousing movie can make your discharge very heavy in the next hour or so that follows.

1743. Does normal vaginal discharge usually occur during ovulation?

Just prior to and during ovulation, the cervix forms a clear discharge that is stringy and aids the passage of sperm. This can pass out of the vagina as a clear mucus discharge. It is different from the scant discharge that occurs from menstruation to ovulation and is also different from the thick, creamy discharge that builds up from ovulation to menstruation.

WOMEN'S DISEASES AND SURGERY: VAGINITIS—CAUSES, TREATMENTS, AND TYPES

1744. What causes vaginitis?

The most frequent cause of a mild vaginitis that disappears within a few days without any treatment is trauma. This means intercourse when you are not lubricated. Other causes of vaginitis, in order of frequency, are: Candida (yeast or fungus infections), Trichomonas, herpes, Gardnerella (Hemophilus), gonorrhea, Chlamydia, and hormone deficiency.

1745. Why do I constantly get vaginal infections, even though I am very clean?

It doesn't matter how clean you are if your sex partners have infections. Infections do not come from being dirty, they come from having sex with someone who has an infection. The only infection that occurs without sex is the yeast or fungus infection, Candida albicans, which can come from being too clean. If you put antiseptic douches into your vagina, you kill the bacteria that hold back the fungus. If you take antibiotics, you also kill the

WOMEN'S DISEASES AND SURGERY: VAGINITIS—CAUSES, TREATMENTS, AND TYPES (Continued)

bacteria in the vagina that hold back the fungus. Being too clean makes a fungus infection more likely to occur.

1746. My doctor says my vaginitis is due to a lack of estrogen. How did that happen?

While breast-feeding, your body produces very little or no estrogen at first, and the vagina becomes very red and tender, making intercourse painful. This is called an atrophic or lactation vulvovaginitis, and it will respond to estrogen cream. Stopping breast-feeding or the return of menstruation will also eliminate the vaginitis. After menopause, whether natural or surgical, you may not have any estrogen unless you take some orally. Vaginal atrophy can occur at this time, unless your fat helps you produce some estrogen. Burning, painful intercourse, itching, burning with urination, and tenderness can occur, even though there is no infection present at all. Spotting can also occur after coitus. Estrogen creams will work to correct these symptoms, and so will oral estrogens, if you decide to use them. If sex has been avoided, dilation of the vagina may be needed, too, because it shrinks with menopause.

1747. After I have a lot of sex, I have a lot of burning and itching, but not extra discharge. Does this mean that I have a vaginal infection?

No. What you are experiencing is called traumatic vaginitis. There is no sexually active woman alive who has not experienced this at some time or other, but some women make a habit of it. These women, like you, may think that they have an incurable yeast infection, when actually they need to learn a better sex technique. Adding a surgical lubricant to your love-making may be a temporary solution, but in the long run you need to defer intercourse until you are lubricated by sexual arousal. The more you want to please, the less you may be willing to wait for entry until you are lubricated. However, you will pay for this dry intercourse with burning and itching the next day. It goes away if you stop having sex for a while, but if you continue the same performance at frequent intervals, you may think you have a constant problem. You do have a problem, but it is not an infection. You need to learn how to make love, not how to please.

1748. I have been told that I have nonspecific vaginitis. What is that?

Nonspecific vaginitis was a term used when doctors could not find the cause of the vaginitis but could show that it was not gonorrhea, Trichomonas, or yeast. Today, however, all causes of vaginitis can be diagnosed by culture or other means, and the term nonspecific vaginitis is no longer acceptable as a diagnosis. The most frequent cause of what was

WOMEN'S DISEASES AND SURGERY: VAGINITIS—CAUSES, TREATMENTS, AND TYPES (Continued)

formerly diagnosed as nonspecific vaginitis is Hemophilus vaginalis, also known by its new name, Gardnerella vaginalis.

1749. Are nylon undergarments to blame for an increase in vaginal infections and diseases? Are cotton panties advisable?

No, nylon undergarments are not to blame. An increase in the change of sex partners may be to blame for sexually transmitted diseases; antibiotics may be to blame for increased yeast infections. Since yeast fungus, Candida, grows in a moist place, cotton panties might be better, because they absorb moisture while nylon does not, and this additional moisture encourages the yeast. However, the vagina is always a moist place and is, therefore, always a good place for yeast to grow if the bacteria in the vagina do not resist it, so it doesn't matter what type of panties you wear. The moisture or sweat present on the pubic hair area or the vulva does not matter at all.

1750. Is there any way to prevent or avoid vaginal infections?

Avoiding intercourse would eliminate all infections except Candida, which is a yeast or fungus infection. Avoiding antibiotics and washing your hands before you use the toilet would prevent most of the fungus infections.

1751. How is vaginitis treated?

Vaginitis often is not treated at all, and eventually it goes away. Lukewarm baths, gentle treatment, avoidance of intercourse, and cortisone ointment can provide comfort. However, to give the proper treatment, you must first diagnose the problem. If your diagnosis is gonorrhea or Chlamydia, then it would be best for you to be professionally treated. If your partner gave you the vaginitis and still has it, you will get it back anyway, and the treatment will be of little help. If you have a fungus, you will have to be treated for a fungus. There are different treatments for the different causes of vaginitis.

1752. What can I do about vaginal itching?

At the first sign of vaginal itching, you can use a cortisone cream to stop the itching. These creams are available over the counter in drugstores or even grocery stores and contain 1 percent hydrocortisone. One brand name is Cortaid. Douching or using a tampon temporarily to remove discharge also brings comfort, as does sitting in a tub of tepid water. Desitin Ointment is soothing, especially if there is a yeast (fungus) infection. However, if the itching persists, you may need a diagnosis from a physician or nurse practitioner. Cultures and microscopes are very helpful in selecting the right treatment for the right diagnosis.

WOMEN'S DISEASES AND SURGERY: VAGINITIS—CAUSES, TREATMENTS, AND TYPES (Continued)

1753. Is it true that eating yogurt will help to prevent vaginal infections?

There is a theory that fungus infections of the vagina come from a fungus, Candida, that grows in the feces. People who believe this think that they get this infection from wiping feces from their rectums into their vaginas. So, if you eat yogurt and keep down the Candida, or fungus, in the colon by loading it up with the Lactobacilli in the yogurt, you would prevent vaginal fungus (yeast) infections. I do not agree with this theory, and find it impractical. Some feminist health clinics have recommended that the yogurt be inserted directly into the vagina daily. This would make more theoretical sense, but, in fact, I still find yeast infections in women who have done this.

1754. Could other diseases develop as a result of a vaginal infection?

This depends on the cause of the vaginal infection. Pelvic inflammatory disease (PID) can result from gonorrhea or chlamydial vaginal infections, and infertility can result from PID. The first time you have herpes, you may become generally sick with a fever and headache. Cancer of the cervix and vulva are more frequent in women who have had herpes genitalis or condylomata (venereal warts). The remaining conditions that commonly cause vaginal infections, such as Trichomonas, Gardnerella or Hemophilus vaginalis, and Candida albicans (yeast or fungus infections), do not affect the rest of the body.

1755. What is Gardnerella or Hemophilus vaginitis?

Gardnerella or Hemophilus vaginalis is a bacterium that causes a sexually transmitted vaginitis, which produces an objectionable odor. There is a gray discharge, but the vagina is not inflamed, tender, or itchy. Odor is almost the entire problem, and it is perceptible to the woman and her partner, as well as to her doctor. It does not affect her body anywhere else and has no long-term, bad effects.

1756. How do you treat Gardnerella or Hemophilus vaginitis?

Metronidazole (brand name Flagyl) in the form of oral tablets is the most effective method of treatment for Gardnerella or Hemophilus vaginitis. Preferably, it is given to all partners. Creams and suppositories are of little value, and other antibiotics, such as ampicillin, have only limited success. Since there is no effect on your body, except odor from your vagina, there is no medical reason to treat the problem besides personal aesthetics. If you are going to continue sex with your partner, then you might as well not bother to treat it at all. Douching at intervals to remove the discharge helps for awhile. Inserting a tampon to remove the discharge along with its odor also helps, perhaps more than douching. Neither of these methods is a cure.

WOMEN'S DISEASES AND SURGERY: VAGINITIS—CAUSES, TREATMENTS, AND TYPES (Continued)

1757. I have been told that I have a trichomonas vaginitis. What is that?

Trichomonas vaginalis is a one-celled protozoan that infects the vagina of women and the urethra and prostate in men. It causes a sexually transmitted disease, trichomonas vaginitis, that does not bother the body anywhere else. The only problem is a yellow, bubbly, odorous, irritating, burning, and itching discharge that can make intercourse painful. Trichomonas vaginitis is diagnosed by looking at a drop of discharge under the microscope and seeing the trichomonads swimming about. They are larger than white cells. It is sometimes also diagnosed by being reported on the Pap smear. Cultures can be done, but they are not too reliable. The most effective treatment is metronidazole (brand name Flagyl), which is an antibiotic available in an oral tablet. Douching, especially with a topical anti-infective, such as Betadine, brings temporary relief, as does using a tampon to remove the discharge. Using creams and suppositories in the vagina also gives temporary relief, but seldom cures the disease. To remain cured you must also treat your partner or stop having sex with him. If he will not take treatment, then you might as well not bother. It is not a medical necessity to treat trichomonas vaginitis because it will not harm your health, but it can be harmful to your sex life.

WOMEN'S DISEASES AND SURGERY: VAGINITIS— YEAST INFECTION

1758. What is a yeast infection, and what causes it?

Yeast infections are caused by fungi called Candida organisms, usually Candida albicans. They are less frequently caused by another fungus, in which case there is milder itching and less discharge. A recent menstrual period, intercourse, early pregnancy, or recent exposure to antibiotics are common conditions associated with the onset of the fungus (yeast) infection. Oral contraceptives have been accused of contributing to the onset of yeast infections, but this is now quite controversial. Most investigators consider that men are more likely to be the receiver of the fungus, rather than the carrier. However, men can harbor the Candida beneath the foreskin of their penises if they are uncircumcised, and on the penises and scrotums, too. This can constitute a reservoir for the infection of women. Some doctors feel that women who have chronic, recurrent cases get it from their own rectums, and they try to clear the infection by prescribing oral fungicidal agents. Sometimes it is a medical puzzle to find the cause of the yeast infection. Taking care of a baby who has a diaper rash exposes women to the yeast. In this case, you should treat the baby and wash your hands. Taking care of other women who are sick and on antibiotics exposes you, too, since many of them

WOMEN'S DISEASES AND SURGERY: VAGINITIS— YEAST INFECTION (Continued)

may have a yeast infection.

1759. Are yeast infections caused by conditions within my body or by something external?

Conditions within your body can be such that the few yeast cells normally present in your vagina begin to grow unchecked by bacteria; such conditions are diabetes, antibiotic therapy, douching with antiseptics, and sometimes just pregnancy. But also a large contamination with yeast (Candida albicans) from the outside can cause a yeast vaginitis even in a healthy woman. Such contamination could be from a baby with an extensive diaper rash of Candida, intercourse with a man who has Candida on the skin around his genitals, nurses working with patients who have severe yeast infections, or girls living in a dormitory where a yeast infection runs through like an epidemic.

1760. Are yeast infections caused by sex?

If your partner has yeast on his genitals and you do not, then sex can be the cause of the infection. However, the symptoms will develop later, not immediately. If you have immediate burning and itching following intercourse and find that you have a yeast infection, then it was already there when you started the intercourse. The sexual activity only brought the symptoms into full bloom.

1761. Can sex aggravate a yeast infection?

Yes, indeed, and a yeast infection can certainly aggravate sex. It is better to discontinue intercourse until the symptoms are gone or until you have finished treatment. This way, you will not turn against sex altogether. Sometimes you really won't know if you are well until you can have sex without burning and itching afterwards.

1762. How do you diagnose yeast infections?

Yeast infections, also called "yeast," fungus, moniliasis, or candidiasis are diagnosed by finding the Candida organisms in a drop of discharge treated with potassium hydroxide (KOH) under a microscope. A laboratory culture also can confirm or reveal the presence of a yeast infection, and it is sometimes reported on a Pap smear. Yeast is always suspected when itching is the primary symptom of the vaginitis.

1763. How common is yeast (fungus) infection with Candida?

Yeast infection is the most common vaginitis among women, as well as among little girls and babies. Hardly a woman goes through life without having a yeast infection at some time or other. You do not always have to be treated to get rid of it, but sometimes it may be necessary. It is also the most

WOMEN'S DISEASES AND SURGERY: VAGINITIS— YEAST INFECTION (Continued)

commonly overdiagnosed vaginitis. Many women think that they have yeast infections when they do not, and lots of doctors tell them they do when, in fact, their laboratory culture proves that they do not.

1764. What are the symptoms of a yeast infection?

Severe itching is the major symptom of a yeast infection. Burning occurs, especially with intercourse. You may have a discharge that is either heavy and similar to cottage cheese curds, or grey-white and milky. Burning with urination occurs on the skin around the vagina, but not in the bladder area. You may also feel the urge to empty your bladder or bowels. Redness around the vulva and even on the skin of the thighs can occur. This will look similar to a diaper rash, which is also a yeast infection with Candida.

1765. How can I prevent or avoid yeast infections?

You should try to avoid antibiotics, but when you can't, use a suppository that guards you against yeast during the days you take the antibiotics. Wash your hands before going to the toilet if you think you have been exposed to yeast. Exposure can come from a baby who has a diaper rash and from associating with someone who has a yeast infection and doesn't treat it. When you treat yourself for a yeast infection, also treat your partner, or avoid sex for a few days. Avoid douching, especially with antiseptics. If you have a chronic, recurrent case, use a fungicide with every menstrual period for six months.

1766. What is the best cure or treatment for a yeast infection?

The best treatment is any of the topical fungicide creams or suppositories, such as clotrimazole (brand names Gyne-Lotrimin or Mycelex), miconazole (brand name Monistat), or nystatin (brand name Mycostatin). In times past, the vulva and vagina of women with yeast infections were painted with a 1 percent gentian violet. Besides staining underclothing, this treatment often caused severe allergic reactions, so it is seldom used anymore. Oral nystatin (brand name Mycostatin) is used when there are recurrences of the infection and it is thought to come from the rectum. If you cannot get a prescription quickly (these medications should all be sold over the counter, but they are not), use a tampon or a douche to remove most of the discharge from your vagina. You can also put a cortisone cream on the vulva. A 1 percent hydrocortisone cream, such as Cortaid, is available over the counter. You also could use Desitin Ointment, just like you would for your baby's diaper rash. Douching with vinegar seems to give temporary relief. These treatments will help the discomfort on the outside, but not the inside. If you wait long enough your own bacteria may again grow and

WOMEN'S DISEASES AND SURGERY: VAGINITIS—
YEAST INFECTION (Continued)

destroy the fungus so that you become comfortable again. Little girls can recover from yeast infections with an external treatment, such as Desitin Ointment or a fungicidal cream, because their vaginas are closed, dry, and not infected. Avoiding yeast infections is easier than curing them. One way to do this is by putting something in your vagina every time you take antibiotics that guards you against Candida fungus. You could also wash your hands a lot.

1767. Is douching the best cure for a yeast infection?

No, but douching may bring temporary relief from the symptoms of yeast infection. This may be all you need to give your body time to build up its own defenses in the form of bacteria to fight the fungus. However, Candida can be grown in vinegar, so vinegar douches will not kill it.

1768. What would cause a yeast infection to occur repeatedly?

Recurring yeast infections can be a real medical puzzle. One cause is incomplete treatment of the first attack, so that the fungus grows again every time you menstruate and provide blood for it to grow on. The repeated use of antibiotics for recurrent sore throats or even bladder infections can cause repeated overgrowths of fungus, or "yeast." Small numbers of Candida organisms are usually present in the normal vagina, but their growth is held back by the bacteria normally there. When you kill those bacteria, the Candida can grow. Douching with antiseptics, such as the Lysol contained in many douche powders, to kill bacteria makes yeast more likely. Taking penicillin sets you up for a yeast infection. Treating your acne with antibiotics for long periods of time puts you at a risk for Candida overgrowth. Associating with someone who has a yeast infection and doesn't treat it, whether an older woman or a young girl, exposes you. Failing to treat the Candida on your partner's genitals makes your own treatment useless. You may have given the yeast to him in the first place, but if he is not treated, he will give it back to you. Most men are circumcised and dry, so they do not keep the Candida growing for more than a day or two; however, some do. Diabetics who have sugar in their urine are very subject to yeast infections of the vagina. At least one research project also showed that women who do not drink very much water or take very much vitamin C are more subject to yeast infections.

1769. Are yeast infections contagious?

Yes, yeast infections are contagious. Usually the contagion is from woman to woman (not sexually, but by hands). It will run through a girl's dormitory like wildfire. It also can be transmitted from babies to women. A

WOMEN'S DISEASES AND SURGERY: VAGINITIS— YEAST INFECTION (Continued)

woman can infect her male partner, but usually he is so dry that the fungus disappears in a few days. If it lingers, he may give it back to her during their next intercourse.

1770. Can a woman give a yeast infection to a man during intercourse?

Yes, a woman can give a yeast infection to a man during intercourse. The man may complain of burning for a day or two, but if he is dry, circumcised, and clean of any other inflammation of the skin (dermatitis), the yeast will usually leave him without treatment. If he has moisture under his foreskin for the Candida to grow on or a dermatitis, such as jock itch, where it can continue to grow, then he can keep it and give it back to the woman later.

WOMEN'S DISEASES AND SURGERY: CYSTITIS (BLADDER INFECTION)

1771. What is cystitis?

Cystitis is an infection of the urinary bladder.

1772. What are the symptoms of a bladder infection, or cystitis?

Urinating frequently, even at night; urgency; pain, particularly at the end of urination; and especially blood in the urine (hematuria) are usually due to a bladder infection.

1773. How common are bladder infections?

Most women have had a bladder infection at some time in their lives. Some have one as often as once a year. If it is more often than that, you may have a special problem that requires study, such as with X-rays, cystoscopy (examination of the bladder with an instrument called a cystoscope), and a urological consultation.

1774. Are bladder infections caused by having sex?

Bladder infections are not sexually transmitted diseases, because women can get them when their partners have no infection at all. Ninety-five percent of cystitis follows sexual intercourse and is caused by it. The problem seems to be caused by the mechanical thrusting of the penis into the vagina during sexual activity. When this thrusting produces pressure on the urethra, pushing it against the pubic bone and rubbing it raw, a bladder infection is likely to occur. When this happens, the bacteria in the glands around the urethra empty into the urethra and even back up into the bladder, causing an irritation and infection. The bacteria normally present in these glands are called Escherichia coli (E. coli). The symptoms of the infection usually appear within forty-eight hours of the sexual activity that brought them about.

WOMEN'S DISEASES AND SURGERY: CYSTITIS (BLADDER INFECTION) (Continued)

1775. What is honeymoon cystitis?

Honeymoon cystitis is a bladder infection that follows first intercourse. It is supposed to occur on your honeymoon (which doesn't happen much anymore). First intercourse, especially if repeated often for the first few days or weeks, produces cystitis very frequently. This is due to the tightness of the virginal hymen, which holds the penis tightly against the pubic bone during intercourse and irritates the urethra. When the opening in the hymen becomes looser and the woman is more relaxed and therefore not tightening her muscles so much, then intercourse stops producing cystitis. Some women, however, never learn to have sex without being tight and getting cystitis.

1776. Are bladder infections more common in women than in men? Why?

Women have far more bladder infections than do men. Men do not have pressure in their pelvises on the base of their bladders or on their urethras during coitus. When they get an infection, it is usually from a contagious disease, such as gonorrhea or chlamydial infection. Another reason for women having more bladder infections than men is that the female urethra is so short. It is a small distance from the outside skin, where bacteria are always present, to the inside of the bladder. Men have a longer route for the bacteria to travel before they can reach the bladder.

1777. What is the best treatment or cure for a bladder infection?

The urine can be examined to see if it shows pus, and then cultured to see what bacteria are present. Various antibiotics can be tested on the bacteria, then the one that is the most effective is selected. Usually this process takes too long, so while it is taking place, some sulfa or other antibiotic that is usually effective against E. coli is started. A dye can be given that relieves the urgency and pain before the infection is cured. This usually is an azo dye (brand name Pyridium). The patient is also encouraged to drink lots of water and cranberry juice. If there is a vaginitis present, it should be treated, too, because it may be the reason for tightness during intercourse and the source of the bacteria that is being pushed into the urethra. All of this takes time and money. It can be done in a doctor's office or clinic, or with a nurse practitioner. A laboratory is needed to do much of the work, but if you have a severe cystitis, it is worth it. Weeks after you are treated, your urine must be rechecked to be sure that the infection is completely cleared.

1778. Can cystitis be treated without the use of drugs?

Yes. Quite frequently if you stop having sex, drink lots of water and

WOMEN'S DISEASES AND SURGERY: CYSTITIS (BLADDER INFECTION) (Continued)

especially cranberry juice, and wait a few days, the signs and symptoms of cystitis will disappear. A subsequent examination of your urine will show that the cystitis has completely cleared. Drugs can speed up your relief, and sometimes they seem absolutely required for a severe, prolonged attack.

1779. How can I prevent cystitis?

Drink lots of water, especially after intercourse. Do not allow your partner to put forward pressure on your urethra or bladder, as is sometimes done by those who are looking for the G-spot (Grafenburg spot). This pressure rubs your urethra against the pubic bone. If you feel an urgency to void right after intercourse, you were allowing the urethra to be rubbed. Don't be too tight, as in vaginismus, a spasm of the muscles around the vagina that holds the penis tightly against the pubic bone. Make sure you are lubricated,because if you are dry you will automatically be tight. Don't have protracted coitus for over twenty or thirty minutes, and don't have sex too many times in one night, especially when you have lost interest and become dry. Be in charge of your body, and do not let it become a toy for someone else to use when you are not even involved in what is going on. Many urologists suggest you get up and urinate shortly after intercourse, so the urine will wash the bacteria in the urethra out instead of letting it go up into the bladder. Some advise a sulfa or antibiotic in the morning after you have had sex. Sometimes nothing seems to prevent cystitis except complete abstinence, and some women have done just that. But it seems to me that it would be better to learn to control the details of the activities in intercourse, rather than give it up altogether.

WOMEN'S DISEASES AND SURGERY: TOXIC SHOCK SYNDROME

1780. What is toxic shock syndrome (TSS)?

Toxic shock syndrome is a bacterial infection associated with a staphylococcus infection somewhere in the body, especially in the vagina. This may be associated with surgical wound infections, deep and superficial abscesses, infected burns, abrasions, insect bites, shingles, tampon use, and even diaphragm use. It is believed that poisons produced by the Staphylococcus aureus bacteria travel into the blood stream and cause the symptoms of the syndrome. The Staphylococcus bacterium is a common skin organism that also causes infections, such as sore throats, sties, and boils. About five hundred cases of toxic shock syndrome have been reported within the last two years; some have been fatal.

WOMEN'S DISEASES AND SURGERY: TOXIC SHOCK SYNDROME
(Continued)

1781. What are the symptoms of toxic shock syndrome?

Typically, toxic shock syndrome begins abruptly with a fever that often rises above 102° F. This is sometimes accompanied by vomiting or watery diarrhea. Complaints of headache, sore throat, muscle aches, and stomach pain are also common. If the illness is severe, there is a rapid drop in blood pressure and shock occurs, although milder cases can occur without these symptoms. Another common symptom is a rash resembling a sunburn that appears on the palms of your hands or elsewhere during the first two days of the illness. This is often followed three to fourteen days later by peeling skin, usually on the palms of the hands and the soles of the feet.

1782. Is toxic shock syndrome new?

Toxic shock syndrome was first discovered in 1978. At that time, it was considered a childhood disease, because it developed in children suffering from any one of a number of common staph infections. In 1980, toxic shock syndrome was first linked with tampon use.

1783. Does anyone know yet what causes toxic shock syndrome?

Most women who have had toxic shock syndrome have had a Staphylococcus aureus cultured from their vaginas. It is theorized that this produces the toxin that causes the shock, fever, and rash symptoms. However, not all Staphylococcus aureus infections produce this toxin, just a certain strain. Toxic shock syndrome is a serious disorder, and some people have died from it. Hospital treatment is required to survive.

1784. What is the relationship between the use of tampons and toxic shock syndrome?

Toxic shock syndrome was first linked to tampon use in 1980. In 1981, 85 percent of the cases of TSS that were reported were associated with menstruation, and 98 percent of these involved tampons. Today, the link between tampon use and toxic shock syndrome is still under investigation. Studies have shown that tampons, especially super absorbent tampons, may produce conditions in the vagina that enable the Staphylococcus bacteria to grow. It is thought that tampons may dry, scratch, or tear the skin of the vagina, which speeds the body's absorption of the toxin produced by the bacteria. Studies are currently being conducted to see if the change from cotton to synthetic tampons is a cause of toxic shock syndrome.

1785. What are the other known causes of toxic shock syndrome, besides the use of tampons?

Surgical wound infections, abscesses, infected burns, abrasions

WOMEN'S DISEASES AND SURGERY: TOXIC SHOCK SYNDROME
(Continued)

(scrapes), insect bites, shingles, and even diaphragms that are left in too long all have been associated with toxic shock syndrome.

1786. Can toxic shock syndrome occur in all women?

Yes, and it also can occur in men. However, it seems only to occur in people who have a staphylococcus infection somewhere in their bodies.

1787. How can I tell if I have a staphylococcus infection in my vagina?

Perhaps 5 percent of all women harbor a Staphylococcus aureus infection in their vaginas, yet only 1 in 25,000 women actually get toxic shock syndrome. A culture of your vagina can tell you if you have a staphylococcus infection. It will not tell you whether it is the strain that produces the toxin of toxic shock syndrome. It is difficult to get rid of the staph by taking antibiotics, so perhaps if you find that you have a staphylococcus infection in your vagina, you should avoid using tampons.

1788. How many women with this Staphylococcus culture in their vaginas will get toxic shock syndrome?

Of the 5 percent of women who have this culture in their vaginas, 1 in 1,000 will get toxic shock syndrome; the other 999 who have it do not get TSS.

1789. Is toxic shock syndrome more likely to occur in younger women?

Yes. Women between the ages of fifteen and twenty-four are more likely to develop toxic shock syndrome than are older women.

1790. How do you diagnose toxic shock syndrome?

To qualify as toxic shock syndrome, you must have a fever, a rash, a drop in blood pressure, and a Staphylococcus aureus infection somewhere in your body. Another infection that would account for the same symptoms, such as Rocky Mountain spotted fever, should not be present. If you develop a high fever and vomiting during your menstrual period, you should contact your doctor immediately, especially if you are using tampons.

1791. Why would certain brands of tampons be more likely to cause toxic shock syndrome than others?

Toxic shock syndrome has been associated with all major brands and styles of tampons. However, the use of high-absorbency tampons seems to increase a woman's chances of developing it. The removal of Rely, a brand of tampons, from the market has not eliminated toxic shock from the nation. Studies are currently being conducted to see if the change from cotton to synthetic tampons is a cause of toxic shock syndrome.

WOMEN'S DISEASES AND SURGERY: TOXIC SHOCK SYNDROME
(Continued)

1792. Should I stop using tampons in order to avoid getting toxic shock syndrome?

I think the advantages of tampons outweigh the remote chance that you will get toxic shock syndrome, but if the threat of TSS worries you too much, don't use them. If you do wear tampons, change them **very** often. Do not wear the same tampon for a long period of time. Women who have already had toxic shock syndrome should **not** wear tampons again, since it can recur with the next menses.

1793. If I wear a tampon to bed at night, does that increase my chances of getting toxic shock syndrome?

Yes, it does. Women are advised **not** to wear a tampon for a whole night of sleeping or for an entire day. Tampons are safer if they are changed very often.

1794. Why have extra-absorbent tampons been linked to toxic shock syndrome?

It is believed that the extra-absorbent tampons become dry when they have soaked up all the blood, and a dry tampon can scratch the vaginal lining more than a wet one. It is therefore advised that women use a tampon that has the absorbency required for their flow, but not more absorbency than they need.

1795. Do you recommend tampons for teenagers?

Yes. The number of women who are going to get toxic shock is small, 1 in 25,000, and the chances of getting it are even less if you wear pads at night. Many teenagers have a hard time learning to insert a tampon. They use them during menstruation when they want to participate in sports, especially water sports. Teenagers are embarrassed by the detectable odor of menstruation and the bulge of pads. With tampons, they are less embarrassed. Tampons also help to improve the life of the teenager during menstruation; their lives are often bad enough without adding pads. However, teenagers are cautioned not to leave tampons in for too long. **It is very important to change tampons frequently.**

1796. How big of a problem is toxic shock syndrome?

By April 1982, a total of 1,660 cases had been reported in the United States. Although it is a rare disease, it is serious because it may cause death in about 5 percent of the cases.

1797. Is it possible to get a slight case of toxic shock syndrome and not know it?

It would be difficult not to know if you are in shock, collapsing, or ex-

WOMEN'S DISEASES AND SURGERY: TOXIC SHOCK SYNDROME
(Continued)

periencing a drop in blood pressure. It would be obvious if you have the sunburn-like rash with peeling, especially on your hands, when you have not been in the sun. More research is really needed, since women who feel ill or are vomiting or feverish with their menses may perhaps be having a partial syndrome. If you have any of these symptoms during menses, you should at least have a culture of your vagina taken to look for Staphylococcus. You should also avoid tampons if you feel ill. In the flu season, with its fevers and vomiting, menstruating women will become even more confused about what to do, and so can their doctors.

1798. How do you treat or cure toxic shock syndrome?

Treatment depends upon the severity of the case. It usually consists of intravenous feeding of fluids to help the body maintain a steady blood pressure, support the heart and other vital organs, and prevent shock. For this reason, most TSS cases require hospitalization and even intensive care facilities. Antibiotics may be used to try to eliminate the staph bacteria and decrease the risk of recurrent infections, but they do not help very much in treating the syndrome. Medicated douches or antibiotic ointments inserted in the vagina are more effective in preventing the spread of toxins.

1799. Could sterility occur as a result of toxic shock syndrome?

No. Toxic shock syndrome does not affect the reproductive organs very much, but if it goes undetected and untreated, TSS can lead to liver trouble, shock, and even death in about 5 percent of the cases.

1800. How can I avoid toxic shock syndrome?

One way to avoid toxic shock syndrome is to avoid tampons. But since it is such a rare syndrome, women are seldom advised never to wear a tampon, although a TSS warning label now appears on tampon packages. If you prefer to use tampons, you can reduce your risk of toxic shock syndrome by using them every other day of your period, especially at the time of your heaviest flow. **Never** wear a tampon during sleeping hours or for an entire day. If you develop fever and vomiting during your menstrual period, contact your doctor.

1801. Are there any long-term effects with TSS?

The worst long-term effect of toxic shock syndrome is that it can recur with each menstrual period. Almost one-third of the patients who have had TSS have a recurrence within six months. Usually the recurrent illness is not as severe as the initial episode of the syndrome. Women who have had TSS are advised not to use tampons following the illness. Liver trouble is another long-term effect that can follow toxic shock syndrome.

WOMEN'S DISEASES AND SURGERY: PROLAPSED UTERUS

1802. What is a prolapsed uterus?

A prolapsed uterus is a uterus that has dropped from its original position in the pelvis into the vaginal area. It may even drop down to and through the opening of the vagina. In its most extreme stage, the uterus hangs completely out of the vagina. The vaginal wall is inverted around it and the uterus hangs between the legs. This can produce discomfort, especially with activity, at the more severe stages.

1803. What causes a prolapsed uterus?

A prolapsed uterus is caused by an inherited condition, in which tissues stretch easily. It is also caused by childbirth, in which the tissues are stretched by a large baby or a long and difficult birth (not a cesarean section, however). An episiotomy helps to prevent this stretching of tissues, but it must be done before the tissues are stretched. Even a tear can help to prevent the stretching.

1804. What can be done for a prolapsed uterus?

A prolapsed uterus can be removed by a vaginal hysterectomy. Suspensions of the uterus have been tried in women who wanted to retain it in order to have more children. However, the condition usually recurs, especially if the woman does have more children.

WOMEN'S DISEASES AND SURGERY: ENDOMETRITIS

1805. What is endometritis?

Endometritis is an infection of the lining of the uterus. In the past, this occurred with tuberculosis. It also occurs when a gonorrhea infection travels into the uterus and then into the tubes. An infected abortion or an infected uterus after childbirth is also endometritis. Sometimes a D & C is required to make the diagnosis.

1806. What is the cure for endometritis?

Endometritis is cured with antibiotics.

WOMEN'S DISEASES AND SURGERY: ENDOMETRIOSIS

1807. What is endometriosis?

Endometriosis is a disease of women in which the lining of the uterus, the endometrium, is found growing in various spots outside of the uterus. It can be found on the ovaries, tubes, ligaments, bladder, rectum, and all over the pelvis. Every time a woman with this disease menstruates, these little spots of tissue menstruate and bleed, too. Since there is nowhere for the

WOMEN'S DISEASES AND SURGERY: ENDOMETRIOSIS
(Continued)

blood to go, they form bloody cysts, called endometriomas. These cysts are usually quite painful and sometimes produce adhesions to the bowel that cause pain at all times throughout the month, not just during menses. The deformities caused by the cysts and adhesions can also cause infertility. Women with endometriosis often are unable to get pregnant because the eggs from their ovaries cannot reach the tubes.

1808. What are the symptoms of endometriosis?

The most common symptom is increased menstrual pain as you grow older than twenty-five. Endometriosis is usually diagnosed between the ages of twenty-five and forty. The second most common symptom is pelvic pain between menstrual periods that is sometimes quite disabling. Another symptom is pain with intercourse, especially with deep penetration. Sometimes infertility, the inability to get pregnant, is the main symptom. You might not feel much pain at all, but could have so much endometriosis that you cannot get pregnant. Twenty-five percent of women who cannot get pregnant have endometriosis.

1809. How do you diagnose endometriosis?

Endometriosis is often diagnosed by listening to the patient's symptoms and performing a pelvic examination, in which tender nodules are felt at the upper end of the vagina behind the cervix. Large endometriomas, "chocolate cysts" filled with blood, may also be felt. To be really sure of the diagnosis, a laparoscopy can be done. In this procedure, a tube is inserted into the abdomen, and with a special light and lens, the areas of endometriosis around the pelvis are actually examined. Sometimes a laparotomy, cutting open the abdomen to operate on the reproductive organs, is necessary to confirm that it is endometriosis and to treat it.

1810. How common is endometriosis?

About 15 percent of the patients in a gynecologist's office have endometriosis. In one study, at least 25 percent of the women who complained of pelvic pain had endometriosis. Also, 25 percent of women who are unable to get pregnant have endometriosis.

1811. Who is likely to get endometriosis?

It mostly occurs in women between the ages of twenty-five and forty, and occasionally younger. It is rare in women who have had many children while they were young and much more common in women who have delayed having children until their later years. It is also much more common in women who do not use contraceptive pills, because these pills help protect women from developing endometriosis by reducing menstrual flow. It also

WOMEN'S DISEASES AND SURGERY: ENDOMETRIOSIS
(Continued)

occurs more frequently in women who have a heavy menstrual flow and more rarely in those with a very scant flow or no menses at all. Endometriosis goes away with menopause.

1812. How do you cure endometriosis?

You can treat endometriosis by hormonal suppression of menstruation, such as with birth control pills that produce a very scant flow. This relieves the pain and also actually reduces the amount of bloody cysts formed in the pelvis. Sometimes these pills are given continuously for nine months, producing a false pregnancy that relieves endometriosis. Often, women are advised to get pregnant, because that will clear up their endometriosis for a while. Danocrine is an androgen, or male hormone, that can be used to suppress menstruation altogether. After taking it for a few months, the endometriosis sometimes subsides for years. When medical therapy does not work, and especially if the woman wants to get pregnant, surgery is done to get rid of the adhesions and cauterize (burn) as many of the bloody cysts as possible. Perhaps the one ovary that is in the worst condition is also removed. The final cure is to remove the uterus, perhaps along with one or both ovaries if they are very badly involved, so that no more menstruation will occur.

WOMEN'S DISEASES AND SURGERY: CERVICITIS

1813. What is cervicitis?

Cervicitis is an inflammation of the cervix in which the cervix is raw, red, and bleeding. A discharge containing pus also occurs. The cervix can bleed and cause pain during intercourse, or it may bleed between periods. Cervicitis can be associated with a vaginitis and have other symptoms, too. It can be caused by having a baby, if it occurs postpartum, but it is usually the result of an infection. Chlamydia is a frequent cause of cervicitis, and herpes is another. Sometimes the cause is very hard to find, because the infection goes away but the cervicitis is still there.

1814. Is there any treatment or cure for cervicitis?

One treatment for cervicitis is to simply give it time, because sometimes it will heal by itself if it is not aggravated again. Antibiotics may be necessary if the cause for the cervicitis can be found. If your Pap smear is abnormal, this must be studied. If it is not, electrocautery (burning) can heal many cervicitis problems, and so can cryosurgery (freezing). Generally doctors do not prescribe treatment for the cervix unless you complain about the problems the cervicitis has created. So, you are in charge of your cervix. If

WOMEN'S DISEASES AND SURGERY: CERVICITIS (Continued)

you want it treated, complain. Ask to see it. Ask what it looks like. And ask for treatment.

1815. Is pain during intercourse a sign of cervicitis?

Yes, but there are so many other causes of pain during intercourse that it is not a sure sign of cervicitis. Bleeding after intercourse is a more significant sign. It is also a sign that your partner is hitting your cervix with his penis, instead of going under it where there is a lot more room and comfort.

WOMEN'S DISEASES AND SURGERY: DYSPLASIA

1816. What is dysplasia?

Dysplasia is an abnormal growth of cells of the cervix in which the cells do not mature properly. They are changing in the direction of actual cancer cells, but have not reached that point yet. By finding dysplasia and treating it with something as simple as cryosurgery, which is done in the doctor's office, cancer of the cervix can be prevented. Some, but not all dysplasia, will eventually become invasive cancer of the cervix if it is not treated. A hysterectomy or even a conization (removal of the mouth of the cervix in a cone-shaped section) are not usually required to get rid of dysplasia, but if the dysplasia is extensive and recurrent, they are sometimes performed.

1817. Is dysplasia a sign of cancer?

No. Dysplasia develops long before cancer, if cancer develops at all. Sometimes dysplasia does not even turn into cancer. Since it is impossible to tell which dysplasias will turn into cancer and which will not, all of them should be treated. The treatment is minor, such as a conization, cryosurgery, or even hot cauterization. More recently, laser therapy has been used to eliminate widespread dysplasia.

WOMEN'S DISEASES AND SURGERY: CYSTOCELE

1818. What is a cystocele?

A cystocele is a bulging wall in the vagina under the bladder that protrudes to or even through the vaginal opening. It may cause discomfort, especially when walking, or it may cause you to lose control of your bladder. Women who have cystoceles often wet their pants when they laugh, sneeze, or stand up suddenly. This is known as stress incontinence. Many women who have had vaginal deliveries do this a little bit, because they have a small cystocele. You can do muscle exercises, called Kegels, to strengthen your control and avoid surgery. Some women have a large cystocele but no loss of urine with activity. These women may still want to have surgery to remove

WOMEN'S DISEASES AND SURGERY: CYSTOCELE (Continued)

the bulge. A cystocele repair is best done when combined with a hysterectomy, because if the uterus is not removed it will act as a weight to push the bladder wall down again, especially if you have a baby.

WOMEN'S DISEASES AND SURGERY: RECTOCELE

1819. What is a rectocele?

A rectocele is a protrusion of the vaginal wall above the rectum. It comes down to or even through the vaginal opening. A rectocele can be uncomfortable because of the bulge, especially when walking, and it may make it very difficult to defecate. The stool gets caught in the bulge and will not come out the anus. Some women have to use their fingers to put pressure on the vaginal wall to get the stool to come out, especially if they are constipated. Rectoceles can be repaired surgically, but this is best done when combined with a hysterectomy. Usually, women who have a rectocele have a cystocele as well. After it is surgically removed, having more babies would produce the rectocele again.

WOMEN'S DISEASES AND SURGERY: TUMORS—WHAT THEY ARE, HOW TO TEST IF THEY ARE CANCEROUS

1820. What is a tumor?

A tumor is a lump that normally is not a part of a person's body. A boil is a tumor, caused by an infection, that will heal and go away. When you are pregnant, the baby is a tumor. Fatty tumors on your back or elsewhere can be removed if they are big and bother you, but they are otherwise no trouble and can be left in place.

1821. What is the difference between a tumor and a cyst?

A tumor can either be solid or cystic, but a cyst can only be a fluid-filled sac; it is never solid.

1822. How reliable are ultrasound scanners in determining if a tumor is cancerous or benign?

The ultrasound scanner, or sonogram, can accurately measure a solid tumor or an ovarian cyst. In the case of a lump in the pelvis, it cannot always identify whether it is on the ovary, tube, or uterus, just that it is in the pelvis. It certainly cannot determine whether or not it is cancerous. Only a biopsy, which involves surgery, can really do that.

1823. Is biopsy the only way to be certain that a tumor is benign?

Yes, that is basically true. However, if the lump goes away, you don't have to biopsy it. If you or your doctor recognize it as something that is always benign, like a little fat tumor, then you don't have to biopsy it either, even though it will not go away.

WOMEN'S DISEASES AND SURGERY: FIBROID TUMORS

1824. What are fibroid tumors? How do they differ from other tumors?

A tumor simply means a lump. A fibroid tumor is a lump of fibrous, or muscular, tissue. It grows in peculiar shapes and sizes within the wall or lining of the uterus, or is attached by a stump to the outer wall of the uterus. Sometimes they are attached to ligaments or found elsewhere in the abdomen. Occasionally, they are free floating because they have become separated. They differ from other tumors in that they are made of the same kind of tissue as the uterus. Although the tissue is changed, they are almost always benign and not cancerous. They can be troublesome because they grow so quickly. They also can make the uterus bleed or cause pain, especially if they degenerate or become twisted. Sometimes they do not make any trouble at all and are not even large. One in eight women will have fibroids, but all of them won't know it. Certainly, all of them will not have to have a hysterectomy. Only if the fibroids get too large or cause trouble will they need to be removed.

1825. In what areas of the body are fibroid tumors likely to occur?

Fibroids only occur in or adjacent to the uterus. There are fibroadenomas that occur in the breasts, but they are not the same as fibroid tumors.

1826. What are the symptoms of fibroid tumors?

The most common symptom of fibroid tumors is bleeding, as with heavy menstrual periods. Enlargement of your abdomen, so that you look as though you are pregnant, is another symptom, while pain is less frequent. Anemia is another sign of fibroids. It sometimes results from the bleeding, but rarely because the tumor itself destroys the blood cells as they pass through its great mass. Inability to get pregnant may also be a symptom. Sometimes large fibroids that women had no idea existed are found during pelvic examinations.

1827. How common are fibroid tumors?

One in eight women who have their uteri could have fibroids. They are one of the most common causes of a hysterectomy.

1828. What are the causes of fibroids? Could a hormone imbalance be a cause of fibroids?

One theory is that fibroids are caused by an excess of the estrogen hor-

WOMEN'S DISEASES AND SURGERY: FIBROID TUMORS
(Continued)

mone over progesterone. Fibroids seem to be hereditary, and so do hormone patterns. They are also more frequent in women who did not have many children when they were young. Perhaps the reason these women did not have many children is that the fibroids interfered with the implantation of a pregnancy, or perhaps it was the hormone imbalance that prevented pregnancy in the first place. The causes of fibroids are difficult to assess.

1829. Do fibroids stop growing after menopause?

If your estrogen level drops very low with menopause and you do not take any hormones, the fibroids usually stop growing. They also may shrink and become so small that they are no longer detectable during a pelvic examination. This is a good reason why women over fifty with small fibroids that do not bother them can wait to see if they will go away. However, if you take hormones for hot flushes, the fibroids will grow, and you will have the same problem again. If you can keep the dosage of hormones small enough that the fibroids won't grow, then you may avoid surgery. One of the largest fibroids I have removed was in a woman who was over seventy years old. She had taken estrogen for twenty years, but had not had a pelvic examination during that time. Her fibroids grew quite large before they were discovered.

1830. Do fibroids in the uterus cause heavy menstrual bleeding?

Fibroids can, and often do, cause heavy menstrual bleeding. However, you can have large fibroids with no heavy menses at all, and vice versa. You also can have fibroids, but find that your heavy bleeding is really due to a uterine cancer or some other disorder.

1831. What are the chances of fibroid tumors being cancerous?

Fibroid tumors are very rarely cancerous. Only in older women does a fibroid occasionally turn into a sarcoma, a muscle cancer. The chances of this happening are so rare that it is not a good reason to remove the fibroids to prevent cancer.

1832. Are women with fibroids in their uteri more likely to develop cancer of the uterus than women without fibroids?

No, women who have fibroid tumors are not more likely to develop cancer of the uterus.

1833. If I have my fibroid tumors removed, will they come back?

Those specific tumors will not return, but new ones probably will form. If you have inherited the tendency to form fibroids and have not had lots of children, which helps prevent them, then there is nothing to keep you from forming more. Only a hysterectomy will keep them from coming back.

WOMEN'S DISEASES AND SURGERY: FIBROID TUMORS
(Continued)

The removal of a fibroid without removing the uterus is called a myomectomy. It only is done when a single fibroid is very large, or there is a desperate attempt to remove enough fibroids so that you can get pregnant. Such removal may make such deep incisions in the wall of the uterus that a cesarean section would have to be done, because the uterine wall can no longer withstand labor. Sometimes a single fibroid has to be removed because of pain, especially in pregnancy.

1834. Why do so many doctors suggest hysterectomy for women with fibroid uteri?

Because hysterectomy is the only treatment available for fibroids. Removing the fibroids without removing the uterus itself is very difficult and usually impossible. The only reason for doing this would be to preserve the uterus for childbearing. Most women who have fibroids discover them in their thirties and have already had all the children they want. Therefore, the preferred treatment is hysterectomy, which means removing the fibroids and the uterus that contains them. Of course, there is also the question of whether or not you should treat them at all. If you are bleeding or in pain, or if the tumor is larger than a four-months pregnancy, you usually will be quite happy to get rid of it and the problems it creates. If you let the size grow larger than a four-months pregnancy, other problems follow. These develop from the pressure that the tumor puts on other organs, such as the bladder and rectum, or even the ureters, which are located between the bladder and the kidneys. Hysterectomy becomes more difficult when the tumor is extremely large. I have seen a tumor that weighed twenty-six pounds. The largest that I have removed in the last few years weighed eight pounds. There is no reason for women to wait until their tumors are that large to have them removed. If they are small and you are near menopause, you might wait and see if they go away with the reduction in hormones of menopause. However, sometimes they grow larger instead.

WOMEN'S DISEASES AND SURGERY: BOILS

1835. What causes boils around my vaginal area and legs?

Most boils are due to a Staphylococcus aureus bacterial infection. This bacteria can occur on the skin, but uses any break in the skin to produce an infection. Shaving the hair on your legs gives them just such an entry. If you are diabetic, such boils get out of control. Washing with an antiseptic soap, like Phisohex or Dial, can keep the bacteria down so that it occurs less often.

WOMEN'S DISEASES AND SURGERY: POLYPS

1836. What are polyps?

Polyps are finger-like projections of soft, velvety tissue, similar to the lining of the cervix or the uterus. They are usually pink in color and contain a lot of blood vessels. Sometimes they also contain fibroids, in which case they are hard and pale.

1837. What is the difference between a polyp, a tumor, and a cyst?

A polyp is a finger-like projection of tissue hanging down in the uterus or in the cervix. It is visible during a pelvic examination. A tumor is a lump, and a fibroid tumor may be found inside of a polyp. A cyst is a sac filled with fluid. Small cysts, called nabothian cysts, can be found on the cervix. You can even feel them with your fingers when you touch your cervix. These are visible during a pelvic examination but are of no importance and need no treatment. A cyst on the ovary is more important. It can be a larger-than-usual cyst related to ovulation that will go away, or it can be a new growth, even a cancer, that will not go away. A cyst at the opening of your vagina can be a plugged Bartholin's gland duct or a clogged Skene's gland if it is around the urethra.

1838. Where are polyps likely to develop in women?

The only polyp that is known only to occur in women develops in the uterus. It is found up in the upper cavity or down in the cervix. Other polyps, such as in the nose, can form in both men and women.

1839. How do you diagnose polyps of the uterus?

Your physician can look at your cervix during a pelvic examination and sometimes see a polyp sticking out. It looks like a little tongue. Other times, nothing is visible but when a curettage of the lining of the uterus is done because of abnormal bleeding, polyps appear in the material that is removed.

1840. Do polyps lead to other diseases?

No, but they may indicate a disease, such as cancer or an overgrowth of the lining of the uterus (hyperplasia of the endometrium). Polyps may need to be controlled with hormones or even by a hysterectomy.

1841. Are polyps ever cancerous?

Yes, polyps can be cancerous; for this reason, they must be removed and examined by a pathologist. This is sometimes the only way that the cancer is found. However, most polyps are not cancerous, just as most breast lumps are not cancerous.

1842. How do you treat polyps?

Polyps can be removed by cutting them off of the cervix and treating

WOMEN'S DISEASES AND SURGERY: POLYPS (Continued)

the stalk so that it won't bleed. A D & C (dilatation and curettage) also can be done with or without anesthesia. Following the D & C, the polyp that was removed as well as the uterine lining are sent to a pathologist to be examined. Women are often pregnant when the polyp is discovered, as polyps are often produced by pregnancy. This is called a decidual polyp. In this case, treatment is usually delayed until after delivery, and often the polyp is gone before delivery even occurs.

1843. Must all polyps be removed?

Yes. Polyps may reveal a cancer; so they must be examined. They can produce cramps as they come through the cervix, causing contractions of the uterus. They may bleed, especially between menstrual periods, and also can plug the cervix and interfere with getting pregnant.

1844. Do polyps come back?

Yes, sometimes new polyps will form. To prevent formation, extra progestins can be prescribed to counteract the growth stimulation of estrogen. Birth control pills do this very nicely.

WOMEN'S DISEASES AND SURGERY: CANCER—WHAT IT IS, INCIDENCE OF CANCER, DIET

1845. What is cancer?

Cancer occurs when cells change from their normal state to abnormal growth that is uncontrolled. They can travel to other parts of the body, called metastasis, and grow there in an uncontrolled fashion.

1846. What are the most common types of cancer in women?

Breast cancer is by far the most serious cancer and causes the greatest number of cancer deaths in women. Next is cancer of the lung. Third place belongs to cancer of the colon, and fourth is cancer of the ovary.

1847. What is the most frequent cause of cancer death in women?

Estimated cancer deaths in the United States for women in 1983 are as follows:

(According to the American Cancer Society)

Breast	37,000
Lung	34,000
Colon	26,000
Ovary	11,000
Pancreas	10,000
Cervix	7,000
Endometrial (uterine lining)	3,000

WOMEN'S DISEASES AND SURGERY: CANCER—WHAT IT IS, INCIDENCE OF CANCER, DIET (Continued)

Due to increased smoking and drinking, the incidence of lung cancer and pancreas cancer among women has increased. Women are becoming equal with men in these diseases. The fastest rising cancer in women is lung cancer; by the end of the 1980s it will surpass breast cancer as the most frequent cause of cancer death in women. Cancer of the cervix is falling off rapidly, probably due to the use of Pap smears and preventive treatment of the cervix. Deaths from endometrial cancer (lining of the uterus) continue to remain low because of its high cure rate by hysterectomy.

1848. Do women's life styles have any effect on the rate of cancer?

Yes, they do. Smoking, for instance, increases the chances of lung cancer. Starting sexual activity early, having babies while you are young, and having many sex partners greatly increases cancer of the cervix. Not having babies increases cancer of the lining of the uterus (endometrial cancer) and also cancer of the ovary and the breast. Taking birth control pills cuts your chances of getting cancer of the ovary and the lining of the uterus in half. Alcoholism increases the risk of cancer of the liver and the pancreas. The extent of the effects of life style on the rate of cancer is lengthy.

1849. What are the warning signs of cancer?

In women, the most important warning sign of cancer is abnormal bleeding anywhere, but especially from the vagina and the nipples of the breasts. A lump that does not disappear and cannot be explained can be a sign of cancer and must be investigated. Any sore that does not heal cannot be ignored. Unexplained weight loss needs to be explained. A mole that itches, grows larger, develops redness around it, or has little satellite moles should be removed. A change in bowel function, especially smaller-shaped stools, can mean a tumor around the rectum. Extreme bruising can be a sign of leukemia.

1850. Is spotting between periods a sign of cancer?

Yes, spotting between periods can be a sign of cancer. It must be investigated and the cause must be found. A D & C (dilatation and curettage) may be necessary. Of course, most spotting between periods is not a sign of uterine cancer. Spotting or bleeding after menopause is a much greater sign. If that occurs, you must have a D & C, unless you know you have produced the bleeding by taking estrogen and progestins.

1851. Can chronic yeast or vaginal infections be an early sign of cancer?

No. Chronic yeast infections can be a sign that you are diabetic, but they are unrelated to cancer. Herpes and venereal warts (condylomata) can cause cancer of the cervix and vulva to occur many years later. These diseases are not a sign of cancer; they are a cause.

WOMEN'S DISEASES AND SURGERY: CANCER—WHAT IT IS, INCIDENCE OF CANCER, DIET (Continued)

1852. Is it true that women who have never had children are more likely to develop cancer of the breast or cervix?

It is true that women who never had children are more likely to develop cancer of the breast, but they are less likely to develop cancer of the cervix. Cervical cancer is more frequent in women who started sex early and had many partners.

1853. Is cancer more likely to occur among women who have smaller numbers of children?

Cancer of the breast, ovary, and endometrium, are more frequent in women with fewer children. They are also more likely to occur in women who had children after they were thirty-five years old and not before. However, if these women took contraceptive pills for at least eight to ten years, they would reduce their chances of cancers of the ovary and uterus.

1854. Are certain forms of cancer more likely to occur in women who have had children?

Cervical cancer is more frequent in women who had pregnancies in their teenage years. Perhaps this is just because they started having sex early. Sex and early pregnancy, however, are a greater risk than sex alone.

1855. Does diet play any role in controlling cancer? Are vegetarians less likely to develop serious diseases, such as cancer, due to the absence of meat in their diets?

The National Academy of Sciences issued a report on "Diet, Nutrition, and Cancer," that showed a strong correlation between diet in affluent societies, like the United States, and cancers of the breast, uterus, and colon. They found people changed their patterns of cancer when they migrated to new countries. They also found that exposure to pollutants in an industrialized society is not a significant cause of cancer, although long-term effects may not yet be clear. According to the report, one-third of cancers could be eliminated by a proper diet, and another third if everyone stopped smoking. The strongest relationship with diet was between cancers of the colon, rectum, and breast and consumption of a high, total-fat diet that included meat and animal protein. They specifically condemned alcohol and foods that are smoked, salt pickled or salt cured. The good foods were found to be fruits, vegetables, and whole-grain cereals.[1] So, if they are right, vegetarians would be better off. This has not been entirely accepted, however, and many scientists think it does not warrant a change in diet even for the prevention of breast cancer.

[1] Gloria Hochman, "The Diet That May Have Licked Cancer," *San Diego Union*, 19 April 1983, p. Dl.

WOMEN'S DISEASES AND SURGERY: CANCER—WHAT IT IS, INCIDENCE OF CANCER, DIET (Continued)

1856. Should I worry as much about cancer if I have had a hysterectomy?

No, you should not. If you had a total hysterectomy, you have prevented cancers of the uterus and cervix. If you had your tubes and ovaries removed, too, you have prevented cancer of the ovary. However, you can worry about your breasts and lungs. These are two of the most frequent areas of the body to develop cancer in women.

WOMEN'S DISEASES AND SURGERY: CANCER—OVARIAN CYSTS, OVARIAN CANCER

1857. What is an ovarian cyst?

An ovarian cyst is a fluid-filled sac located on the ovary. During every menstrual cycle, women form at least one small cyst, called a follicle cyst. When the cyst is about one inch in size, the ovary releases its egg. At that time, the cyst fills with blood and forms a corpus luteum, which is a yellow, more solid body. Sometimes these are very, very large, as much as five or ten inches in diameter. They can be felt during a pelvic examination or revealed by ultrasound and may cause pain. Sometimes the pain is so severe that surgery is required. They also may bleed so badly inside the abdomen that surgery is required to stop the hemorrhage. There are other kinds of cysts on the ovary, too. The follicle cysts and corpus luteum cysts are called functional cysts, because their function is to ovulate.

1858. What are the symptoms of ovarian cancer?

The first signs may be just a vague discomfort in the lower part of your abdomen, persistent indigestion, or a bloated feeling after eating a little food. A rapid enlargement of your stomach so that you can't wear your normal clothes might be a warning sign.

1859. How do you treat an ovarian cyst?

If there is severe pain or evidence that there is internal bleeding, emergency surgery may be needed to stop the pain and bleeding. This is necessary, even if it is a functional cyst that would go away in time. If there is not much pain and the woman is at an age where she is still ovulating, then it is wise to wait for a menstrual period to see if it goes away. Hormones also could be given to be sure it will go away quickly. This is usually the case between the ages of fifteen and forty. If it remains, then surgery must be planned to remove the cyst, even if it means removing the ovary. If it is cancer, then both ovaries and the uterus probably will be removed, and bowel surgery might even be necessary. Ovarian cancer will require intensive chemotherapy, as well.

WOMEN'S DISEASES AND SURGERY: CANCER—OVARIAN CYSTS, OVARIAN CANCER (Continued)

1860. How is ovarian cancer detected?

It is very difficult to find ovarian cancer before it spreads to other pelvic organs. To detect it early, it would be necessary to find an enlarged ovary during a pelvic examination. Any mass found on the ovary needs to be surgically explored to see if it is cancerous.

1861. If the ovarian cyst is cancer, what are the chances for a cure?

Twenty-five years ago, almost no one survived from ovarian cancer. Now, with extensive and repeated surgery and intensive chemotherapy, as many as 30 percent survive for at least five years. If detected early, five-year survival rates are quite high.

1862. What causes ovarian cancer?

It is not known exactly what causes ovarian cancer. However, what is known is that women between the ages of fifty and sixty and women who have never had children or who have an infertility problem are more likely to get it.

1863. If the cyst doesn't go away with my menstrual period or when I take hormones, what kind of cyst could it be?

The problem with an ovarian cyst that doesn't go away is that it could be a cancer. Ovarian cancer is a very difficult cancer to cure, and it is fatal if left untreated. So any cyst that doesn't go away has to be surgically removed, if only to be sure that it is not cancer. However, there are other ovarian cysts that are benign. A common one is a dermoid cyst. This is an odd one because it often contains many kinds of tissues, including a real tooth that shows up on an X-ray. Some ovarian cysts and tumors produce female hormones that are high in estrogen, even in little girls. Some produce the male hormone testosterone. They can cause the little girl to mature early, or they can make a woman become masculine in appearance. There also can be an endometrioma, a "chocolate cyst" of endometriosis that may not shrink, even with hormone therapy. There are twenty-five kinds of ovarian cysts and tumors, all of which must be removed. Even twenty- and thirty-year-old women can have malignant ovarian cysts. After menopause, since ovulation no longer occurs, cysts are always considered to be some kind of abnormal growth, and they are frequently malignant. You can ask for tests, such as a sonogram, to measure the cyst. You also can wait for a menstrual period to see if it goes away, or you can ask for hormonal suppression. But if it is still there in a few weeks, taking charge of your body means removing the ovarian cyst. If it is benign, removing it may allow some of the ovarian tissue to still function, if there is any left.

WOMEN'S DISEASES AND SURGERY: CANCER—OVARIAN CYSTS, OVARIAN CANCER (Continued)

1864. Is there any way to shrink an ovarian cyst through the use of medication?

Yes. If the cyst is a functional cyst, a follicle or corpus luteum related to ovulation, you can shrink it by taking hormones, such as birth control pills, to prevent the ovary from completing its function. In time, this kind of cyst will shrink anyway, usually after a menstrual period or two, but suppressing it with hormones hastens the process. This speed is important if you are considering surgery in case the cyst does not go away. If the cyst is something other than a functional cyst, it will not go away.

WOMEN'S DISEASES AND SURGERY: CANCER OF THE LINING OF THE UTERUS (ENDOMETRIAL CANCER)

1865. What are the warning signs and symptoms of cancer of the lining of the uterus?

Bleeding between periods; bleeding heavily with periods, especially if it does not stop or continues longer than ten days; bleeding that occurs a year or more after menopause has been completed; and, rarely, a Pap smear that shows abnormal endometrial cells are all warning signs of cancer of the lining of the uterus, also simply called uterine cancer.

1866. Are there any known causes of uterine cancer?

Yes, there are many known causes of uterine cancer (cancer of the lining of the uterus). Taking estrogen without taking progestins increases the incidence of uterine cancer ten times. Women who do not ovulate have estrogen without progesterone, and they have a higher incidence of uterine cancer. Women who are overweight and produce estrone (an estrogen) in their fat from their adrenal hormones have a higher rate of uterine cancer. These women often are also diabetic and hypertensive. There seems to be an inherited tendency to develop uterine cancer, along with obesity, high blood pressure, and diabetes. If your mother and grandmother had uterine cancer, you are at a high risk and should pay more attention to any abnormal bleeding. Having children seems to reduce the probability of uterine cancer, so by default, not having children becomes a cause of it, too. Birth control pills, taken for at least eight or ten years, reduce the incidence of uterine cancer by half. Uterine cancer also is more likely if you live until an old age.

1867. How do you diagnose cancer of the uterus? Does a Pap smear help?

Cancer of the lining of the uterus (endometrial carcinoma) can only be diagnosed by a curettage in which a sample of the lining of the uterus is sent to the pathologist and examined. A Pap smear is not a reliable method of

WOMEN'S DISEASES AND SURGERY: CANCER OF THE LINING OF THE UTERUS (ENDOMETRIAL CANCER) (Continued)

finding cancer of the lining of the uterus because it will miss the cancer most of the time. However, if the Pap smear is abnormal and suggests that such a cancer is present, a D & C then should be used to find it, and that sequence of events does occur. So a Pap smear can help, but it is not to be depended upon. Usually uterine cancer is found when abnormal bleeding is investigated by doing a D & C or an endometrial biopsy.

1868. Will uterine cancer spread to other parts of my body?

If you do not treat it in time, uterine cancer will spread to other parts of the body.

1869. Is uterine cancer common among women today?

Uterine cancer is more common today than it was thirty years ago, but it is less common than it was prior to 1975 when more women were taking only estrogen for menopause. The number of uterine cancers has decreased since the use of estrogen has decreased; yet it is still the sixth most common cancer in women. Approximately 37,000 women will get uterine cancer each year.

1870. How many women will develop uterine cancer in their lifetimes?

About 1 in 1,600 women will actually develop cancer of the lining of the uterus, endometrial cancer, in their lifetimes. If you are taking only estrogen for your menopause, your chances are increased about ten times, to 1 in 160. This means that 37,000 women each year are diagnosed as having endometrial cancer of the uterus. However, only 3,000 women die from the disease each year.

1871. How many cases of uterine cancer (endometrial cancer) occurred because women took estrogen?

Between 1970 and 1975, there were approximately 15,000 excess cases of uterine cancer due to women taking estrogen without taking progestins.

1872. Does breast-feeding reduce the chances of getting uterine cancer?

Having children reduces your chances of having uterine cancer, whether you breast-feed or not. There have been studies that indicate breast-feeding in the United States does not help to reduce the chances of uterine cancer. Perhaps, studies also would show that women in the United States don't breast-feed long enough for it to have an effect.

1873. Can women with cancer safely take hormones?

Women with breast or endometrial cancer whose cancers are sensitive to estrogen cannot safely take estrogen. If estrogen were given, some of the cancer cells that had spread to other parts of the body might grow. Other

WOMEN'S DISEASES AND SURGERY: CANCER OF THE LINING OF THE UTERUS (ENDOMETRIAL CANCER) (Continued)

cancers are not affected by estrogen. Cervical cancer patients can and do take estrogen, especially after their ovaries have been removed surgically or by radiation. Colon cancer has no relationship to female hormones at all.

1874. Since cancers of the breast and uterus take a long time to develop, how do I know I am not speeding them up by taking estrogen before I discover the cancers?

That is theoretically possible, and it is a real consideration in the decision to take estrogen. It is a good reason to get a mammogram to be sure you do not already have breast cancer and a good reason to do a D & C or endometrial biopsy to be sure that no endometrial cancer is present when estrogen is started. Another way to be relatively safe is to take a progestin in a cyclic fashion along with the estrogen. This protects you from endometrial cancer, and some large studies indicate that it also reduces your chances of developing breast cancer. If you are going to take the "hormones of youth," take both of them: estrogen and progesterone.

1875. Does the likelihood of uterine cancer increase after menopause?

Yes, in fact, most uterine cancer occurs after menopause, even if hormones were never taken for menopause. The incidence of uterine cancer is ten times more frequent in women who take only estrogen for menopause. There is no increase in frequency in women who take progestin along with the estrogen.

1876. If I were to discover that I had uterine cancer, could I safely conceive and carry a child before having my uterus removed?

No. It would not be safe to delay treatment of a cancer of the lining of the uterus that is beginning to penetrate the muscle of the uterus itself. Since this cancer seldom occurs in young women, there is seldom the consideration of another pregnancy.

1877. How do you treat uterine cancer?

Uterine cancer (endometrial carcinoma) is cancer of the lining of the uterus, but not the cervix. The primary treatment is a hysterectomy, combined with removal of the tubes and ovaries. This is done because hormones from the ovaries would make any metastatic cancer from the uterus grow and also because ovaries are one of the first places to which the cancer spreads. Sometimes this treatment is combined with radiation, if the cancer is a very active one, if it has penetrated far into the muscle, or if the uterus is quite large. Radiation after surgery also is done if lymph nodes are involved. If the cancer has already spread to the lungs, as shown by an X-ray taken before surgery, then nothing is done except a D & C to diagnose what kind of

WOMEN'S DISEASES AND SURGERY: CANCER OF THE LINING OF THE UTERUS (ENDOMETRIAL CANCER) (Continued)

cancer it is. Chemotherapy or hormone therapy with strong-acting progestins, like Depo-Provera, can be used to supress the cancer but will seldom eradicate it completely. In some cases, all of these methods are used.

1878. Is hysterectomy always necessary in cases of uterine cancer?

If you are going to have a cure, hysterectomy is always necessary. Radiation increases the chances of a cure, but is not a cure by itself. A hysterectomy would not be done if a cure is not possible, as when the cancer has already spread to the lung or the woman is so old or in such poor medical condition that she cannot withstand surgery and anesthesia. In that case, radium or radiation alone is used.

1879. How effective is the cure for uterine cancer?

The rate of cure for the cancer caught while still in the in situ state, not yet invasive, is almost 100 percent. If it has not spread beyond the uterus at the time of surgery, the cure rate for uterine cancer is above 90 percent, especially if surgery is combined with radiation. Even if it has spread, the control with chemotherapy and hormones is so good that most of the time life can be prolonged for more than five years. The kind of uterine cancer that was caused by estrogen did not add to the mortality rate from uterine cancer, even during the years when it occurred most often. This is because the cure rate by hysterectomy is so high.

1880. What is the cure rate for cancer of the uterus?

The cure rate for endometrial cancer, cancer of the lining of the uterus, is 85 percent if diagnosed early, and 75 percent for all cases, whether diagnosed early or late.

WOMEN'S DISEASES AND SURGERY: CERVICAL CANCER

1881. What is cancer of the cervix?

It is a scale-like cell growth at the mouth of the cervix that invades deeply into the tissue and can spread to different parts of the body. It also can spread locally and cause death by shutting off the ureters, the tubes that lead from the bladder to the kidney.

1882. What are the signs and symptoms of cervical cancer?

Today, the most frequent sign of cervical cancer is an abnormal Pap smear. Symptoms really are absent until it is too late to cure the cancer easily. These symptoms include bleeding, especially between periods; a very abnormal discharge; pelvic pain; and weight loss. Such late cervical cancer symptoms are only found in women who go for years without a pelvic ex-

WOMEN'S DISEASES AND SURGERY: CERVICAL CANCER
(Continued)

amination or a Pap smear. If all women had Pap smears and pelvic examinations, even every three years, cervical cancer never would get to that stage before treatment.

1883. How do you diagnose cervical cancer?

A biopsy is necessary to diagnose cervical cancer. An abnormal Pap smear can lead your doctor to do a biopsy. Your doctor also could see something on the cervix that looks suspicious even without a microscope. In both situations, he or she then would do a biopsy in that area and find a real cancer of the cervix. A Pap smear that is abnormal can best be investigated by colposcopy in the doctor's office. In this procedure a binocular microscope on a stand is used to examine the cervix through the vagina. This can show the doctor where the most abnormal spot is that is shedding the suspicious cells on the Pap smear, and a biopsy is taken there. The tissue is always sent to the pathologist who examines and diagnoses it. If cancer of the cervix cannot be found this way, then a cold conization of the cervix is done, usually under anesthesia in a hospital. In this procedure the mouth of the cervix is removed in a cone-shaped section. It is then thoroughly studied to find if there is a cancer.

1884. How effective is a Pap smear in detecting cervical cancer?

The Pap smear is a very effective means for detecting cancer of the cervix. It is so effective that deaths from cancer of the cervix actually have been reduced in recent times, and it is no longer one of the top three cancers in women. Through the use of the Pap smear, cancer of the cervix is a preventable disease. If you have the Pap smear at least once every three years and, certainly, if you have one every year; if you follow up any abnormal Pap smear with office examinations, colposcopy, biopsies, or hospital conizations; and if you treat any of the many precancerous conditions that are found, you can avoid the actual diagnosis of cancer of the cervix. It progresses slowly from the precancerous to the cancerous stage and gives you a lot of time to find it before it is a problem to cure. In the precancerous stage, called dysplasia, treatment may be an office procedure called cryosurgery (freezing the cervix) or a conization, which is a minor hospital surgery. Hysterectomy is reserved for very early cancers, called carcinomas in situ, that are not growing into the tissues (invasive). Hysterectomy also may be sufficient if there is minimal invasion.

1885. How many women will get cervical cancer in their lifetimes?

About 1 in 4,800 women will get cervical cancer in their lifetimes. This means that each year 16,000 women are diagnosed as having cervical cancer,

WOMEN'S DISEASES AND SURGERY: CERVICAL CANCER
(Continued)

and about 7,000 women die each year from the disease.

1886. What is the cure rate for cancer of the cervix?

The cure rate for cancer of the cervix is 81 percent if it is diagnosed early. The overall cure rate is only 57 percent for all cases, regardless of whether they were diagnosed early or late.

1887. Is it true that sex can be a cause of cervical cancer?

Yes, this is true. Virgins do not need Pap smears because they will not get cervical cancer, **unless** their mothers took DES (a synthetic estrogen) while they were pregnant with them. Hopefully, that cause will disappear with time. Catholic nuns have a very low incidence of cervical cancer, and they have been the subject of intense examination to find out why. Of course, there have been a few cases of cervical cancer among nuns, and virginity is not a requirement to be a nun in all orders. However, the highest rate of cervical cancer is among prostitutes. It also is high among poor people. It is higher when sexual activity began at a young age, especially when this was associated with pregnancies and multiple changes in partners. There are thought to be several causes. The herpes virus seems to increase the chances of getting cervical cancer. The condyloma virus (warts on the vulva) also increases the incidence of cervical cancer. However, cervical cancer can occur without either of these diseases being present, perhaps because sperm itself can enter the cervical cells and combine with the nucleus to form an abnormal cell that becomes cancerous. It can do this in the laboratory, so perhaps it also does it in women. To avoid cervical cancer, you would have to avoid all sexually transmitted diseases, such as genital herpes and warts, and avoid all sperm. So far, abstinence seems to be the only solution. Since this is not practical, Pap smears are relied upon to find cervical cancer before it even is really a cancer, and cure it in the office by minor procedures. Women have a right to know that early sexual activity, especially with pregnancy and many partners, increases their chances of getting cervical cancer. This information has not been well publicized.

1888. Is it true that I could develop cervical cancer as a result of having sex with more than one partner when I was a teenager?

Yes. Cervical cancer is more prevalent in women who started sex early, especially if they got pregnant and had several partners. It is increased if they had herpes genitalis or venereal warts. It is unfair that this information is not made available to junior high school girls.

1889. Is cervical cancer less likely to occur in Jewish women?

Yes, cervical cancer is less likely to occur in Jewish women. Extensive

WOMEN'S DISEASES AND SURGERY: CERVICAL CANCER
(Continued)

studies have been conducted to try to find a cause of cervical cancer and to discover why Jewish women don't have it as often. The answer is not yet clear. But it is clear that it is not because their Jewish husbands are circumcised, because Jewish women married to uncircumcised men still do not have as much cervical cancer and non-Jewish women married to circumcised men still have a lot more cervical cancer. Perhaps Jewish women really do not have as much sexual activity in their teens, and they do not have as many sexual partners as non-Jewish women. Cervical cancer does occur in some Jewish women, especially in those who have been sexually active from an early age and who have had many changes in partners.

1890. Will cervical cancer spread to the rest of my body?
Yes. It is the nature of cervical cancer to spread to other parts of the body if it goes untreated or if it is not treated in time to stop the spread.

1891. How do you treat cervical cancer?
Previously, invasive cervical cancer (cancer that is growing into the tissues) was treated mostly by radium, and sometimes this was followed by a hysterectomy. Today young women often are treated by a radical hysterectomy. The ovaries are left in, but are placed in an area that will not be harmed by the radiation that is given to the pelvic area after surgery. A simple hysterectomy alone is not good enough to cure cervical cancer, except in the very early stages before it has become invasive (carcinoma in situ). Chemotherapy is only used in the later stages when the cancer has already spread to other parts of the body. Sometimes very radical surgery, such as removing the entire bladder, rectum, and even the vagina, is done to try to rid the body of a local spread of cervical cancer. This has been successful in some cases, but the danger and complications of the surgery are great. Such radical surgery is only done when the cancer has spread into the bladder and/or rectum before treatment.

WOMEN'S DISEASES: NAMES OF SEXUALLY TRANSMITTED DISEASES; WHERE TO GO FOR CONFIDENTIAL HELP

1892. What are the names of all the different diseases that are transmitted by having sex?
That is a large order. Some are: syphilis, gonorrhea, Chlamydia, herpes genitalis, Gardnerella or Hemophilus vaginalis (nonspecific vaginitis), trichomonas vaginitis, Candida albicans, vulvovaginitis (yeast infection or fungus), chancroid, venereal warts, lymphogranuloma venereum, molluscum contagiosum, scabies, lice (crabs), hepatitis, and AIDS.

WOMEN'S DISEASES: NAMES OF SEXUALLY TRANSMITTED DISEASES; WHERE TO GO FOR CONFIDENTIAL HELP
(Continued)

1893. Where can I go for confidential help if I think I have VD?

All contacts with physicians are confidential. Even if the disease is reported to the public health department, it is still confidential. All laboratories are required to report to the public health department a positive test for syphilis or gonorrhea, but not most of the other sexually transmitted diseases. Most cities have a communicable disease department that runs a clinic where you can go for free diagnosis and treatment if you think you might have VD. You can pick up the phone and dial TELMED, which is available in many cities. On the phone, you will hear tapes with information on sexually transmitted diseases, so that you can learn what you want to know before you even visit a doctor, or perhaps a nurse practitioner, in a clinic or office. The free clinics for poor people always are equipped to test for VD, as well as treat the disease. All medical care is confidential.

WOMEN'S DISEASES AND SURGERY: SEXUALLY TRANSMITTED DISEASES AMONG TEENAGERS

1894. As a teenager, if I suspect that I have a venereal disease, where can I go for help without telling my parents?

In California, you can go anywhere, because there is a special law that permits treatment of teenagers without parental knowledge when VD is suspected. Most other states have a similar law, but not all of them. You can find out from Planned Parenthood clinics whether this is true in your state. You also could call your Public Health Clinic, and there are even hotlines available especially for teenagers. Your school counselor can help you, too.

1895. Is venereal disease the greatest danger for the sexually active teenager?

No. Teenage girls are twice as likely to get pregnant as they are to get venereal disease. Surveys in this country and others show that among teenage girls, nineteen and under, there are twice as many pregnancies as there are cases of venereal disease.

1896. Is the teenager very likely to get VD?

The teenager is definitely very likely to get VD, since there can be so many changes of partners. Barrier contraceptives, such as a diaphragm, foam, jelly, or condom, may help reduce VD, but they are harder for the teenager to arrange to use at the time of coitus. They also lead to many more pregnancies in this very fertile group.

WOMEN'S DISEASES AND SURGERY: SEXUALLY TRANSMITTED DISEASES—GENERAL QUESTIONS (HOW ARE THEY TRANSMITTED, HOW CAN I TELL WHO HAS ONE, etc.)

1897. If I have one steady partner who I am sure is not "cheating," what are my chances of getting a venereal disease?

If your partner is not "cheating" and has never had sex with anyone before you, you are 100 percent safe. If your partner has had previous partners, then some disease, such as recurrent herpes genitalis, syphilis, Gardnerella, or Trichomonas still could be around to infect you. Gonorrhea and Chlamydia usually are over in six or eight weeks, but some men are carriers. Only 100 percent monogamy for life makes you safe from sexually transmitted diseases. An interval between partners of a few weeks, especially with a medical checkup for such diseases in between partners, might help.

1898. Are there any sexually related diseases that could be passed from woman to woman?

The diseases of homosexual women have not been nearly as well studied as the diseases of homosexual males. Homosexual males have a greater incidence of sexually transmitted diseases because the germs are found in the ejaculate that is placed in other men's rectums. Since women have no ejaculate filled with germs, the transmission is surface only. This would permit rapid transmission of herpes genitalis, since this is a surface disease. Warts also could be easily transmitted. It has been difficult to study sexual diseases among women homosexuals.

1899. Is it possible to have sex with a person who has VD and not get it from them?

Yes. Only 80 percent of women will get herpes when their partner has an open sore. If your partner wears a condom, if you use a contraceptive cream or foam, or if all the sex is oral-genital, then the rate of transmission is reduced for most of the sexually transmitted diseases. But that still does not make it safe.

1900. Is is possible to get VD from a public bathroom?

No. If toilets transmitted diseases, then if one member of your household had VD, everyone at home would get it from using the single toilet, and that does not happen.

1901. Can I catch VD by simply touching, kissing, or being close to someone who has it?

No, you will not catch VD that way. This is evidenced by the fact that

WOMEN'S DISEASES AND SURGERY: SEXUALLY TRANSMITTED DISEASES—GENERAL QUESTIONS (HOW ARE THEY TRANSMITTED, HOW CAN I TELL WHO HAS ONE, etc.) (Continued)

a mother who has VD does not give it to her children whom she holds closely and kisses. Only if you kiss the penis could you get a transmission to your mouth.

1902. If I have oral sex with someone who has VD, will I still get VD? Will I get VD sores in my mouth?

Yes. If you have oral sex with someone who has VD, you can get the VD sores in your mouth. VD can be transmitted by oral sex.

1903. How can I tell if my partner has VD?

Mostly, you can't tell if your partner has VD, but if he has sores on his penis, a dripping, white discharge from the end of his penis, or if he cries out in pain when he urinates, then you might be suspicious. If he tells you that he has VD, believe him. If he says nothing, you should be brave enough to ask. However, he may not know that he has VD, because there are so many sexually transmitted diseases that he could give you when he has no symptoms at all. If he speaks of having many partners, you have a right to worry.

1904. How can I tell if my daughter has a venereal disease?

You probably cannot tell if your daughter has VD, but if she walks around doubled over and holding her stomach in pain, and does not have appendicitis, you should suspect that she has a venereal disease. This symptom would be especially suspect if it were not the first day or two of her menses.

1905. Were venereal diseases less common in earlier days when there was not so much sexual permissiveness?

Yes, but there also were very few successful treatments, so the results were far worse.

1906. Can I develop an immunity to any of the sexually transmitted diseases?

Herpes produces an immunity for the strain that you have, but not for other strains or types. Venereal warts only occur once. When finally cleared, they will not return. You cannot get them again from someone else because the virus and its antibodies remain in your system. Other sexually transmitted diseases have no immunity.

1907. What specific hygienic precautions can I personally take in order to avoid contracting a venereal disease?

First, try to select partners who do not have many other partners. Use

**WOMEN'S DISEASES AND SURGERY: SEXUALLY TRANSMITTED
DISEASES—GENERAL QUESTIONS (HOW ARE THEY
TRANSMITTED, HOW CAN I TELL WHO HAS ONE, etc.)**
(Continued)

a contraceptive foam (even if you are on pills) that helps kill the various
germs of VD, and insist that your partners wear a condom as well. Both of
these methods will help reduce disease transmission, but they do not make it
safe to have intercourse with someone who already has a disease.

1908. Could I have a venereal disease and not know it?
Yes, you could have VD and have no symptoms. In this case, you are
a carrier. That is true of almost all of the various diseases that are transmitted sexually.

1909. Can I get VD more than once and still succeed in healing it?
Yes. The only venereal disease that is less likely to heal with repeated
attacks is pelvic inflammatory disease that is the result of gonorrhea or
Chlamydia. The infection can be cured, but the damaged tubes can make
trouble for the rest of your life until they are removed.

**1910. How long will it take after I have contracted a venereal disease for the
symptoms to appear?**
It takes at least three days for the symptoms to appear. However, this
varies for each disease. Of course, sometimes you never get the symptoms,
even though you have the disease.

**1911. Can a venereal disease go dormant for a while after it is contracted,
before the symptoms begin to show?**
It may seem to be dormant because, at first, there may be no symptoms. This happens when there is gonorrhea in the vagina. The pain and
misery come weeks later when it becomes pelvic inflammatory disease.

**WOMEN'S DISEASES AND SURGERY: SEXUALLY TRANSMITTED
DISEASES—SYPHILIS**

1912. What is syphilis?
Syphilis is a disease that first appeared in the fifteenth century. It is
caused by a small organism called a spirochete that is transmitted by intercourse and also congenitally, which means that an infected mother can give it
to her unborn child. Syphilis can affect all of the organs of the body. It is a
very slow disease and may cause death after many years.

1913. What are the symptoms of syphilis?
Several weeks to months after being infected with syphilis, a rather
large ulcer with rounded edges appears on the vulva around the vagina or in-

WOMEN'S DISEASES AND SURGERY: SEXUALLY TRANSMITTED DISEASES—SYPHILIS (Continued)

side the vagina. It is not tender and later heals and disappears. In three months, a rash that looks somewhat like measles may appear all over the body, but also may disappear. The liver can be affected, causing hepatitis, jaundice, and skin rash. This stage is called secondary syphilis. But, perhaps, no symptoms appear until the nerves are affected years later. Then the nerves to the legs, particularly in the knee joint, are so deficient that injuries go unnoticed. As a result, a widened, deformed knee joint forms. The eyelids droop, and the pupil does not react properly. This is all called tabes dorsalis. Further deterioration can result in brain deterioration or dementia. Blood vessels can be affected, forming an aneurysm (a weakened arterial wall), especially close to the heart in the aorta. This is called tertiary syphilis and can occur twenty or thirty years after the first attack. To get to this stage, you would have to avoid all antibiotics, especially penicillin, because this would stop the progress of the disease. Few people ever get to tertiary syphilis anymore. Congenital syphilis means the disease is given to newborn children by their mothers. This causes deformities, such as pointed teeth, and deformed bones and nasal septum. Yet, the babies live. If treated with penicillin, they can be cured, but will still have some of the deformities. State laws require that pregnant women be tested for syphilis, so this will not happen. If the mothers are treated in the first few months of pregnancy, their children will be all right.

1914. How is syphilis diagnosed?

If you have a large, slow-healing ulcer on your genital area, you should let a doctor take a sample from the ulcer and look at it under a dark-field microscope. If you have syphilis, the spirochetes can be seen swimming there. At this point, the blood test for syphilis will still be negative. Later, after three months, the blood test will be positive, and sometimes it will stay that way for the rest of your life. This blood test is required for marriage in many states. It also was required for food workers at one time. However, there are so few cases of VD found by this method that most states are removing these laws. The few cases that are found this way do not justify the enormous amount of money spent on testing everyone. A VDRL (Venereal Disease Research Laboratory) blood test also can be done that will find if you are positive for syphilis. Sometimes this result is confused with other things, and then a special fluorescent treponemal antibody-absorption test (FTA-ABS) can be done to prove it really is syphilis and not just a false positive test due to something else. The rash that develops with syphilis really is not diagnostic. It is a skin rash that is raised and red on the trunk and arms, or entire body, and looks like many other rashes. But if a rash is pres-

WOMEN'S DISEASES AND SURGERY: SEXUALLY TRANSMITTED DISEASES—SYPHILIS (Continued)

ent, a test for VD should be run to be sure. The late signs of syphilis are due to nerve involvement, and at that time a spinal tap will be positive. These tests are done on the spinal fluid. Sometimes diagnosis also is made by liver and skin biopsies.

1915. How does syphilis differ from herpes?

Syphilis and herpes only are alike in that they both produce an ulcer, both are sexually transmitted, and both can be transmitted to a newborn baby. The germs that cause them are different, and so are the rest of the symptoms. The main difference between the diseases is that syphilis is easily cured with penicillin, or other antibiotics if you are allergic to penicillin. After treatment for syphilis, you no longer are contagious to other people. However, your blood test (VDRL) may remain positive, even though you are well and not contagious. This becomes a social problem only when you have to have a blood test for marriage or pregnancy.

1916. Can a person really go insane from syphilis?

Yes. The organic deterioration of the brain that occurs from syphilis can appear to be insanity. Once this stage is reached, treatment with penicillin cannot restore the normal function of the brain.

1917. Is syphilis more common in men or in women?

Previously, all venereal or sexually transmitted diseases were more common in men than in women. This was because men got them from prostitutes who had been with many men. Now that sexual freedom distributes partners more equally, the numbers of men with syphilis or other sexually transmitted diseases are not much greater than the numbers of women who have them.

1918. Is syphilis the most common form of venereal disease?

No, it almost has become rare. This is due to the efforts of public health departments and the ability of the blood test to diagnose the disease. Doctors report patients with syphilis to the health departments. The health departments investigate, find, and treat all of the people with whom the patient has had sexual contact. Their thoroughness has reduced the incidence of syphilis to one of the less frequent venereal diseases.

1919. If I discover that I have VD, do I really have to tell all of the people with whom I have had sex?

If you have syphilis, it will be reported to the local public health department, and they will contact you and ask you for all these names. Then they will contact these people and make sure that they are tested and treated. Your name will not be given; you will be referred to by a code number. This

WOMEN'S DISEASES AND SURGERY: SEXUALLY TRANSMITTED DISEASES—SYPHILIS (Continued)

also is done for gonorrhea, but there are so many cases of venereal disease that it is not always possible to contact everyone. With other venereal diseases, it is not even attempted. For your own sake, you should tell the partner with whom you are going to have sex again that you have VD, so that person can be cleared and will not give it back to you. It is up to your own system of ethics whether you tell all the rest. It is hard to know how long you have been exposing partners to VD before you had a diagnosis.

1920. Is it common for a woman who has VD to suffer psychological problems, such as feeling unworthy of sex, as a result?

The most common reaction to VD is rage against the person who gave you the disease. Today, with herpes, there are many men and women who feel they no longer have a right to have sex because at any moment they might be contagious and not realize it. If you were taught in childhood that monogamy is the only way to have a sexual relationship, you may feel that VD is a punishment for not being monogamous; therefore, you may feel guilty and depressed. If you were brought up to feel that you have an inalienable right to sexual activity with a partner, come what may, then you will not feel guilty. You also will be more able to forgive and tolerate the infidelity of the partner that brought about the sexually transmitted disease. This is probably the hardest task of all. It seems to be part of human nature, particularly of women's, to tolerate infidelity, or a partner with multiple partners, until that arrangement brings about a disease that was sexually transmitted. Then most people suddenly become very condemning and demand monogamy. There are contradictory attitudes of approving of sexual freedom but not approving of sexually transmitted diseases.

WOMEN'S DISEASES AND SURGERY: SEXUALLY TRANSMITTED DISEASES—GONORRHEA

1921. What is gonorrhea?

Gonorrhea is one of the most common sexually transmitted diseases today. It is caused by a bacterium, named gonococcus vaginalis. It infects the vagina and cervix in the female and then can spread to the uterus, tubes, and ovaries. It infects the urethra of the male. Occasionally it even spreads to many of the joints, such as the wrist, ankle, or knee. It also can infect the eyes of newborn babies and cause blindness, if the mothers have it at the time of delivery. This is why drops of silver nitrate or antibiotic cream must be put into the eyes of newborn babies within two hours of birth.

WOMEN'S DISEASES AND SURGERY: SEXUALLY TRANSMITTED DISEASES—GONORRHEA (Continued)

1922. What are the symptoms of gonorrhea?

In the female, there are no symptoms about 25 percent of the time, yet you are contagious to your partner. When there are symptoms, they may only be an odorous, unpleasant discharge. In the male, symptoms possibly may be painful urination. However, in females after a menstrual period occurs, the infection spreads via the menstrual blood into the uterus and up into the tubes and ovaries. Then severe pain, cramps, and heavy bleeding occur that worsen as the menstrual period goes on. These cramps are different from menstrual cramps, because with menstruation, the cramps are worse at the beginning of your period. If you have worse cramps at the end of your period, you should consider the possibility of gonorrhea. If neglected, abscesses can form in the tubes and ovaries. These can rupture and even cause death. There may or may not be a fever. Occasionally, after the vaginal infection, the disease spreads to the joints of the body, instead of the tubes and ovaries. Then you have a hot, red, tender wrist, knee, or ankle, as well as a fever. This is called gonorrheal arthritis, and it is rather rare.

1923. Are there sores with gonorrhea?

No, there are no sores with gonorrhea.

1924. Can gonorrhea be transmitted by kissing?

It is possible to develop gonorrhea in the mouth, especially from oral sex. If so, it is possible to give it to someone else in the mouth by kissing or, better yet, again with oral sex. It also is possible to get gonorrhea in the rectum from anal sex. Mouth gonorrhea is not very frequent because the germs already in the mouth take over and resist the gonorrhea. This also is somewhat true of the rectum. The vagina is the most defenseless area to get gonorrhea. However, in one study, half of children who suffered sexual abuse from family members and friends had gonorrhea of the throat (pharyngeal gonorrhea) without having any symptoms.

1925. Is gonorrhea painful?

In the early stage, when gonorrhea only has infected the vagina, it is not painful. But when it has become pelvic inflammatory disease, the pain can be very severe. Typically, you cannot walk without bending over and holding your stomach. After the infection is gone, the scarred tubes and adhesions may be extremely painful. When this happens, you will be unable to lead a normal existence until you have all your reproductive organs surgically removed.

1926. How common is gonorrhea?

Gonorrhea is near epidemic proportions, especially among young

WOMEN'S DISEASES AND SURGERY: SEXUALLY TRANSMITTED DISEASES—GONORRHEA (Continued)

people today. It is still the most frequent cause of pelvic inflammatory disease, with its subsequent sterility, although Chlamydia trachomatis is now becoming a close second.

1927. How is gonorrhea diagnosed?

Most of the time, gonorrhea is diagnosed in the female by taking a culture from the vagina. This usually is done because her partner has told her that he has it. He is far more likely to have symptoms, like painful urination and a white dripping discharge from the end of his penis in an early stage, than she is. If an early diagnosis is made, gonorrhea is easily cured by the right antibiotic. Usually the antibiotic is given even before the culture is reported. The diagnosis is more difficult after a menstrual period has sent the infection up into the pelvis, uterus, tubes, and ovaries. It may have even left the vagina altogether, although a culture from the cervix still can show it there. A laparoscopy (a procedure in which a tube with a special light and lens is inserted into the abdomen) may have to be done to catch drippings from the end of the tubes to culture the gonococcus just to be sure. Since this is a very expensive procedure, diagnosis usually is made based on the symptoms of severe pain, tenderness, signs of abdominal inflammation, enlargement of the tubes and ovaries, and a special test for high white blood count and high sedimentation rate of the blood. There is not always a fever, so the doctor diagnoses the disease on clinical grounds. A negative culture later does not prove that the doctor was wrong or that you do not have gonorrhea. Treatment with antibiotics at this stage is essential because the gonorrhea has become pelvic inflammatory disease.

1928. Does gonorrhea only occur in women?

No. Gonorrhea is sexually transmitted, so it occurs in both men and women.

1929. How will I know if I have contracted gonorrhea?

The best way to know if you have contracted gonorrhea is for your partner to tell you when he has been diagnosed for the disease. He will, of course, have it first. The chances of your getting it from someone who has it are high, so you should be treated if your partner has it. It is impractical to have every slightly different discharge cultured for gonorrhea. Certainly if you have severe pelvic pain, especially if menstruation is over and if the menstrual flow was worse than usual, you should suspect that pelvic inflammatory disease is developing as a result of gonorrhea. This is definitely worth a visit to a physician for cultures and for treatment, regardless of the results of the cultures.

WOMEN'S DISEASES AND SURGERY: SEXUALLY TRANSMITTED DISEASES—GONORRHEA (Continued)

1930. How do you treat gonorrhea?

If gonorrhea is diagnosed in the stage of vaginal infection, it clears up quickly with penicillin, ampicillin, or tetracycline taken orally. However, it could be one of the penicillin-resistant gonococci that produces a substance that destroys the penicillin! Then spectinomycin or some other antibiotic may be used to effect a cure. This particular strain of gonorrhea has recently entered the United States from the Far East by way of the West Coast. The possibility of having a penicillin-resistant gonococcus always makes it very necessary to go back and get a second culture to be sure you are really cured by penicillin. If the diagnosis is not made until the uterus, tubes, and ovaries are infected, treatment is more prolonged and difficult. Other bacteria join the gonococcus in producing abscesses in the pelvis, especially one called Bacteroides fragilis. Then strong, new antibiotics, often intravenous types, and even hospitalization may be needed. Surgery also may be required, and the uterus, tubes, and ovaries might have to be removed because a ruptured abscess can be fatal. This is called pelvic inflammatory disease.

1931. Is gonorrhea completely curable?

Yes. If treated in the early stages, gonorrhea can be cured with no damage to the body at all. If it has reached the tubes and ovaries before it is cured, 10 percent of the time it leaves severe scars on them. If gonorrhea reaches the tubes and ovaries twice, the chances of this happening are 20 percent. The scars on the tubes and ovaries really are not curable, and sometimes they produce so much trouble and pain in later years that the only cure is to surgically remove the tubes and ovaries. However, that is still a cure.

1932. Is hysterectomy ever necessary in cases of gonorrhea?

Yes, hysterectomy can be necessary in cases of gonorrhea. More frequently, it is the removal of tubes and ovaries that is required because of abscesses (pockets of pus), old scars, and adhesions that completely deform the ovary and tube and cause adhesions to the bowel as well. The adhesions also affect the uterus, and in the past it was thought that you might as well remove the uterus if the tubes and ovaries were gone because there was no way to get pregnant. Now, with the possibility of test-tube babies and donor mothers for ova, perhaps it is not impossible, and perhaps the practice of removing the uterus will change. There has been at least one woman, in Australia, who had a uterus but no ovaries that became pregnant by in vitro fertilization.

1933. What is the difference between gonorrhea and syphilis?

In the early stages of syphilis, there is a sore, an ulcer, while gonorrhea

WOMEN'S DISEASES AND SURGERY: SEXUALLY TRANSMITTED DISEASES—GONORRHEA (Continued)

has almost no symptoms, except a little discharge and pain on urination. Syphilis can last a lifetime if it goes undetected and untreated. It can cause deterioration of the entire body in old age. Gonorrhea is an acute disease in women. It leads to pelvic inflammatory disease, which is extremely painful, that leads women to treatment. It does not last long, even as a contagious condition. Syphilis can be contagious for a much longer time. Gonorrhea is much harder on the female than the male and leads to sterility. Syphilis may affect children that are born while the mother has the disease but does not lead to sterility. Syphilis is caused by a spirochete, and gonorrhea is caused by a bacterium.

1934. What is the difference between gonorrhea and herpes?

Gonorrhea can be cured with penicillin or other antibiotics rather easily; herpes cannot. Gonorrhea is contagious for a relatively short time, while herpes can recur and be contagious for life. Herpes has spontaneous recurrences without a new infection. Gonorrhea does not recur. If you get it again, you have a new infection from a new partner or from the same partner who never got treated.

1935. If I get gonorrhea, what are my chances of never being able to have children?

This depends upon how quickly you treat the gonorrhea. If you treat it while it is still in the vagina, there is no harm to your ability to have children. If you do not catch it until it has traveled into your tubes, causing pelvic inflammatory disease, then 10 percent of the time your tubes will be so scarred that you can no longer have children. If you have pelvic inflammatory disease a second time, the figure is 20 percent. If you have it ten times, you are 100 percent certain of being unable to have children, because your tubes have become scarred and blocked.

1936. How long must I have gonorrhea before it makes me sterile?

Long enough for it to go up into your tubes, which it does at the time of menstruation. If you get gonorrhea just before menses, this will not be more than a week. If you get it right after menses, it may take four weeks. Each time your tubes are infected, you have a 10 percent greater chance of becoming sterile.

WOMEN'S DISEASES AND SURGERY: SEXUALLY TRANSMITTED DISEASES—PELVIC INFLAMMATORY DISEASE (PID)

1937. What is PID?

PID is pelvic inflammatory disease, also sometimes referred to as in-

WOMEN'S DISEASES AND SURGERY: SEXUALLY TRANSMITTED DISEASES—PELVIC INFLAMMATORY DISEASE (PID)
(Continued)

flamed ovaries. It is an infection of the fallopian tubes, ovaries, and surrounding tissues, as well as the uterus. In severe cases, PID causes large abscesses, pockets of pus, to form in the pelvis. These can break and spread all over the abdomen. PID can be fatal.

1938. What are the symptoms of PID?
   The symptoms of PID usually start with a menstrual period. The pain and flow of menstruation will seem to be more pronounced than usual, and they will become worse as the menstruation progresses. After the bleeding stops, the pain gets even worse, and you may walk bent over and have to hold your abdomen. If you press in on your abdomen with your hands, it is tender, but if you remove your hands suddenly, then the motion makes it hurt even worse. The pain can sometimes also be felt in the shoulders. You may have a fever, but not always. It is especially painful to have intercourse. It also hurts to run and jump. You may become so ill that you collapse.

1939. What causes PID?
   In the United States the most common cause of PID is the sexually transmitted disease, gonorrhea, and the next most common cause is Chlamydia trachomatis. In Sweden, it is just the opposite, and that may soon happen here. Rarely, the infection may come from a ruptured appendix, an infected abortion or delivery of a child, or even an infected surgery in the pelvis. IUDs aggravate the infection, but they do not actually cause it. Birth control pills tend to help prevent the disease or make it better, but they are not a complete prevention.

1940. Can IUDs be a cause of PID?
   The presence of an IUD in the uterus makes the PID far worse than if nothing were there, but it does not actually cause the PID.

1941. How common is PID?
   Pelvic inflammatory disease (PID), also called salpingitis or adnexitis, annually affects thirteen out of every one thousand women who are fifteen to thirty-nine years old. It is most common in women who are twenty to twenty-four years old, affecting twenty out of every one thousand women in this age group each year. There were twice as many women with PID in 1980 as there were in 1960. Most PIDs are caused by sexually transmitted diseases, like gonorrhea or chlamydial infection, and only a small fraction of PIDs are due to tuberculosis or infected abortions. Ectopic pregnancies are increased 25 percent in women who had PID, accounting for 50 percent of all ectopic pregnancies in 1980. Forty percent of female infertility is due to PID, a rise

WOMEN'S DISEASES AND SURGERY: SEXUALLY TRANSMITTED DISEASES—PELVIC INFLAMMATORY DISEASE (PID)
(Continued)

of 60 percent since 1960.

1942. How is PID diagnosed?

The diagnosis of PID mostly is made from the symptoms that are present and the examination of the woman, especially her pelvic area. One major problem in diagnosing PID is that the symptoms are very similar to those of acute appendicitis, so it is difficult for the doctor to tell the difference. Blood counts and sedimentation rates are helpful, but not final. Cultures taken from the cervix also are helpful, but not final. Treatment with the right antibiotics and finding improvement in the symptoms help to prove the diagnosis of PID. Appendicitis will not get better with antibiotics.

1943. Is PID easily treated?

Some milder forms of PID, especially those caused by Chlamydia, respond quickly to oral tetracycline or even erythromycin, both of which are antibiotics. PID cannot be treated with penicillin, especially if it was caused by Chlamydia. Rest is helpful, especially pelvic rest. This means avoiding intercourse and not being physically active, which means no running or jumping. Heat helps to clear the infection, and so warm baths are comforting. Pain medication certainly relieves the pain, and also slows you down so that you will have a chance to get well. Treating your partner or partners so you will not get it again when you are well enough to have sex is especially important. Of course, you do not have to have two partners to get PID, but your partner does. With severe cases of PID, hospitalization may be needed, along with strong antibiotics given intravenously and absolute bed rest. Surgery may be required, especially in repeated cases and in the later stages, particularly if it has been going on for years.

1944. Are hysterectomies ever necessary in cases of PID?

If you develop scars on your tubes and ovaries, and chronic infection and pain, the only final cure for your PID may be to remove all of your reproductive organs, including the uterus. Otherwise, you can become a "pelvic cripple," whereby you would be too tender to have intercourse or do any other physical activity.

1945. How can I prevent PID?

To prevent PID, you must treat your gonorrhea or chlamydial infection before it travels into your fallopian tubes. To do this, your partners will have to tell you quickly that they have a sexual disease, so you will have to show them that you are ready to receive the information without prejudice. If you are going to blow up when they tell you, they will not tell you. Then

WOMEN'S DISEASES AND SURGERY: SEXUALLY TRANSMITTED DISEASES—PELVIC INFLAMMATORY DISEASE (PID) (Continued)

your vaginal infection will progress to a PID before you get it treated. You also could demand monogamy, but that doesn't mean you will get it.

WOMEN'S DISEASES AND SURGERY: SEXUALLY TRANSMITTED DISEASES—CHLAMYDIA TRACHOMATIS

1946. What is Chlamydia trachomatis?

Chlamydia trachomatis is a small bacterium that acts almost like a virus. It produces a sexually transmitted disease that is very similar to gonorrhea. It infects the urethra and cervix, and if it is not treated, spreads up into the uterus, tubes, and ovaries and becomes pelvic inflammatory disease. Chlamydia trachomatis is almost as frequent a cause of PID as gonorrhea. It is a fast-rising, epidemic venereal disease that is hard to handle. It causes a great deal more sterility than does gonorrhea, because the symptoms are not quite as severe as gonorrhea when it becomes PID, so it is neglected longer. If a mother has Chlamydia trachomatis when her baby is born, it can get into the baby's eyes and cause blindness, just as gonorrhea can. Erythromycin ointment placed in the baby's eyes will prevent this.

1947. How is Chlamydia trachomatis diagnosed?

Chlamydia trachomatis is difficult to culture because it must be grown within another cell, and most cities do not have the facilities to do this. Diagnosis is based on the absence of gonorrhea in a patient who has all the symptoms of gonorrhea, but the diagnosis can be difficult to prove. Blood tests can show a rise in the level of antibodies (titer), but these must be done two weeks apart.

1948. Is there any treatment for the infection caused by Chlamydia trachomatis?

The best treatment for chlamydial infection in men and in women is tetracycline or erythromycin, both of which are antibiotics.

WOMEN'S DISEASES AND SURGERY: SEXUALLY TRANSMITTED DISEASES—HERPES: WHAT IS IT? WHO GETS IT?

1949. What is herpes?

Herpes is a virus belonging to the herpes simplex family of viruses, including type I and type II. Type I is usually associated with cold sores, blisters, and ulcers of the lips of the face, also called fever blisters, because they often flare up when you have a fever. Type II virus occurs in women in

WOMEN'S DISEASES AND SURGERY: SEXUALLY TRANSMITTED DISEASES—HERPES: WHAT IS IT? WHO GETS IT? (Continued)

the vagina, the cervix, and the labia (the lips around the vagina). When it is in the vagina and cervix, no pain occurs, but when it is on the labia, severe pain usually results. First, small vesicles (blisters filled with clear fluid) appear for a day or so. These break and form ulcers that last seven to ten days on a first attack. Burning, itching, pain on urination, and extreme tenderness may last for two to six weeks. Both types of herpes can cause problems.

1950. Is herpes simplex the same as genital herpes?
Genital herpes is one form of herpes simplex infection. Another form is the herpes that is found on the lips of the face, called herpes facialis. Many children and adults have this type of herpes over and over again.

1951. What are the symptoms of genital herpes?
The symptoms of genital herpes are burning, itching, pain on urination, and extreme tenderness.

1952. What does genital herpes in women look like?
Genital herpes starts as a small blister on the vulva. It also can be several small blisters together. If the blisters are in the vagina and cervix you cannot see them and they do not hurt. After twenty-four to thirty-six hours, the blister breaks and leaves a very small ulcer with a little redness around it. It really looks rather unimportant, but it feels important.

1953. Are the sores I get in my mouth a form of herpes simplex?
Sores in your mouth usually are not herpes. They are canker sores that are caused by a different and milder virus. Cold sores on your lips are herpes, usually type I in this country, whereas genital herpes is usually type II. In Japan, it is the other way around.

1954. Has herpes always been a problem, or has it just recently become widespread?
Genital herpes has just recently become a widespread problem. Twenty-five years ago it was hardly ever diagnosed or seen on the vulva in women. Eighty percent of the population had had cold sores on their faces by the time they were adults. This made them somewhat immune to genital herpes. Now fewer adults have had cold sores on their faces; therefore, they are not at all immune to an attack of herpes on the genitals. There also is much more sexual activity and change of partners today than there was fifty years ago, and there is more oral-genital sexual activity.

1955. What percentage of people will contract herpes during their lives? What percentage of people already have herpes?
This depends on where you live. In Colombia, virtually all of the

WOMEN'S DISEASES AND SURGERY: SEXUALLY TRANSMITTED DISEASES—HERPES: WHAT IS IT? WHO GETS IT? (Continued)

population have type II herpes from their childhoods on. In a private gynecologic practice in Houston, about 10 percent of the patients have had the disease, while in the county (charity) hospital there, 25 percent of women have it.

1956. Is herpes more common among men or women? Are men or women the most common carriers of herpes?

There is no known difference. However, it is a more serious problem for women to have herpes, because if they have an outbreak at the time of labor, their babies can be infected with the disease.

1957. Is herpes more common among single or married people?

Herpes is more common among single people. This is true because it is more common among younger people and those who have many partners.

1958. I've heard that herpes simplex of the genitals can cause cancer of the cervix. If I've had herpes on my vulva, am I more at risk for cancer of the cervix? Should I have Pap smears more often?

You are correct; genital herpes can cause cancer of the cervix. The first study to indicate this showed that 80 percent of women with cancer of the cervix had a higher level of antibodies (titer) to herpes type II in their blood than the average population. Later the virus was demonstrated in the cancer cells. It also corresponds with the finding that early sex and having many partners increases the chances of getting cancer of the cervix. It does not mean that you have to have Pap smears more often. It just means you have to have them regularly, and you should take action if the Pap smear turns out abnormal.

WOMEN'S DISEASES AND SURGERY: SEXUALLY TRANSMITTED DISEASES—HERPES: HOW ONE GETS IT, DIAGNOSIS

1959. How do I get herpes?

You usually get oral herpes, of the lips of the face, by kissing someone who has a cold sore that is open at the time. Children and babies get it from adults this way. Herpes genitalis, of the vulva or penis, comes from sexual intimacy with someone who has an open sore or is shedding the virus at the time.

1960. Is genital herpes only contagious when the sores are open?

Unfortunately, no. The vagina can shed the herpes virus for at least a week after the sore has healed. Two percent of women can shed the virus from their vaginas with no sores at all. Researchers do not yet admit that

WOMEN'S DISEASES AND SURGERY: SEXUALLY TRANSMITTED DISEASES—HERPES: HOW ONE GETS IT, DIAGNOSIS
(Continued)

men can shed the virus without sores, but eventually they probably will.

1961. Is genital herpes transmitted by any way other than through sexual contact?

No, not really. In this day of great sexual freedom, why do people continue to try to prove that the disease was not sexually transmitted? Transmission of herpes requires intimate contact, and intimate contact is classified as sexual. Kissing transmits herpes of the lips of the face, cold sores. Oral-genital contact can make the cold sores appear in the genital area. That is sexual contact, even if it is not intercourse.

1962. Will a child delivered vaginally to a woman with genital herpes also develop herpes?

Yes. The newborn infant passing through an infected vagina and open herpes sores can develop a serious and widespread infection that is 70 percent fatal and causes severe neurologic damage in survivors. Medical advice is to do a cesarean section if the woman has active herpes sores on her vulva or has had a primary attack of herpes, but has had no sores for the last two weeks. However, if her membranes have been ruptured for over four hours, a cesarean section will not help because the baby still can be infected. One-half to two-thirds of babies affected by herpes are born to mothers who have no history of herpes at all. Fortunately, the total number of such babies is not very many, although four or five have been born in each large city.

1963. If I have had herpes genitalis, can I safely deliver a child vaginally?

If you have had no primary attack for four weeks, no recurrent attack for two weeks, and no visible lesions at the time of labor, you can safely deliver vaginally. Often obstetricians take cultures of the vagina in the last month to try to be sure that there is no virus present.

1964. Can I get herpes from using public bathrooms?

Bathrooms are not a source of herpes infection, not even in your own home. Sexual intimacy is the source.

1965. Can I have herpes sores around my mouth and not on my genitals, and vice versa?

Yes. A good, strong case of cold sores around the mouth will give you some immunity against having a severe case on the genitals, even if the herpes is type II instead of type I.

1966. Can oral herpes be transmitted by using another woman's lipstick who has it?

Yes, if the lipstick is quickly used just after she uses it. You would get

WOMEN'S DISEASES AND SURGERY: SEXUALLY TRANSMITTED DISEASES—HERPES: HOW ONE GETS IT, DIAGNOSIS
(Continued)
it more easily if you kissed her on the lips.

1967. How do I know if I have herpes?
     If you have one or more very small, slightly red ulcers on your vulva that first appeared as blisters and that are not more than 1 to 5 mm in diameter (largest measures 1/5th of an inch), and if they are very tender, in all likelihood, you have herpes simplex of the genitalia, the vulva. If you want to be certain, you can get the experienced opinion of a physician. Most doctors, as well as nurse practitioners, know immediately if you have herpes because they have seen so many cases. If you must be more certain, a culture can be done, but this costs money. In addition, you can take blood tests that will show a rise in the blood measurement of antibodies (titer) to herpes. However, if you have had cold sores on your facial lips in the past, there will be no rise because these antibodies show up on the titer, too.

1968. Will my doctor be able to tell me if I have herpes when I go in for my annual check-up?
     Your doctor only will be able to tell if you have herpes if you have open sores at the time of your checkup. After these sore spots are gone, there is no way for your doctor to be able to tell.

1969. How is herpes diagnosed?
     Herpes sores can be so typical that the disease can be diagnosed just by looking at them. If not, or if you want to be sure, a culture can be taken from the sore spot or from the vagina and cervix within three or four days of the onset of the problem. If you wait any later than three or four days, the culture will be negative. Blood tests for measurements of antibodies can be done on two occasions, two weeks apart. If the measurement rises, then it is a first-time herpes attack. If the measurement stays the same, you've had it in the past, and this may be a recurrence. If you have no measurement at all, it is not herpes, and you have never had it. A more rapid way to diagnose herpes is to examine scrapings of cells from the ulcers for the typical giant cells of herpes.

WOMEN'S DISEASES AND SURGERY: SEXUALLY TRANSMITTED DISEASES—HERPES: RECURRENT ATTACKS, SEXUAL ACTIVITY

1970. If I had herpes at a young age, could it go dormant for a long time and then reappear again later?
     It can, but it is unlikely to recur if you have had no recurrence for six

WOMEN'S DISEASES AND SURGERY: SEXUALLY TRANSMITTED DISEASES—HERPES: RECURRENT ATTACKS, SEXUAL ACTIVITY (Continued)

months. One of the problems of transplant patients, such as those with transplanted kidneys, is that the immunosuppressive therapy that they must undergo to prevent rejection of the transplanted organ sometimes allows their dormant herpes to flare up. This also is true of patients who are on chemotherapy for cancer. Such patients can have widespread herpes if they do not have help. Intravenous acyclovir, an antiviral agent, is now available to use in these cases.

1971. Once I have had herpes, will I always get recurrent attacks?

Only about one-half of the people who have herpes get attacks later on. These attacks are shorter (they last days instead of weeks), and they become milder and milder. However, you are still contagious during an attack. After two or three years, the attacks may stop entirely. Most of them are provoked by certain physical or emotional factors, such as fever, irritation of the skin from something else, or stress.

1972. Is it true that once I get herpes, I will always have it?

You will always have the herpes virus in your body, along with the antibody that inactivates it. This is true of many, many viral diseases, such as measles, chickenpox, hepatitis, and polio. The problem isn't that you always have the virus, but that 50 percent of the people with herpes have recurrences of the open sores that shed the virus and are contagious again.

1973. Should I refrain from having sex if I have herpes?

When you have a sore on your genitals, you should refrain from sex. You will not give it back to the one who gave it to you, but you can pass it on to someone else. If you have changed partners since you got herpes, you should not have sex while you have an open sore or for a week after it heals. You can still do sexy things, but do not allow intimate touching of the sore. If you have a cold sore on your mouth, you can have sex, but do not use your mouth for similar reasons.

1974. Before having sex with a new partner, should I tell him or her that I have herpes?

You only **have** herpes when you have an open sore or right after you have had an open sore, not all the time. So the question becomes, should I tell him or her that I **had** herpes? Would you tell your partner that you had hepatitis? I personally do not believe that you are obligated to tell your partner that you have had herpes of the lips or the genitals unless you have an active sore. It is not a severe danger to a man's health. It only is a danger to the health of a woman's unborn child if she has an open sore at the

WOMEN'S DISEASES AND SURGERY: SEXUALLY TRANSMITTED DISEASES—HERPES: RECURRENT ATTACKS, SEXUAL ACTIVITY (Continued)

moment of birth, which is an unlikely coincidence. So if you are a man and have a female partner, perhaps you should tell her. Recurrent herpes is only a minor annoyance, not a severe disease. If you go about telling your dates that you have herpes, you probably won't have too many dates. People recoil from disease and contagion, and they will recoil from you even if they, themselves, have had herpes. People are not always logical.

1975. Is it safe to have intercourse with a partner who has herpes?

If your partner has an open sore, you have an 80 percent chance of getting herpes, if you have not already had herpes. If your partner has had herpes in the past, but has no open sore at the time of intercourse or the week before, you are safe, unless you are among the 2 percent of women who have sex with a partner who has herpes and is shedding the virus without having a visible open sore! If your partner has herpes on the lips of the face, cold sores, you are safe to have intercourse, but not to kiss.

1976. If I have herpes sores on the lips of my mouth, is it possible to transfer these to my partner's genital area through oral sex?

Yes, but only if your partner is not already immune by having had cold sores on the lips, too.

WOMEN'S DISEASES AND SURGERY: SEXUALLY TRANSMITTED DISEASES—HERPES: TREATMENT AND CURE

1977. Are there any drugs available that are useful in treating herpes?

Yes. A primary case, or the first attack, can be treated with a cream called acyclovir (brand name Zovirax Ointment) that is obtained by prescription. It will reduce the time that you are infective and also the time you have the open sore. If you have a severe systemic case, with fever and headaches, you can be treated with intravenous acyclovir, an antiviral agent, which will ease and shorten the disease. This is especially necessary for people who have a poor immunity system, such as cancer patients on chemotherapy or transplant patients on suppressive therapy. It is not useful for the ordinary recurrent sores of the subsequent herpes attacks, and it will not prevent them. That kind of treatment is what most people really need, and it has not yet been found.

1978. What treatments are presently available for people with herpes?

If it is your first attack, it may be worthwhile for you to go to a physician or clinic and get the acyclovir cream. But for recurrent attacks, there is

WOMEN'S DISEASES AND SURGERY: SEXUALLY TRANSMITTED DISEASES—HERPES: TREATMENT AND CURE (Continued)

no need to go to a physician unless you are not sure of what you have, because there is no medical treatment that shortens the course of the disease or prevents recurrences. You can do whatever makes you feel most comfortable. The easiest treatment is an anesthetic ointment of the caine type of drugs, available over the counter everywhere. Apply this regularly to reduce the pain and to keep urine from burning the area. Any ointment will keep urine from burning the area, but the caine ointments are somewhat numbing. Keeping the area clean, but not aggravating it with rough treatment, is advisable. Lysine (an amino acid sold in health food stores), ether, red dyes, and BHT (a food preservative) have all been shown to be completely ineffective. The sores always eventually heal and recurrences become less and less frequent no matter what you do, so you really don't have to do anything, if you don't want to.

1979. Why can't a cure for herpes be found?
Herpes is a viral disease, and there is no known cure for any viral disease. There are no general antiviral agents that are effective in curing these. Vaccines only act as preventives. The herpes virus lies dormant along the nerve where it first infected, and it comes down the nerve to the skin when it is reactivated. There is not enough known about this process to intervene. However, a lot of research is currently going on to discover a cure.

1980. How can the spread of herpes genitalis be prevented?
The usual advice is not to have any sexual contact during the time when you have any symptoms of the disease, especially open sores, and for a week after all symptoms have disappeared. However, 2 percent of women actually shed the virus when they have no symptoms of herpes. It is denied that men shed the virus without symptoms. Use of a condom also appears to protect somewhat against viral transmission.

WOMEN'S DISEASES AND SURGERY: SEXUALLY TRANSMITTED DISEASES—VENEREAL WARTS

1981. What are venereal warts?
They are warts that are found in the genital area. They usually are transmitted by sexual contact with someone who has the wart virus, but does not necessarily have the warts. Venereal warts can appear on the labia, anus, vagina, and cervix.

1982. What do venereal warts look like?
Venereal warts look like any other wart on your hand or elsewhere. They are pointed, hard, and rather white. They vary from small to large and

WOMEN'S DISEASES AND SURGERY: SEXUALLY TRANSMITTED DISEASES—VENEREAL WARTS (Continued)

may be singular but usually are multiple. Sometimes, when they are old, they are a little flat on the end. They grow in clusters around the vulva and the anus.

1983. How do they differ from ordinary warts?

They look the same, but their location is different. They are caused by a different virus from the one that causes warts on the hand or other areas of the body. Warts on your hand will not cause warts on your vulva.

1984. Are warts similar to cold sores?

No. Warts stick up and grow larger and larger. Cold sores start out briefly as blisters, but quickly form shallow holes (ulcers).

1985. Are venereal warts contagious?

Yes. All warts are contagious because they are caused by viruses. But just as there are two types of herpes viruses, there are two wart viruses. Genital warts, or venereal warts, come from a virus that is different from the virus that causes warts on your fingers. Venereal warts usually are contagious by sexual contact, so that is how they got their name.

1986. How do venereal warts differ from other venereal diseases?

Once venereal warts are gone, they are gone for good, unless you develop an immune deficiency state, such as with chemotherapy.

1987. Are venereal warts curable?

Yes, but often with great difficulty. Sometimes the wart you treat goes away, but a new wart forms somewhere else. Sometimes the wart has to be treated over and over before it will go away entirely, even if it is surgically removed.

1988. How are venereal warts treated?

The most common treatment, and perhaps the most effective overall, is to paint them with an oxidating agent known as podophyllum. This is a brown liquid that also is used on warts found elsewhere on the body. It should not be used in pregnancy because some of it is absorbed and may affect the placenta. Silver nitrate also is sometimes successful in treating warts. Sometimes persistent warts are frozen with cryosurgery, but each one has to be frozen separately, and each takes a few minutes. They also can be surgically removed, but this leaves more scarring than other methods. If you leave them alone, they eventually will go away, just as warts on your hand will, but sometimes this takes one or two years, and few people are patient enough to wait. They do not cause pain or itching, but they feel and look ugly. If you do have pain and itching, you probably have some other

WOMEN'S DISEASES AND SURGERY: SEXUALLY TRANSMITTED DISEASES—VENEREAL WARTS (Continued)

vaginitis infection, and should treat that. Treating an irritating vaginitis can sometimes make the warts go away, too.

1989. Can venereal warts have any long-term effect on a woman?

Yes, the condyloma virus, or wart virus, has been held responsible for an increase in cancer of the cervix, as well as cancer of the vulva. When you have warts on your cervix, it may not only look like cancer, but your Pap smear may become quite abnormal. A biopsy may be the only way to make certain that you do not need treatment for cancer of the cervix, just treatment for warts. Later, the changes induced by the virus really may develop into cancer of the cervix. If you are pregnant and have an active wart virus at the time your baby is delivered, the baby could develop warts on its vocal cords, which is a rare but very serious problem.

WOMEN'S DISEASES AND SURGERY: ACQUIRED IMMUNE DEFICIENCY SYNDROME (AIDS)

1990. What is the newly discovered disease, AIDS?

AIDS means acquired immune deficiency syndrome, and it is now classified as an epidemic. It occurs in previously healthy individuals who suddenly acquire all kinds of infections, as well as cancers, that are unusually severe. It first was seen in homosexual men and intravenous drug abusers. Now it also is found among Haitian and other Caribbean immigrants to the United States, as well as in patients with a blood disease called hemophilia. Of the seven hundred cases that have been reported in the United States, half were in New York City; the rest were in Miami, San Francisco, Los Angeles, Chicago, and Boston. Widespread herpes simplex, candidiasis (yeast), toxoplasmosis (usually a mild disease associated with animals), and parasites have been found growing rampant in these people. Kaposi's sarcoma (a cancer caused by a virus) occurs in the skin and intestines. It was thought that homosexuals were contagious through rectal intercourse, the drug abusers through shared hypodermic needles, and the hemophiliacs through blood transfusions. All cases of AIDS are to be reported to public health departments so that the new problem can be solved.

1991. What is AIDS caused by?

Some evidence suggests that AIDS is caused by an agent that is spread by blood or blood products.

1992. Is there a treatment or cure for AIDS?

Prolonged treatment for infections shows only temporary improvement. The patient usually gets worse, loses weight, and dies with multiple in-

WOMEN'S DISEASES AND SURGERY: ACQUIRED IMMUNE DEFICIENCY SYNDROME (AIDS) (Continued)

fections. A lot of research is currently being done to learn more about AIDS.

WOMEN'S DISEASES AND SURGERY: DIETHYLSTILBESTROL (DES)

1993. What was DES?

Diethylstilbestrol (DES) was the first oral estrogen. It became available in the 1920s and was used for many different purposes for which estrogen was thought to be helpful, including the replacement therapy of menopause.

1994. Why did women take DES?

Women mainly used DES for menopause. In Boston, there was a group who thought DES given to pregnant women who were diabetic would produce a better outcome for the baby, and many women were treated in this way. Throughout the country, DES was used to try to stop the bleeding of pregnant women, in the hopes that a miscarriage could be prevented. It also was used as a morning-after pill, and was about 95 percent effective in preventing a pregnancy when taken after unprotected intercourse.

1995. How did DES affect the women who took it?

DES worked very well in replacing estrogen when it was deficient, as in menopause. Today, it is not considered helpful to diabetic pregnant women. It stopped bleeding in some women, but it did not prevent a miscarriage. Since the 1960s it has not been used much for this purpose. DES did not harm the women who took it any more than any other estrogen would; however it did harm their daughters. Although it was cheaper than conjugated estrogens, such as Premarin, it caused much more nausea.

1996. What problems do DES daughters face?

The most serious problem that DES daughters face is that between one hundred and two hundred of them have been found to have a very rare cancer of the vagina, called adenocarcinoma of the vagina. This cancer first appeared in the girls when they were quite young, between the ages of fifteen and twenty-five, and some cases were fatal. Others were treated with rather extensive surgery in which their reproductive organs were removed. Even though the numbers were small, it is significant that a drug given to mothers could cause cancer fifteen to twenty years later in their daughters. In addition to the cancer, there were deformities found in the cervix, lumps of glandular formation (adenosis) in the vagina that were benign, and deformities of the uterus that decreased the fertility of some of the daughters. It was thought at first that those daughters who did not have cancer when they first

WOMEN'S DISEASES AND SURGERY: DIETHYLSTILBESTROL (DES) (Continued)

were examined might develop cancer later, but so far they have not. The deformities of the cervix actually improve with age, and the vagina grows more normal instead of becoming malignant. Nevertheless, each case has been followed very carefully, and all the tests, examinations, and fright it has caused in the daughters has clouded their lives. Of course, DES no longer is given to pregnant women.

WOMEN'S DISEASES AND SURGERY: PAP SMEARS

1997. What is a Pap smear?

A Pap smear consists of a sample of cells from your cervix taken from the edge of the mouth of the uterus and a little bit inside. It is done in your doctor's office while you are lying down and takes just a few minutes. This sample is then put on a slide and studied to look for abnormal cells that are changing in the direction of cervical cancer. A Pap smear also can report the effect of estrogen on the cells; evidence of infection, especially Trichomonas and yeast; and, occasionally, even abnormal cells from the lining of the uterus. It is named after Dr. George Papanicolaou who, with Dr. Herbert Traut of the University of California at San Francisco, developed the smear technique. Women now demand that Pap smears be taken, because they have learned that Pap smears can protect them from cancer of the cervix by finding it early enough to treat it easily.

1998. If my Pap smear is abnormal, what is the next step I should take?

If the abnormality is so mild that it only suggests a change due to infection, then it is all right to treat the infection or just wait until it goes away. The Pap smear can be repeated the following year. But do not wait three years if your Pap smear is abnormal. If it is more than mildly abnormal, suggesting dysplasia (a precancerous stage), the next step is to study the cervix by biopsies. These are best done when directed by colposcopy, a microscope adapated to studying the cervix through the vagina. The entire procedure can be done in the doctor's office or clinic. Only if an invasive cancer is found does radiation or a hysterectomy have to be done. If this technique does not find the abnormal spot or the spot extends up into the inside of the cervix, then a surgery called a conization is done under anesthesia in a hospital. In this procedure, the central section of the cervix is removed and studied. What is left of the cervix is stitched back to form a new cervix. This procedure has more complications of bleeding and it can interfere with carrying a pregnancy to term, so it is avoided if possible. If a small, noninvasive cancer (carcinoma in situ) is found on the biopsies, then sometimes a conization will be done to see if there is more cancer. If no cancer is there, the cervix

WOMEN'S DISEASES AND SURGERY: PAP SMEARS (Continued)
can be treated by freezing (cryosurgery).

1999. Will a Pap smear detect all diseases that might be present in a woman's sexual organs?
No. A Pap smear is designed only to detect cancer of the cervix and the changes, such as dysplasia, that occur prior to cancer of the cervix. The smear sometimes is read for estrogen deficiency or evidence of infection, such as Gardnerella, Trichomonas, or fungus. Sometimes herpes, or even cancer of the uterus, is found as the result of a Pap smear, but it is not designed to do these things. It is just meant to detect cancer of the cervix.

WOMEN'S DISEASES AND SURGERY: CHEMOTHERAPY, RADIATION, NEW CANCER TREATMENTS

2000. What is chemotherapy?
Chemotherapy is a cancer treatment using chemicals that attack the cancer cells more than they attack other cells in the patient's body. These chemicals are poisons, but they are more poisonous to the cancer than to the person. They are still poisonous, however, and often cause vomiting, hair loss, and other toxic effects on the heart and nerves of the person taking them. People on chemotherapy also are more subject to infection.

2001. What are the long-term effects of chemotherapy?
A small percentage of people taking some form of chemotherapy are more likely to develop leukemia ten or more years later. Of course, without the chemotherapy they might not have lived ten years.

2002. What are the long-term effects of radiation?
Sometimes the surface burns caused by radiation turn into scars and tissues that do not heal well and this becomes a long-term problem. Sometimes the irritation of the bowel and bladder continues to produce diarrhea and urinary frequency. There always is the fear that the radiation will produce a cancer later, especially leukemia. This is evidenced by the fact that long ago radiation was used on women to stop menstruation, but later these women developed more cancer of the uterus.

2003. Are there any relatively new cancer treatments available to women?
Various forms of chemotherapy are still the newest cancer treatments available to women. Also in research are promising methods of producing very specific (monoclonal) antibodies that are fashioned to attack the person's cancer cells and nothing else. These are not yet available, but they provide hope and might eventually make some of the other cancer surgeries obsolete.

WOMEN'S DISEASES AND SURGERY: DILATATION AND CURETTAGE (D & C)

2004. What is D & C?

D & C is an abbreviation for dilatation and curettage. With a D & C, the opening in the cervix is dilated or widened until it will admit an instrument called a curette. The lining of the uterus is then scraped with the curette until it is empty.

2005. How is a D & C performed?

Some D & Cs are performed under general anesthesia, with the patient completely asleep. In this procedure the cervix is grasped with an instrument to hold it steady. Dilators of increasingly larger sizes are inserted into the cervix to widen it. Then a curette, either a sharp metal loop or a plastic tube with a sharp end connected to a suction machine, is inserted into the cavity of the uterus. The curette is moved around, in and out, until everything that will come loose with the curette has been removed from the uterus. A D & C also can be performed in the doctor's office under a local anesthesia. The anesthesia usually consists of some injections of a caine solution, called paracervical block. In this procedure dilation usually is avoided and a much smaller plastic suction currette attached to a vacuum (either a machine or a large syringe) is inserted. It is moved in and out and around the uterus until all the material is obtained. This type of D & C is still somewhat painful, in spite of the paracervical block. Sometimes other drugs are used to sedate, but not completely anesthetize, the patient.

2006. Why is a D & C done?

The most common reason for performing a D & C today is as an abortion. This is done in the first two or three months of pregnancy, either in the doctor's office or in the hospital. The next most common reasons for having a D & C are to diagnose abnormal bleeding, such as very heavy menstrual flow, especially if it will not stop; intermenstrual bleeding; and too frequent bleeding. This procedure often works as a cure as well as a diagnosis. As the result of having a D & C, a polyp that may have been causing the bleeding or a thick lining will be removed. Then steps are taken to prevent a recurrence of the problem, such as hormone therapy. A D & C is necessary to diagnose cancer of the uterus. It is done when a woman bleeds after menopause with no explanation. A D & C also may be done to investigate a Pap smear that shows abnormal endometrial cells suggesting uterine cancer. It may be used to investigate why a woman is having trouble getting pregnant. With a D&C, the doctor can find out if the woman ovulates properly and makes a good lining in her uterus for implanting a pregnancy. Another more frequent purpose for a D & C is to complete a spontaneous abortion or a miscarriage. It removes the rest of the pregnancy from the uterus and stops the bleeding in a

WOMEN'S DISEASES AND SURGERY: DILATATION AND CURETTAGE (D & C) (Continued)

woman who has lost part of her pregnancy, but not all of it. In this case, a D & C may be necessary as a life-saving emergency procedure.

WOMEN'S DISEASES AND SURGERY: HYSTERECTOMY

2007. What is a hysterectomy?

A hysterectomy is the surgical removal of the uterus, that muscle in the pelvis that menstruates and carries babies. It can be performed through the abdominal wall (the tummy), or it can be done through the vagina in some cases. A hysterectomy does not include the removal of ovaries and tubes, or the plastic surgery repair of the vagina, although these may be combined with a hysterectomy. After a hysterectomy you cannot menstruate or carry babies. Nothing else changes.

2008. Is eighteen years of age too young to have a hysterectomy?

There is no consideration of age when the medical problem that requires a hysterectomy is life threatening. The desire for children is the primary consideration when the problem is not life threatening, just miserable. It becomes a balancing of how much misery you can put up with in order to keep your childbearing equipment until you have had all the babies you want. If you are bleeding to death and nothing controls it; if you have severe abscesses that already have destroyed your ability to have children, as in some pelvic inflammatory disease; or if you have cancer that will kill you before you ever get to be a mother, then you should have a hysterectomy at eighteen or any other age. You give up your ability to have children in order to stay alive. If you can control your problem by some means other than a hysterectomy until you have finished having children, then you delay the hysterectomy until that day. The decision to have a hysterectomy is something that women should take part in with more clarity as to the problems. Childbearing is the problem, not age. If you have six children by age eighteen, you may very well pray for a hysterectomy for any minor problem, such as a prolapsed uterus and vagina. If you are thirty-eight, childless, and sincerely want a child, you may be willing to put up with a lot of misery and a lot of danger to have a baby in the following year. It is your choice to have children, and your choice to keep your uterus so you can do this. The choice does not need to be based on age. Of course, the younger you are, the less anyone thinks you know your own mind.

2009. When is a hysterectomy really necessary?

There are degrees of necessity. A hysterectomy can be needed as an emergency life-saving measure, as a means of getting rid of symptoms that

WOMEN'S DISEASES AND SURGERY: HYSTERECTOMY
(Continued)

make life miserable, as a prevention of a future severe or life-threatening disease, or simply as a way of making life more pleasant and comfortable. Most medical centers and insurance programs do not approve of a hysterectomy that is done simply for sterilization, because it is more dangerous than a tubal ligation. Emergency situations that could require a hysterectomy might be an enormous hemorrhage that occurs right after delivery, after a surgery, such as an abortion, or as a complication of fibroids. This type of hysterectomy must take place within hours of the problem if no other solution is found. Most hysterectomies, however, are not emergencies. They are done to keep life from being miserable, as with fibroids that bleed heavily each month and make a woman anemic or fibroids that grow so large that the woman looks like she is pregnant. It might also be done in cases of severe menstrual pain, pelvic pain between menses that does not respond to medical treatment, as a late result of pelvic inflammatory disease, and especially as a result of endometriosis. Cancer of the cervix, uterus, ovaries, or even fallopian tubes requires hysterectomy to save a woman's life, even if she is not yet miserable. Precancerous conditions of the cervix, uterus, and ovaries also may need preventive surgery that includes a hysterectomy. If a dropped uterus, bladder, and/or rectum makes life uncomfortable and inhibits physical activity, hysterectomy and repair of the loose tissue is justified. It greatly improves the life of the woman who has these problems, even though they did not threaten her health. In this case, happiness is necessary, too.

2010. What diseases in women would necessitate a hysterectomy?
There are many diseases in women that would require a hysterectomy. One of the most frequent is called by many names, such as pelvic relaxation, prolapse of the uterus, cystocele, rectocele, or even enterocele. With this condition, the fibrous tissues and ligaments that support the uterus within the pelvis have stretched and become so weak that everything (uterus, bladder, and rectal wall) is dropping down and even protruding from the opening of the vagina. This may not affect a woman's health, but it is annoying and uncomfortable. A less frequent reason for hysterectomy is fibroids, also called leiomyomata. These are noncancerous tumors of the uterus that bleed, grow large, or produce pain. Endometriosis (small cysts) and adenomyosis (endometriosis of the uterus) are becoming even more frequent causes of hysterectomy. Severe infections and abscesses of the ovaries, as in pelvic inflammatory disease, lead to hysterectomy as well as removal of tubes and ovaries for chronic pain. In the past, if tubes and/or ovaries had to be removed, then the uterus was removed, too, because there was no way to have a baby after that. With the test-tube baby program, maybe the uterus

WOMEN'S DISEASES AND SURGERY: HYSTERECTOMY
(Continued)

still will be left intact in women who want to try this new way to get pregnant.

2011. Are there any kinds of diseases or disorders that are more likely to develop in women who have had hysterectomies?

No, unless you develop a depression over not being able to have children. With the hysterectomy alone, it is possible that you could develop adhesions in your internal organs that could lead to pain or even bowel obstruction and that would require another surgery. You also could develop a complication of surgery, such as a cut ureter, bladder, or rectum. This could cause problems if it is not properly treated and if it does not heal properly.

2012. What is a total hysterectomy?

A total hysterectomy is the removal of the entire uterus but not the ovaries or tubes. It means taking out the whole uterus, including the cervix or mouth that is so subject to cancer. It is technically more surgically difficult to remove the cervix along with the uterus, because of its attachments. Fifty years ago this was not done because it prolonged the surgical time. When surgery became safer, it became important to remove the cervix to prevent cervical cancer.

2013. What is a partial hysterectomy?

This is a bad term because the meaning is not clear. "Partial" should mean that all of the uterus was not taken out. Most women, however, use this term to mean that the entire uterus was removed but not the ovaries. It would be better not to use this term at all and say just exactly what was removed.

2014. What is a subtotal hysterectomy?

A subtotal hysterectomy is when the uterus is removed, but the cervix is left in. It is done when the entire surgery is very difficult and long, and it is not worth the extra time required to get the cervix out, too. This would be the case when the patient is in poor condition, as in an emergency hysterectomy for a severe hemorrhage. Subtotal hysterectomy also is performed when surgery for cancer, especially ovarian cancer, makes it difficult to remove the cervix, and it heals better if the cervix is left in. These are all technical surgical problems in which you have no choice.

2015. What is a panhysterectomy?

Panhysterectomy is removal of the uterus, tubes, and ovaries. It is an old-fashioned term. The modern term for this is hysterectomy with bilateral salpingo-oophorectomy. "Bilateral" means both sides, "salpingo" refers to

WOMEN'S DISEASES AND SURGERY: HYSTERECTOMY
(Continued)

the fallopian tubes, "oophor" refers to the ovaries, and "ectomy" means removal.

2016. What percentage of women suffer mental disorders, such as depressions, as the result of having a hysterectomy?

Studies show that there is no increase in the incidence of depression in women who have had hysterectomies. As women get older, there is a higher percentage who have depressions, but the percentage is not higher among those who have had hysterectomies. Actually, most women feel relieved of the problem for which they had the surgery. In addition, they are released from the fear of pregnancy. There is greater freedom for activity, including sexual activity, simply because there is no longer the normal menstrual flow and pain. Women who have had hysterectomies can discard pads and tampons, as well as contraceptives. Most of them rejoice!

2017. Does a hysterectomy affect menstruation?

Yes, hysterectomy completely eliminates menstruation forever.

2018. Does a hysterectomy affect sexual performance or desire?

There is no medical or physical reason why hysterectomy should have any effect on sexual performance or desire. Psychologically, most of the effects are positive. The surgery may have eliminated painful problems that interfered with sex, the fear of pregnancy, the need for contraceptives that interfered with sex, and the heavy bleeding. The actual process of intercourse is not different, since the vagina is the same. The newfound freedom that accompanies hysterectomy often increases sexual desire and activity. Only if a woman grieves over the loss of her ability to have children or feels that she is not a desirable woman if she cannot get pregnant, does she have a decrease in sexual desire and activity. Of course, if her husband or partner also agrees that without the possibility of getting pregnant sex is no fun, then there is a definite problem. Counseling can sometimes modify this reaction.

2019. How is the operation of hysterectomy performed?

The operation varies depending upon why the hysterectomy is being done. You should always discuss it with your surgeon prior to operating, because you may have a choice in the matter. In general, a vaginal hysterectomy leads to a more rapid recovery than does an abdominal one. This is because there is less pain when the incision is in the vagina, rather than in the abdominal wall. Also, while you are healing after surgery, activity does not produce as much pain when the incision is in the vagina. But if the uterus is too large to deliver through the vagina or if there are problems in the tubes and ovaries, the incision must be made in the abdomen. In this case, you can

WOMEN'S DISEASES AND SURGERY: HYSTERECTOMY
(Continued)

discuss with your surgeon whether you will have a midline vertical incision, from your navel (umbilicus) to your pubic hair, or a crosswise (transverse) incision where your bikini would end. A large tumor or a cancer that requires a radical surgery may require the midline, but most hysterectomies can be done through the transverse incision. This not only looks nicer, but is stronger and less likely to come apart. Anesthesia must be used. It can be regional, like a spinal, or general, such as gas and intravenous drugs. Essentially, the supporting structures of the uterus and its attachments to the ovaries, the tubes, the blood vessels, and the vagina around the cervix are cut, tied, and all layers are closed with sutures. The procedure can take from one-half hour to two or three hours, depending upon the difficulty of the problems and the experience of the surgeon.

2020. I had a hysterectomy when I was relatively young, under thirty-five, and continued to have premenstrual symptoms. After I reached my forties, I even had hot flushes. Why?

Your ovaries were left in to continue to work for you. It is the hormones from the active ovaries that gave you the menstrual feelings. The only symptom you are guaranteed of not having is cramps. When the ovaries failed, sometimes in your forties, but usually in your fifties, you began to have hot flushes and other symptoms of estrogen deficiency. The only thing that was removed when you had your hysterectomy was your uterus. The only things you lost were the bleeding, the cramps with menses, and the ability to have babies.

2021. I had a hysterectomy around thirty-five and my doctor gave me hormones to take after that. Why do I need hormones?

If you had your ovaries taken out when you had your hysterectomy, then you needed to take hormones. If you do not take hormones and your ovaries are gone, you will have menopausal symptoms, such as hot flushes, dry vagina, urgency with voiding, and the special aging that comes with menopause. I hope that there was a very good reason for you to have your ovaries removed, such as tumors, infections or endometriosis.

2022. How does my body compensate after a hysterectomy?

After a hysterectomy, you no longer bleed, so you do not become anemic anymore. The space that was occupied by your uterus is now occupied by a loop of bowel, so your tummy is a tiny bit flatter. Unless your uterus was very large, you won't notice this. There is no other compensation required by the body after a hysterectomy. The function of childbearing cannot be performed by anything else, nor can the function of bleeding. Since there is no physical requirement that you have babies or bleed, you just stop

WOMEN'S DISEASES AND SURGERY: HYSTERECTOMY
(Continued)

doing those things.

2023. What happens to my hormones after a hysterectomy? Does my body continue to produce them?

Your ovaries produce your female hormones, and they are not removed as part of a hysterectomy. If they are removed in **addition** to a hysterectomy, then you also had a bilateral salpingo-oophorectomy. That means that your tubes and ovaries were removed as well as your uterus. If these are removed you will have menopause. If they are not removed, your ovaries will continue to produce hormones just as well after a hysterectomy as they did before. If there is nothing wrong with them, it may be your choice as to whether your ovaries are removed or not. It is essential that you know the difference.

2024. My doctor said if I didn't have my ovaries out with the hysterectomy, I might have to come back later and have them out. Does a hysterectomy cause that?

No. If there is nothing wrong with your ovaries at the time of your hysterectomy, the surgery will not cause problems in your ovaries later. But there is no guarantee that they will not develop problems later. If you are young or just not yet in menopause, you may prefer to take your chances and possibly have a second surgery for any problems that might develop later, including cancer of the ovary. This may seem better to you than having a surgical menopause and having to struggle with taking hormones beginning right after surgery. The United States is a wealthy country, and most people can afford to finance the cost of a second surgery if it should become necessary. If you are in reasonable health, a second surgery is not all that dangerous. If you are past menopause, then it probably is wise to remove the ovaries, since they are nonfunctioning and still can form cysts and cancer. You lose nothing, since the ovaries do nothing for you after menopause anyway.

2025. Why do doctors remove ovaries with a hysterectomy if there is nothing wrong with them?

Over forty years ago, many surgeons removed ovaries because it was technically easier than leaving them in. Many gynecologic surgeons still remove them today, even in a young woman, but their motive is to prevent cancer of the ovary in later years. Cancer of the ovary occurs in one in every one hundred women at some time in their lives. Other surgeons feel it is wrong to do this in a young woman of thirty-five, because she then has a surgical menopause that includes hot flushes, dry vagina, and bone

WOMEN'S DISEASES AND SURGERY: HYSTERECTOMY
(Continued)

deterioration. Without her ovaries, she needs hormones, so she has to buy and take them, or suffer the consequences. For the one women who is going to get ovarian cancer, it is a very good idea to remove the ovaries, but for the other ninety-nine it is not so good. Most physicians will remove normal ovaries if the woman is around forty-five years of age or older, since she would be in menopause in five or ten years anyway. Others never remove the ovaries unless the woman has demonstrated that she already has gone into menopause, whatever the age. This is something you should discuss with your surgeon before the hysterectomy, so that you can understand and help make the choice.

2026. When is it required to remove the ovaries along with the uterus at the time of hysterectomy?

If you have cancer of the uterus, the ovaries are removed to take away the hormone that promotes the cancer. They also are one of the first places to which the cancer spreads. Often the ovaries are removed with hysterectomy for cancer of the cervix because a very wide radical surgery must be done. There are newer techniques today to preserve the ovaries and even move them out of the way of any radiation that may be done for cervical cancer. If the ovaries are left in, the woman will not have a surgical menopause and will not have to take hormones. Of course, you have to remove ovaries if they are diseased and are the reason for your surgery. Cancer of the ovaries, endometriomas (tumors) of the ovaries with endometriosis (small cysts), painful scars and adhesions of old infection around the ovaries, acute abscesses of the ovaries, or tumors, such as dermoids, that already have grown large and destroyed the ovaries are all diseases that would necessitate removing the ovaries. The list of other diseases is long.

2027. My doctor says it is easy and inexpensive to take hormones to replace those made by my ovaries, so he might as well take out my ovaries when I have a hysterectomy. Is it easy to take hormones?

No, it is not always a simple matter to give a woman the right female hormones that will make her feel as well as she did when her ovaries were producing them. They also cost more money than birth control pills do, and they make trips to the doctor necessary more often than if you were not in a surgical menopause. It probably costs more money for the hormone replacement therapy in women who have had their ovaries removed as a preventive measure than it would cost for the few women who develop problems in their ovaries to pay for a second surgery later. Men can develop cancer of the testicles, but you do not see them removing their testicles and taking testosterone to replace the hormones after they want no more children. They

WOMEN'S DISEASES AND SURGERY: HYSTERECTOMY
(Continued)

know how to stand up for their rights. Women should learn.

2028. Is sexual performance affected if I have a repair of a loose vagina along with a hysterectomy?

Yes, it may be improved. Repairs of the vagina are called many things: cystocele, rectocele, and anterior or posterior repair. If you were so loose that before surgery, your partner could hardly keep his penis in your vagina, then after surgery it will feel much tighter. A problem could develop if the vagina is made too tight. There may be pain on entry until it is stretched. Stretching by sexual activity is effective, but if this is difficult, dilators and creams may be used to enlarge the vagina and its opening again. If you are past menopause and do not have sex for a long time after the repair, your vagina could shrink so much that intercourse would be impossible. The best treatment for this is to have sex as soon as it is allowed after your surgery or to use dilators. If you have not yet gone through menopause at the time of the repair, then there is no shrinkage.

2029. How does hysterectomy affect the aging process?

Hysterectomy alone does not affect the aging process at all, except to prolong a life that was threatened by the disease for which the hysterectomy was done. It is only the removal of ovaries at the time of hysterectomy that produces the special aging process of menopause. When female hormones are gone because the ovaries are gone, hot flushes begin in most women. The vagina becomes dry and tender, voiding acquires a special urgency, and bones become thin and deteriorate, which leads to fractures in ten or fifteen years. Bones become particularly painful with this process. This condition is called osteoporosis. It is especially painful in the ribs at the front of the chest, a condition called radiculitis. Some women are not aware that their ovaries were removed, and although the surgeon gave them hormones to take after surgery, after a while they just stop taking them. Ten years later they may be very sorry.

Chapter 9

Menopause

I know that lately you
have been having problems
and I just want you to know
that you can rely on me for anything
you might need
But more important
keep in mind at all times
that you are very capable
of dealing with any complications
that life has to offer
So
do whatever you must
and keep in mind at all times
that we all
grow wiser and
become more sensitive and
are able to enjoy life more
after we go through
hard times

— Susan Polis Schutz

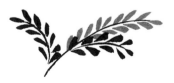

MENOPAUSE

Aging women and men are often extremely capable and productive people who have wonderful lives. After menopause women have a new freedom from concern about reproduction and society's rules about it. They are no longer burdened with infant care, and can turn their energies to politics, creative arts, or re-entering the work force. In India this is dramatized by women removing the veils that hid their faces, and coming out of their seclusion after they reach menopause. For the first time they can socialize and work with men. No wonder the women of India welcome menopause. We, too, can welcome being valued for ourselves, and not our reproductive capacity.

The special type of aging that women endure, which includes the thinning of bones leading to thousands more hip fractures in women than in men, has not received serious public concern. Geriatrics, medicine for the aging, is still in its infancy, and a lot of research needs to be done. There is no general medical decision as to how the majority of women should treat menopause. This indecision gives you the freedom to seek all the information you need and make your own choices. Who cares most about the bodies of women over fifty years of age? It must start with the women themselves. You must care very much. Even if you have never taken charge of your body before menopause, the change of life can be an opportunity to control the last third of your life.

MENOPAUSE: WHAT IT IS AND ITS SYMPTOMS

2030. What exactly is menopause?

Menopause is the time of ovarian failure, when your ovaries have no more eggs to form follicles and secrete the hormones that produce menstruation. During this time you may have symptoms of hot flushes, night sweats, dry vagina, bladder urgency, and irritability if there is lack of sleep. When these symptoms stop, it is called postmenopause. Most people determine when their menopause occurs by when menstruation stops, but if you have had a hysterectomy and your ovaries were left in, then menopause occurs when your ovaries stop functioning. If there are no symptoms, menopause is hard to detect.

2031. What are the symptoms of premenopause?

Premenopause is marked by a change in the pattern of the menstrual flow, usually skipping periods and having a few hot flushes, or worse, menstruating more often with a longer and heavier flow. Both patterns occur because you are not ovulating regularly anymore.

2032. How will I know for sure that I'm going through menopause?

There is no simple way to be sure, except looking backward a year later. Even medical testing is not absolute. Blood tests can show a low estrogen level, typical of menopause, and a high level of the pituitary hormones FSH (follicle stimulating hormone), which indicate that your ovaries are failing; yet three months later you can have another menstrual flow and your hormones will change again. When you've had no menses for a year, especially with hot flushes, you can be sure. If a doctor agrees with you, that is even better. If you have hot flushes that disappear when you take estrogen, you can also be sure of menopause.

2033. Does an unusually heavy menstrual flow signal the beginning of menopause?

Sometimes women stop ovulating, but still menstruate like teenagers do, with a heavy flow and variation in pattern. However, the problem is that other conditions, such as a miscarriage, a polyp in the uterus, overgrowth of the uterine lining (hyperplasia), or even cancer of the uterus, can also cause a heavy flow. Sometimes a D & C (dilatation and curettage) or at least a biopsy of the lining of the uterus is necessary to be sure repeated heavy flows are not due to other causes like these, because they need to be treated.

2034. How can I tell if someone (like my mother) is going through menopause?

The best way is to ask her. If you see her turn red and sweaty, obviously having a hot flush because there is no other reason to be warm, that is a fairly telltale sign. Sudden embarrassment or upset can also make her blush,

MENOPAUSE: WHAT IT IS AND ITS SYMPTOMS (Continued)
however. Do not use irritability as a sign of menopause, because so many other things can cause it. Ask her if she is sleeping well, and if not, why. If night sweats are the reason, you can be fairly sure that she is going through menopause.

2035. Why does menopause occur?

Menopause occurs because the ovaries have run out of eggs and therefore can no longer produce estrogen or progesterone, which are the hormones that produce menstruation. Women are born with about 100,000 eggs (ova) in their ovaries, but make no more as long as they live. The eggs are constantly being destroyed; some are ovulated and some even produce children. When they are all gone, menopause occurs. No other animal outlives its ability to ovulate, or its ability to produce hormones, except the macaque monkey and a few other primates. Men continue to produce sperm and testosterone even after they are one hundred years old.

2036. What are the different phases of menopause?

The first phase usually occurs when you are in your forties. This is the time when your ovaries fail now and then, and you do not ovulate as regularly as you did before, resulting in an irregular and sometimes very heavy menstrual flow. By the age of forty-seven, very few women ovulate well enough to even get pregnant. These are called premenopausal years. After you are fifty years old, you will begin to skip periods, usually two or three months at a time for a year or two, often having symptoms of hot flushes when your periods are skipped. Finally, the last menstrual flow occurs, and you have no more bleeding at all. This is menopause. After cessation of menses, most women have occasional hot flushes for more than a year and less than five years. When these stop you are postmenopausal.

2037. Do all women go through the same stages during menopause?

No. Some women apparently ovulate and have menstruation that is perfectly regular until suddenly they stop and bleed no more. They have no symptoms of menopause, so they are postmenopausal when menses stop. Their menopause was perhaps one month long!

2038. Is menopause primarily a mental phase that women go through as they grow older, or are there physical factors involved?

Menopause is primarily a physical hormonal change that sometimes has an effect on the mind. Both men and women sometimes adjust poorly to the process of aging, but this is really quite unrelated to menopause and may occur at a much earlier or a much later age. Some women have no mental changes with menopause at all.

2039. What role does the pituitary gland play in menopause?

The pituitary gland does not cause menopause; the ovaries do.

MENOPAUSE: WHAT IT IS AND ITS SYMPTOMS (Continued)

However, by producing hormones called gonadotropins that try very hard to stimulate the ovaries to action, the pituitary does cause the symptoms of hot flushes. These hormones, especially FSH (follicle stimulating hormone), can be measured in the blood. If they are found to be very high, then that is a good sign of ovarian failure.

2040. Does menopause feel similar to menstruation?

No. It is not a pelvic sensation at all.

2041. Is it possible to go through menopause and not know it?

Yes. Of course, if you still have your uterus, you will notice when you stop bleeding entirely. If you have had a hysterectomy and have not had menses for years or do not have hot flushes or night sweats, you may not know when your ovaries fail and menopause occurs.

2042. Is normal menopause in a healthy woman virtually symptomless?

No, general good health is not an indicator of how menopause will be. Overweight women are not considered to be very healthy, but they seem to have an easier time with menopause than other women. That is because their fatty tissue converts adrenal hormones into estrone, an estrogen. But this does not happen with all women who are overweight. Emotional stability and the ability to cope with problems, especially physical ones, are more indicative of how you will handle the symptoms of menopause, but not whether they will occur.

2043. Will I have cramps during menopause?

Sometimes during the last few menstrual periods before menstruation completely stops, you will have more cramps than in previous years. Perhaps this is because there are large clots to pass or the hormone balance is poor, as it is in the teenage years. Not everyone has cramps, however, and after menstruation has stopped there are no more cramps at all.

2044. Will I have heavy discharges during menopause?

No, definitely not. The vaginal discharge becomes lighter and lighter as the hormone levels become lower and lower.

2045. Is nausea a common symptom of menopause?

No. If you have nausea, there is some other cause.

2046. Will I feel weak and tired all of the time during menopause?

No, unless the night sweats are so severe that you never get enough sleep. If you are sleeping well, you should look for another cause of fatigue; it is not due to menopause.

2047. Will my breasts enlarge during menopause?

No, not unless you gain weight or take estrogen. The decrease in

MENOPAUSE: WHAT IT IS AND ITS SYMPTOMS (Continued)

estrogen that comes with menopause usually makes your breasts decrease in size and become dense, with less support and turgor as well.

2048. Will my voice deepen as a result of menopause?

Many older women do develop a deeper voice, but not all. The reason for this could be explained by the absence of estrogen and the continued production of androgens and testosterone (male-type hormones) from the remaining ovaries and similar ones from the adrenal gland. Androgens can certainly make the voice deeper. If you make your living with your voice, estrogen therapy could help to keep this from happening.

2049. Are calcium deposits in any way associated with menopause?

Calcium deposits are only associated with menopause in that they become worse as you grow older.

2050. Is tension a big problem during menopause?

If tension has been a problem for you all along, it can become a bigger problem in menopause, particularly if you lose sleep with night sweats. If you don't have night sweats or hot flushes, and if you are not usually tense, you probably will not have tension. Even without menopause, tensions can mount in a mid-life crisis.

2051. Is it true that my personality will change when I start menopause?

No, it is not true. Your personality is not based on hormones.

2052. Is disorientation a common symptom among menopausal women?

No, it is not. Aging is sometimes associated with Alzheimer's disease, which is an organic deterioration of the brain characterized by confusion, disorientation, and loss of memory, and actually occurring in men more often than in women. Changes in brain function should be investigated by a psychiatrist and not attributed to menopause. A severe depression should also be treated, not ignored or just treated with hormones.

2053. Will I gain weight during menopause?

You have control of that by whether you eat more and exercise less, or eat less and exercise more. There is nothing inevitable about weight gain during menopause, but it is common. Eating more and exercising less is also common.

2054. Why is menopause so often referred to as the "change of life"?

Because it really does change your life to some extent. You no longer need tampons or pads and can completely discard any contraception. Fear of pregnancy is demolished. There is no more premenstrual syndrome. It is a definite change, even if your only symptom is cessation of menses.

MENOPAUSE: WHAT IT IS AND ITS SYMPTOMS (Continued)

2055. Is an increase in illnesses a symptom of menopause?

No. You are not more subject to infectious illnesses during menopause, but cancer becomes more frequent, as do heart disease and high blood pressure, when you are fifty or older.

MENOPAUSE: HOW IT AFFECTS THE BODY AND ITS FUNCTIONS

2056. What are some of the things that are likely to happen to my body when I start going through menopause?

About 75 percent of women experience hot flushes, a sudden feeling of heat starting around the neck and head but spreading further, with perspiration, sometimes a speeding up of the heart, and faintness. It only lasts one to three minutes. Irregular menstruation may precede real menopause by about two years. A heavier and more painful flow is not uncommon. After menstruation has stopped for some time, estrogen deficiency can produce tender tissues around the vagina, as well as dryness. This deficiency can also cause bladder urgency, so that you have to hurry to the bathroom. The skin can become drier as well. If hot flushes occur at night and ruin your sleep, you may show signs of sleep deprivation, such as irritability or lack of concentration. Fifteen or twenty years later you may break a bone with a mild fall, if you have developed osteoporosis (thinning of the bones). This condition can be prevented with hormones, calcium, and exercise. But some good symptoms occur, too. Migraine headaches that appeared at puberty usually disappear, premenstrual syndrome becomes rare, since you do not cycle anymore, and all the bleeding and cramping of menstruation stops!

2057. What bodily functions are affected by menopause?

Reproduction is eliminated. When the ovaries have completely failed, pregnancy is no longer at all possible. Sexual activity continues as before, unless the tender, dry vagina interferes. It usually takes longer to lubricate with sexual arousal, but it still occurs satisfactorily. The nervous system remains the same, unless hot flushes and sweats produce sleep deprivation. Most bodily functions, such as respiration and digestion, remain in the same condition they were in until osteoporosis causes the bones to break easily.

2058. Does my physical condition in any way determine the effects menopause will have on my body?

If you exercise regularly you will be less likely to have severe osteoporosis than if you lead a sedentary life. If you are not overweight and have regular exercise, your chances of having a heart attack are not as greatly increased by menopause as they would be if you were overweight and seden-

MENOPAUSE: HOW IT AFFECTS THE BODY AND ITS FUNCTIONS
(Continued)

tary. If you are emotionally stable, you will be less disturbed by menopausal symptoms, but the hot flushes, bladder urgency, and tender vagina can occur anyway, unless prevented by estrogen replacement therapy.

2059. How will menopause affect my physical appearance?

No one will notice any changes immediately, except for the occasional hot flush that may make you turn red for a moment or two and perspire. Your breasts will have less tone, and will not stand up as much as they did before. They should also become less fibrocystic. Most other changes are due to aging, not menopause. If osteoporosis sets in five, ten, or fifteen years after menopause, the collapsed vertebrae in your spine may make you look hunched over and smaller.

2060. What happens to my ovaries during menopause?

They become smaller, no longer forming follicles or cysts, until they can hardly be felt in a pelvic examination. The cells remaining in them may continue to produce some testosterone and other androgens (male-type sex hormones) but no estrogen. They can still form a tumor, like an ovarian cancer, so they must still be examined at intervals and certainly investigated if you have pain in that area.

2061. What changes occur in my uterus and vagina during menopause?

Your uterus becomes firm and smaller in size, even if it contains fibroids, which also shrink. Your vagina produces less and less discharge and tends to shrink in size, becoming tender as well. The lips that surround your vaginal opening (labia) become thinner and smaller, decreasing in length.

2062. Is a prolapsed uterus (a uterus that has dropped from its original position in the pelvis into the vaginal area) a problem during menopause?

Yes. The tissues around the vagina become weaker when estrogen disappears, so the supporting structures of the uterus can become less efficient and a prolapsed uterus more annoying.

2063. Does menopause create any vitamin or mineral deficiencies?

Yes. There is less requirement for iron, because you no longer bleed. There is a greater requirement for vitamin D in order to absorb and use calcium in greater amounts. You lose calcium in greater amounts; therefore, you should eat or take calcium and vitamin D in greater amounts.

MENOPAUSE: AGE

2064. At what age does menopause usually occur?

The average age that the last menstruation occurs is between fifty and fifty-four in the United States.

MENOPAUSE: AGE (Continued)

2065. What is the youngest age that menopause can occur?

Less than 1 percent of women have menopause before forty. Ovarian failure, or premature menopause, has occurred at all ages—in the forties, thirties, twenties.

2066. Is it really true that women have been known to start menopause as early as age thirty-five?

Yes, and even earlier. Surgical menopause will occur at any age when the ovaries are surgically removed. Sometimes women in their thirties miss a few periods, perhaps because they are running a lot, and they call this menopause. But unless they have hot flushes or tests to show no further function of the ovaries, it is just temporary amenorrhea (absence of menstruation), and menses can return later, as well as fertility.

2067. Are there any problems that frequently occur in women who go through menopause early?

Yes. The first one is the loss of the ability to have children, which is a personal tragedy if women want to have children. If they are not on estrogen replacement therapy, they develop severe bone loss (osteoporosis) at an earlier age than those women who have menopause later. They age more rapidly in the breasts, skin, vagina, and vulva. This is why the practice of routinely removing ovaries with a hysterectomy in young women has fallen into disrepute. Removing ovaries to save women from possible ovarian cancer is not worth the early and severe surgical menopause they go through, not to mention the small fortune and time spent in doctors' offices seeking relief by hormonal and other therapy.

2068. Does menopause tend to occur later, the healthier you are?

Yes, and the later menopause occurs, the greater your chances are of living longer. Better health is the reason that this generation has menopause two years later than the previous generation. When menopause occurs late, you have fewer postmenopausal hormone deficient years. Hormone deficiency can lead to hip fracture and its complications. Also, heart attacks are more frequent in women after menopause, so if menopause is later, heart attacks are deferred, too.

2069. Is it better for menopause to occur at an early age or a later age?

It is usually better for menopause to occur at a later age, because this delays the problems of bone loss or heart attacks, and menopause occurs later in people who seem destined for longevity. Occasionally if a woman has fibroids or endometriosis (lining of the uterus found growing outside of the uterus), which will subside with menopause, it may be better if it comes early

MENOPAUSE: AGE (Continued)

in order to avoid surgery.

2070. What would cause me to go through menopause early?

If your ovaries run out of eggs at an early age, then you will go through menopause early. No one knows what causes this. Removing both ovaries will do this immediately, but removing one does not make you have menopause sooner, because the destruction of ova in that ovary does not depend upon whether there is another one on the other side. Recent studies have shown that women who smoke enter menopause early, so heavy smoking may be a cause.

2071. Is there any kind of test that I can undergo to determine at what age menopause will occur?

No. You would probably have to count the ova left in your ovaries, and calculate the rate at which they are disappearing. No one can do that now. However, heredity is important, so you could find out when your mother or aunts had menopause.

2072. At what age should I begin to worry if I haven't started menopause?

At age sixty, but there is still no need to worry unless your periods consist of abnormal bleeding instead of regular menstruation. Describe them to and discuss them with your physician. Less than 5 percent of women go beyond the age of fifty-four before menopause occurs.

2073. Does the average age that women start menopause vary from country to country?

Yes, it does. In developing countries the age is usually younger, and in countries with a high standard of living, it is later. Folklore says that certain tribes in the Himalayas have a very late menopause, but the age is hard to prove, since records are primitive. It is not clear whether the factors that make it sooner or later are genetic or environmental.

2074. Does menopause increase my aging process?

Yes, it accelerates it in a special way that does not occur in men. The cessation of the protective estrogen leaves women more vulnerable to heart attacks, while men are vulnerable when they reach thirty-five. The loss of hormonal support allows the skin to become dry and lose its turgor, forming wrinkles. The lack of estrogen allows the bones to lose their calcium and collapse and fracture easily, contributing to the aging appearance. In men this happens much later and more gradually. Hormone replacement can prevent or delay all of these effects in women.

2075. Is the onset of menopause all part of the aging process?

No other animal has this as part of its aging process, except the

MENOPAUSE: AGE (Continued)

macaque monkey and other primates; all others remain fertile to the end of their lives. Men do not have a sudden dramatic decrease in their sex hormone, testosterone, with symptoms to match. They decline gradually, but continue to produce hormones until well past one hundred, if there is no disease or surgery to affect their testicles. So menopause is a special aging process for women.

2076. Does the age at which I had my first or last child affect the age that I will begin menopause?

No. This has been proven in studies of identical twins, where one had children and the other did not.

2077. Do women who have had abortions tend to experience an early menopause? What about women who have had one or more miscarriages?

The numbers of abortions or miscarriages, or for that matter full-term deliveries, have no effect on the age of menopause.

2078. Is it likely that I will experience menopause at the same age as my mother did?

There seems to be a genetic control of how long the ovaries last, but you will probably be about two years later than your mother because of generally better health conditions. Today menopause occurs two years later than it did thirty years ago.

2079. Do twins usually begin menopause at the same time?

Identical twins will usually begin menopause at the same time, unless surgical removal of the ovaries changes things. In a pair of identical twins, if one has six children and the other has none, menopause still occurs at the same age. Non-identical twins are only as much alike as sisters might be.

MENOPAUSE: LENGTH OF MENOPAUSE

2080. How long does menopause usually last?

Since menopause is the time you have symptoms from ovarian failure, it lasts one to five years for most women.

2081. Does the length of menopause vary from woman to woman?

Yes, greatly. One-fourth of women seem to have no symptoms at all, so they are hardly in menopause at all. Another fourth have hot flushes that last for less than one year, and then they feel fine. Another fourth have symptoms that last up to five years, but then subside. In the remaining fourth, the flushes may never stop, even into the eighties and nineties, or for as long as they live.

MENOPAUSE: LENGTH OF MENOPAUSE (Continued)

2082. Are there any drugs I could take to shorten the length of my menopause?

If you take hormones, you can eliminate the symptoms of menopause, but when you stop taking them, the symptoms come right back unless you take them for as long as the symptoms last. So drugs cannot really shorten the length of your menopause; it is unpredictable.

MENOPAUSE: VAGINAL DRYNESS

2083. How can I prevent dryness in my vagina during menopause?

If you continue to be sexually active before, during, and after menopause, your vagina will not shrink as much or become as tender and dry as it will if you are sexually inactive. You can also use a surgical lubricant jelly (such as K-Y, H-R, or Lubafax) just prior to coitus. But the most effective prevention is taking estrogen. This can be in the form of an estrogen cream applied to your vagina two or three times a week, or the more standard oral estrogen pills, combined with a progesterone-type of hormone for part of the cycle. Estrogen shots or any other form will also work to decrease vaginal dryness.

2084. What causes my vagina to dry up during menopause?

The decrease in the estrogen hormone production causes your vagina to lose its lubricating discharge and makes the texture of the lining and the lips surrounding your vagina (labia) thin and tender. When you are a little girl, before puberty, your vagina is dry and has no discharge. It gets like that again after menopause.

MENOPAUSE: HOT FLUSHES

2085. How frequently do hot flushes usually occur?

Most women have about ten or fifteen hot flushes per day during the first year of menopause. "Hot flashes" is a slang term for hot flushes.

2086. What is the safest and most effective medication for controlling hot flushes?

The most effective medication is not always the safest one. The most effective medication for controlling hot flushes is estrogen, and the next most effective is some form of progesterone. Usually both of these are used, since using the progesterone overcomes some of the problems of using estrogen. Tranquilizers have been used, but they are not very effective. They are also habit forming and may have other personality effects that are disturbing. Medications that affect blood vessel contraction and dilation have also been used, but are not as effective as estrogen.

MENOPAUSE: HOT FLUSHES (Continued)

2087. Will taking hormones control hot flushes?

If enough estrogen is taken, it will control a genuine hot flush. If you use too little, it may not. If your hot spell is really due to a fever or nervousness, estrogens will not do anything at all. Check your temperature to be sure it is normal.

2088. What are the newest findings in regard to estrogen and the control of hot flushes?

The newest finding is that you can use estrogen safely for control of hot flushes, if you use it in a cyclic fashion and take progesterone for at least ten days of the cycle. When you add progesterone, or any of the progestogen-like compounds, then you do not increase your chances of having cancer of the uterus (endometrial cancer). When you cycle in this way you also produce a withdrawal bleeding similar to menstrual flow. In some major studies there have even been fewer cancers of the breast and uterus when progesterone is used with estrogen than normally expected, even if no hormones were taken.

2089. Will vitamin E help relieve hot flushes?

Since most women's hot flushes reduce in frequency and disappear after a while, whatever they are using to control them will be given credit for their relief. Dr. Evan Shute of Canada believes that vitamin E helps, because it acts as a mild estrogen.

2090. Can other vitamins help control hot flushes?

No. If you are vitamin deficient, vitamins can help you to have better health, but they do not stop flushes.

MENOPAUSE: BREAST TUMORS AND CYSTS

2091. What causes fibrous breast tumors in menopausal women?

Since fibrocystic breasts are probably a reaction to estrogen, menopausal women may develop this condition when they are producing only estrogen prior to menopause, and their chances of developing it increase if they use only estrogen after menopause. If they do not take estrogen or they only take small dosages, their fibrocystic breasts should improve and usually do.

2092. Are women more prone to tumors and cysts during menopause?

Yes, tumors and cysts of the breasts are frequent just prior to menopause. Cancer of the breast also becomes progressively more frequent with age, but it is not related to menopause. These breast conditions are not more frequent in young women who have gone through surgical menopause.

MENOPAUSE: OSTEOPOROSIS (Thinning of Bones)

2093. Is there a connection between menopause and osteoporosis? If so, what is it?

Osteoporosis is the loss of density of bones, in which both the calcium and the actual structure of the bone (matrix) are reduced. Bone is constantly being destroyed and built up throughout your life, but with osteoporosis it is destroyed faster than it is rebuilt. The most common cause of osteoporosis is loss of estrogen, as in menopause. This is aggravated by bed rest, smoking, poor calcium intake, and vitamin D deficiency. Other less-frequent causes are too much cortisone (a hormone), hyperthyroidism, and advanced age (eighty-five or older). At that age, osteoporosis even occurs in men.

2094. How can I find out if I am developing osteoporosis (thinning of the bones)?

Tests are available at many medical centers now that can actually measure the density of your bones, and then compare that to normal bone. Bone densitometry is a relatively easy and inexpensive test that measures the bone density in your wrist. A CAT scan (computerized axial tomography) is a more expensive and elaborate test, but it is a more accurate method of X-ray that measures the concentration of bone in your spine. These tests can be repeated every year or two to see if you are holding your own, or if you are losing bone faster than normal. They have also been used in studies to show that estrogen prevents the loss of bone.

2095. Can osteoporosis be prevented if measures are taken before or during menopause?

Yes, menopause is the time when treatment must be started if osteoporosis is to be completely prevented. If bone loss is allowed to occur for several years before treatment is started, it can never be replaced, even though further loss can be prevented by estrogen, calcium, vitamin D, and exercise. The average loss is 1 percent per year, although some women lose as much as 3 percent each year.

2096. How serious is osteoporosis?

Osteoporosis is a serious killer of women. Every year in the United States 600,000 women break their hips, and 10 percent of them die from complications that result from the injury, such as pneumonia. So 60,000 women per year die from breaking their hips because they did not take hormones to prevent osteoporosis. Letting your back become curved or fracturing your wrist is not as deadly as breaking your hip, but it is certainly a painful problem. Of women without hormone therapy, 25 percent will get a fracture due to osteoporosis by the age of eighty, and many women will live that long.

MENOPAUSE: MENSTRUATION AND MENOPAUSE

2097. If I began menstruation at an early age, is it true that I will also begin menopause early?

No. Computerized studies have shown that there is no correlation between the age of menstruation and the age of menopause.

2098. I always had a hard time with menstruation. Does that mean that I will also have a hard time during menopause?

No, there is no correlation, but you will be relieved when you no longer have menstruation.

2099. What percentage of women over the age of fifty still menstruate?

About 90 percent of women over the age of fifty still menstruate, if they still have a uterus. Of course, if they have had a hysterectomy, they do not.

2100. What sorts of changes in my menstrual flow would indicate the onset of menopause?

Irregular menses that occur two or three weeks apart or skip two or three months at a time and sometimes a heavier flow can be signs of approaching menopause. These symptoms indicate that ovulation is inconsistent or else has stopped completely.

2101. Will my menstrual period stop abruptly when I start menopause, or will it decline gradually?

No one can predict that for you. Both situations can occur.

2102. Are very irregular periods a sign that I am going through menopause?

Not always. Teenagers, dancers, and runners have irregular periods, too. However, if you are in your late forties, they could be a sign of menopause.

2103. Will I continue to menstruate during menopause?

If you are menstruating regularly, you are probably not in menopause. If you are bleeding a lot and having hot flushes, too, your bleeding may be abnormal and an investigation by a D & C (dilatation and curettage) may be necessary to find the cause. Women usually do not menstruate in menopause.

2104. How does menopause compare to puberty? Are there any similarities? Differences?

It is amazing how similar they are. Both teenagers and women in their forties frequently fail to ovulate, and as a result they have irregular and occasionally very heavy menses. The difference is that the older woman must have a D & C to be sure her bleeding is not caused by cancer, whereas the teenager rarely requires a D & C, except to stop a hemorrhage. Both may

MENOPAUSE: MENSTRUATION AND MENOPAUSE (Continued)

ovulate poorly and produce inadequate progesterone, so that they have very painful cramps and pass clots. Both skip periods, but only the older woman has hot flushes when this happens. They are both relatively infertile. The teenager is going to become more regular, and the older woman is going to stop menstruating entirely. Thus both problems are temporary.

2105. I've heard that women who are close friends frequently have their menstrual periods at the same time. Is the same true for menopause?

No, but since menopause occurs in women between the ages of fifty and fifty-four, one-fourth of women in this age group will have menopause in one of those four years, and they might be friends.

2106. What is the average time that I should expect to have irregular periods before they stop completely?

You will probably have irregular periods for about two years.

2107. I have had irregular menstrual cycles all of my life. How will I know when menopause starts?

You should suspect that the irregularity is due to menopause if you are having some hot flushes. If you are not having hot flushes, you will know it is menopause only after you have stopped menstruating altogether. The rule is: if you go one year without menstruating and with menopausal symptoms, then you should bleed no more. If you do bleed, it could be abnormal and must be investigated.

MENOPAUSE: HYSTERECTOMIES AND MENOPAUSE

2108. Can menopause occur if I have had a complete hysterectomy?

If your ovaries, as well as your uterus, were removed when you had your hysterectomy, then menopause will occur immediately. When ovaries are surgically removed, symptoms of hormone deficiency occur in a few days. Surgical menopause is an inevitable consequence of removing ovaries, but it can be treated with replacement hormones.

2109. I have had a hysterectomy, so how will I know when I start menopause?

If your ovaries were left in when you had your hysterectomy, they will continue to produce hormones for you until they fail because they have run out of eggs. You will probably notice hot flushes and night sweats, usually between fifty and fifty-four years of age. If you are one of the lucky women who has no symptoms, you may simply ask your doctor to check your hormone level; if your estrogen level is low, you are likely to be going through menopause. A Pap smear report may repeatedly show you are low in estrogen, and this is an inexpensive way to find out.

MENOPAUSE: HYSTERECTOMIES AND MENOPAUSE
(Continued)

2110. I had a partial hysterectomy. Am I likely to have an early menopause?

No. If even one ovary is left in, menopause will probably come at the average age.

2111. Does a hysterectomy prevent or lessen some of the symptoms of menopause?

Having your uterus removed prevents the irregular bleeding that can occur around the time of menopause, but the other symptoms are the same.

2112. Is it common for women who have a hysterectomy to go right into menopause?

If their ovaries are removed along with their uteri, then they will indeed go right into menopause, because the surgically removed ovaries are no longer there to make hormones. If the ovaries are not removed, then menopause will occur at the normal age, fifty to fifty-four.

2113. What is surgical menopause?

Surgical menopause is ovarian failure caused by the surgical removal of the ovaries.

2114. Why do so many doctors recommend hysterectomy during menopause?

It is during the late forties and early fifties that uncontrollable hemorrhages occur, fibroids grow large, and cancer of the endometrium (the lining of the uterus) develops. These are all good reasons for a hysterectomy.

2115. Can I undergo a hysterectomy during menopause?

Yes, of course. Menopause does not worsen your health or condition for surgery.

2116. I am fifty-two years old and have not yet reached menopause. Should I have a hysterectomy as my doctor suggests?

Your doctor should give you a reason for the hysterectomy. If the lining of your uterus is changing in the direction of cancer or you are hemorrhaging and becoming anemic, you might take your doctor's suggestion. If you don't know why your doctor suggests a hysterectomy, you should find out. Perhaps it is because you complain that it feels like your uterus is falling out, or you cannot control your urine.

2117. Is a hysterectomy always necessary in cases of heavy bleeding during menopause?

No. If tissue obtained from the lining of your uterus by a D & C (dilatation and curettage) shows there is no cancer or precancer changes, you may be able to control bleeding with a hormone, such as progesterone, until

MENOPAUSE: HYSTERECTOMIES AND MENOPAUSE
(Continued)

menopause occurs. If you do not get anemic, perhaps because you take iron, then the bleeding is just inconvenient rather than harmful to your health. It can be your choice in that case whether to have a hysterectomy or not.

MENOPAUSE: SEX AND MENOPAUSE

2118. Will menopause affect my sex drive?

Changes frequently occur during menopause that both increase and decrease your sex drive. The freedom from fear of pregnancy and even the freedom from menstrual days can increase your sexual activity and often does in many women. If you are suffering severely from hot flushes or especially if your vagina becomes dry and tender and makes intercourse uncomfortable, your activity level may decrease. A few women feel that the need for sex is over when they are sterile; this is especially true if sex was always uncomfortable for them.

2119. Will my attitude about sex change during this time?

Your attitude toward sex may improve, and it may get worse. After menopause, many people begin to work on their sex problems more than ever before, simply because they have more time. Their children are raised and gone, and their marital relationship becomes more focused on itself.

2120. Do any sexual problems accompany menopause?

Not necessarily. If intercourse becomes painful because the vagina is dry and tender, hormone therapy can eliminate the problem entirely. Lubrication and gentleness, with time and attention given to arousal, can also help to solve the problem if hormones are not advisable.

2121. What percentage of women experience an increased sex drive during menopause?

Less than half experience an increase in sex drive at menopause. Many woman adopt the cultural attitude that after they no longer menstruate, they are asexual. They respond to this by ceasing to speak of sexual matters or show sexual interest.

2122. Do women with relatively inactive sex lives go through menopause earlier than woman with active sex lives?

No, sexual activity seems to have no effect on the onset of menopause. However, sexually active women seem to experience a delay in the time when their vaginas shrink (become atrophic), or become dry and tender. "Use it or lose it" is applicable here.

MENOPAUSE: SEX AND MENOPAUSE (Continued)

2123. How can I get comfortably through menopause and still feel sexually attractive?

If you never stop your sexual activity for any long period of time, it is not likely to deteriorate. Maintain a normal weight and stay physically fit, and you will feel more energetic and sexually attractive. If you have severe symptoms, or perhaps even if you do not, consider hormone therapy. Discuss it with your physician. If vaginal dryness develops, use external lubrication, such as a surgical jelly.

2124. Is there any time during menopause when I should refrain from sex?

No, there is no prohibition of sex in menopause, but you should not force yourself to have sex when you don't want it.

MENOPAUSE: MENOPAUSE AS CONTRACEPTION

2125. At what stage of menopause can I safely have sex without having to worry about pregnancy or birth control?

If you are over fifty years old, you can probably safely omit birth control, if you are certain that you are in menopause. It is dangerous to stop birth control just because your periods have become a little irregular and you have had a few hot flushes. Menopause is not certain until you have not had a period for a year and have had hot flushes. Without those symptoms, you should have a doctor's opinion before you stop birth control. There are other causes, besides menopause, for menstruation to stop.

2126. If I stop using birth control during menopause, what are my chances of getting pregnant?

The answer depends upon your age and whether the menstrual irregularity you are experiencing is truly menopause. Hot flushes would be reassuring. If you are forty-seven years old or older, you have less than a 1 percent chance of getting pregnant. This approaches 0 percent at fifty-eight. It also approaches 0 percent if it has been one year since your last menses.

2127. Do the hormones contained in birth control pills affect the time of onset and/or degree of difficulty a woman will have during menopause?

No, but the hormones in birth control pills will prevent you from knowing that you are in or past menopause until you stop taking them. They completely replace any hormone deficiency you may have, and you will menstruate for as long as you take them. Your natural menopause will occur at the same age it would have without any pills. If they were not considered dangerous for older women to take, birth control pills might be a lovely way to eliminate the whole problem of menopause.

MENOPAUSE: MENOPAUSAL PREGNANCIES AND THEIR PRECAUTIONS

2128. If I have a child during menopause, will it stop the process?

No. Most women who had a child during what they thought was menopause simply had some irregular periods and believed the irregularity to be menopause. They were probably only forty-three or forty-five years old, and after their pregnancy, they continued to have regular periods because they were nowhere near menopause. No way has been found to stop the process of menopause.

2129. Are there any complications that tend to occur in children who were born of menopausal women?

Yes, the occurrence of Down's syndrome (also known as Mongolism) increases as the age of the mother increases. Children born with this syndrome have forty-seven chromosomes, instead of forty-six, and are severely mentally retarded. Amniocentesis is a test that can detect Down's syndrome in the unborn fetus. It is advisable for any woman who is over thirty-five, but especially for any woman over forty-five, because the chances of having a baby born with Down's syndrome at that age increase to about one in fifty or more.

2130. How common are menopausal pregnancies?

Very few children have been scientifically determined to have been born of menopausal women. The term "menopausal pregnancy" mostly comes from the women themselves who thought they were in menopause because they were over forty and their periods were irregular, but they were probably not in menopause at all. In ten years in the United States, only sixteen children were born to women over fifty.

2131. Are there extra precautions that I should take to reduce the chances of pregnancy during this time?

The rhythm method is hard enough to follow when your periods are regular, but it becomes almost impossible when they are very irregular at the time of menopause. Continuing to use the same contraceptive you have been using is a good idea, because it gives you security and confidence. You are not more likely to get pregnant during menopause; you are much less likely to get pregnant, especially if you are over fifty. People who speak of having menopausal babies usually had them in their early forties and thought that a few irregular periods meant menopause, but it did not. However, pregnancies that occur at forty-seven or older are rarer than contraceptive failures in young people. Being older than forty-six is 99 percent contraceptive in itself.

MENOPAUSE: WHEN TO SEE A DOCTOR

2132. What discomforts during menopause would be considered severe enough that I should see a doctor?

You should see your doctor about the discomforts of menopause when you want to consider treatment to remove the discomforts, not because there is any danger that the doctor can avert. The discomforts that can be eliminated or relieved are hot flushes, night sweats, vaginal dryness and tenderness, and urinary urgency that may possibly be due to the estrogen deficiency of menopause.

2133. What would be considered abnormal symptoms during menopause?

Any problem other than hot flushes, night sweats, sleeplessness associated with irritability, tender and dry vagina, or urinary urgency would not really be a symptom of menopause. Any depression, confusion, disorientation, panic, or other emotional disturbance should be diagnosed and treated by your physician, perhaps with the assistance of a psychiatrist. It should not be neglected because you think it is a symptom of menopause.

2134. Is there a simple method for detecting cancer of the ovary and uterus in menopausal women?

No, there is no simple method, like a Pap smear that can detect cancer of the cervix. If you are uncomfortable and suspect cancer of the ovary, your doctor can perform a pelvic examination. However, it can only be definitely diagnosed by surgery. Cancer of the uterus may be suspected if there is abnormal bleeding, but can only be detected by taking a sample of the lining of the uterus by an endometrial biopsy or a D & C (dilatation and curettage).

2135. With the technology of today, why must we suffer the symptoms of menopause?

You need not suffer at all! No one can make you fertile, but all the other symptoms of menopause can be alleviated. You should see your doctor if you want these symptoms relieved. Hormones taken in cycles can come close to the normal state of hormones your ovaries used to produce. The problem is that many women have been frightened out of using hormones for fear the hormones will produce cancer, or else they feel they should just be natural and take nothing at all.

MENOPAUSE: DELAYING MENOPAUSE

2136. Is there any way to delay menopause?

No. It is not known how to keep the eggs from being destroyed.

2137. Why would a women want to delay menopause?

Some women would like to delay it because they want another child; others are too busy to tolerate the symptoms or their treatment.

MENOPAUSE: DELAYING MENOPAUSE (Continued)

2138. Can certain vitamins delay or reverse menopause?
Not so far as is known today.

2139. I am very active in athletics. Will conditioning of this sort delay the onset of menopause?
No, athletic conditioning will not delay the onset of menopause.

MENOPAUSE: FALSE MENOPAUSE

2140. Is there such a thing as "false menopause"?
"False menopause" is a long time of not menstruating associated with hot flushes, followed by the return of menstruation. If you are young, the cause of "false menopause" should be found. If you stop menstruating after thirty-five, some people will call it menopause, but if menstruation returns, it was not menopause.

2141. Could emotional stress and shock cause a women to go into menopause?
Stress and shock can cause menstruation to stop temporarily, but not because the ovaries failed. The ovaries still have eggs (ova), estrogen is still produced, the pituitary is not releasing a high level of FSH (follicle stimulating hormone) or gonadotropins, and you have no hot flushes. Under those circumstances, fertility pills or pituitary hormones could return ovulation and menstruation. Of course, if failure to menstruate due to shock lasts until you are old enough for menopause, one kind of amenorrhea (absence of menses) might run into another. The only way you could tell if menopause had occurred would be the presence of hot flushes. Prolonged hypotension, which is medical shock rather than emotional shock, especially if connected to hemorrhage in pregnancy, can destroy the pituitary gland. Menses then will stop, since pituitary hormones are needed for menstruation. If such pituitary hormones are supplemented externally, menses will return. Since it is not the ovaries that have failed, this is not really menopause.

MENOPAUSE: USE OF HORMONES TO TREAT MENOPAUSAL DISCOMFORTS

2142. How do hormones help?
Hormones replenish the deficiency of hormones, which is called menopause. They eliminate all the problems of menopause, except infertility; they do not enable you to have a baby. If you take both estrogen and progesterone, which are the hormones that you produced all your adult life before menopause, you will completely replace the deficiency. Given in a cyclic fashion, they will also produce regular withdrawal bleeding, like menstruation, just as birth control pills do.

MENOPAUSE: USE OF HORMONES TO TREAT MENOPAUSAL DISCOMFORTS (Continued)

2143. When would hormones be advisable?

Hormones would be advisable as soon as a clear and permanent hormone deficiency can be established. They are especially important in relieving disturbing symptoms of menopause, but must be started within a year or so after menopause, even if there are no symptoms, if you are to prevent bone loss (osteoporosis). Of course, certain aspects of your health, such as fibroids that might grow large or severe fibrocystic breasts needing biopsies, might make it unwise for you to take hormones right away. If given time, these conditions may subside, and hormones can then be started later. If you have diabetes, breast cancer, or uterine cancer, you possibly should not take them at all. This is a medical decision to discuss with your doctor.

2144. What amount of hormones will I need?

You will need enough hormones to control the symptoms that are caused by the hormone deficiency of menopause, such as hot flushes. However, too much hormone will cause your breasts to become very tender. If you are taking estrogen and progesterone in a cycle, your menstrual flow can be a reflection of the dosage of the hormones and their balance. The more estrogen, the more you will flow; but the more progesterone, the less you will flow. You should also keep your bones as strong as they were when you started taking hormones. Some studies have suggested that bones get thinner, unless you take at least 0.625 mg of conjugated estrogens (natural estrogen compounds). These studies found that 0.3 mg keep the bones only half as dense. For a few years the attitude was to take as little hormones as possible and to stop taking them as soon as possible. Many doctors still agree with this, and it appeals to many women. But it may not really be effective enough to prevent bone loss (osteoporosis). Any dangers of estrogen do increase with higher doses, especially if not combined with progesterone. So you and your doctor need to find just the right dosage and balance for you. The average menopausal woman today takes 0.625 mg of conjugated estrogens for twenty-five days a month, and 10 mg of medroxyprogesterone (a synthetic progesterone compound) for ten days a month.

2145. Why are hormones so often prescribed for women who are going through menopause?

Most women really need hormones for their physical comfort, for freedom from hot flushes and night sweats, for restful sleep and its resultant emotional well-being, for continued sexual activity without pain, for bladder control, and for general well-being. At least one-fourth of women must have

MENOPAUSE: USE OF HORMONES TO TREAT MENOPAUSAL DISCOMFORTS (Continued)

hormones to prevent osteoporosis, a bone loss that leads to serious hip fractures from which 10 percent of women die. Sixty thousand women die each year in the United States from complications of hip fractures. This is worth preventing, even in women who have no menopausal symptoms.

2146. Why doesn't my doctor tell me to use estrogens for my menopause and post-menopausal years?

Physicians are taught in their training and in their literature that there is no general recommendation to be made concerning the use of estrogen during menopause and postmenopausal years. A "Consensus Development Conference on Estrogen and Postmenopausal Women" was held at the National Institutes of Health in 1979. The Conference concluded that no general recommendations concerning estrogen therapy can be given until the natural course of the menopause, the optimal way to provide estrogens, and all of the beneficial and adverse effects of the compounds are understood. Typical advice to doctors is contained in one paragraph from the book *Menopause in Modern Perspective,* by W. H. Utian, 1980: "Long-term therapy cannot yet be recommended for all women after menopause. It is not, however, justifiable to withhold such treatment from a normal informed patient who requests it on an individual basis, provided there are no contraindications and the patient agrees to regular checkups." This means that women are expected to take charge of their own bodies, become informed, and ask for the hormonal therapy. Doctors are not taught to offer it to you. At the present time, surveys show that only about 15 percent of women ever ask their physicians about help with menopause.

2147. How many women stopped using estrogens after learning that they could produce endometrial cancer?

In 1975, twenty million prescriptions for the various estrogen compounds were filled, meaning about two-thirds of the thirty million menopausal women were using estrogens. Some women may have filled several prescriptions, but others filled none because they obtained their estrogen in shots from their physicians. After 1976, when the studies about endometrial cancer were widely publicized, about half of these women stopped taking estrogen, and fewer new prescriptions were started. Surveys show that the older doctors did not stop prescribing estrogen, but the middle-aged and younger ones dropped to a very low level of prescribing estrogens. The number of women on estrogen dropped to about half of what it had been in 1975 for five years or more. More recently the problem of bone loss (osteoporosis) has received fresh attention, and estrogen replacement therapy is being revived by all ages of physicians to prevent it. This year

MENOPAUSE: USE OF HORMONES TO TREAT MENOPAUSAL DISCOMFORTS (Continued)

Ayerst Laboratories, the makers of Premarin (the most commonly prescribed estrogen for menopause), announced that their volume of sales has finally reached the level it was in 1975. There has been no decrease or increase in deaths from cancer of the uterus during this time.

2148. How many women developed cancer of the uterus because they took estrogen?

Between 1970 and 1975, over 15,000 women developed uterine cancer because they took estrogen without taking progestins.

2149. Is it too expensive to treat all postmenopausal women with estrogen to prevent osteoporosis and bone fractures?

Some people think it is. A study in 1980 showed that the total amount spent annually on estrogen in Great Britain would be about $183,000,000 for prevention of osteoporosis in postmenopausal women. This would be in addition to the cost of medical services necessary to get the hormones, which would equal another $132,000,000 per year. In contrast, they estimated that treating the hip fractures and wrist fractures that occur in women because of osteoporosis in Great Britain would be about $20,000,000 per year. In the United States, hip fractures cost a total of $1 billion each year.

2150. Can the emotional problems associated with menopause be treated with hormones?

Yes, partially. When emotional problems in a woman occur at the same time as menopause, it is wise and practical to treat her with hormones to find out how much of her problem will be relieved. Then psychotherapy can treat the rest of the problems that are purely emotional. It is dangerous to treat with just hormones, because a real depression may eventually lead to suicide without additional help.

2151. What percentage of women take hormones during menopause?

Following the widespread publicity of the research showing that taking estrogen alone (without progesterone) could lead to cancer of the uterus (endometrial cancer), the percentage of women taking hormones for menopause fell to a new low, even among women who had no uterus to become cancerous. Today, that percentage is increasing. About twenty million, or over one-half of women, take hormones during menopause.

2152. What percentage of women go through menopause without taking hormones?

Approximately one-half of all women go through menopause without taking hormones.

MENOPAUSE: USE OF HORMONES TO TREAT MENOPAUSAL DISCOMFORTS (Continued)

2153. Do most doctors routinely prescribe hormones?

No. Hormones have only been available for doctors to prescribe for a little over fifty years. Thirty years ago, women had to complain frequently and bitterly to get hormones instead of a sedative, like phenobarbital, for their menopausal problems. In the 1960s, enthusiasm for remaining young and "feminine forever" reached a peak, and doctors prescribed high doses of estrogen alone, often starting before menopause really occurred. In the 1970s, studies indicating that this could produce cancer of the uterus (endometrial cancer) frightened women, who stopped taking hormones, and doctors, who stopped prescribing them. The pendulum is now swinging back toward treatment with both hormones, estrogen and progesterone, which prevents an increase in cancer but brings back menstrual flow. Many women still refuse this therapy, because they dislike menses so much. Of course, many women do not menstruate with hormone treatment.

2154. Why do some doctors prescribe hormone injections to counteract depression during menopause while others prescribe hormone pills?

Hormone injections are not really prescribed to counteract depression, but to treat a hormone deficiency. Shots act quickly and can last for as long as three weeks. They also keep the hormone from bothering your digestive tract or your liver. However, they require a visit to the doctor once a month, are far more expensive than pills, and if you are given too much, the dosage cannot be modified for a month. Pills are much less expensive, free the patient from dependence on the doctor's office, except for an annual visit to renew the medicine, and the dosage can be adjusted easily. They are also easier to take in a cycle with a progesterone pill to prevent uterine cancer.

2155. Is estrogen the only kind of hormone that is prescribed for menopausal women?

Today many doctors prescribe a progesterone-like medication along with the estrogen, to prevent the risk of developing cancer of the lining of the uterus. Some studies report a better effect on the breasts when this combination is used. Testosterone used to be prescribed in combination with estrogen, but it is unpopular now due to its masculinizing effects, such as facial hair and a deeper voice.

2156. What kinds of treatment, besides estrogen therapy, are available today?

Progesterone therapy is available for women who should not take estrogen for reasons such as already having cancer of the uterus. There are

MENOPAUSE: USE OF HORMONES TO TREAT MENOPAUSAL DISCOMFORTS (Continued)

both pills and injections available that are sometimes quite effective in controlling flushes and even bone deterioration, but these are usually not as effective as estrogen. Testosterone, the male hormone, has also been used and is quite effective for treating symptoms of menopause, but side effects, such as hair growth and a lower voice, are displeasing to women. Tranquilizers, drugs that constrict blood vessels, and others have been found so ineffective that they are not usually recommended if a hormone can be used.

2157. Are estrogen shots new?

No, estrogen shots have been in use for at least fifty years.

2158. How long can I safely take estrogen without the risk of any side effects?

You always have a risk of side effects, even the first month you take estrogen, so the answer to your question is really unknown. Ten years of taking a high dose of estrogen without any cycle of progesterone has been found to increase the chances of cancer of the lining of the uterus (endometrial cancer). If estrogen is taken with progesterone, this risk is eliminated. Other suspected risks, such as gallbladder stones, diabetes, or fibrocystic breasts, are harder to evaluate. Remember, research into this subject is only recent since menopause is only recent. Most women did not live long enough one hundred years ago to have menopause.

2159. What would indicate that I am taking too much estrogen?

Severe breast pain and enlargement, swelling of the legs, and/or a heavy menstrual flow after the progesterone portion of your cycle indicate that you should try a lower dose. Continued hot flushes and a dry vagina suggest that you should try a larger dose.

2160. Will estrogen really keep me looking and feeling younger longer?

If you have ever seen a woman of thirty-five who had her ovaries removed at twenty with no hormone therapy, you would believe that estrogen keeps you looking and feeling younger. Certainly the vagina and vulva look younger with estrogen, but few people will see them. The skin generally retains more fluid and fat under it when you take estrogen, and therefore looks less thin and dry. Breasts are more likely to stay turgid, firm, and uplifted when hormones are taken. A straight back with no collapsed vertebrae due to bone loss (osteoporosis) certainly contributes to looking younger. Feeling young is much more complicated, but a sexually functioning vagina and a good night's sleep without night sweats can certainly help. The bones and joints are also less painful with estrogen, even if you have arthritis, and pain makes you look older.

MENOPAUSE: USE OF HORMONES TO TREAT MENOPAUSAL DISCOMFORTS (Continued)

2161. Are the benefits of estrogen greater than the disadvantages?

If most fatal hip fractures could be reduced, this alone would justify the use of hormones after menopause. If hormones could be given only to women who really need them, and combined with progesterone to reduce possible risks from uterine cancer, the total result would be the best. One research study showed that women who took estrogen had fewer breast cancers than women who took no hormones; there were even fewer breast cancers in women who took both estrogen and progesterone.

2162. Is there less danger in taking estrogen today than there was in years past?

Yes. The dosage generally prescribed has been reduced from the amount usually prescribed ten years ago, and the addition of progesterone (or progestogens) has reduced the occurrence of cancer of the lining of the uterus (endometrial cancer). Oral medication allows for a fine adjustment of the dosage to the individual woman and is now more frequently used. Shots are less frequently prescribed.

2163. How many doctors have stopped prescribing estrogen?

About one-half of doctors stopped prescribing estrogen as the result of reports that linked it to endometrial cancer. Today, more doctors are once again prescribing it for menopausal discomforts.

2164. I've heard that in some cases estrogen can cause bladder problems. Is this true? If so, what are the symptoms and does it occur suddenly?

Estrogen does not cause bladder problems, but it can relieve them, especially urgency whereby you have to rush to the bathroom when you first get the urge to void or else lose control. This can be relieved simply by an application of estrogen cream in the vagina once or twice a week.

2165. How do you combine progesterone in a cycle with estrogen for the treatment of menopause?

There are many routines, but a common one is to take estrogen pills from the first to the twenty-fifth day of the calendar month. You add the progesterone (usually medroxyprogesterone) daily from the sixteenth to the twenty-fifth day of the month, and then take nothing until the end of the calendar month. This may produce some withdrawal bleeding, or menstrual flow, but it should be light and scant. If it is heavy, the dosages can be adjusted to lighten the flow. If there is no flow, that is all right, too. You have still accomplished what you wanted to by adding the progesterone and preventing cancer of the uterus, and you are helping the condition of your breasts as well.

MENOPAUSE: USE OF HORMONES TO TREAT MENOPAUSAL DISCOMFORTS (Continued)

2166. I've heard that estrogen can lessen or eliminate bone and spinal problems in older women. Is this true?

Yes, it is true. Research has shown a complete elimination of bone loss due to osteoporosis if women take at least 0.625 mg of conjugated estrogens from the onset of menopause and do not stop taking them. Less estrogen only partially protects against bone loss. Calcium, vitamin D, and exercise also partially protect against bone loss.

2167. How will the use of hormones affect my skin?

Estrogen helps retain the water under the skin that gives a woman a softer touch than a man. The skin becomes more dry and itchy without estrogen. Wrinkles and dryness can also develop from exposure to the sun, so protection from the sun will give you a more youthful look than estrogen can.

2168. Are natural hormones better than the synthetic ones?

Natural hormones are the ones most frequently used and therefore the ones with which women and doctors have the most experience. They are well tolerated. Some older synthetic hormones are more nauseating, like DES (diethylstilbestrol), which was the first available estrogen. Many programs are now using synthetic ones to find out if they are better. More research on the treatment of menopause is needed.

2169. Should I take hormones just as I feel I need them or regularly?

If you are going to take hormones at all, you should take them on a regular basis, especially if you still have a uterus. If you take them irregularly, you may bleed irregularly as a result, but because irregular bleeding can be a sign of cancer, you would need a D & C (dilatation and curettage) to investigate the irregular bleeding. If you only bleed on the portion of the cycle when you are not taking the pill, as planned, then there is little cause for alarm and surgery is avoided.

2170. If my doctor prescribes hormones for me to take during menopause, what would happen if I decided to not take them?

In the last few years, many doctors have prescribed hormones and women have decided not to take them, especially if they read the package insert that comes with the pills. If you decide not to take them, you will continue to have menopausal symptoms for a while and then may develop bone loss (osteoporosis) and hip fractures. Today, sixty thousand women per year die of hip fractures and only three thousand women per year die because of cancer of the lining of the uterus (endometrial cancer). Most of the women who die from this form of cancer were not using estrogen.

MENOPAUSE: USE OF HORMONES TO TREAT MENOPAUSAL DISCOMFORTS (Continued)

2171. If I take hormones during menopause, will I have to keep taking them after menopause?

Taking hormones during menopause does not make it any more necessary to take them after menopause. When you stop taking them, you will be just like you would have been if you had not taken them at all. Your bones will be better for a year or so, but they will lose substance quickly when you stop. It is true that if you are very symptomatic during menopause, your hormones are probably very deficient, and they will continue to be this way if you stop using hormones. Some symptoms, such as hot flushes, may disappear in the few years that you use hormones.

2172. When can I safely stop taking hormones after menopause?

You are never safe from developing bone loss (osteoporosis) if you stop taking hormones. A bone densitometry, or CAT scan (computerized axial tomography) of the spine, can be done yearly to see if you are losing bone fast or slowly. If you want to be safe from symptoms of menopause, you will really have to stop taking the hormones to find out if you still have symptoms. You could stop estrogens five years before you know you are going to die, because it takes about that long for their effect on the bones to wear off. But who knows when they are going to die?

2173. Is it possible to delay menopause through the use of hormones?

Hormones cannot delay ovarian failure, which is what menopause really is. They can cover up all the symptoms of menopause, so that you do not know that you are going through it until you stop the hormones. Women have taken birth control pills into and beyond menopause; these are more than adequate to hide the symptoms of menopause until they are stopped. Some women want to take them until menopause to be sure that they do not get pregnant, but they must stop taking them to find out if they are in menopause. Or would it be better to take them and not know? Most physicians think the dose of hormones in contraceptive pills is too high for treatment of menopause, and therefore there is a risk of heart attack (coronary artery disease). Some women insist that they feel better on birth control pills than they do on the estrogen and progesterone cycles that are used to treat menopause.

2174. Is the "middle-aged spread," as it is called, due to the hormones women take during menopause, or do the hormones help to prevent this from happening?

The "middle-aged spread" is due to weight gain and reduced exercise, in both men and women. Women frequently gain weight right after meno-

MENOPAUSE: USE OF HORMONES TO TREAT MENOPAUSAL DISCOMFORTS (Continued)

pause, perhaps because they feel better when the fat produces estrogen for them. Taking hormones adds water retention weight as well as some real body weight. It's a tossup as to who gains more weight, those people on hormones or those off.

2175. What is Premarin? Should I take this during menopause?

Premarin is a brand name for conjugated estrogen, the estrogen most widely used for menopause. It is made from pregnant mares' urine, which contains lots of different estrogens, but mostly one called estrone. Whether you should take this is a philosophical and medical question. Philosophically, if you believe in using all that science has to offer to make life good and enjoyable, then you will decide to use estrogens for menopause. If you believe nature cannot be and should not be improved upon, then you will let it take its course, no matter how uncomfortable you might be. Medically, if you have had your uterus taken out by a previous hysterectomy and therefore have no risk of developing estrogen-induced uterine cancer, and if you are in good health without diabetes, breast cancer, high or low blood pressure, or heart disease, you should not be refused estrogens when you request them. If you do have problems, there must be an individual discussion of the dangers and advantages before a decision is made. If you still have a uterus, you can avoid uterine cancer by adding progesterone to the cycle.

MENOPAUSE: HORMONE TREATMENT—ADVERSE AND LONG-TERM SIDE EFFECTS

2176. What are the long-term effects of hormones?

The long-term effects of estrogen and progesterone are: the bones are preserved in their normal adult state, the breasts are preserved in the middle-aged state, the vagina and labia (vaginal lips) remain in a well-nourished pink and functional state, the uterus continues to wax and wane in a cyclic fashion with perhaps withdrawal menstrual flow, the ovaries are suppressed and inactive, the skin ages but retains some thickness and turgor, and hip fractures are reduced. Other long-term effects are: gallstones are perhaps increased, breast cancer grows more rapidly if it occurs, endometrial cancer bleeds more heavily if it occurs, diabetes is worsened if it occurs, and high blood pressure may rarely be aggravated. Heart attacks may be more frequent if progesterones are used as they reduce high-density lipoproteins that should protect you when you take estrogen.

2177. What are the known adverse side effects of hormone shots and pills?

The most publicized side effect of hormone shots and pills is that the

MENOPAUSE: HORMONE TREATMENT—ADVERSE AND LONG-TERM SIDE EFFECTS (Continued)

risk of getting cancer of the lining of the uterus (endometrial cancer) increases eight to ten times. (This is not to be confused with cervical cancer.) It is estimated that about 1 in 160 women on estrogen alone will develop this. The cure rate of this cancer runs better than 80 percent by hysterectomy, but that is still a serious side effect. Without hormones, 1 in 1,500 women develop this cancer. The main effect of progesterone is to prevent endometrial cancer, but at the same time it decreases the level of high-density lipoproteins in the blood and, as a consequence, increases the chances of heart attacks. Minor side effects of estrogen are water retention, weight gain, increase in gallstones, aggravation of diabetes, and high blood pressure in less than 5 percent of women.

2178. What are the adverse side effects of estrogen use for menopause?

Estrogens can induce the production of a type of bile that causes gallstones. The incidence of gallbladder disease almost doubles with estrogen users. Estrogen taken orally goes through the liver and can affect lipoprotein metabolism, blood coagulation, and other liver processes, but there is no convincing evidence that estrogens taken in customary doses increase the risk of blood clots that travel, stroke, or heart disease in women who have undergone natural menopause. The worst side effect of estrogen is the increase in the growth of the lining of the uterus, called hyperplasia of the endometrium. This is considered to be a precancerous condition and an actual cancer of the lining of the uterus. Newer studies report that the use of progestins for several days of each cycle decreases the incidence of this type of cancer.

2179. Does estrogen cause breast cancer?

The National Institutes of Health Consensus Development Conference in 1979 on estrogen replacement therapy, after a careful review of the epidemiological data, including large numbers of case-controlled studies from various locations in the United States, concluded that there was no association between breast cancer and previous estrogen use. The numbers of breast cancers did not go up and down according to estrogen use like endometrial cancer did. There are some studies showing a lower incidence of breast cancer when progestogens are used with the estrogen. This may be a future trend.

2180. Since cancers of the breast and uterus take a long time to develop, how do I know I am not speeding it up by taking estrogen before I discover the cancer?

That is theoretically possible, and a real consideration in the decision

MENOPAUSE: HORMONE TREATMENT—ADVERSE AND
LONG-TERM SIDE EFFECTS (Continued)

to take estrogen. You should have a mammogram to be sure that there is no breast cancer already there, and you might also have a D & C or endometrial biopsy to be sure that no endometrial cancer (cancer of the lining of the uterus) is present when estrogen is started. Another method of being relatively safe is to take a progestin in a cyclic fashion along with the estrogen. This protects you from endometrial cancer and, as some major studies have shown, also reduces your chances of having breast cancer. If you are going to take the hormones, take both of them: estrogen and progesterone.

2181. Can women with cancer safely take hormones?

Women with breast cancer or endometrial cancer (cancer of the lining of the uterus, not the cervix) whose cancers are high in estrogen receptors (sensitive to estrogen) cannot safely take estrogen. Some of the cells might grow better in the breast cancer metastases (area where the cancer has spread) if estrogen were given. Other cancers are not affected by estrogen. Cervical cancer patients can and do take estrogen, especially after their ovaries have been removed surgically or by radiation. Colon cancers have no relationship to female hormones at all.

2182. Is all of this fear over hormones really justified?

The fear was justified because the dose and method of using estrogen really was increasing cancer of the lining of the uterus, so that many women were getting hysterectomies that they could otherwise have avoided, and some women, though few, were dying. However, stopping hormones out of fear has caused more women to die from bone loss (osteoporosis), which leads to serious fractures of the hip resulting in a high death rate. The good result of this fear has been that the dosage of estrogen has been reduced and progesterone has been added, at least for those women with a uterus and perhaps for all women, since it may also protect against breast cancer.

MENOPAUSE: NATURAL WAYS TO RELIEVE
MENOPAUSAL DISCOMFORTS

2183. What natural ways are there to ease the discomforts of menopause?

All women fan themselves or throw off the covers with hot flushes and night sweats because they feel better if they do. Most women gain weight after menopause, perhaps because it really does make them feel better. You need to allow some fat on your body, even if that involves weight gain, because the fat can convert your adrenal hormones into estrone, an active estrogen. Of course, a good, nutritious diet always helps your nerves as well.

MENOPAUSE: NATURAL WAYS TO RELIEVE
MENOPAUSAL DISCOMFORTS (Continued)

2184. Are there any vitamins I can take to lessen the discomforts of menopause?

It is always important to include vitamins in your diet, but there are no special ones that alleviate the discomforts of menopause.

2185. Are there any specific exercises that might relieve the discomforts of menopause?

No. In general, recreational exercise is good for your entire nervous system and will make you tolerant of distracting annoyances, like hot flushes.

2186. Can the symptoms and discomforts of menopause be controlled without drugs?

The symptoms and discomforts of menopause can disappear, and frequently do with time, but that does not mean they are controlled without drugs. Good health, exercise, and a fulfilling life can help you to forget them, but they are still there. Poor health and a depressing life can exaggerate the symptoms and discomforts, but that does not mean they are mental in origin. They are really there.

MENOPAUSE: MEDICATION DURING MENOPAUSE

2187. How many women need tranquilizers during menopause?

As people become older, they have relatively more emotional difficulties that may be helped by tranquilizers. Tranquilizers do not really stop hot flushes although they can help you to ignore them. Many have been prescribed based on the idea that you have hot flushes because you are nervous, but this is not true. If you are unable to use estrogen, you may want to try them. However, you can become addicted to tranquilizers, or they can become habit forming.

2188. Is it safe to take thyroid or blood pressure medicine during menopause?

Yes, it is safe, and if you have hypothyroidism or high blood pressure, it is much safer to continue taking these medications.

MENOPAUSE: HOW WILL I FEEL? WHAT KIND OF
ADJUSTMENTS WILL I NEED TO MAKE?

2189. How will I feel during menopause?

You will not always follow your mother's pattern, but it is at least interesting to know how she felt during menopause. Your emotional reaction to no longer being fertile and to a sign of aging will depend on your total ad-

MENOPAUSE: HOW WILL I FEEL? WHAT KIND OF ADJUSTMENTS WILL I NEED TO MAKE? (Continued)

justment to life and your feelings of self-esteem. If they are based entirely on your youthful good looks, you are in trouble. If your life is wrapped up in your children and they leave you at this time, you will also be in trouble. If you look forward to freedom from menses, contraception, and child care, you may enjoy this period more. If you have a lot of interests and you are planning activities in advance for your new-found freedom, you will be in good shape.

2190. What part does menopause play in the middle-age crisis?

Everyone experiences a middle-age crisis: that time when people look back on their lives and wish they had done something differently. Some may make drastic and frequently unwise changes in their lives. Women have the additional reminder of their state of infertility by the cessation of menses, and perhaps the annoying features of hot flushes, night sweats that produce sleeplessness and irritability, and a dry vagina that can make intercourse uncomfortable. Under such stress, every day may mean a new crisis.

2191. Why are so many women scared by this time in their lives?

In our country, aging itself is viewed as a frightening state, and menopause is definitely a symbol of aging. Women are not really afraid of the hot flushes, the dry vagina, or even the bone loss and fractures; they are afraid of becoming old. Men are afraid of aging, too, but there is no particular time when they must acknowledge it.

2192. What kinds of adjustments will I need to make during the menopause stage of my life?

If you have no symptoms, you may need no adjustments at all. If you still want children, then you will need to adjust to sterility. If you are very symptomatic, miserable with hot flushes and night sweats, irritable from sleep deprivation, and are avoiding intercourse because it hurts, then you may have to accept hormone treatment for your problems.

2193. Is menopause usually the most trying time of a woman's life?

No. Caring for small babies with a husband who works at two jobs and still doesn't make enough money or raising children as a divorced woman who lacks the skills needed to make a living cause more trying times.

2194. Do most women view menopause as a sad occurrence in their lives because it signals the end of their ability to have children, or are most women happy to be done with the inconvenience of menstruation?

Many women have both views at the same time, but perhaps most women are happy, not sad, that they can no longer have children.

MENOPAUSE: HOW WILL I FEEL? WHAT KIND OF ADJUSTMENTS WILL I NEED TO MAKE? (Continued)

2195. Do some women look forward to menopause?

Yes. Women with migraine headaches that started when they began menses look forward to them stopping when they stop menses, which often does happen. Women with fibroids or endometriosis who are trying to avoid surgery hope for menopause soon so it will solve their problems. Women who have never allowed themselves to use contraception look forward to the security of menopause. Unfortunately, many women who do not enjoy intercourse look forward to menopause as an excuse to eliminate sex. But the majority of women who look forward to menopause have uncomfortable, messy menstruation that they will be happy to part with.

2196. Has the menopausal stage of women's lives changed over the years as a result of changes in lifestyles, such as the increase in the number of women who are working outside of the home?

The only noteworthy change is that there is less depression associated with menopause in women who work outside the home. The time of menopause and other symptoms are the same.

2197. Can I still maintain an active, busy life during menopause?

You can be even more active and busier than you were before menopause, because you do not have days in which heavy menstrual flow or pain inhibits your activities. There is nothing about menopause that decreases your strength or energy, except when its symptoms cause sleep deprivation.

2198. How will the fact that my mother is going through menopause affect my relationship with her as her daughter?

She might become a little envious of your youthful looks and your obvious fertility, and the comparisons may become painful to her. She may also become irritable if she has many uncomfortable symptoms that go untreated. Your relationship will survive if you can tactfully emphasize her assets and encourage treatment of her symptoms.

2199. Is menopause easier for women today than it was in the "old days"?

Menopause has not really changed very much, except that it comes at a later age than it did in the "old days." Since the 1930s, estrogen preparations have been available for treatment, although they were not always used by the majority of women. More recently, women have been frightened out of using any treatment at all. Without medical treatment, menopause is no easier than it was. With medical treatment for those who need it, it can be very much improved. Psychologically, women are much less depressed

MENOPAUSE: HOW WILL I FEEL? WHAT KIND OF ADJUSTMENTS WILL I NEED TO MAKE? (Continued)

because they have many more options for activities that maintain their self-esteem.

2200. Are emotional outbreaks or depression common among women who are going through menopause?

Yes, they still do occur with moderate frequency, but such outbreaks or depression also occur with men in the mid-life crisis at about the same age range. Unfortunately, many emotional outbreaks in women seem to be attributed to menopause even when women are nowhere near menopause. Treating symptoms of menopause may not help the emotional crisis at all when menopause is not the cause.

2201. Will I cry more during menopause?

If you have a depression that coincides, but is not caused by menopause, you will probably cry more. If you have severe night sweats that wake you up every hour or so, you will develop symptoms of sleep deprivation, including irritability and crying easily. These will disappear if you take hormones that stop the night sweats. If you put off having children too long, you may cry over the loss of fertility; however, most women celebrate this.

2202. How can I avoid being depressed during menopause?

You can use the same techniques you use to avoid being depressed at any other time in your life. Menopause does not, in itself, cause depression. People who have struggled with depressions in the past have usually developed some techniques of their own to combat this. They can also be helped by psychotherapy and psychiatric assistance, including antidepressant medications.

2203. What is the "empty nest syndrome"?

The "empty nest syndrome" is depression and a feeling of uselessness experienced by women, whose whole lives were devoted to bearing and raising children, after their children are grown and gone. There is a void of activities and goals that needs to be filled by something else. Centuries ago, this didn't happen because women did not survive that long. Now they do. We can no longer bring up little girls to expect to spend their lives raising children. They cannot get pregnant after forty-six years of age, and the children will go to college or elsewhere by the time they are sixty-four or sixty-six. Then they still have ten or fifteen years to fill. Most women have all their babies by the age of twenty-six, and the children are gone by forty-six. Then what do they do? They must raise their self-esteem and become involved in activities that interest them.

MENOPAUSE: LIFE AFTER MENOPAUSE

2204. Is there life after menopause?

There is about twenty-five years of life remaining for most women. If we allow these years to be miserable and of poor quality, we will have cast aside one-third of our lives. If we assume responsiblity for their quality and take action to make them good, they will be good.

2205. Dr. Carson, were you happy to have menopause occur? Why?

Not really. I knew that longevity was more likely with a late menopause, and I wanted to live forever. My menopause occurred at fifty-four. I had always had a persistent desire to have a fourth child, and menopause meant that it was absolutely not to be. I never wanted to be sterilized, because that was so final. Menopause is also final. But most annoying, I had all the severe symptoms you can imagine: hot flushes ten and twenty times a day that interrupted my sleep even more than phone calls from my patients. I perspired so much that it ruined my hairstyle. My curiosity made me want to see how long these would last, but after a year or so I suppressed them with Premarin and Provera, the estrogen and progesterone routine cycles. To wait longer could have compromised my bones. I was not depressed. I had a relatively new husband, three small children of my own, and older children of his, as well as a very satisfying and ego-building medical practice to keep me involved and happy.

2206. Will I have to cut down on my physical activities after menopause?

No, physical activity helps prevent bone loss (osteoporosis). Activity may be reduced by such things as heart disease, arthritis, fractures, and lung disorders.

2207. Will the shape of my body be different after menopause?

Both men and women develop a little pot belly as they age, even if they are not overweight. But women who are not on estrogen replacement therapy often develop a painful curvature of their spines that causes them to be humped over. Of course, some are worse than others, and good posture and exercise can help.

2208. Will I gain weight after menopause?

You probably will gain weight, but it is not absolute. Your metabolism is generally slower and your activity is less, so you should reduce your caloric intake to stay the same weight.

2209. Will I feel better after menopause is over?

Yes.

2210. Are there any special health care requirements that I will have after menopause?

Calcium loss is great and should be increased in your diet, or you

MENOPAUSE: LIFE AFTER MENOPAUSE (Continued)

should take 1200 mg of calcium with vitamin D to help your bones (unless you have kidney stones and are advised against it).

2211. What causes bleeding after menopause?

Bleeding after menopause is considered to be caused by cancer, until proven otherwise by a medical examination and tests, including surgery. It can be due to thin, fragile tissue in the vagina or even in the uterus, called senile atrophy. It may also be caused by a polyp or an overgrowth that is not yet cancer, called hyperplasia. Use of estrogen can be a cause, too.

2212. Are women more susceptible to female diseases and disorders after menopause?

The diseases and disorders change and become more serious, but they are not really more frequent. Menstrual disorders, benign ovarian cysts, fibroids, endometriosis, pregnancy, and contraceptive problems are all gone. Pelvic inflammatory disease is almost unheard of! Problems of the prolapsed uterus, bladder, and rectum are increased. Cancers of the uterus and ovaries are increased, but cancer of the cervix decreases greatly after sixty. If you are not on estrogen replacement therapy, you will probably need your gynecologist less and your internist more, although ideally you should see both of them regularly.

2213. How many women suffer from depression after menopause is over?

Many more women suffer from depression after menopause than before, because depression increases in frequency and severity with age.

2214. Is heart disease more likely after menopause?

Heart disease is much more likely in women after menopause. Until this time, men have many times more heart disease than women, but after menopause women begin to catch up. This is true for coronary artery disease (narrowed arteries in the heart), arteriosclerosis (hardening of the arteries), and heart attacks but not for other types such as rheumatic or congenital heart disease, which occur in young people. Estrogen replacement therapy can reduce this increase in heart disease.

2215. Will I be more or less sexually active after menopause?

The probability is that your sex life will decrease due to a general decrease in energy level, the specific discomforts of menopause unless they are treated, and the decrease in number of possible partners as age progresses.

MENOPAUSE: WHEN TO SEE THE DOCTOR AFTER MENOPAUSE

2216. How often should I see my gynecologist for checkups after menopause?

After menopause, a yearly checkup is advisable for checking your

MENOPAUSE: WHEN TO SEE THE DOCTOR AFTER MENOPAUSE
(Continued)

breasts and having a mammogram, regardless of whether or not you are on estrogen replacement therapy. Pap smears become less important, but a pelvic examination for ovarian cancer becomes more important.

2217. Should I stop having Pap smears after menopause?

The American Cancer Society advises that you can stop having Pap smears after the age of sixty-five if all previous Pap smears have been normal. The Consensus Panel on Pap Smears of the National Institutes of Health advises a Pap smear every three years, but when two have been normal after age sixty, you can stop. Some women continue to have Pap smears to find out the estrogen effect in their vagina. The American College of Obstetricians and Gynecologists recommends that a yearly Pap smear and pelvic exam be continued, as well as breast examinations.

MENOPAUSE: DO MEN HAVE A SIMILAR CHANGE?

2218. Do men have a physical and emotional period in their lives similar to menopause?

Men do not have a sudden hormonal change at any age, except when they have an injury or surgery that results in the removal of their testicles. The decline in testosterone is very gradual and lasts well beyond one hundred years of age. However, just as women experience a mid-life crisis that is unrelated to hormonal menopause, men also frequently have a mid-life crisis, which is psychological and social, mostly based on the realization that they are aging and have not done all they have wanted to do. "Male menopause" is also used as a term to mean impotence. Impotence may be based on a disease, like diabetes, or on psychological factors, but it is not due to a decrease in testosterone, nor is it corrected by dosages of testosterone.

MENOPAUSE: CURRENT RESEARCH

2219. What sort of research is currently being done in regard to menopause?

Efforts are being made to find a drug that would prevent menopause altogether. One such drug is bromocriptine (Parlodel), which inhibits prolactin. Other projects are testing various doses and combinations of hormones for treatment and preventive treatment of other health disorders of postmenopausal women.

2220. There is such a long period of time between the time that women are finished having babies and the onset of menopause. Why doesn't it occur earlier in life?

A few years ago, surveys showed that most women in the United

MENOPAUSE: CURRENT RESEARCH (Continued)

States had finished having their babies by the age of twenty-six. Since menopause comes twenty-five years after that, your question is a valid one. However, in recent years women have been having babies at later ages. Some women really want babies after forty, and most are annoyed when menopause and the infertility that precedes it prevents this. But the real answer is that if menopause came at twenty-six, then our bones would deteriorate by age forty, and we would have an increase in heart attacks at an earlier age as women do after menopause. We would then not live as long or as well. In the distant past, women had to have ten or twelve babies in order for three or four to live, so for the survival of mankind, women had to be able to get pregnant past the age of twenty-six. Now that babies survive well, it is not as necessary for that purpose.

Chapter 10

Body Abuse

BODY ABUSE

There are times when control of your body is completely lost and you feel helpless, powerless, and vulnerable. This is the case with rape, incest or child sexual abuse, alcoholism, drug addiction, bulimia, anorexia nervosa, or even a heavy habit of cigarette smoking. But you can survive and you can regain control of your body and take charge once more. You may need help from others—family, friends, agencies, and professionals—to do this. Use them all to your advantage.

This chapter is not an exhaustive study of the causes and treatment of various abuses. Help for all these problems can be found in the front of the phone book under "Emergency Calls" or "Crisis Intervention Agencies." Numbers for a child abuse hotline, a crisis team, or even a poison control center are often listed. "Community Services Numbers" also list services under "Abuse," such as Adult Protection Service, Battered Women, Child Protection Service Hotline, or Drug Abuse. These are usually twenty-four-hour service lines for emergencies.

BODY ABUSE: RAPE

2221. What is rape?

Rape is forcible penetration of a body cavity (vagina, mouth, or rectum) with the penis against your will. Statutory rape is such penetration with a girl who is too young to give consent, even though she does. If there is no penetration, it is child sexual abuse. If the rape is by a father or brother, it is incest.

2222. Does rape only happen to attractive, provocative women?

No, rape victims include elderly women, children, men, and babies, in all social classes, races, and life styles. Only in the mind of the rapist do victims provoke the attack.

2223. Aren't rape reports sometimes phony? Don't women cry rape to get back at their boyfriends?

No. Less than 10 percent of rape reports are unfounded, according to the Law Enforcement Assistance Survey. This is no higher than for other crimes. In fact, only 10 percent of rapes are ever reported. In 1968, 31,000 rapes were reported. This has grown to 82,000 reported rapes in 1982.

2224. Aren't rapists always put behind bars for a long time?

Less than 2 percent of reported rapes end in a court conviction of the rapist for rape.

2225. Why are some women afraid to report being raped to the police?

They are afraid of the medical examination and the legal process. In the past, the medical examination was not done with great sensitivity, and during the legal process the woman's character seemed to be on trial. Now laws have changed, and the medical handling of rape has improved. There should be less fear and more reporting and prosecution if rape is ever going to be stopped. One of the reasons women are afraid to report rape is that they feel guilty, just as victims of incest and child abuse and battered women also feel guilty, as if they were somehow responsible. Women have been led to think that if they smile or act friendly or walk in a suspect place, then anything that happens to them after that is their fault. It is not! A friendly gesture, getting into a car with a man, going to dinner with a man, even going to his room does not confer upon him the right to rape. People must stop agreeing with those who believe rape is a woman's fault for not avoiding such things for their own safety.

2226. What should I do after I am raped?

Call the police and report the rape as soon as possible. To be able to convict the rapist, you must have a medical examination within two to six hours. The police will take you to a medical center where you will have all the proper examinations. You will need follow-up examinations for venereal

BODY ABUSE: RAPE (Continued)

disease and pregnancy. You can also ask for a rape counselor while you are at the medical center, or you can call and make arrangements to have a rape counselor with you later during the medical and legal process. Every city has a rape-counseling service. If you can't find it in the phone book, just ask the police to contact them for you, or ask the telephone operator for a rape hotline. Trained counselors are waiting for your call.

2227. What kinds of tests and treatments are given to rape victims?

The medical examination is a crucial part of the sexual assault investigation, although it seems to be one of the most frightening aspects to the woman who is going through it. This is why a rape counselor from a crisis center will accompany her through the ordeal, which is done as soon as possible. A thorough physical examination of the whole body, looking for bruises, injuries, or other signs of trauma, is performed first. Then a pelvic examination is done on a table with the woman's legs in stirrups, just as in a gynecologist's office. The examiner looks first for swelling or bleeding of the vulva. Then a speculum is inserted to see the inside of the vagina and the cervix to look for injuries or tears. Material is taken from the vagina, cervix, and later from the rectum to put on slides and in tubes, which will be checked for sperm or fluid from the attacker's prostate gland. This fluid can be tested and used to identify the rapist. Cultures are taken for disease. Clothing will be carefully saved for evidence. Samples of saliva, hair, pubic hair, rectal swabs, oral swabs, and even scrapings from under the victim's fingernails where she may have scratched the rapist are all taken as evidence to indict the rapist.

2228. How can I prevent pregnancy from rape?

If you were not using birth control at the time of the rape, you may want to have an IUD inserted within the five days that follow the attack. This will prevent implantation of a fertilized egg. You could also take DES (diethystilbestrol) for five days, but it is very nauseating. Most women wait two weeks and take a pregnancy test, and then they have an abortion if they are pregnant. Abortion for rape was approved long before abortions were generally legal. About 4 percent of rape victims become pregnant. The time to have a pregnancy test is about the same time as a culture for gonorrhea and a blood test for syphilis are recommended. Even though you want to forget the rape, follow-up care is very important for your health.

2229. If I call the police, does that mean that I will have to testify in court?

You can always decide against prosecution later, but if you do not call the police, you will have little chance of prosecution. The best decision would be to call the police, partly so you can have the best medical care and examination for evidence right away, and also so you can report the crime

BODY ABUSE: RAPE (Continued)

while you remember all the details. Then if you decide later that you cannot tolerate a court proceeding, you can back out. Maybe the attacker will plead guilty, and you won't have to bother, but at least you will have a chance to prosecute. If you don't preserve the evidence or report the crime until much later, you will have a poor case and the rapist will certainly fight it in court. With overwhelming evidence, you have a better chance of winning without much of a court appearance.

2230. Where else could I go, besides the police, for help after I have been raped?

It is natural to go to a good friend or close family member for help. You should let them call the police to give a report on the rape and also take you to a medical facility within one or two hours for an examination for evidence of rape. Crisis centers and rape hotlines, listed in the phone book, will provide counseling on what to do, as well as provide a sensitive, sympathetic rape counselor who will help go through the process with you. They will also advise you of the legal process and provide counseling to help you recover afterwards.

2231. Can internal injuries occur in a woman who has been raped?

Injury from rape is more likely to occur in children, but it has happened to women, especially with the kind of rape that occurs in war. Surgery was performed in field hospitals on German women raped by American servicemen in World War II, where their vaginas and even their bladders and rectums were ruptured. In the Bangladesh-Paskistani war, 200,000 Bengal women were raped.

2232. How does a woman deal with rape?

There are as many ways to deal with rape as there are women. There are also many different degrees of rape. Today any woman who considers that she has been raped can ask for and receive police protection, examination for injury and evidence of rape, and counseling from specialized groups who will also assist her through a court procedure against the rapist.

2233. If a woman has an understanding husband or boyfriend, can't she get over rape more quickly?

An understanding friend of either sex can help, but over half of all stable relationships break up one year after a rape. The loved ones may be angry that the victim was damaged or changed, they may not believe the victim resisted enough, or they may feel guilty that they were unable to protect the victim. These ideas may not be expressed, but the breakup occurs.

2234. Do most rape victims need psychological counseling before they are able to return to a normal life?

Psychological counseling would certainly be helpful in dealing with

BODY ABUSE: RAPE (Continued)

any stress, but it is not always available. Support and the counsel of friends is sufficient for many women to be able to return to normal life.

2235. How can I prevent rape?

Unfortunately, attacks cannot always be prevented. There may be several attackers, the victim may be very young or old, or very fearful. In 85 percent of cases, there is a weapon or physical abuse from choking or brutal beatings. It is the fear of rape that keeps women from behaving as though they are free and really in control of their bodies. It keeps them at home and off the streets at night. It keeps women passive and makes them fearful that they may be thought of as being provocative. But some women are learning to defend themselves, by learning karate or how to shoot guns. Women will not be free until the atmosphere of violence is ended. To end that, the nature of male behavior must change. In the meantime, there are some concrete things women can do to avoid rape.

2236. What precautions against rape can I take at home?

Have lights in all entrances. Use dead-bolt locks. Lock windows, and have curtains or blinds. Use only your initials on your mailbox and in a phone book. Get a peep hole in your door and/or a chain lock. Identify repairmen before they are allowed to enter. Make the phone call for a stranger who wants to use your phone; don't let him in. If you find an intruder in your home, throw something through a window. Call the police if you have a problem.

2237. How can I take precautions in my car?

When you are in your car alone, lock your doors. Of course, lock the car when you leave it, and check the back seat before you get back in. Park in a well-lit area, or near the entrance of a shopping area. If you must pick up hitchhikers, pick up only women, reducing rape for them and for yourself. If you have car trouble, raise the hood and lock your doors. If someone stops, ask them to call for assistance. If you are being followed, drive to a busy place or a police station.

2238. How can I be safe walking?

Walk in well-lit, well-populated areas. Walk near the curb or in the street, away from bushes and alleys. Look like you know where you are going. Don't look timid or disoriented, as if you would be easy prey. Wear shoes that you can run in. If you feel danger, run to the nearest well-lit place, and scream all the way.

2239. Can I be safe hitchhiking?

No. The odds are against you. If you must hitchhike, stay with a com-

BODY ABUSE: RAPE (Continued)

panion or accept rides only from women. Do not get into a car with more than one person.

2240. What if I think a friend or acquaintance is about to rape me?

Trust your feelings and get away. Always carry money to take a cab home. Don't become drunk or high with someone you don't trust. Assertiveness training or self-defense courses may help you here. Some men are scared away by a struggle; some are turned on. Kicking, screaming, pulling hair, and biting can stun an attacker. Weapons have to be handy and can be used against you. A lit cigarette is a useful weapon. Keys or a ring between your fingers can be used to scrape his face. It's easier to avoid a dangerous situation than to resist an attack, and in some situations, submission may be the best way to avoid injury.

2241. If I stay home at night and don't talk to strangers, will I avoid rape?

Studies show that one-third to one-half of all rapes occur in the victims' homes. In over half, they are by friends and acquaintances.

2242. How can I avoid more violence if I am being raped? Should I fight back or not?

It depends upon how you perceive the rapist. If he is turned on by your fighting, then your resistance will make him more violent, unless you can overpower him. If he is looking for an easy prey, then a scream or violent reaction on your part may scare him away. Not all rapists are alike in their motives and reactions.

2243. Do you advise women to take self-defense courses?

Yes. It is good for their self-image and self-confidence. It also makes them realistically aware of their limitations, and prudent in what they may attempt to do. To be in charge of your body, you may have to defend it, sometimes in situations other than rape.

2244. What sort of person is a typical rapist?

A study from the Bridgewater Treatment Center in Bridgewater, Massachusetts classifies them as four kinds: 1) The aggressive rapist wants to hurt the victim, punish, defile, and cause agony out of rage. He is employed, has the highest IQ among rapists, and pretends to be friendly until he reaches an area where the victim is vulnerable. He is the most curable of the rapists, usually requiring one to two years of treatment. 2) The sexual-aim rapist wants to prove he isn't feminine or homosexual; he fantasizes that the female will like being raped. He is more easily scared away by screams and resistance and is not very successful in the rest of his life. 3) The sadistic rapist is impotent unless there is resistance and is frequently married to a sadomasochistic wife. He is the most dangerous rapist and the least treatable. 4) The date

BODY ABUSE: RAPE (Continued)

rapist simply assumes that women are not equal to men. They think women never mean "no" when they say it. If he takes a woman on a date and pays for the outing, he expects sexual payment in return. These are the least likely rapists to be reported, because the women feel guilty for having had the poor judgment to date the man in the first place.

2245. Are rapists sick and perverted?

According to studies, most rapists have socially acceptable sexual personalities but they express violence and rage more often. In one study, 85 percent of the rapists surveyed had been arrested for a crime before, and 35 percent had been arrested for rape before.

2246. Why do men rape? Are they sex starved and unable to control their passion?

Forty percent of rapists already have available sex partners. Rapists say their need was to express violence and gain power, not really sex.

2247. Does rape occur on impulse?

A major study found that 75 percent of rapes were planned in advance. In cases where three or more men raped together, 90 percent were planned in advance.

2248. Do most rape victims know their attackers?

Some studies indicate that most rape victims do know their attackers. What women fear more is being raped by a stranger in an area with no protection or help nearby.

2249. What percentage of rapes are interracial?

According to the National Commission on the Causes and Prevention of Violence, 10 percent of rapes are interracial. Of those, most were committed against black women by white men. This means that 90 percent were intraracial, black against black, white against white.

2250. Can a husband be accused of raping his wife?

No. There is no state where the law allows a man to be convicted of raping his wife. However, he can be convicted of other bodily assault and injury. Battered wives have some protection, but not sexually abused ones. Most cities have shelters for battered wives and their children.

2251. Don't women fantasize rape?

No. Our culture conditions women to enjoy submitting to men, and women fantasize about overpowering men, but not rape. No woman enjoys the reality of rape. It hurts.

BODY ABUSE: RAPE (Continued)

2252. Should I carry Mace, a gun, or some other weapon to protect myself against rape?

Before you can legally carry Mace, you have to take a course in its use. It cannot be taken on airplanes. You have to register a concealed gun to obtain a permit to carry it. If you are trained to use a weapon, it could help to protect you from rape; however, most people are not trained in this.

BODY ABUSE: BATTERED WOMEN

2253. Who are battered women?

They are women who are physically abused by their husbands or by the partners with whom they are steadily living. This can include forced sexual intercourse, but it is not rape if the persons forcing it on them are their husbands.

2254. Do most women report their abuse to the police?

No, probably only a small portion who are desperate make a report to the police.

2255. Is it a large problem today?

Yes, and it seems to be growing, but perhaps it is just being recognized and reported more today than in the past.

2256. What percentage of women are battered?

One estimate is that in one out of every two households, a woman will be battered sometime in her lifetime. Another estimate is that a woman is battered once every fourteen seconds in the United States. Statistical evidence on wife-battering comes from domestic disturbance calls to police, complaints by wives, hospital emergency room rosters, and crime reports. A survey in Chicago showed that police response to domestic disturbance calls in which wife-beating occurred exceeded the total responses for murder, rape, aggravated assault, and other serious crimes. Legal experts think that wife-abuse is one of the most underreported crimes in the country. In one year in New York, 14,167 wife-abuse complaints were handled in Family Court. Nationwide, it is estimated that battered wives number over one million. Boston City Hospital reports that 70 percent of the assault victims received in its emergency room are women who have been attacked in their homes, usually by their husbands or lovers. One-third of female homicide victims in California were murdered by their husbands.

2257. What can these women do to escape abuse?

They can and should report the abuse to the police, obtain a restraining order against the men who are abusing them, and prosecute them. They can also go with their small children to shelters for battered women where they will receive counseling and legal aid. Most cities have one or two of

BODY ABUSE: BATTERED WOMEN (Continued)

these, and they are always overflowing with victims. Their location is kept secret from the public, so the battering husbands cannot find their wives there.

2258. Are very poor women more likely to be battered?

Very poor women are more likely to stay with a partner who batters them, because they are so dependent upon that partner that they cannot afford to leave.

2259. Why don't these women do something about their situation, like report it to the police?

They feel guilty, as if they brought it on themselves, just as children feel guilty if they are punished (even if they were innocent). Women feel guilty for having made their husbands so mad at them, even if their husbands were drunk at the time. They are attached to their husbands and feel the only right course of action is to stay with the men they marry, no matter how much abuse the men give them. They are often religious about this.

2260. Do men ever complain of being battered by women?

Yes, but in 75-95 percent of assault cases, it is the woman who complains. In homicides, husbands are the victims almost as often as the wives (48 percent husbands, 52 percent wives). However, women who commit murder are usually motivated by self-defense seven times as often as male offenders.

2261. What should I do if my husband starts hitting me?

The best thing to do is leave. Then you can both meet later and get marriage counseling to try to solve the problem. However, if you have small children, leaving is not easy, since you feel you must take them with you because he may abuse them, too. Most women go home to their mothers with their children during this time. Then negotiations start about a reconciliation. If there is no place to go, call the police and hope your town has a shelter for battered women and their children. Legal action will then be combined with counseling to see if his behavior can be modified, perhaps with a change in your behavior, too. Jobs and economic independence make women less likely to tolerate battering, but some women still do. They think divorce and separation would be worse. Studies on child abuse show that men who physically abuse children are likely to abuse their wives also.

2262. Are there any books I can read about battered wives?

There are many books on this subject, and I urge you to read at least one, such as Del Martin's *Battered Wives*. The Battered Wives Service Group has recently published a workbook entitled *Getting Free* for women who are battered and trying to work their way out of the dilemma.

BODY ABUSE: INCEST AND CHILD ABUSE

2263. What is the definition of incest?

According to Webster's Dictionary, incest is sexual intercourse between two persons who are too closely related to be legally married. In this country, that means sexual intercourse between parents and their children, or brothers and sisters.

2264. What is the difference between incest and child sexual abuse?

Incest means intercourse between relatives of the first degree, usually a girl with her father or brother. When it is with anyone else, like a stepfather, family friend, or uncle, it is child sexual abuse, which also includes fondling and sexual acts other than intercourse.

2265. Why does a girl allow incest or sexual abuse?

Young children are taught to be obedient to adults, especially relatives or someone they know well. Force is seldom involved, but secrecy is always taught to them. Secrecy makes them feel guilty, so they are afraid to tell anyone of the abuse. Also, real threats of family breakup, the father being put in jail, or the mother's nervous breakdown may be used on older children. Sometimes the occasional sexual pleasure they feel can make them feel even more guilty. They may also feel they are the only ones in the world with this problem. The sexual abuse often occurs over a long period of time.

2266. What percentage of families have incidences of incest?

The amount of incest varies in different economic, social, and geographic areas, but is probably higher than most people suspect. Some surveys indicate that 10 percent of families have incidences of incest.

2267. What might cause a person to commit incest?

The cultural taboo against incest is strong, but when something breaks down the effectiveness of that taboo, incest can occur. The attraction and opportunity for incest are always there; only the taboo prevents incest. It breaks down more easily in step-parent and step-sibling situations.

2268. Are there any signs that would indicate this could be happening in the family?

Some physical signs in a girl are: loss of appetite, difficulty in urinating, bladder infections (cystitis), vaginal infections, or, of course, pregnancy. Behavioral signs are: withdrawal, unwillingness to go a certain place or with a certain person, suddenly failing in school, or being singled out for special attention by the father or brother.

2269. How can the child be helped?

Believe the child. Reassure her that she won't get into trouble for telling about the abuse this time or any other time. Protect the child from the of-

BODY ABUSE: INCEST AND CHILD ABUSE (Continued)

fender. Get counseling for the offender. Every city has a department for the protection of children with this problem. They are listed under Children's Protective Service. Call them for help.

2270. What can the girl do to stop it?

She can tell her mother, although often the mother does nothing for fear that the family will break up. She may have to tell a relative outside the home, a trusted grandmother, or a teacher or counselor at school. Hopefully, they will believe her and seek help for her.

2271. How does a bad sexual experience early in life, such as rape or incest, affect a woman's sex life later?

If it is one episode and it is handled well by her family with support and protection, it does not leave much effect. If it is prolonged over a period of years and the offender is a person whom the woman should be able to trust, the effect is greater. She may need counseling in her adult life to adjust to more normal relationships. She needs to know she is not the only person to whom this has ever happened. She may distrust men altogether.

BODY ABUSE: ALCOHOLISM

2272. What is alcoholism?

According to the dictionary, alcoholism is the condition of habitual drunkards who are poisoned by alcohol. The key words are habit and poison. People who cannot stop drinking have a strong habit, and some people seem to be more poisoned by alcohol than others. Practically speaking, alcoholism is present whenever the need to drink alcohol interferes with your life, your job, your relationships, or your health.

2273. How big a problem is alcoholism in the United States today?

It is estimated that fifteen million Americans are problem drinkers, and 25-50 percent of them are women. This means four to seven million women are alcoholics. Alcoholism is the single greatest drug abuse in the United States. It interferes with the health and happiness of the alcoholics and their families. It is also involved in at least half of the fatal automobile accidents.

2274. Is alcoholism common in women?

The great majority of identified alcoholics are men, so most treatment centers are designed for men. Because of their jobs, their drinking is obvious. Women alcoholics are not identified as early as men, because they are often hidden drinkers, hiding at home where no one notices how much they are drinking. They are not as dangerous, because they are less likely to drive, commit crimes of violence, or become public drunks. But they ruin their own

BODY ABUSE: ALCOHOLISM (Continued)

lives, as well as the lives of their families, and they suffer all the same physical consequences of alcohol.

2275. Is alcoholism hereditary?

There are some studies, all done on men only, that tend to show that alcoholism is indeed hereditary, inherited from father to son. These studies have been able to identify the boys who will become alcoholic. This could be useful, because if the identified person knew he was liable to become an alcoholic, he could avoid ever taking a social drink and therefore never have the problem.

2276. Does alcoholism have any long-term effects on my body?

There is an extensive list of possible long-term effects. Whether you reach them depends upon the quantity of alcohol consumed, the time over which it was taken, your general diet, activities, and perhaps inheritance, as well as other factors that are individual. The most serious result is liver damage (cirrhosis), which can be irreversible and fatal. Related to this are dilated blood vessels of the esophagus (esophageal varices), which can cause fatal bleeding. Brain deterioration that affects alcoholics in a special way and is irreversible is next in seriousness. Numbness in the hands and feet (peripheral neuritis) can be reversed if drinking stops and nutrition starts. Skin ulcers of the legs are the result of alcohol and poor nutrition. Stomach ulcers (gastric ulcers), inflammation of the esophagus (esophagitis), weight gain, aggravation of diabetes, heart disease, high blood pressure, and just vitamin deficiency problems can be reversed if alcoholism is cured. Inflammation of the pancreas (alcoholic pancreatitis) is a long-term result. Cancer of the pancreas may occur, and in the United States, cancer of the liver. Of course, the injuries sustained in falls and accidents while drunk may stay with you forever.

2277. Is it true that once you are an alcoholic, you are always an alcoholic?

Present medical theory agrees with that and warns that alcoholics can never become social drinkers. Although they stop drinking, they must still be considered alcoholic, because they can never drink without a problem. This is probably because the condition is inherited.

2278. What is the difference between a social drinker and an alcoholic?

A social drinker can drink with others on an irregular basis on social occasions, yet stop drinking at any point. An alcoholic cannot stop at a safe point. A social drinker does nothing to harm his own life, job, family, or health. The alcoholic damages all these things but continues to drink anyway.

BODY ABUSE: ALCOHOLISM (Continued)

2279. Am I an alcoholic if I have one or two drinks before dinner every night?

If you really have to have those drinks, you may be an alcoholic, especially if they have become harmful to your health or any part of your life. Try stopping and see.

2280. What should I do if a member of my family is a heavy drinker?

Get professional help for them if you can. Of course, your relationship with the drinker controls what you can do. A child cannot do much for her father, but a wife can contact Alcoholics Anonymous, attend meetings by herself, and learn how to involve her husband in the program. She also may be able to convince him to see a doctor or enter an alcohol rehabilitation program. Family influence can be strong when it is united.

2281. Can alcoholism be cured?

Alcoholics can be helped to stop drinking, and some of the physical results on their bodies, such as gastritis, pancreatitis, ulcers, cirrhosis of the liver, peripheral neuritis, and mental changes, particularly D Ts (delirium tremens), can be treated. You can see your doctor for medical problems, but may have to go to a residential treatment center for alcoholics to stop drinking.

2282. Where can alcoholics and their families go for help with alcoholism?

A.A. (Alcoholics Anonymous) is one of the most effective programs known to keep alcoholics from drinking. There is also an A.A. organization for spouses of alcoholics called Al-Anon, and for children of alcoholics, called Al-Teen. Family treatment is important in the rehabilitation of the alcoholic if he or she is to return to the family environment without drinking. There is a special organization to fight the accidents caused by drunk drivers called MADD (Mothers Against Drunk Driving).

2283. Can treated alcoholics learn to drink socially with moderation?

The answer is definitely no. There was one study that claimed to show this was possible, but it turned out to be a fraud. The inherited difference between alcoholics and other people is that they cannot drink in moderation.

BODY ABUSE: DRUG ADDICTION

2284. What is meant by addiction to drugs?

Drug addiction means that you require more and more of the drug to get the same effect and that if you stop, you have withdrawal symptoms.

2285. How many women are addicted to drugs?

Only 26 percent of the people in treatment programs for drug addiction are women, but it is likely that women do not enter the programs easily,

BODY ABUSE: DRUG ADDICTION (Continued)

and there are really more who should. It is estimated that 80 percent of people on tranquilizers and antidepressants (psychotropic drugs) by prescription are women. It is also estimated from some surveys that 50 percent of all women have taken a psychotropic drug at some time in their lives. One of the efforts of the feminist organizations, such as the National Organization for Women (NOW), is to encourage women to stop taking tranquilizers and actually change the world to suit themselves, rather than trying to change their psyches to suit the world. As long as they are tranquil, there will be no changes made.

2286. How big a problem is addiction to tranquilizers, such as Valium, among women today?

It is a bigger problem than among men. The National Organization for Women complained that drug companies always advertise their tranquilizers to doctors by showing a picture of a distraught woman. Doctors were conditioned to give women more tranquilizers, instead of helping them to solve their problems. Perhaps our culture has more problems that make women distraught. But tranquilizers keep them adjusted to the situation, instead of allowing them to make a change. This is what NOW wants them to do. Preventing agitation in women can save marriages and prevent child abuse. Tranquilizers can also make them more depressed and lead to suicide.

2287. How many women commit suicide each year from drug overdoses?

Women attempt suicide by drug overdose many more times than men, but they usually do not succeed. Sleeping pills take a long time to kill you, so women are usually found and revived before death occurs. As a result, the actual suicide rate for men is three times greater than that of women. The overall suicide rate in the United States is 12.7 successful suicides per 100,000 people; but for men it is 19 per 100,000, and for women 6.3 per 100,000. This rate does not vary much in different age groups. The trend in recent years is for women to use more violent methods for suicide, such as knives or guns. With these they are more successful in committing suicide than with pills. If this trend continues, the rate of women's suicides will rise. As the age of women increases, the relative rates of suicide for women also increase, so that men's suicides are only twice as numerous as women.

2288. How many women are addicted to prescription drugs?

Of course, if you need insulin, thyroid, heart medicine, or blood pressure medicine, that is not considered addiction, and you should not try to stop. Addiction problems are caused by mood-changing drugs. The first such drug was phenobarbital, given to nervous women. The Drug Enforcement Agency (DEA) maintains control over these prescription drugs and investigates any use that appears to be excessive. Doctors who prescribe them

BODY ABUSE: DRUG ADDICTION (Continued)

excessively may lose their licenses to practice. If women get them from several doctors, it is still noted by the pharmacist and the DEA. Women often put great pressure on doctors to get the drugs, but the number who are addicted is really not known.

2289. I have been addicted to prescription drugs for years. What can I do?

You can ask your doctor or a hotline in your community for help with your drug addiction. Many groups are organized to help. They are called by different names in different communities. Some are national in scope and include rehabilitation programs. Look in the classified section of your phone book under "Drug Abuse" and "Addiction Information and Treatment Centers" for your community.

2290. Are diet pills safe?

No. They have the capacity to make you need more and more of them to achieve the same mood-elevating effect, and they give you a real drugged feeling when you stop taking them, including withdrawal symptoms. There are safer ways to lose weight. Today diet pills are only used for something like narcolepsy (a sleep disorder in which the person can't stay awake).

2291. Is it possible to be addicted to over-the-counter medications?

No. They can become a habit, but they are not truly addicting. If they were, they would be placed on the controlled drug list of the DEA. Even caffeine is habit forming and causes some withdrawal headaches when you stop using it, but you don't need more and more of it to achieve the same effect.

2292. When should I resort to antidepressants?

You should use all the techniques you know to relieve a depression when you realize you have one. This can just be having a soda, as the caffeine gives you a lift. But when your methods have failed and you are close to losing your job, your family, or your life, you should seek professional help. Doctors know when to prescribe antidepressants, but psychiatrists know best of all. Antidepressants can save you from wasting a year and a half of your life in a deep depression or from being hospitalized to prevent suicide. They are not addicting, but you may need to take them for more than a year until your depression lifts. Tranquilizers are far more likely to be addicting.

2293. How can I know if I am getting addicted?

If you find yourself taking more of a drug than was prescribed and if getting that drug becomes the most important thing in your life, you should suspect addiction. Trying to stop taking the drug is a more difficult test for addiction, because you may really need the drug. Consult the doctor who prescribed it for you.

BODY ABUSE: DRUG ADDICTION (Continued)

2294. What are the most common drugs that have addiction possibilities?

Heroine is the most addicting drug known, and it is illegal for any use for that reason. Yet, it will addict only 10 percent of people who use it. Smoking opium is a famous addiction. Morphine is more addicting than Demerol; it is especially a problem to doctors and nurses who find it available to them. Excessive cocaine use for a long period can be both addicting and damaging. Benzedrine and amphetamines are certainly less addicting than cocaine, but they are seriously abused in the streets today. Codeine addiction is rather rare, but does occur with heavy usage in some people. All the tranquilizers, starting with phenobarbital; all sleeping pills; Valium; Librium; meprobamate; and phenothiazines can be mildly addicting or at least habit forming. Primarily they prevent the users from solving the problems bothering them. Marijuana is not addicting, but may be habit forming. It is mostly a legal problem, but you can cause accidents when you are high or stoned. Alcohol is a very separate but similar problem.

BODY ABUSE: SMOKING CIGARETTES

2295. Is smoking cigarettes an addiction?

No, it is habit forming. You can smoke at the same rate for years, with the same effect. Stopping causes withdrawal symptoms, but not severe ones like drug addiction. It is difficult to break the habit.

2296. Does smoking really cause lung cancer?

Yes. Lung cancer is the most frequent cause of cancer death in men, and by 1990 it will be the most frequent cause of cancer death in women, if the same rate today holds. It is now the second cause of all cancer deaths, causing 25,000 deaths in women per year, second only to breast cancer. Smoking is increasing among women, although it is not as high as in men.

2297. What else does smoking do to your health?

Smoking is a major cause of heart attacks, even if you are not taking birth control pills. Smoking can cause stomach ulcers, bladder cancer, circulation problems that can lead to amputations of your hands and feet, as in Buerger's disease, bronchitis (the smoker's cough), and emphysema. It can also cause you to be underweight.

2298. Is smoking particularly bad for women?

Yes it is, in two ways. One is that smoking in older women increases osteoporosis (thinning of the bones) that leads to compression fractures of the spine and hip fractures. The other is that in young women who are pregnant and smoke as much as ten cigarettes per day, there is an increase in premature deliveries, in small babies who do not do well, and in placental in-

BODY ABUSE: SMOKING CIGARETTES (Continued)

sufficiency, placentas that separate accidentally and do not nourish the baby well. Smoking can also interfere with the mother's good nutrition, but even if she eats well, she still has smaller, premature babies. There is a need for a national program to help pregnant women stop smoking. The nausea of pregnancy can cause women to stop smoking, but when that is over, women often resume. Smokers are usually nervous and slightly nauseated, so they do not enjoy the taste of food. That is why some women smoke, to be slender.

2299. How can I stop smoking?

If you have tried and can't stop on your own, call or write your local chapter of the American Cancer Society. They will have information on the Schick program, Smokenders, and other new and innovative groups that can help you.

BODY ABUSE: TRYING TO BE TOO THIN—BULIMIA, ANOREXIA NERVOSA

2300. What is bulimia?

Bulimia means recurrent episodes of compulsive, obsessive binge eating usually followed by self-induced vomiting. Binge eating involves the rapid consumption of large amounts of food in a short time period, such as ten thousand calories in twenty minutes or over a five-hour period, with vomiting between and after courses. The frequency of this usually ranges from twice a week to five times a day. Most bulimics become adept at vomiting and drinking water at the end of a binge. They choose easily regurgitated foods.

2301. What is the cause of bulimia?

The reason for the vomiting is to keep from becoming fat. The reason for the binge eating is compulsive behavior; food serves as a substitute for gratification or is a response to boredom, anxiety, or depression. The people doing this are usually secretive, hiding any evidence of bulimia, and are ashamed about it all.

2302. What are the bad effects of bulimia?

There are several physical side effects as well as psychological ones. Teeth and gum recession with enamel breakdown occurs from vomiting. The esophagus can get irritated, causing heartburn. Vomiting leaves you dehydrated and low in potassium, which can make you feel weak and faint; this makes an irregular heartbeat likely. The dryness can enlarge the parotid gland, under the ear. Mood swings can reflect the changing level of blood sugar. Your eyes become red right after vomiting.

BODY ABUSE: TRYING TO BE TOO THIN—BULIMIA, ANOREXIA NERVOSA (Continued)

2303. Who has bulimia?

Thirteen percent of the college population is estimated to have bulimia; 85-90 percent of them are women. Some researchers say it affects two million American women. It started with upper-middle-class adolescent girls, but now it is spreading to many socio-economic classes. The age of onset is thirteen to twenty-two, but it can last until the person is sixty. People have it for two to sixteen years.

2304. How is bulimia different from anorexia nervosa?

Both concentrate on food, diet, and weight. Both develop a habit of overestimating body size in a self-depreciatory way. Bulimics are much less likely to starve themselves to death. They recognize their behavior as abnormal, whereas the anorexic does not. Bulimics are less dependent upon their parents, more sexually and socially mature, and more functional. They have more ego strength and a better chance of getting over it entirely. Some bulimics have been anorexic in the past.

2305. What is the effective treatment for bulimia?

Unlike anorexia nervosa, bulimics usually do not need to be hospitalized, unless they are very dehydrated or suicidal. Psychotherapy is usually difficult due to the wide range of underlying problems and personality styles encountered. Group therapy is helpful afterward to prevent a relapse. Common misconceptions about eating, dieting, and fat content of the body require re-education in nutrition. Goals for changing eating habits must be gradually set and tolerable to the patient. It may be necessary to adjust the girl to the possibility of gaining weight before overcoming bulimia. If she is in college, she can ask her college counselor for a referral, probably on campus. Or she can ask her doctor, clinic, or local hospital for a referral to a psychologist who has a special interest in the problem.

2306. What is anorexia nervosa?

It is an eating disorder, usually occurring in teenage girls, in which they eat less and less. They think they are fat, even when they are skinny, and they try to diet to lose more weight. They usually stop menstruating altogether.

2307. Can anorexia nervosa be fatal?

Yes. If unchecked and untreated, the girl can lose so much weight that all her body systems fail and she dies a slow death of emaciation. Psychiatric intervention may be lifesaving.

BODY ABUSE: TRYING TO BE TOO THIN—BULIMIA, ANOREXIA NERVOSA (Continued)

2308. Why do the girls stop eating?

They want to be slender. It usually begins in early teens, when girls reject the bulging of breasts and hips that makes them female. Some chance remark about their development or that they are getting fat starts them off. Even their menses goes away. Clothes seem to be designed for undeveloped young men, instead of healthy teenage girls. If girls have to be very slender, it is far healthier to achieve it by exercise than by anorexia nervosa.

2309. Can anorexia nervosa be cured?

Yes, but even psychological counseling that involves the whole family may not be enough. If anorexia nervosa continues for six months, the help of a psychiatrist should be sought, and the girl may have to be hospitalized to impress her with the need for change.

Author Biographies

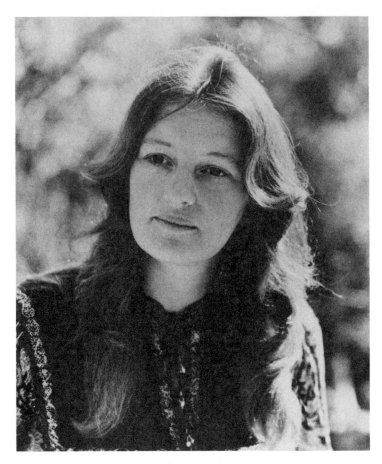

Susan Polis Schutz

For Susan Polis Schutz, *Take Charge Of Your Body* is the fulfillment of a need she personally recognized—easy-to-understand answers to all the questions a woman has about her body, gathered together in one volume.

The author of seven books of poetry, Susan is no stranger to the literary world. More than five million books and 100 million notecards containing Susan's poems have been sold. With the coauthoring of *Take Charge Of Your Body,* Susan enters a dimension that she has always been very close to—science and the right of women to be in charge of their lives.

Susan's poetry featured throughout this book takes a woman through her fears, questions, anxieties, and joys in a soothing manner. She has always written about women taking charge of their bodies and minds. Because so many people identify with Susan's ideas, she has become one of the world's most popular poets.

Susan grew up in a small country town, Peekskill, N.Y., and began writing at the age of seven. She graduated from Rider College majoring in English and biology. After studying physiology in graduate school in New York City, Susan was a social worker, a teacher, and a writer for magazines and newspapers. In 1965, Susan met Stephen Schutz who, at the time, was studying drawing and calligraphy in addition to physics. He received a Ph.D. in theoretical physics in 1970 from Princeton University.

Stephen and Susan were married and moved to the mountains of Colorado in 1969. Inspired by the beauty of the West, they became key contributors to the creative revolution that was blossoming. Working together—Stephen's illustrations accompanying Susan's poetry—they sold their work from the back of their van to support themselves.

In 1972, *Come Into The Mountains, Dear Friend,* Susan's first book of poems with Stephen's illustrations, was published. The public acceptance of this book was phenomenal, and history was made in the process. It became apparent that people readily identified with Susan's poetic words and Stephen's mystical illustrations. By the end of that year, their joint career, combined with a very special love, became their way of life.

In addition to Susan's books of poetry, many of her poems have been published on notecards and prints, in magazines and text books, and she has edited books by other well-known authors. She is also writing an autobiographical novel.

Susan and Stephen's works have been translated into Spanish, German, Hebrew, Japanese, Afrikaans, and Finnish, and have been published throughout the world.

The conviction with which Susan expresses feminist ideas does not preclude an equally intense commitment to her family. She has two children and is about to have her third child at the age of thirty-nine. Her efforts to weave together a modern female independence with the classical idea of love is a source of harmony in her work. *Take Charge Of Your Body* expresses these attitudes.

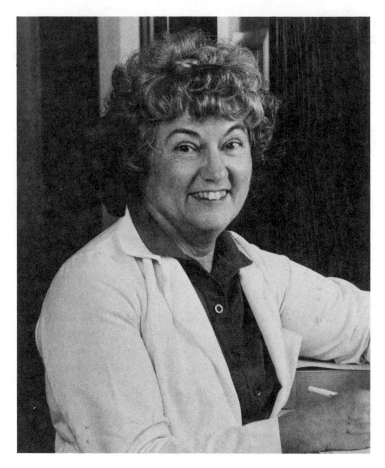

Katherine F. Carson, M.D.
F.A.C.O.G.

To Dr. Katherine Carson, *Take Charge Of Your Body* represents one of the high points in a medical career that spans almost thirty years of medical and personal accomplishments. She is the first woman to be chief of the Department of Obstetrics and Gynecology at Sharp Hospital in San Diego and has received many prestigious awards for her efforts toward providing women's health care.

Take Charge Of Your Body has provided Dr. Carson with a vehicle to reach more women than ever before with her ability to communicate her knowledge of the female body.

Dr. Carson graduated from medical school (University of California, San Francisco) in 1954 when only 7 percent of all medical students were female. She did her residencies at Stanford University Hospital and Kaiser, and has been on the staff in Obstetrics and Gynecology at Mercy, Sharp, Grossmont, Scripps, and University Hospitals since 1960.

Dr. Carson is considered a friend by her patients; she is easygoing and soft-spoken. But this belies her reputation as a "gutsy lady and a fighter," which is how her colleagues describe her. She has lobbied on behalf of natural childbirth, abortion rights, contraception for teenagers, and fathers' presence in delivery rooms. She has marched in Washington, D.C. to protest government funding cuts for abortions for poor women and military wives, and she has opposed efforts to require teens to have parental consent for abortion or birth control.

Dr. Carson has delivered over 6,000 babies and counseled over 25,000 women patients and is herself a mother of three. Despite such an active career, she is devoted to her daughters and to her husband, George West.

Dr. Carson is a fellow of the American College of Obstetricians and Gynecologists. In 1964, she became a Diplomate of the American Board of Obstetrics and Gynecology, and was recertified in 1978. In 1981, she was elected vice-chairperson of District IX of this organization, which consists of California obstetricians. She hopes to be elected its chairperson. She is chairperson of a national task force for the Advancement of Women Fellows in the American College of Obstetricians and Gynecologists. In 1982 she was elected to membership in the prestigious Pacific Coast Obstetrics and Gynecology Society, the first woman in forty years to be so honored. Dr. Carson has served as the first woman president of the San Diego Gynecological Society. In San Diego she has served as the chairperson of the Service Committee of the American Cancer Society, the Medical Advisory Committee of the Planned Parenthood Association, and the Public Relations Committee of the San Diego County Medical Society.

CAUTION: IMPORTANT NOTICE

This book is not a substitute for medical care. Since health is a highly individualized matter and new information is constantly being discovered which may have a bearing on your health, it is important to consult with your physician before acting on any information contained in this book. Failure to do so may cause or aggravate health problems.

If you have any questions which are not answered in this book, please send them to the address below. We will not be able to answer your questions individually, but we will try to incorporate your questions into future editions of this book.

Blue Mountain Press, Science Division
Post Office Box 4549
Boulder, Colorado 80306

Index

a woman to
be respected
a woman who
knows what she wants to do
and has the will
a woman who
dares enough
to speak out for what she believes
a woman who
is kind and good and giving
yet wants for herself also
a woman who
has high goals for herself
and achieves them
a woman who
is beautiful on the outside
and inside
a woman who
understands her body and
is in complete charge of her body
a woman who
is a success at work
and with those she loves
a woman who
is caring yet sensitive
strong but gentle
a woman
who believes in
a strong
equal future
a woman
who is
. . .
a human
. . . woman. I am human?